Clinical Sonography

ClinicalSonography

A PRACTICAL GUIDE

Third Edition

Editor

Roger C. Sanders MD, MA, BM, Bch (Oxen), MRCP, FRCR

Medical Director
Ultrasound Institute of Baltimore
Lutherville, MD
Clinical Professor of
Radiology and Obstetrics
University of Maryland
Baltimore, MD

Assistant Editor

Nancy Smith Miner RT(R), RDMS

Associate Professor of Diagnostic Ultrasound
New Hampshire Technical Institute
Concord, NH

with

Joan Campbell, RT (R), RDMS
John Casey, RT (R), RDMS
Joyce Cordier, BS, RT (R), RDMS
Oscar Del Barco, RDMS
Barbara Del Prince, BA, RDMS
Gretchen M. Dimling, BS, RDMS

Sandra L. Hundley, RDMS, RVT
Patricia May Kaplan, RT (R), RDMS.
Mary McGrath Ling, BS, RT (R), RDMS
Dan Miner, MD
Joe Rothgeb, RT (R), RDMS

Gail Sandager
Mimi Maggio Saylor, RT (R), RDMS
Lisa Simons, RT (R), RDMS
Deroshia B. Stanley, RN , C
Sandy Steger, RT (R), RDMS
Irma Wheelock Topper, RT (R), RDMS

LIPPINCOTT WILLIAMS & WILKINS
A **Wolters Kluwer** Company
Philadelphia • Baltimore • New York • London
Buenos Aires • Hong Kong • Sydney • Tokyo

Acquisitions Editor: Lawrence McGrew
Sponsoring Editor: Holly Chapman
Project Editor: Erika Kors
Senior Production Manager: Helen Ewan
Senior Production Coordinator: Nannette Winski
Design Coordinator: Doug Smock

3rd Edition

9   8   7   6   5   4   3

Library of Congress Cataloging-in-Publication Data

Clinical sonography : a practical guide / editor, Roger C. Sanders;
   assistant editor, Nancy Smith Miner, with Joan Campbell ... [et
al.]. – 3rd ed.
       p.   cm.
   Includes bibliographical references and index.
   ISBN 0-781-71556-3 (alk. paper)
   1. Diagnosis, Ultrasonic.   I. Sanders, Roger C., 1936-
II. Miner, Nancy Smith.
   [DNLM: 1. Ultrasonography.   WN 208 C6405 1998]
RC78.7.U4C585   1998
616.07'543–dc21
DNLM/DLC
for Library of Congress   97-33686
                                                    CIP

Care has been taken to confirm the accuracy of the information presented and to describe generally accepted practices. However, the authors, editors, and publisher are not responsible for errors or omissions or for any consequences from application of the information in this book and make no warranty, express or implied, with respect to the contents of the publication.

The authors, editors, and publisher have exerted every effort to ensure that drug selection and dosage set forth in this text are in accordance with current recommendations and practice at the time of publication. However, in view of ongoing research, changes in government regulations, and the constant flow of information relating to drug therapy and drug reactions, the reader is urged to check the package insert for each drug for any change in indications and dosage and for added warnings and precautions. This is particularly important when the recommended agent is a new or infrequently employed drug.

Some drugs and medical devices presented in this publication have Food and Drug Administration (FDA) clearance for limited use in restricted research settings. It is the responsibility of the health care provider to ascertain the FDA status of each drug or device planned for use in their clinical practice.

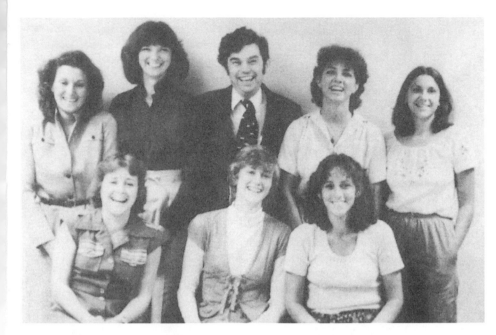

Standing (L-R): Susan Guidi, Irma Wheelock Topper, Roger Sanders, Joan Campbell, Nancy Smith Miner
Sitting (L-R): Patricia May Kaplan, Mary Silberstein, Mimi Maggio Saylor

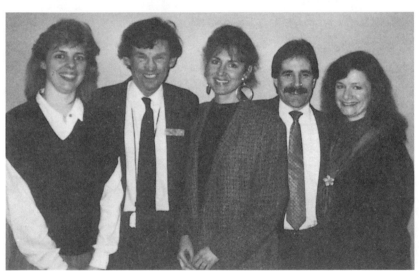

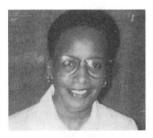

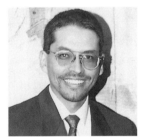

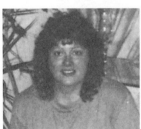

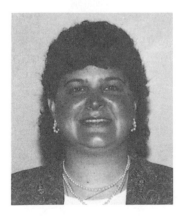

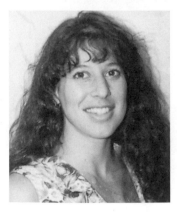

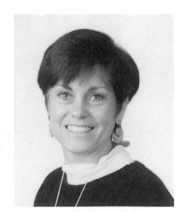

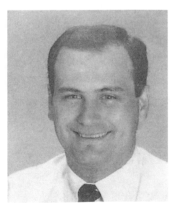

Clockwise (L-R): Gretchen Dimling, Roger Sanders, Kari Steurer, John Casey, Mary McGrath Ling, Deroshia Stanley, Oscar Del Barco, Sandra Hundley, Joe Rothgeb, Gail Sandager, Lisa Simons, Sandy Steger

PREFACE TO THE THIRD EDITION

The third edition of *Clinical Sonography: A Practical Guide* follows the mission statement of its two predecessors—to provide practical guidance to sonographers and to those physicians who are involved in hands-on scanning. *Clinical Sonography* is designed to be the book a sonographer counts on to provide creative solutions to difficult situations. This continues to be the book's strength—it dispenses practice-tested techniques and solid information on areas like report-writing to help the sonographer achieve excellence in today's difficult managed-care environment.

As in previous editions, the chapters start with a statement of the diagnostic problem to be considered and a brief overview of the place of ultrasound in the context of the clinical problem. Anatomy and technique are then described, and the pathological appearances of the area in question are discussed. Pitfalls are specified and areas for further examination of pathologic findings are suggested.

The third edition has been thoroughly updated to reflect the latest developments in sonography. For the first time, we included color flow images to demonstrate those scanning situations where color makes a diagnosis possible. We added chapters on intracranial vascular problems, ultrasound-guided procedures, arterial problems in the limbs, and rectal wall masses. New appendices were provided to be used as a reference source for the practicing sonographer. In addition, we expanded sections on infertility, fetal anomalies, pelvic mass, vaginal bleeding, pelvic pain, and imaging of the breast. The introduction describes the rationale behind these revisions.

It is our belief that the third edition will continue to be the book that is kept by the machine in the ultrasound lab.

PREFACE TO THE SECOND EDITION

The first edition of *Clinical Sonography* clearly filled a need, but new developments such as color flow Doppler, the vaginal and transrectal transducers, and the demise of the B-scanner have made the first edition out of date. In the second edition we continue to discuss the B-scan approach at the end of each chapter, although this technique is essentially unused in the U.S.A. B-scanning remains widely used in developing countries where our book is very popular. However, the new edition is geared to a realtime only approach. New areas covered in this edition are infertility, the prostate, fetal echocardiography, infant spine, hip joints and shoulders, fetal well-being assessment, and a much more detailed look at fetal anomalies.

Sonographers are in short supply. We hope that our book will help to alleviate the shortage by providing everyday practical guidance in the laboratory for those who are learning on the job. However, we know from teaching in residency programs and ultrasound schools that those who are in a formal course find material in this book that is not covered elsewhere. We feel that sonographers are a different breed from the technologists who work in other imaging modalities such as CT, MRI, or x-ray. To quote from Monica Bacani, "The notion that a sonographer is a minor variation of a radiologic technologist has been discarded in the same fashion as the idea that a child is nothing more than a diminutive adult. The production of a radiograph is not dependent on the technologist's ability to recognize pathology. Radiologic personnel evaluate their images for technical quality. The sonographer evaluates images for diagnostic content. The collection of diagnostic images is dependent on the sonographer's ability to recognize the appropriate information.

Performing an ultrasound examination is akin to fluoroscopy. The role of the sonographer is not merely to image but to utilize clinical and technical knowledge to gather the proper information that will provide the physician with images containing the diagnostic information necessary for an accurate interpretation." (*Administration Radiology* 1987)

While this book is intended as a practical guide for sonographers, it has proved very popular with physicians, especially radiology and obstetrics residents who themselves learn to scan. Scanning ability is an essential component of the competent sonologist, so this book is also dedicated to "sonologists." A recent issue of *JDMS* is devoted to a profile of the sonologist. Here are some quotes from descriptions by sonographers of the perfect sonologist.

"My idea of the perfect sonologist encompasses the following attributes.

1. One with a warm welcome, a smile, the occasional handshake as one enters the scanning room, realizing that the patient is the reason we are there.
2. A hard worker. I respect those who work as hard as I do.
3. An excellent teacher. If I am wrong, correct me. If I am right, praise me. If I do not know, teach me. Assume no knowledge when teaching me a new specialty—begin with the basics.
4. One with a sense of humor. Life is misery without it.
5. One with extensive knowledge and a scanning ability that seems almost magical; the person the other doctors go to if they are having trouble. One's scans and measurements should be consistently as good or better than mine.
6. One who is sensitive and friendly to the staff, from the orderly on up.
7. One who is polite to referring physicians, keeping interdepartmental conflicts to a minimum as well as the patient load high.
8. One who is not above helping push machines and gurneys."

"A sonologist has the following:

Brain: Housing the intelligence to trust his sonographer's scanning abilities and impressions.

Eyes: The vision to recognize a good scan.

Ears: Capable of listening and discovering departmental needs.

Nose: Able to sniff out even the most subtle echoes and findings.

Mouth Ready to speak and capable of smiling and displaying friendliness.

Thyroid: Functioning adequately to keep him going . . . active, alert, and stable.

Voice: To speak clearly about his needs in order to make a good diagnosis; to speak out when compliments as well as criticisms are appropriate.

Lungs: With the capacity to take in a deep breath whenever things go wrong and not shout at the staff.

Heart: Big enough to love his patients and his profession and to genuinely care about his peers and colleagues.

Stomach: To "take it" if he misses a diagnosis.

Guts: To speak up for his sonographers whenever necessary.

Bladder: Capacity relatively normal...so that he can appreciate what patients have to go through during an extended examination.

Legs: To get him back and forth between the examining and reading rooms and still permit him to scan during the sometimes eight-hour-plus workday."

Most of the new illustrations for this book were produced on a Mac II computer. Kati Steurer, R.T., R.D.M.S., drew many of the best images. Zahid Pasha, M.D., contributed some of the charcoal images.

R.C.S.
N.S.M.

PREFACE TO THE FIRST EDITION

Our motive for writing this book was the feeling that existing sonographic texts use an organ (e.g., liver) or disease (e.g., pancreatitis) approach rather than focusing on the clinical problem (e.g., right upper quadrant pain) as it presents to the sonographer. Most books are geared to physicians rather than sonographers and do not tackle the nuts and bolts of how to run a sonography department on a day-to-day basis.

The group of sonographers and sonologists at Johns Hopkins has been together for some years, and we felt that pooling the technical approaches that we have evolved might help others who are just beginning to become sonographers. Other sonography textbooks often describe pathologic, physiologic, or anatomic processes that cannot be seen visually or that have no ultrasonic impact. We decided to put our book squarely into a clinical context by describing only those phenomena that have an ultrasonic aspect. The reader, therefore, will not find details of pancreatic enzyme physiology or how the exchange mechanism in the kidney functions, but you will find out why there are little white marks all over the picture one morning or how to obtain decent views of that pancreas that seems so inaccessible.

We would like to think that our book is the sort of book that will be used in the lab as the patient is being examined rather than studied at night for theoretical knowledge before the registry exam (although we hope it will have value in that area as well).

Numerous individuals have helped with the production of this book. We feel particularly grateful to Ed Krajci, M.D., who went through much of the book with a fine-tooth comb making editorial changes; to Joan Batt, who devoted hours of her time to the typing of innumerable versions; to Ed Lipsit, M.D., Mike Hill, M.D., Frank Leo, B.S.E.E., Natalie Benningfield, R.D.M.S., and George Keffer, R.T.(R), who helped eliminate some of the errors, both in text and ideas; and to our artists, Tom Xenakis, assisted by Ranice Crosby, who have been very patient and inventive with numerous diagram versions.

R.C.S.

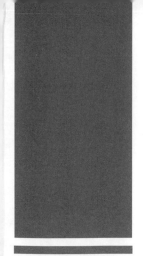

ACKNOWLEDGMENTS

Billie J. Fish has been, as usual, an outstanding Girl Friday in the production of this book. I cannot think of how long it would have taken had I been using a standard secretarial aid at the typical academic institution. Ted Witten, Kevin Barry, Dr. Wendy Berg and Dr. Jade Wong reviewed chapters and made many helpful suggestions. Kati Steurer has contributed artistic work for the book and has been responsible for many of the finest images.

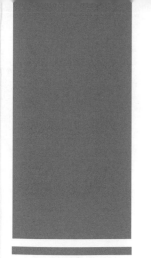

CONTENTS

Clinical Sonography

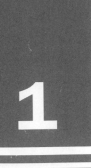

1

Introduction

ROGER C. SANDERS, NANCY SMITH MINER

The attributes of a sonographer are increasingly being defined, as befits a growing profession. Criteria for accreditation of ultrasound laboratories are being established, guidelines for virtually all sonographic examinations have been laid out (see Appendix 35), and the Society of Diagnostic Medical Sonographers (SDMS) has approved a Code of Ethics, which we have included as Appendix 36 in this edition. As welcome as all these additional guidelines are, they fail to convey that "extra something" that is the intangible essence of the quality sonographer. Managed care may be requesting speed at the expense of competence—indeed, a good sonographer has both—but a quality sonographer can accomplish an efficient examination without sacrificing intellectual curiosity. What separates a great sonographer from the average? The *real* diagnosis, one that may require creative scanning that goes beyond a hastily filled-out requisition. True sonographers, given a patient with right upper quadrant pain, do not stop at an empty gallbladder and normal duct crossing the portal vein. They keep looking until they find the mass in the bowel or the lobar pneumonia. They pursue pathology aggressively. They are detectives on the trail of a diagnosis.

This has always been our approach. The tools available, of course, continue to change. Life is a little easier with color, for instance, although not much. There are a few places where color makes a diagnosis we could not have made before; for the most part, it is just an adjunct which makes the diagnosis faster and more definitive. In our quest to keep this book affordable, we have included only a few color images, in situations where color was invaluable.

We have endured much disapproval for including B-scans in our last edition. B-scans were still in use in some countries and our text is used globally; we have many enthusiastic readers in the third world. However, recent travel has convinced us that the B-scanner has finally become extinct. In the western world, other imaging modalities have become the preferred method for some areas of study, such as the liver, adrenals, and pancreas, but in other parts of the world ultrasound remains the primary imaging technique. There are occasions when ultrasound still gives the answer after those other modalities fail. Because of this, and because incidental pathology is uncovered in these regions during other ultrasonic examinations, these chapters remain in the text.

A number of new areas have come to be important over the last few years, most of which are included in the book. Dysfunctional bleeding is now a common indication for a sonogram, and adnexal masses can be usefully categorized with ultrasound. Pelvic masses no longer represent a "Take me out!" situation for gynecologists; many can be managed conservatively or by laparoscopic surgery. Masses in the endometrium can now be outlined by hysterosonography (see Chapter 10). We have greatly expanded the fetal anomaly section. We have added vascular Doppler interrogation of the intracranial arteries (see Chapter 43) and of arteries in the limbs (see Chapter 46). The transplant section has been expanded to include the pancreas and liver.

There are various other areas we could have included, such as endoluminal, transesophageal, gastrointestinal endoscopic, and ophthalmic ultrasound. We did not because these procedures are performed almost exclusively by physicians rather than sonographers. The focus of this book continues to be on the sonographer, although we know this text is read by those physicians who are involved in hands-on scanning. This book is dedicated to all those who go beyond the merely adequate.

Basics

Physics

ROGER C. SANDERS

SONOGRAM ABBREVIATIONS

Bl   Bladder

D   Diaphragm

Gbl Gallbladder

K   Kidney

L   Liver

P   Pancreas

Th   Thyroid

Ut   Uterus

KEY WORDS

Acoustic Impedance. Density of tissue times the speed of sound in tissue. The speed of sound waves in body tissue is relatively constant at approximately 1540 meters per second.

Amplitude. Strength or height of the wave, measured in decibels.

Attenuation. Progressive weakening of the sound beam as it travels through body tissue, caused by scatter, absorption, and reflection.

Beam. Directed acoustic field produced by a transducer.

Crystal. Substance within the transducer that converts electrical impulses into sound waves and vice versa.

Cycle. Per second frequency at which the crystal vibrates. The number of cycles per second determines frequency.

Decibel (dB). A unit used to express the intensity of amplitude of sound waves; does not specify voltage.

Focal Zone. The depth of the sound beam where resolution is highest.

Focusing. Helps to increase the intensity and narrow the width of the beam at a chosen depth.

Fraunhofer Zone (Far Field). Area where transmitted beam begins to diverge.

Frequency. Number of times the wave is repeated per second as measured in hertz. Usable frequencies, except in the eye where higher frequencies can be used, lie between 2.5 and 13 million per second.

Fresnel Zone (Near Field). Area close to the transducer where the beam form is uneven.

Hertz (Hz). Standard unit of frequency; equal to 1 cycle per second.

Interface. Occurs whenever two tissues of different acoustic impedance are in contact.

Megahertz (MHz). 1,000,000 Hz.

Piezoelectric Effect. Effect caused by crystals (such as zirconate and titanate) changing shape when in an electrical field or when mechanically stressed, so that an electrical impulse can generate a sound wave or vice versa.

Power (Acoustic). Quantity of energy generated by the transducer, expressed in watts.

Pulse Repetition Rate. The number of times per second that a transmit-receive cycle occurs.

Resolution. Ability to distinguish between two adjacent structures (interfaces).

Specular Reflector. Reflection from a smooth surface at right angles to the sound beam.

Transducer (Probe). A device capable of converting energy from one form to another (see *Piezoelectric Effect*). In ultrasonography, the term is used to refer to the crystal and the surrounding housing.

Velocity. Speed of the wave, depending on tissue density. The speed of sound in soft tissues is between 1500 and 1600 meters per second. Velocity is standardized at 1540 meters per second on all current systems.

Wavelength. Distance a wave travels in a single cycle. As frequency becomes higher, wavelengths become smaller.

PHYSICS FOR SUCCESSFUL SCANNING

In order to obtain the best image possible, basic fundamentals of ultrasound wave physics must be understood and applied.

Audible Sound Waves

Audible sound waves lie between 20 and 20,000 Hz. Ultrasound uses sound waves with a far greater frequency (i.e., between 1 and 30 MHz).

Sound Wave Propagation

Sound waves do not exist in a vacuum, and propagation in gases is poor because the molecules are widely separated. The closer the molecules, the faster the sound wave moves through a medium, so bone and metals conduct sound exceedingly well (Fig. 2-1).

Effect on Image

Air-filled lungs and bowel containing air conduct sound so poorly that they cannot be imaged with ultrasound instruments. Structures behind them cannot be seen. A neighboring soft-tissue or fluid-filled organ must be used as a window through which to image a structure that is obscured by air (Fig. 2-2). An acoustic gel must fill the space between the transducer and the patient, otherwise sound will not be transmitted across the air-filled gap. Bone conducts sound at a much faster speed than soft tissue. Because ultrasound instruments cannot accommodate the difference in speed between soft tissue and bone, current systems do not image bone or structures covered by bone.

The Pulse-Echo Principle

Because the crystal in the transducer is electrically pulsed, it changes shape and vibrates, thus producing the sound beam that propagates through tissues. The crystal emits sound for a brief moment and then waits for the returning echo reflected from the structures in the plane of the sound beam (Fig. 2-3). When the echo is received, the crystal again vibrates, generating an electrical voltage comparable to the strength of the returning echo.

Effect on Image

Gray scale imaging shows echoes in varying levels of grayness, depending on the strength of the interface. Some liv-

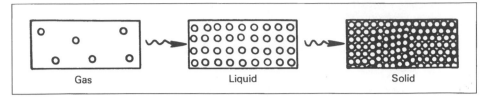

FIGURE 2-1. Sound propagation is worse in gas because molecules are widely separated. It is better in liquids and best in solids.

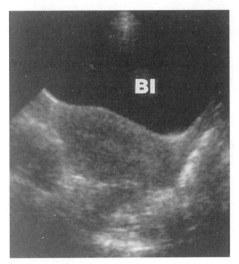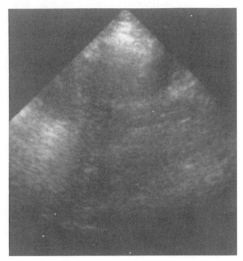

FIGURE 2-2. Sound propagation: effects on image. (**A**) A distended urinary bladder (Bl) serves as a window for the uterus. (**B**) With an empty urinary bladder the uterus cannot be seen.

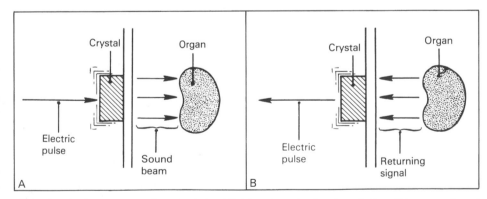

FIGURE 2-3. The pulse-echo principle. (**A**) The electrical pulse strikes the crystal and produces a sound beam, which propagates through the tissues. (**B**) Echoes arising from structures are reflected back to the crystal, which in turn vibrates, generating an electrical impulse comparable to the strength of the returning echo.

ers are homogeneously echogenic when fat is deposited. On the other hand, in acute hepatitis, overall echogenicity is lowered so that the portal vein's borders stand out more brightly.

Beam Angle to Interface

The strength of the returning echo is related to the angle at which the beam strikes the acoustic interface. The more nearly perpendicular the beam, the stronger the returning echo; smooth interfaces at right angles to the beam are known as specular reflectors (Fig. 2-4A). Echoes reflected at other angles are known as scatter (Fig. 2-4B).

Effect on Image

To demonstrate the borders of a body structure, the transducer must be placed so that the beam strikes the borders at a more or less right angle. It is worthwhile attempting to image a structure from different angles to produce the best image. Some smaller echoes that return from structures which are not at right angles to the beam help to define the borders and contents of an organ or lesion (Fig. 2-5).

Tissue Acoustic Impedance

The strength of the returning echo also depends on the differences in acoustic impedance between the various tissues

in the body. Acoustic impedance relates to tissue density: the greater the difference in density between two structures, the stronger the returning interface echoes defining the boundaries between those two structures on the ultrasound image.

Effect on Image

Structures of differing acoustic impedance (such as the gallbladder and the liver) are much easier to distinguish from one another than structures of similar acoustic texture (e.g., kidney and liver) (Fig. 2-6).

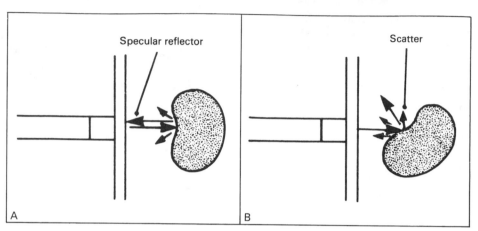

FIGURE 2-4. Angle of sound beams. (**A**) When the sound beam is perpendicular to the organ interface, specular echoes are produced. (**B**) When the sound beam is not perpendicular to the organ interface, scatter is seen.

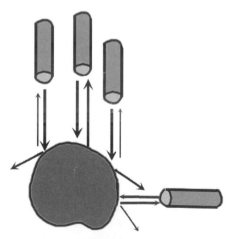

FIGURE 2-5. It is important, when visualizing a structure, to scan at several different angles to find the best possible interface (thick arrows). Only a few echoes return from the interfaces at an oblique angle to the beam—specular reflections (thin arrows). Most of the echoes are scattered.

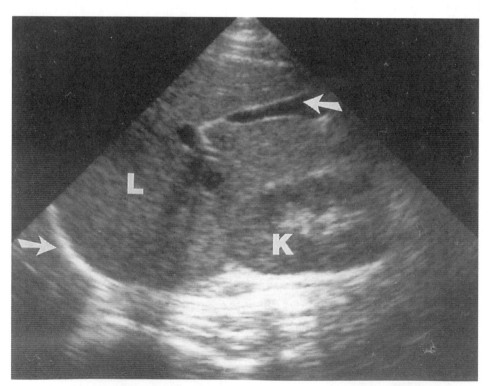

FIGURE 2-6. Tissue acoustic impedence. The bright interfaces at the gallbladder (right arrow) and the diaphragm (left arrow) are due to large differences in acoustic impedance (density) compared with the liver (L). The kidney (K), which is similar in texture to the liver, is not as easy to see.

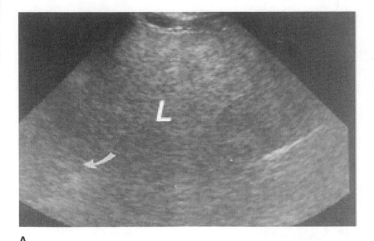

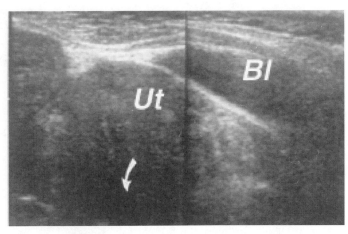

A

B

FIGURE 2-7. Absorption and scatter. (**A**) A longitudinal scan of a fatty liver; the diaphragm is not seen (arrow). (**B**) Posterior borders of a large fibroid uterus are not well delineated (arrow).

Absorption and Scatter

Because much of the sound beam is absorbed or scattered as it travels through the body, it undergoes progressive weakening (attenuation).

Effect on Image

Increased absorption and scatter prevent one from seeing the distal portions of a structure. In obese patients, the diaphragm is often not visible beyond the partially fat-filled liver (Fig. 2-7A). Fibroids may absorb so much sound that their posterior border may be difficult to define even though no sizable mass is present (Fig. 2-7B).

Transducer Frequency

Transducers come in many different frequencies—typically 2.5, 3.5, 5, 7, and 10 MHz. Increasing the frequency improves resolution but decreases penetration. Decreasing the frequency increases penetration but diminishes resolution.

Effect on Image

Transducers are chosen according to the structure being examined and the size of the patient (Fig. 2-8). The highest possible frequency should be used because it will result in superior resolution. Pediatric patients can be examined at 5 to 7.5 MHz. Lower frequencies (e.g., 2.5 MHz) permit greater penetra-

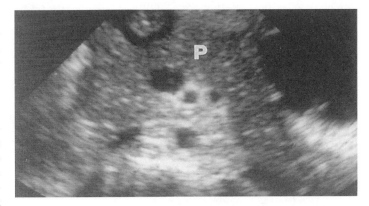

A

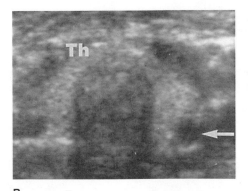

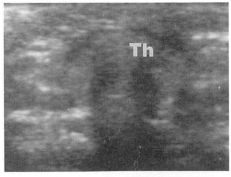

B

C

FIGURE 2-8. Transducer focal zones. (**A**) A superficial pancreas (P) is seen well using a 5-MHz short-focus transducer. (**B**) A thyroid (Th) scan using a 5-MHz short-focus transducer. Note carotid artery (arrow). (**C**) A less-detailed thyroid (Th) scan with a 3.5-MHz medium-focus transducer; this frequency is inappropriately low for such a superficial structure.

tion and may be needed to scan larger patients (Fig. 2-9).

Beam Profile

The sound beam varies in shape and resolution. Close to the skin, it suffers from the effect of turbulence, and resolution here is poor. Beyond the focal zone the beam widens (Fig. 2-10).

Effect on Image

Information that appears to be present in the near field may really be an artifact. Structures beyond the focal zone are distorted and difficult to see. A structure as small as a pinhead may appear to be half a centimeter wide (Fig. 2-11).

Transducer Focal Zone

Sound beams can be focused in a similar fashion to light. Most systems use electronic focusing, which permits the transducer to be focused at one or more variable depths. The focus level can be altered electronically by the sonographer.

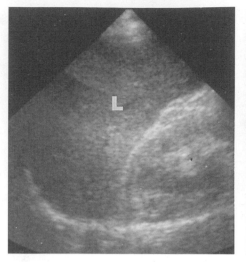
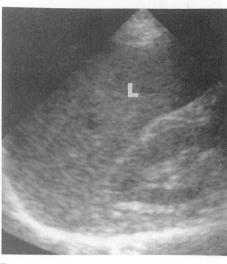

A   **B**

FIGURE 2-9. Low-frequency transducers. (**A**) A longitudinal scan using a 3.5-MHz transducer does not penetrate to the posterior aspect of the liver (L). (**B**) A 2.5-MHz transducer penetrates adequately in the obese patient.

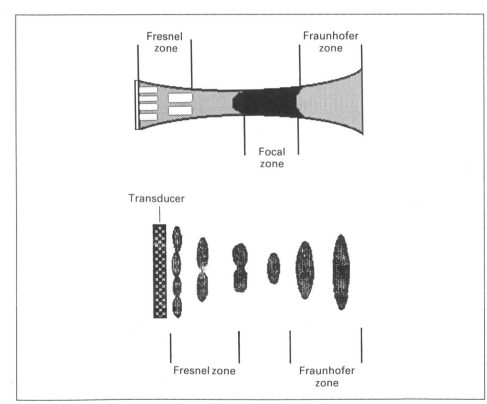

FIGURE 2-10. Diagram of the waveforms in a sound beam. Unequal waveforms in the near field (Fresnel zone). Widening of focal beam (Fraunhofer zone) beyond the focal zone.

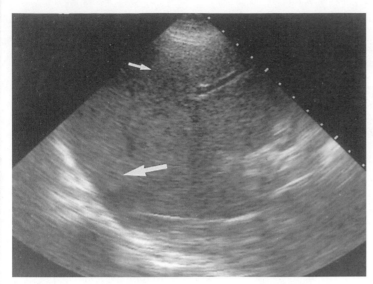

FIGURE 2-11. Longitudinal view of liver. Information is lost in the first 4 cm of the liver (small arrow). Pinpoint structures are distorted in the far field (large arrow).

Effect on Image

To achieve high resolution, one must select a transducer with the proper focal zone or use electronic focusing set at the right depth for the study. For example, imaging the thyroid with a 3.5-MHz transducer using a focal zone set at 10 cm would give poor quality images (see Fig. 2-8B and C).

SELECTED READING

Edelman, S. *Ultrasound Physics.* EST, Inc., 1994.

Hykes, D., Hedrick, W., and Starchman, D. *Ultrasound Physics and Instrumentation.* New York: Churchill Livingstone, 1995.

Kremkau, F. W. (Ed.). *Diagnostic Ultrasound: Physical Principles and Exercises* (4th ed.). New York: Grune & Stratton, 1993.

McDicken, W. N. *Diagnostic Ultrasonics: Principles and Use of Instrumentation* (3rd ed.). New York: Churchill Livingstone, 1991.

Zagzebski, J. *Essentials of Ultrasound Physics.* St. Louis: CV Mosby, 1996.

3

INSTRUMENTATION

MIMI MAGGIO-SAYLOR, ROGER C. SANDERS

KEY WORDS

A-Mode (Amplitude Modulation). A one-dimensional image displaying the amplitude strength of the returning echo signals along the vertical axis, and the time (and, therefore, the distance from the transducer) along the horizontal axis (see Fig. 3-1).

Annular Array. A type of phased array transducer utilizing several concentric ring-shaped elements. Not commonly used in modern equipment.

Axial. Depth axis. The resolution is best in an axial direction. It is accurate to a fraction of a millimeter.

B-Mode (Brightness Modulation). A method of displaying the intensity (amplitude) of an echo by varying the brightness of a dot to correspond to echo strength (see Fig. 3-2). Real-time scanners are based on B-mode.

Backing Material. See *Damping Material* (see Fig. 3-4).

CRT (Cathode Ray Tube). The term used to describe the monitor on which the image is displayed.

Curved Linear Transducer (Curved Array). Linear array transducers with a curved scan head. Focusing is electronically controlled. Useful in abdominal and OB/GYN imaging (see Fig. 3-13).

Damping Material. Material attached to the back of the transducer crystal to decrease *ring-time* (continued vibration of the crystal after the internal responses; see Fig. 3-4).

Dynamic Focusing. The ability to select focal zones at different depths throughout the image. As the number of focal zones increases, the frame rate decreases.

Dynamic Range. The range of signals the components of a system can process. Unit of measure is decibels (dB).

Electronic Focusing. Each element, or group of elements, within a transducer is pulsed separately to focus the beam at a particular area of interest. Used in array technology of all types.

Endorectal Transducer. High-frequency transducer which is placed into the rectum to evaluate the prostate and rectal wall. Some probes have both longitudinal and transverse transducers mounted on the same probe head.

Endovaginal Transducer. A high-frequency probe which is introduced into the vagina for evaluation of the pelvic organs.

Focusing. The act of narrowing the ultrasound beam to a small width. Accuracy of image increases within narrowed region.

Footprint. Portion of the transducer that is in contact with the patient.

Frame Rate (Image Rate). Rate at which the image is refreshed in a real-time system display. Usually 30 times per second, but slows if a wide field of view is used.

Freeze Frame. Control that stops a moving real-time image for photography or prolonged evaluation.

Linear Array. A transducer with many small electronically coordinated elements oriented side by side, producing a rectangular image. Useful in obstetrics, small parts, intraoperative, and vascular imaging. The long bar shape interferes with imaging between the ribs, making abdominal imaging difficult.

Matching Layer. Minimizes the difference in acoustic impedance between the transducer crystal and skin (see Fig. 3-4).

Mechanically Steered System. The physical movement of the element or mirror that causes the sound beam to sweep through the tissue, providing a real-time image.

Monitor. Term used for the TV display.

Multihertz. The ability to cycle between two or more sending frequencies within a given transducer.

Oscilloscope. The TV display screen.

Phased Array. Electronically steered system where many small elements are electronically coordinated to produce a focused wave front. Utilized in curved linear, linear, sector, and phased array transducers.

Real-Time (Dynamic) Imaging. Type of imaging in which many frames are run together to create a cinematic view of the tissue.

Ring-Time. Length of time that a transducer crystal vibrates after it has been activated.

Scan Converter. A device that gathers all of the signals and organizes them on the basis of their location to give a two-dimensional display.

Sector Scanner. Transducer with a small head which produces a pie-shaped image. May be a mechanical, curved linear, or phased array (see Figs. 3-9 and 3-13C).

Transrectal Transducer. See *Endorectal Transducer*.

Transvaginal Transducer. See *Endovaginal Transducer*.

Vector Array. Small-footprint transducer which utilizes the entire transducer face to form the image. Produces a trapezoid image with a larger field of view than the traditional sector (see Fig. 3-13B).

TYPES OF
ULTRASOUND DISPLAY

A-Mode

In A-mode (amplitude modulation or mode), the most basic form of diagnostic ultrasound, a single beam of ultrasound is analyzed. The distance between the transducer and the structure determines where an echo is seen along the time axis. The time elapsed from the transmission to the return of the signal is converted to distance. An echo (sound wave) is assumed to travel at a constant speed of 1540 m/sec in soft tissue; thus the time it takes for the echo to return to the transducer represents a distance. Isolated use of the A-mode is almost obsolete, however, it may be helpful to differentiate a cystic lesion from a solid lesion on some equipment. A cystic lesion will appear as a flat line with a prominent back wall echo (Fig. 3-1).

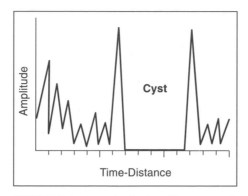

FIGURE 3-1. A-mode display. The strength of the acoustic interface is shown by the size of the echo. Note that no echoes are seen where there is fluid in the cyst.

B-Mode (Brightness Mode)

An A-mode signal can be converted to dots which vary in brightness depending on the strength of the returning echo (amplitude). A stronger (high amplitude) echo will display a brighter dot than a weaker (low amplitude) echo (Fig. 3-2). The depth of the reflector is displayed by the location of the dot. Multiple B-mode images may be displayed together to form a two-dimensional B-scan.

FIGURE 3-2. B-mode. The amplitude of an echo is displayed as the brightness of a dot comparable to the echo strength on the A-mode display.

M-Mode (Motion Mode)

In M-mode, a series of B-mode dots is displayed on a moving time base graphing the motion of mobile structures. M-mode imaging formed the basis of echocardiography prior to real-time (Fig. 3-3). M-mode is currently used in conjunction with real-time imaging in adult, pediatric, and fetal echocardiography.

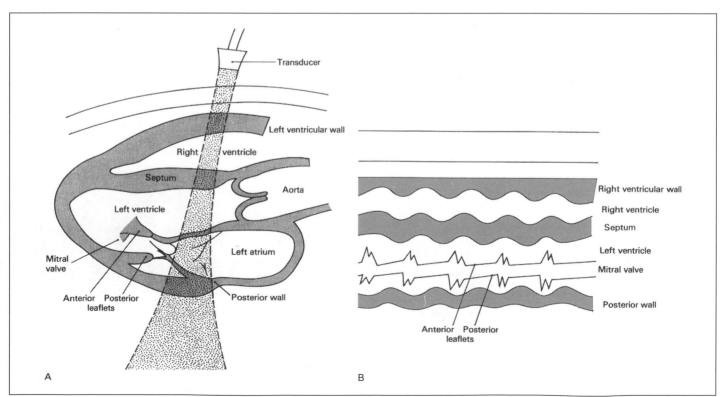

FIGURE 3-3. M-mode. (**A**) Diagram demonstrating the sound beam angled through specific heart structures. (**B**) The M-mode readout of those structures within the sound beam.

B-Scan (Static Scan)

The B-scan utilizes a series of B-mode images to "build" a two-dimensional view of the tissue. The transducer is attached to an articulated arm which provides the ultrasound system with information on transducer position and orientation. This type of imaging is not used in modern equipment owing to the numerous disadvantages. These disadvantages are as follows:

1. Scanning motion and planes are limited because of the articulated arm.
2. Examinations are lengthy and require much patient cooperation.
3. A high level of operator skill is required.
4. Movement cannot be displayed.
5. Equipment is large and unwieldy. A portable examination cannot be performed.

Real-Time, B-Scan

Real-time systems provide a cinematic view of the area being evaluated by displaying a rapid series of images sequentially. The following are advantages of real-time scanning:

1. Scanning planes that best demonstrate the area of interest can be easily found.
2. A rapid examination can be performed because there is constant visual feedback on the display screen.
3. Extended structures such as vessels can be followed, allowing them to be traced to their origin.
4. Movement observation may aid in organ identification (e.g., mass versus bowel).
5. Infants, children, and uncooperative patients can be examined easily.
6. Critically ill patients and those with acute conditions can be studied portably.
7. Pulsed and color flow Doppler can be performed coincident with the real-time examination.

REAL-TIME IMAGING

All modern systems use a real-time approach. Real-time B-scan ultrasound systems use a transducer which contains a crystal that can convert ultrasound impulses into electrical impulses. These signals are integrated by a computer, known as a scan converter, into a two-dimensional image. A description of the components of the basic system follows.

Scan Converter

This is the portion of the imaging system in which the image data are stored and converted for display on the cathode ray tube (CRT). Analog scan converters are the oldest form and are not used in modern equipment. An electron gun is used to fire electrons on a grid which stores the charges and then displays the information on the CRT. Digital scan converters, now found in all new systems, use computer memory to digitize the image and transfer it to the display monitor.

Preprocessing and postprocessing of the image information occurs in the scan converter. The brightness level for an electronic signal derived from an ultrasound echo can be varied, depending on whether strong or weak signals need to be emphasized.

Transducers

The transducer assembly consists of five main components: the transducer crystal, the matching layers, damping material, the transducer case, and the electric cable (Fig. 3-4).

1. The transducer crystal is composed of a piezoelectric material, most commonly lead zirconate titanate. The transducer crystal converts the electrical voltage into acoustic energy upon transmission, and acoustic energy to electrical energy upon reception.
2. The matching layers lie in front of the transducer element and provide an acoustic connection between the transducer element and the skin. Some loss of sound transmission (impedance) occurs at this layer. Decreasing the difference in acoustic impedance will decrease the amount of acoustic reflection back into the body from the transducer and, therefore, aid in the transmission of the sound beam.
3. Damping material such as rubber is attached to the back of the transducer element to decrease secondary reverberations of the crystal with returning signals. Decreasing the ring-time results in an increase in depth (axial) resolution.

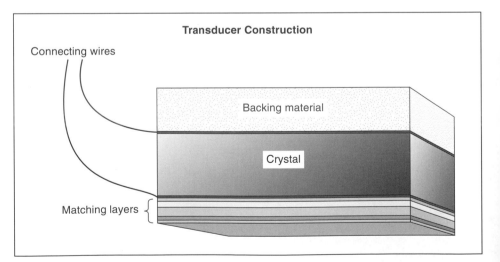

FIGURE 3-4. Diagram showing transducer construction. Matching layers of material decrease the size of the main bang acoustic interface that occurs between the crystal and the skin. Backing material acts as a damping tool to stop secondary reverberations of the crystal. The crystal is constructed of piezoelectric material which can convert electrical impulses into sound waves and vice versa.

4. The transducer case provides a housing for the crystal, a damping material layer, and insulation from interference by electrical noise.

5. The electronic cable contains the bundle of electrical wires used to excite the transducer elements and receive the returned electrical impulses. There must be an individual wire for excitation and for reception of each individual transducer element.

Several types of transducer elements exist:

1. *Mechanical Transducers.* The transducer crystal is physically moved to provide steering for the beam. Most of these probes provide a sector image with a fixed focus. Mechanical steering is not commonly used in modern equipment.

   a. Rotary Type (Wheel). In mechanically steered systems using a rotary type transducer, one or more transducer elements are arranged in a wheel like housing that moves the beam through an arc-shaped sector (Fig. 3-5). The small size of the transducer face allows intercostal access for scanning organs such as the liver and heart.

   b. Oscillating Transducer (Wobbler). The drive motor and transducer element are housed in a small container in mechanically steered systems using an oscillating transducer. The motor drives the transducer element back and forth, producing a sector image (Fig. 3-6).

   c. Transducer With Oscillating Mirror. In this type of mechanically steered system, the transducer element is stationary but the beam is moved by oscillating a mirror that reflects the sound (Fig. 3-7).

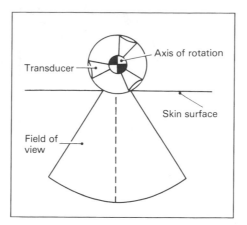

FIGURE 3-5. Mechanical rotary sector scanner.

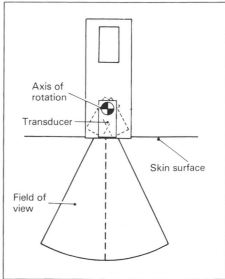

FIGURE 3-6. Oscillating transducer (wobbler).

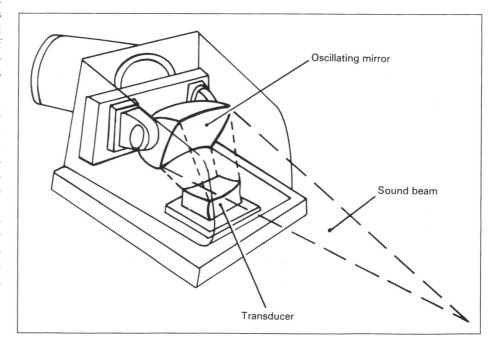

FIGURE 3-7. Stationary transducer with oscillating mirror.

2. *Electronically Steered Systems.* In this type of transducer, multiple piezoelectric elements are used. A separate electrical supply is provided for each element. Steering and focusing occur by sequentially exciting individual elements across the face of the transducer. Focusing is controlled electronically by the operator. The images are displayed in a sector, vector, linear, or curved linear format.

   a. Linear Sequenced Arrays. Multiple transducer elements are mounted on a straight or curved bar. Groups of elements are electronically pulsed at once to act as a single larger element. Pulsing occurs sequentially down the length of the transducer face, moving the sound beam from end to end (Fig. 3-8).

   b. Phased Array. The phased array consists of multiple transducer elements mounted compactly in a line. All elements are pulsed as a group with small time delays to provide beam steering and focusing. The resulting image is in a sector or vector format and is particularly useful in cardiac, intercostal, and endocavitary imaging (Fig. 3-9; see Fig. 3-13C).

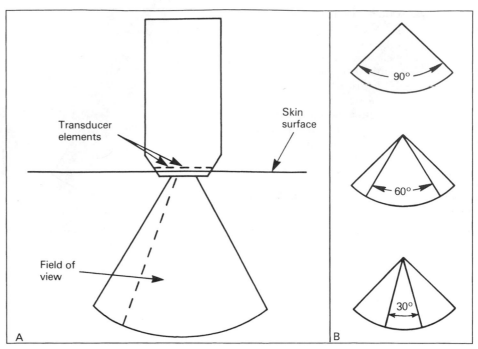

FIGURE 3-9. Wedged-shaped field. (**A**) Phased (steered) array. (**B**) Different size fields of view. Smaller fields give better resolution.

   c. Annular Array. The annular array system employs crystals of the same frequency arranged in a circle. The circular transducers are electronically focused at several depths (Fig. 3-10). The beam may be reflected off an oscillating acoustic mirror into a water bath.

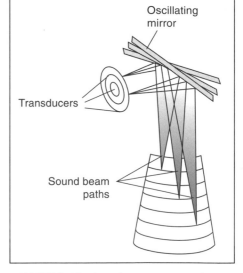

FIGURE 3-10. Annular array transducer.

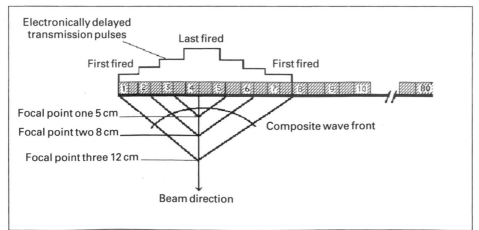

FIGURE 3-8. Linear sequenced array. Multiple transducer elements are pulsed in groups. Time differences in the delay of the returning signal allow focusing at different depths.

SPECIALIZED ULTRASOUND SYSTEMS

Small Parts Scanners

Small parts scanner systems usually utilize real-time probes capable of high resolution, for example, a 7.5- or 10-MHz transducer in a water or oil bath. All types of real-time systems have been used as small parts scanners. They are designed for visualizing the fine detail of superficial structures, usually at a depth of less than 4 cm from the skin surface (e.g., thyroid, carotid arteries, testes, breast, or structures in an infant).

Endoultrasound Systems

The transducer—which can be a linear, phased array, or mechanical sector scanner—is placed on the end of a rod. This rod is inserted into the rectum, vagina, or esophagus (Fig. 3-11). Even smaller transducers on the end of catheters can be introduced into vessels, the biliary duct, or the ureter (transluminal transducers).

Operative Systems

Standard ultrasound systems are modified so they can be used in a sterile fashion in the operating room. Special high-frequency ultrasound probes are used for this purpose.

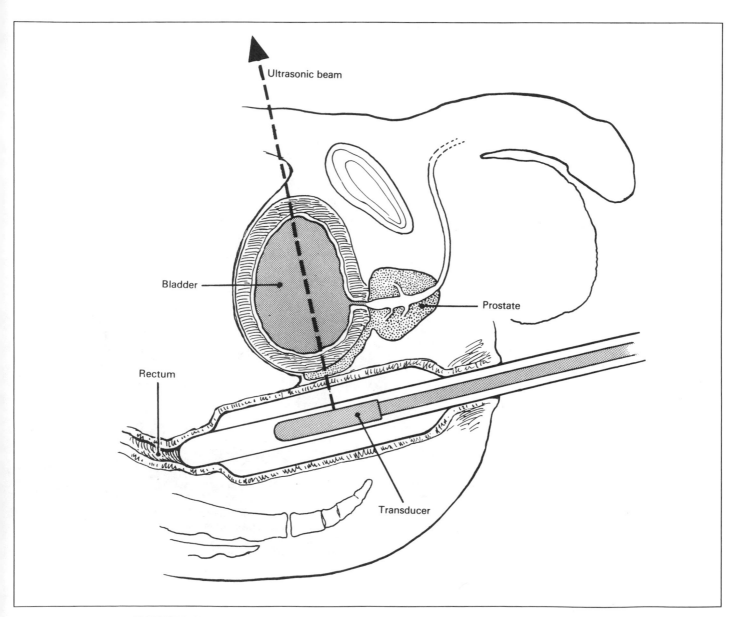

FIGURE 3-11. Rectal scanner. An ultrasound probe in a balloon filled with water is placed in the rectum adjacent to the prostate. The probe is moved or rotated to create an image of the prostate and bladder.

Special Transducers

Special transducers (Fig. 3-12) have been produced to help view specific areas:

1. Small parts (5.7, 5, and 10 MHz) transducer
2. Rectal transducers in longitudinal (linear) and transverse (radial) configurations
3. Endovaginal transducer
4. Biopsy transducer
5. Doppler probe
6. Intraoperative probes for access to small orifices (e.g., imaging the brain via burr holes) or for imaging flat organs (e.g., linear arrays for the liver)
7. Endoluminal transducers for accessing vessels, ureter, and the common bile duct

Transducer Formats

There are four basic types of transducer formats. These are linear, vector, sector, and curved array. The linear format provides a rectangular image (Fig. 3-13A). This transducer is most useful in obstetrics, small parts, and vascular imaging. A vector format provides a trapezoidal image (Fig. 3-13B). This small footprint transducer is often used in abdominal, gynecologic, and obstetric applications. The sector image is pie-shaped and is commonly used in cardiac, abdominal, gynecologic, obstetric, and transcranial imaging (Fig. 3-13C). A curved array transducer will provide a large field of view with a convex near field (Fig. 3-13D). This transducer is most commonly used in obstetrics, however, other applications include abdominal and gynecologic imaging.

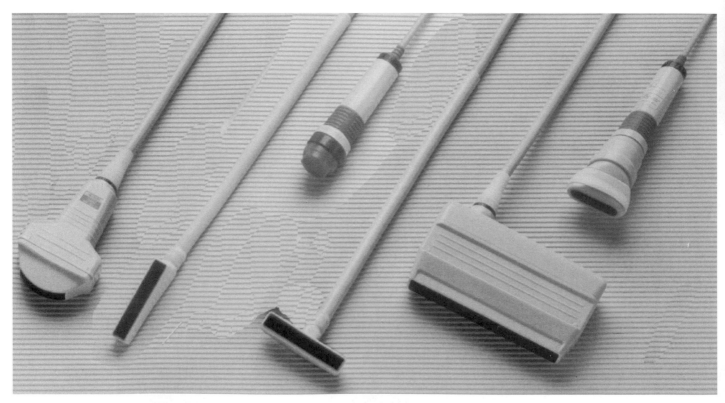

FIGURE 3-12. A variety of transducers are available for specific purposes. The transducers shown on this image are, from left to right: a curved linear array, a sagittal transrectal probe, a mechanical wobbler, a transverse intraoperative linear array, an abdominal linear array and a small footprint cardiac transducer for use between ribs.

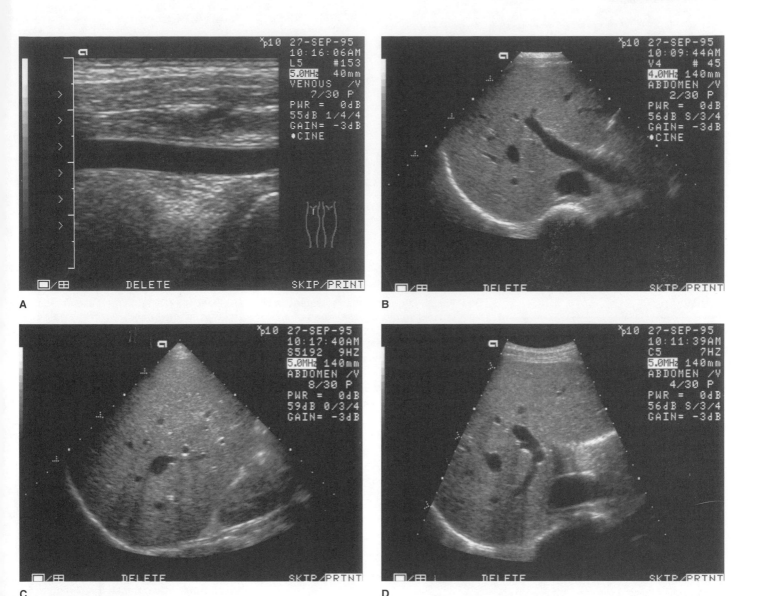

FIGURE 3-13. Transducer formats. (**A**) Linear image. (**B**) Vector image. (**C**) Sector image. (**D**) Curved array image.

SELECTED READING

AIUM/NEMA. Safety standard for diagnostic ultrasound equipment. *JUM* 2:4, 1983.

Edelman, S. *Ultrasound Physics.* EST, Inc., 1996.

Hykes, D., Hedrick, W., and Starchman, D. *Ultrasound Physics and Instrumentation.* New York: Churchill Livingstone, 1995.

Kremkau, F. W. (Ed.). *Diagnostic Ultrasound: Physical Principles and Exercises* (4th ed.). New York: Grune & Stratton, 1993.

Zagzebski, J. *Essentials of Ultrasound Physics.* St. Louis: CV Mosby, 1996.

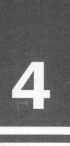

4 KNOBOLOGY

MIMI MAGGIO-SAYLOR, BARBARA DEL PRINCE

KEY WORDS

Acoustic Power/Transmit Power. A control that varies the amount of energy the transducer transmits to the patient. Power should be used at the lowest level consistent with satisfactory image production.

Alternate Color. A control that switches between various forms of color (e.g., color Doppler and color Doppler energy).

Annotation Keys. Allow labeling of the image. May consist of preprogrammed keys or a keyboard for typing.

B-Color. Colorizes the gray scale.

Body Markers. Provide a drawing of the specific area being examined (e.g., abdomen, pelvis, breast) to aid in labeling of the image.

Calipers. Measurement tool.

Caps Lock. Allows either lower case or upper case characters to be typed.

Caret. Arrow along vertical axis of image denoting the location of the transmit zone or focal zone.

Cine Loop/Playback. The system memory stores the most recent sequence of image frames before the freeze button is pressed. The sequence of images can then be reviewed by the operator.

Color Doppler. Activates the color Doppler mode of the system.

Delay. Sets the depth at which the TGC (time gain compensation) slope commences; used to depress artifactual echoes in the near field. Not commonly found on modern equipment.

Depth Range. Varies the depth to which the echoes are displayed. The maximum depth varies depending on the transducer used.

Dual Image. Allows the display screen to be split in order to display two views of an image or to compare the anatomy of the abnormal side with that of the normal side. One image will be frozen while the other is active in real time.

Dynamic Range/Log Compression. The range of intensity from the largest to the smallest echo that a system can display.

Ellipse. Measurement tool used in circumference measurements.

Field of View. Gives four or five choices to the sonographer to make maximal use of the screen's potential resolution and yet display all of the relevant area (e.g., 1:1, 2:1, 3:1, 4:1, 5:1 imaging display).

Freeze. All display data (real time image frames) start and stop with this control. An image cannot be printed or measured until it is frozen.

Gain. Regulates the degree of echo amplification (the brightness of the image).

Knee. Region of the time-gain curve where the slope changes markedly. Not commonly found on modern equipment.

M-Mode. Activates the motion mode (M-mode) used in cardiac imaging to trace movements of the cardiac tissue.

Multihertz. Allows the user to choose between different sending frequencies of the transducers.

Near Gain. The amplification of echoes returning from the near field are regulated by this knob. Not commonly found on modern equipment.

Needle Guide (Biopsy Guide). Activates graphics on the display screen corresponding to the intended path of the needle during invasive procedures.

Oscilloscope (CRT). Screen used to display the B-scan image and TGC (*time gain compensation*) characteristics.

Persistence. Control that allows the accumulation of echo information over a longer period. Subtle texture differences can be enhanced using this control.

Postprocessing. This control may be adjusted in real time or while the image is frozen. The postprocessing alters image aesthetics by placing more or less emphasis on specific echo levels.

Preprocessing. Control which adjusts edge enhancement of image pixels. It is used prior to scanning.

Print. This control activates the camera to document the image on the screen.

Pulsed Wave Doppler. Activates the spectral Doppler mode.

Recall Application/Recall Set/Program Select. Pre-established parameters which are specific for the different studies performed. Preprocessing, persistence, and postprocessing are among the preset parameters.

Slide Pots. TGC (*time gain compensation*) controls can be adjusted in short segments with the use of slide pots.

Slope Rate. The rate at which echoes are suppressed or amplified as the depth varies.

Time Gain Compensation (TGC), Time Compensation Gain (TCG), Depth Gain Compensation (DGC). Control which compensates for the loss (attenuation) of the sound beam as it passes through tissue.

Trace. Measurement tool which allows the user to trace the outline of an area being measured. Often used to obtain circumference measurements.

Trackball/Joystick. Controls the movements of the annotation cursor, calipers, focal zone carets, and cine loop.

Transducer Choice. Permits the activation of the different transducer ports.

Transmit Zone/Focal Zone. The transmit zone enhances the resolution of an area in the image by electronic focusing. The frame rate is lowered when this control is used.

Triplex. Allows the simultaneous use of gray scale imaging and spectral and color Doppler.

USE OF KNOBS

The basics of knobology are interchangeable between different types of real-time systems. Controls specific to Doppler technology are described in Chapter 5 (Doppler and Color Flow Principles). Learning to use the knobs effortlessly is an important part of the art of ultrasonic scanning.

Gain

The system gain controls the degree of echo amplification, or brightness of the image. The gain control is usually measured in decibels, an arbitrary measurement of sound amplitude (Fig. 4-1).

Care must be taken with the use of gain. Too much overall gain can fill artifactual echoes into fluid-filled structures, whereas too little gain can negate real echo information.

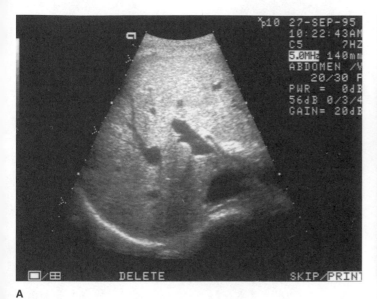

A

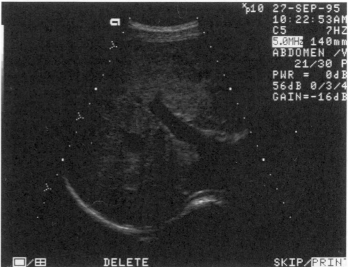

B

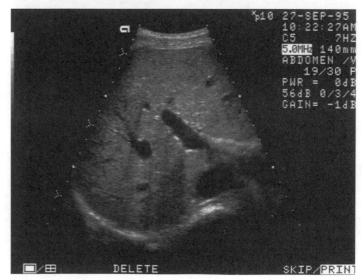

C

FIGURE 4-1. Overall gain. (**A**) Too much overall gain in the near field. (**B**) Too little overall gain. (**C**) Correct gain setting.

Depth Gain Compensation (DGC)

The DGC attempts to compensate for the acoustic loss by absorption, scatter, and reflection and to show structures of the same acoustic strength with the same brightness no matter what the depth. Individual controls for small segments of the display, known as slide pots, are available from most manufacturers. The DGC and gain controls should be used together to provide a uniform image (Fig. 4-2).

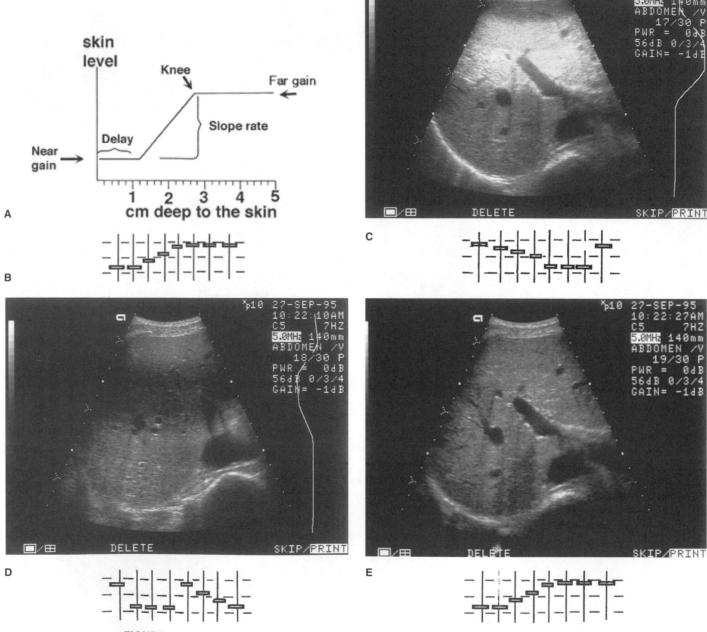

FIGURE 4-2. (**A**) Diagram showing the components of the time gain compensation curve. (**B**) Slide pots are used in modern systems rather than separate controls. Often the slide pots are prearranged to compensate for tissue attenuation and are all set at the same level. (**C**) DGC curve: Too much emphasis on mid-field echoes. (**D**) DGC curve: Too little emphasis on mid-field echoes. (**E**) Correct DGC setting.

Log Compression (Dynamic Range)

The log compression (dynamic range) is the range of intensities from the largest to the smallest echo that a system can display. Changing the log compression does not affect the number of gray shades in the image—instead it varies the brightness. For example, a signal will appear more sonolucent at a lower log compression than the same amplitude signal at a high log compression setting. The log compression may be used to remove reverberation artifacts from cystic structures or to enhance the display of low-level echoes such as gallbladder sludge or soft plaque (Fig. 4-3).

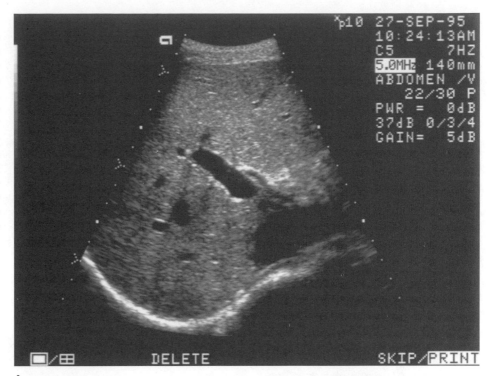

FIGURE 4-3. Log compression (dynamic range). (**A**) Low log compression of 37 dB creates a more contrasty image. (**B**) High log compression of 60 dB.

Preprocessing (Edge Enhancement)

The preprocessing control alters the edges of the image pixels to accentuate the transition between areas of different echogenicities. Altering the preprocessing may aid in performing measurements by making borders sharper (Fig. 4-4).

Persistence

Persistence is a frame-averaging function that allows the accumulation of echo information over a longer period of time. By increasing the persistence, subtle tissue texture differences will be enhanced. Decreasing the persistence allows the user to evaluate moving structures more easily.

Postprocessing

Postprocessing alters image aesthetics by placing more or less emphasis on specific echo intensities. Changing the postprocessing map may aid the user in evaluating pathology, (e.g., emphasizing bones in obstetric patients) or in the evaluation of technically difficult patients. Postprocessing is the only function which may be changed after the image is frozen (Fig. 4-5).

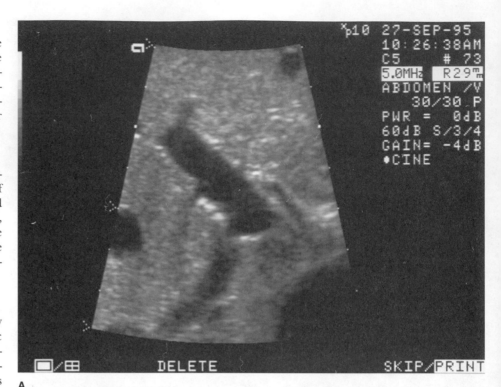

A

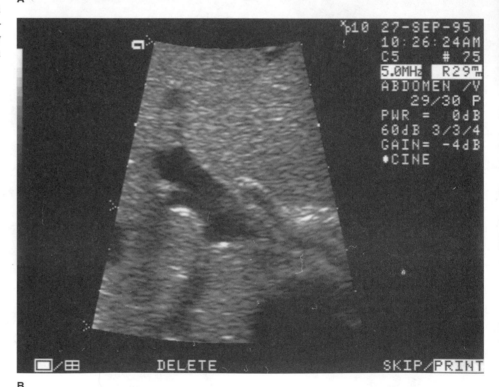

B

FIGURE 4-4. Preprocessing (edge enhancement). (**A**) This setting on this machine provides fuzzy pixel borders. (**B**) This setting on this machine provides crisp pixel borders.

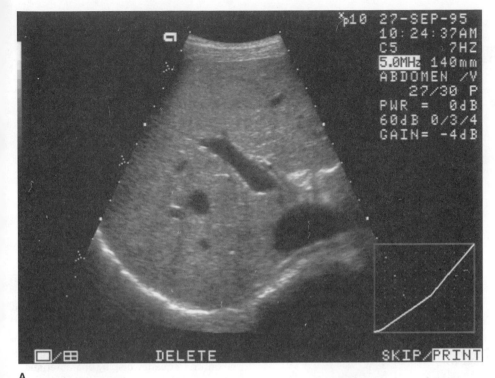

A

B

Zoom

The zoom function allows for magnification of the image by increasing the pixel size, however, this results in image degradation.

Write Zoom (RES)

With write zoom a box is placed on the screen and the area seen within the box can be expanded to fill the screen. The number of scan lines remains the same and the lines are reallocated so that the image is a true magnification of the area under examination.

Video Invert

The video invert feature allows one to select a "positive" or "negative" image (i.e., a white or black background). Negative polarity (black background) is most commonly used because it allows better detection of subtle abnormalities in texture.

Transducer Selection

This feature allows the user to activate the transducer of choice.

Calipers

Caliper markers are available to measure distances. An added feature in some units is the ellipsoid measurement. A dotted line can be created around the outline of a structure to calculate either the circumference or the area.

SELECTED READING

Edelman, S. *Ultrasound Physics.* EST, Inc., 1996.

Hykes, D., Hedrick, W., and Starchman, D. *Ultrasound Physics and Instrumentation.* New York: Churchill Livingstone, 1995.

Zagebski, J. *Essentials of Ultrasound Physics.* St. Louis: CV Mosby, 1996.

FIGURE 4-5. Postprocessing. (**A**) This postprocessing setting de-emphasizes mid-level echoes, as seen in graph in lower right hand corner, providing a soft image. (**B**) This postprocessing setting provides equal emphasis of all echoes resulting in a more contrasty appearance.

5

DOPPLER AND COLOR FLOW PRINCIPLES

BARBARA DEL PRINCE, MIMI MAGGIO SAYLOR, ROGER C. SANDERS

KEY WORDS

Aliasing. A technical artifact. The frequency change exceeds the measurable range because signals are being sent too frequently. One signal returns after a second signal has been sent. The waveform wraps around so that peak signals appear at the bottom of the display. The problem is corrected by decreasing the pulse repetition frequency (i.e., increasing the gap between pulses).

Diastole. The second half of the spectral waveform and of the cardiac cycle, when lower velocities are seen. At this time, the heart muscles are relaxing and the ventricular chambers fill with blood.

Duplex Imaging. The simultaneous display of the B-scan image and the Doppler waveform.

Frame Rate. The number of times per second that the image is refreshed.

Frequency Shift. The amount of change in the returning frequency as compared with the transmitting frequency when the sound wave hits a moving target such as blood in an artery.

Hepatofugal. Flow away from the liver, seen when pressure within the liver portal system is increased to the point where flow cannot enter the liver through the portal vein and instead goes to the heart via collaterals.

Hepatopetal. Portal vein flow toward the liver.

Intima. The inner lining of an artery. The adventitia and media are the other components of the arterial wall.

Laminar. Normal pattern of blood flow in a vessel; the flow in the center of the vessel is faster than at the walls.

Linear Steering. Some units offer this feature with linear array transducers. The angle of the sound beam can be obliqued independently in all three different modes (B-scan image, Doppler, and color) (i.e., the gray scale image can be obliqued to the left while the Doppler image is steered to the right).

Parvus and Tarda Flow Changes. Flow patterns seen distal to arterial obstruction. There is a slow ascending systolic flow signal with overall decreased signal amplitude.

Pulse Repetition Frequency (PRF). Also known as *flow velocity range*. This control sets the number of pulses of ultrasound transmitted per second for a given viewing depth. The deeper the depth or the slower the velocity range, the lower the PRF since more time must be allowed for a returning signal. With a shallow depth, a higher velocity range and higher PRF can be used. Many systems program the PRF for a selected structure or depth. PRF can be adjusted with the *velocity range control* knob. Use of a PRF that is too high for a given depth gives rise to aliasing.

Resistance. As arterial flow enters an organ such as the kidney, the density of the tissue creates pressure against the flow. When the pressure is abnormally increased, as in organ rejection or arterial stenosis, a high-resistance flow pattern develops. High-resistance flow patterns can be normal in some locations (e.g., femoral artery). A high-resistance pattern has high systolic peak and low diastolic flow levels. Low-resistance flow has low systolic levels and much flow in diastole.

Sample Volume (Gate). The sample site from which the signal is obtained with pulsed Doppler. The size and position of the line which outlines the site, known as the gate, can be varied.

Spectral Analysis/Waveform. Evaluation of the entire frequency display characteristics. The systolic frequencies display higher velocity systolic peaks when compared to the lower diastolic flow level.

Spectral Broadening. Echo fill-in of the spectral window proportional to the severity of the vessel stenosis (see Fig. 5-7). It may also result from poor technique or with too much gain or too large a sample volume.

Spectral Window. The area that is being sampled by the Doppler system.

Systole. The first half of the spectral waveform and of the cardiac cycle; high velocities are seen. This signal reflects the contraction of the heart muscle as it propels blood to the body.

Velocity. Speed of blood flow in a vessel.

Velocity Display Mode. This function allows the operator to adjust the displayed colors to correspond to the desired flow velocity range to be measured.

DOPPLER

Doppler physics as it relates to diagnostic ultrasonography concerns the behavior of high-frequency sound waves as they are reflected off moving fluid, usually blood (Fig. 5-1).

The Doppler Effect

When a high-frequency sound beam meets a moving structure, such as blood flow in a vessel, the reflected sound returns at a different frequency. The speed (velocity) of the moving structure can be calculated from this frequency shift (Fig. 5-2). The returning frequency will be increased if flow is toward the sound source (transducer) and decreased if flow is away from the sound source. The frequency of the returning wave can be converted to an audible signal. The Doppler effect is responsible for the variation in the pitch of the sound wave from an ambulance siren as it moves toward and away from you. The siren pitch becomes higher as the ambulance approaches and lowers as the vehicle departs.

Clinical Correlation

The Doppler effect is helpful in localizing blood vessels and determining optimal sites for velocity measurements. Typically veins have a low-pitched hum, whereas arteries have an alternating pattern with a high-pitched systolic component and low-pitched diastolic component.

Continuous Wave Doppler (CW)

The sound beam is continuously emitted from one transducer and received by a second. Both transducers are encased in one housing. Since this is a simple system, it is cheap, but it can only be used when superficial vessels are examined.

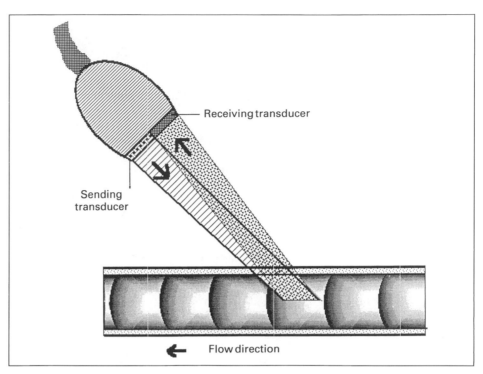

FIGURE 5-1. Diagram of a pulsed doppler transducer demonstrating the direction of the transmitted sound beam toward the flow of blood (black arrow) and the receiving sound beam back to the transducer (gray arrow).

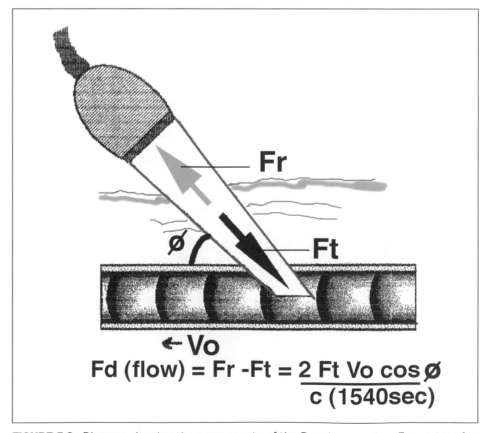

$$Fd \text{ (flow)} = Fr - Ft = \frac{2\,Ft\,Vo\cos\varnothing}{c\,(1540sec)}$$

FIGURE 5-2. Diagram showing the components of the Doppler equation. Fr = return frequency. Ft = sending frequency. $\varnothing$ = angle of insonation of a vessel. Vo = flow rate in centimeters per second.

Clinical Correlation

Vascular surgeons use continuous wave Doppler to check for the presence of flow in superficial arteries. Continuous wave Doppler is also sometimes used to monitor umbilical artery flow. Since the cord lies in the amniotic fluid, no other confusing vessels are within the ultrasonic beam.

Pulsed Doppler

A Doppler sound beam is sent and received (pulsed) over a short period of time (Fig. 5-3). Since the time that the Doppler signal takes to reach the target can be converted to distance, the depth of the site sampled is known.

The pulsed sound beam is "gated." Only those signals from a vessel at a known depth are displayed and analyzed (see Fig 5-3). The size of the gate varies the volume of waveform data that is retrieved. A larger gate is not necessarily better since it diminishes the sensitivity of the signal detection. To obtain the highest velocity in a stenotic vessel, move a smaller gate through the vessel and listen for the highest audible sound. However, when a large clot is present in a vein, using a large sample volume may help detect some area of flow within the vein.

Clinical Correlation

Pulsed Doppler is used to detect the presence of blood flow in a select vessel at a given depth when there are several vessels within the ultrasonic beam. For example, if the right renal artery shows no flow, an occlusion can be diagnosed even though the portal vein and inferior vena cava lie close to the right renal artery because the gate does not include those vessels. Since clots can appear echo-free, a real-time image may erroneously appear to show a normal vessel even though it is occluded. Doppler will detect no flow. Flow from other vessels is not analyzed, since only the gated area is examined. Pulsed Doppler can be used to differentiate between the hepatic artery and the common bile duct as these structures lie anterior to the portal vein. (The hepatic artery can reach the size of a pathologically dilated common bile duct). Doppler confirmation of flow within arteries and no flow within bile ducts is helpful when dilated ducts create confusion.

Flow Direction

The direction of blood flow can be discovered by seeing whether the frequency of the returning signal is above or below the baseline in a suspect vessel. Flow toward the transducer is traditionally displayed above the baseline, and flow away from the transducer is shown below the baseline (Fig. 5-4). Flow direction can also be established by comparing the flow pattern in a vessel in which the flow direction is known with the flow pattern in a neighboring vascular structure in which the flow might be in either direction. Note of caution: the spectral display can be reversed by using a knob on the machine. Be sure it is set correctly before suggesting pathologic reversed flow.

Clinical Correlation

Flow in the portal vein is sometimes reversed when pressure in the liver increases in portal hypertension; flow away from the liver is known as hepatofugal and indicates that the portal pressure is so high that flow has been reversed. Flow toward the liver is known as hepatopetal. Flow direction analysis allows the diagnosis of the abnormal hepatofugal flow.

Flow Pattern

The pattern of flow can be assessed with Doppler ultrasound. Typically a vein shows a continuous rhythmic flow in diastole and systole and emits a lower-pitched signal than arterial flow. Arterial flow has an alternating high-pitched systolic peak and a much lower diastolic level (see Fig. 5-4).

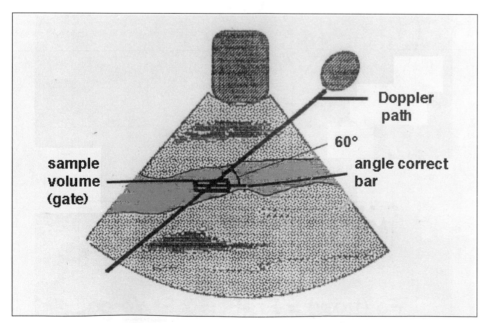

FIGURE 5-3. Real-time image displaying the gate (sample volume) and the angle correct bar within the blood vessel. Note the 60° angle of the beam to vessel flow. Only timed signals from the area within the gate are displayed and analyzed in the Doppler signal.

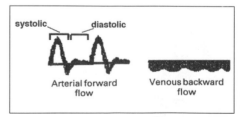

FIGURE 5-4. Arterial waveform demonstrating flow above the baseline; venous flow displayed below the baseline (flow in the other direction). Note phases of systole and diastole in arterial pulse.

Clinical Correlation

Veins may be confused with arteries on real-time. For example, if the patient has portal hypertension, it may be difficult to decide whether the hepatic artery is patent because many venous collaterals are seen alongside the portal vein. The hepatic artery and venous collaterals are, however, easily distinguished using pulsed Doppler.

Flow Velocity

The velocity of blood flow can be deduced from the arterial waveform. If the peak systolic flow frequency and the angle at which the beam intersects the vessel are known, a simple formula allows the deduction of velocity (see Fig. 5-2). The machine performs this computation. The velocity calculation formula is only accurate if the angle of the Doppler beam to the interrogated vessel is less than 60 degrees (see Fig. 5-3). At a 70-degree angle, the velocity error is 25 percent and it is proportionately larger as the angle is increased up to 90 degrees.

Clinical Correlation

Velocity is an important factor in calculating the severity of carotid stenosis. Generally, the more tight the stenosis, the greater the velocity through the narrowed vessel. However, as the vessel becomes critically occluded, flow velocity will diminish.

Low-Resistance Versus High-Resistance Flow

Doppler flow analysis allows the detection of two types of arterial flow, a high-resistance (Fig. 5-5A) and a low-resistance (Fig. 5-5B) pattern. The high-resistance pattern has a high systolic peak and a low diastolic flow. Low-resistance arterial systems demonstrate a biphasic systolic peak and a relatively high level of flow in diastole (see Fig. 5-5B). Resistance is commonly calculated using a simple formula:

$$\text{Resistance Index (RI)} = \frac{\text{Systolic pressure} - \text{Diastolic pressure}}{\text{Systolic pressure}}$$

An alternative technique, known as the pulsatility index, evaluates the diastolic flow in a different fashion. A cursor is run along the superior aspect of the systolic and diastolic flow and the mean is calculated by the system.

$$\text{Pulsatility Index (PI)} = \frac{\text{Systolic velocity} - \text{Mean flow}}{\text{Systolic velocity}}$$

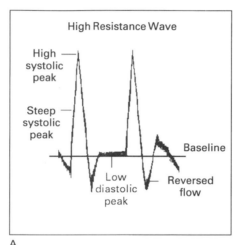

Clinical Correlation

If a high-resistance pattern is seen where there is normally a low-resistance appearance, such as in the common carotid or renal artery, vessel narrowing is present. For example, a completely occluded internal carotid artery may create a high-resistance waveform in the common carotid artery. Increased resistance is also a feature of a number of renal diseases such as rejection and hydronephrosis. Quantifying the severity of the resistance helps in clinical management.

A high-resistance pattern is usually seen in the vessel supplying the ovaries in the proliferative phase of the cycle. If a low-resistance pattern is seen within an ovarian mass, carcinoma is more likely.

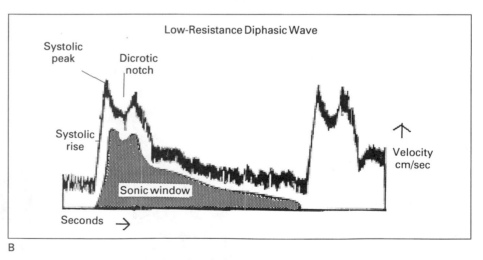

FIGURE 5-5. (**A**) The arterial spectral waveform in a high-resistance bed. Note low diastolic flow. (**B**) The arterial spectral waveform in a low-resistance bed. Note relatively high diastolic flow.

Flow Pattern Within a Vessel (Laminar Flow)

In a normal vessel the velocity of blood is highest in the center of a vessel and lowest closer to the wall. This is termed *laminar flow*. When there is a wall irregularity or the artery is angled, the flow is distorted and may be greatest closest to the wall of the vessel. Stenosis markedly increases the flow velocity through an area of narrowing, whereas vessel dilatation decreases the speed of flow (Fig. 5-6).

Clinical Correlation

To accurately measure the flow velocity in a tortuous carotid artery, place the sample volume (the area that is gated) at the center of the highest flow. Listening to the audible signal is very useful in determining the site for optimal measurement. A high-grade stenosis will have a shrill, chirping sound.

Flow Distortion

Normal laminar flow at and immediately beyond an area of wall irregularity or stenosis is disturbed, resulting in abnormal spectral waveforms. Flow distortion (nonlaminar) is characterized by high velocities in both systole and diastole. The presence of many echoes within the sonic "window" is termed *spectral broadening* and may indicate considerable flow disturbance. Eddies occur because the high-velocity jet suddenly hits flow in an undisturbed vessel (Fig. 5-7). Gray scale visualization of soft echo-free plaques, as the source of a wall irregularity, may be limited. If high velocities are seen without flow distortion or wall irregularity, the Doppler gain may be too low.

Clinical Correlation

Flow disturbance in an artery such as the carotid may be an indication of pathologic atheromatous changes (see Pitfalls later in this chapter).

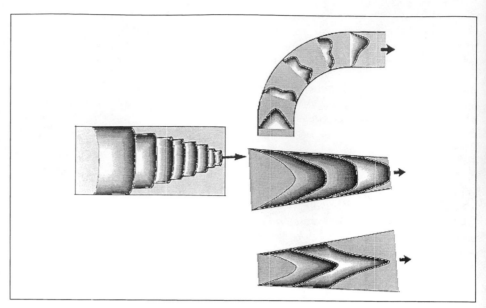

FIGURE 5-6. Because of the narrowing of the vessel lumen, the tortuosity, or the diameter of the vessel, the blood flow pattern will vary.

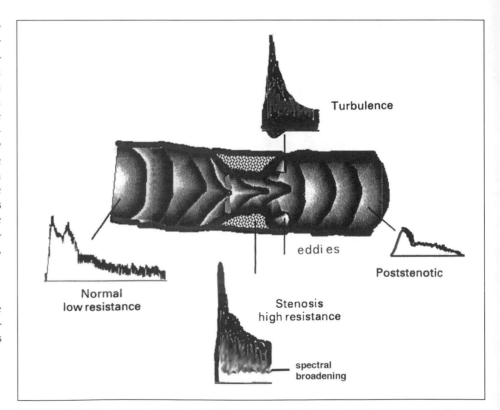

FIGURE 5-7. Diagram showing typical flow pattern before, at, just beyond, and distal to an arterial stenosis. Note that at the level of the stenosis, there is a high systolic and diastolic flow with much spectral broadening. Just beyond the stenosis, there is considerable turbulence with a continued relatively high systolic level and beyond the stenosis in a poststenotic region, there is a slow ascent to the systolic pulse with a low amplitude flow.

Flow Changes Beyond a Narrowed Area (Poststenotic Changes)

Poststenotic changes in arterial flow may be seen in the next few centimeters beyond a narrowed area. When there is severe stenosis, the systolic peak in the poststenotic area will be lower (more rounded) with lower velocities throughout diastole (see Fig. 5-7). The acceleration slope of the systolic peaks (peak systole) will be diminished. This pattern is known as the parvus and tarda abnormality. In less severe obstruction the spectral waveform may resume the normal high or low resistance flow appropriate for that artery.

Clinical Correlation

Detection of a poststenotic pattern is particularly valuable in evaluation of the renal arteries, since the usual site of stenosis, adjacent to the aorta, is rarely seen owing to the presence of bowel gas. Poststenotic changes may also be seen in the common carotid artery, when the stenosis involves the origin of the common carotid. A dampened signal may be displayed (Fig. 5-8). Keep in mind that this dampened signal may be the result of an overall systemic problem (e.g., low cardiac output). The waveform of the other common carotid should be evaluated for comparison. Large calcified plaques may obscure the area of stenosis, so one may be dependent on poststenotic changes to decide on the severity of the narrowing.

Flow Volume

The flow volume through a given vessel can be calculated if the velocity of flow and the vessel diameter are known using the formula shown in Figure 5-2.

Clinical Correlation

The calculation of flow volume is important in situations where a low level of flow is associated with inadequate function (e.g., penile arterial flow).

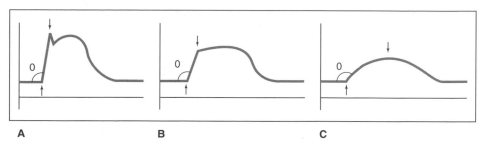

FIGURE 5-8. Flow alterations distal to an area of stenosis. (**A**) Normal steep slope to systole (between arrows). (**B**) Moderate stenosis with less steep angle (between arrows). (**C**) Slow upswing and smooth peak with severe stenosis (between arrows).

Aliasing

If there is a marked frequency shift with a high measured velocity, the signal may return after the next pulse has started (Fig. 5-9). This is called *aliasing*. To compensate for aliasing, increase the velocity range. Most machines will allow one to freeze the real-time image and a wider measurable range of velocities can then be obtained on the spectral waveform. Lower the velocity range (PRF) to display slower velocities accurately. Lowering the baseline may also prevent aliasing.

Clinical Correlation

If aliasing is present, the peak signal will be inaccurately measured as lower than it really is and the severity of the stenosis will be incorrectly measured.

Color Flow Imaging

Color flow assigns different hues to the red blood cells in a vessel depending upon their velocities and the direction of the blood flow relative to the transducer. This allocation is based on the Doppler principle, therefore, some of the same guidelines will apply to both techniques. This color assignment to the flow velocities is performed very rapidly, so a real-time image is generated.

Clinical Correlation

The site of maximum flow can be visualized quickly so that the pulsed Doppler gate can be inserted where the flow is highest. This prevents a tedious hunt with conventional Doppler. Aliasing (see Pitfalls) is readily visible, since there will be a color change with higher velocities.

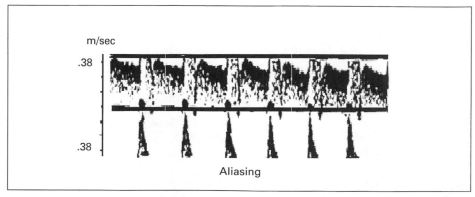

FIGURE 5-9. In this demonstration of aliasing, the velocity is too high to be displayed above the baseline; those velocities that exceed the set scale are therefore projected below the baseline.

Color Flow Display and Direction Within a Vessel

In most systems, flow toward the transducer is allocated red and flow away from the transducer is allocated blue. The flow velocity is displayed with faster velocities in brighter colors and slower velocities in darker colors (Color Plate 5-1). The fastest velocity may be displayed in yellow or white. Turbulent flow will demonstrate a mixture of colors. Usually the operator is given several choices of color scale in the menu for the velocity display mode. As with pulsed Doppler, optimal images are only obtained at an oblique angle. If a vessel runs a straight course, flow at 90 degrees to the color box will not be displayed. The angle of the color box, ROI (region of interest), can be adjusted to the left or right when linear steering is available; otherwise, the probe can be manually angled to provide the angle needed to receive the returning signals (Color Plate 5-2). Keep in mind that if the vessel still does not fill in with color, you may need to widen the dynamic range, allowing lower velocities to be displayed. It should then be fairly straightforward to determine the degree of lumenal stenosis. Scanning the vessel in the transverse plane allows for the most accurate calculation of lumen diameter stenosis.

Clinical Correlation

Soft plaque may be missed on gray scale, but a flow void will be seen using color flow. Sometimes soft plaques may show no changes on gray scale (Color Plate 5-3). Once correct color allocation has been made, normal vessels will fill with color.

KNOBOLOGY: DOPPLER AND COLOR FLOW

Range Gate Cursor (Sample Volume)

The Doppler sample volume is displayed on the B-scan image (see Fig. 5-3). This cursor, which may be presented as a box or two parallel bars, indicates the depth and area from which the Doppler signal is obtained. The size of the box can be varied, depending upon the volume of blood to be evaluated.

Region of Interest (ROI)

This box is utilized to restrict the color display of a blood flow image and to eliminate an unnecessary display of color (see Color Plate 5-1).

Inversion and Direction of Flow and Its Relation to Baseline (Doppler)

When blood flow is moving toward the transducer, sound waves of high frequency are reflected and positive signals are seen above the baseline (see Fig. 5-4). Blood cells that are moving away from the transducer appear as negative signals below the baseline (see Fig. 5-4). Both veins and arteries can show flow in either direction, since the interpretation of flow direction is dependent upon the angle of the vessel to the transducer.

Color Inversion

The display color can be inverted. With the invert on, flow coming toward the probe is blue and flow away from the probe is red. This should be noted so that it is clear to a person who may be interpreting the film or tape at a later time.

Color Flow Baseline

Blood flow toward the transducer will be shown within the measurable range of colors (usually red) above the color bar baseline. Blood flow away from the probe will be displayed in the range of colors below the baseline, usually blue (see Color Plate 5-1). If the range of velocities is too high, reversed colors will appear within the color image. This can be corrected by lowering the baseline, so the color display will remain above the baseline and the highest velocities will be displayed in white or yellow.

Velocity Scale/Velocity Range/PRF (Doppler)

The range of velocities that can be seen in the spectral display is determined by the PRF (pulse repetition frequency) value. A superficial structure (e.g., carotid) requires a high PRF, therefore the velocity range should be increased. For deep structures such as the IVC, a low PRF is used.

PRF (Color Flow)

The range of velocities used in color flow is lower compared to the spectral waveform because the average Doppler shift frequency is displayed, rather than the peak velocity. With lower PRF values there will be a shift to a different color, representing a slightly higher velocity flow (i.e., white or yellow).

Sweep Speed (Doppler Only)

The rate at which the spectral information is displayed can be adjusted using the sweep speed controls. A slow speed (e.g., 25 mm/sec), a moderate speed (e.g., 50 mm/sec), or a fast speed (e.g., 100 mm/sec) can be selected. A slow sweep speed is easier to measure, and a fast sweep speed allows more cycles to be sampled.

Filter (Doppler)

Blood flow signals which are not wanted can be eliminated by using the filter. For example, pulsatile signals from the vascular wall and artifact from respiration can be filtered out by increasing the filter. However, if the filter setting is too high, the flow signal itself may also be deleted. A lower wall filter setting will display more information in the Doppler signal. This is helpful when evaluating venous flow, a slower flow state.

Filter (Color Flow)

A phenomenon called color flash, caused by cardiac or peristaltic motion, or by transducer movement, produces a flash of spurious color in an area where there is no real flow. The area of interest can be concealed by the flash artifact. This may be unavoidable, but check the color filter to see if this condition can be corrected by increasing the filter level.

Gain (Doppler and Color Flow)

The gain controls alter the spectral waveform and the color flow image. Inadequate gain results in an image in which the vessel is incompletely filled with color or in which no conventional Doppler signal can be obtained in areas of slow flow. When too much color gain is used, the color display image and the neighboring tissue will be saturated with color noise, and pixels of color will appear throughout the image. Correct this by lowering the color gain so there is no artifactual flow outside the vessel and a range of colors will be seen within the vessel. Too much Doppler gain will fill in the "sonic window" with echoes and create artifactual spectral broadening.

Angle Correct Bar (Flow Vector)

An angle correct bar is situated within the range gate cursor (see Fig. 5-3). This bar should be aligned with the direction of blood flow. The angle created by the ultrasound beam and this bar must be known if the flow velocity is to be deduced from the frequency of the returning Doppler signal. The angle should be less than 60 degrees. A quantitative calculation of velocity is especially important when evaluating the carotid, since velocity changes have been correlated with degree of stenosis and are used in patient management. Changing the angle (linear steering) helps one achieve the optimum angle in color flow and pulse Doppler mode. At the same time, one can obtain an optimal B-scan image.

Coarse Gain (Doppler)

This knob amplifies returning signals on the spectral waveform. It may be useful when scanning thicker structures such as the carotid artery in a patient with a large neck.

Dynamic Range (Color Flow)

A wide range of velocities can be displayed by changing the dynamic range (e.g., H-high to M-medium). The artery will fill with more color, with more velocities being displayed. Remember some individuals have lower velocities (lower cardiac output) in their arteries.

Power Color Doppler

Movement is visualized, but no attempt to display direction is made. Flow in all directions can be visualized. This technique is more sensitive for subtle flow than conventional color flow Doppler. It is particularly useful in seeing low flow or small subtle vessels (e.g., in an ovarian mass). Clutter and flash artifacts are also more obvious with this technique.

Audio Volume

The Doppler sound will be heard from the built-in speakers. Usually there are independent speakers for both forward and reverse flow. The control varies the volume of the Doppler sound.

Cursor Movement Control

The cursor (range gate cursor and region of interest) movement can be manipulated by means of a trackball or joystick.

Measurements

The standard measurement unit used in displaying the spectral waveform is velocity (m/sec or cm/sec). When dealing with a high-grade stenosis, obtain maximum velocities at and just beyond the area of lumen narrowing.

PITFALLS

Incorrect Angle

A waveform that appears to indicate a distal obstruction is displayed in a vessel; however no plaque is seen in the vessel.

CORRECTION TECHNIQUE. Check the position of the angle bar. If the angle is greater than 60 degrees, then the velocity is not being accurately calculated and an abnormal waveform is created (see Fig. 5-3). This abnormal waveform may mimic a high-resistance waveform (see Angle Correct Bar).

Little or No Doppler Signal in an Artery

The spectral waveform shows apparent low systolic flow and minimal diastolic flow.

Explanation A

There may be a severe obstruction proximal to this area and in an area too difficult to evaluate with the ultrasound beam (e.g., origin of the common carotid artery).

Explanation B

This patient may have diminished cardiac output. In order to document this condition, scan the corresponding vessel on the other side and document the symmetry of the waveform abnormality.

Explanation C

The sample volume (gate) may not be placed where maximum flow is present.

CORRECTION TECHNIQUE. Do not depend solely on the visualization of the vessel. Color flow highlights the higher velocities in the artery and helps in gate placement, but a keen ear is more sensitive. A higher velocity may be evident as one angles the sound beam slightly off the center of the stream.

Explanation D

The sample volume is too large for the small amount of flow.

CORRECTION TECHNIQUE. A larger sample size may be needed when scanning to locate the site of flow, but to obtain a more precise measurement of flow within an artery, decrease the gate size.

Explanation E

The wall filter is set at too high a level.

CORRECTION TECHNIQUE. The wall filter should be set at the lowest setting that does not introduce artifacts, especially when scanning a vein (a low-flow state). Adjust the Doppler gain and volume as you lower the filter.

Explanation F

Try the following maneuvers before giving up.

1. Change to another acoustic window or different incident angle.
2. Open up the gate setting.
3. Lower the velocity range.
4. Use a lower-frequency transducer. The patient may be too obese for a higher frequency transducer.

A High-Resistance Waveform in a Low-Resistance Bed

Explanation

There may be soft plaque distal to this area. If the B-scan gain is too low, soft plaque may be missed. Use color flow to outline the true patent lumen (see Color Plate 5-3).

Aliasing

A tight stenosis causes such high velocities at the site of flow and immediately distal to the narrowed area that flow is seen above the baseline and at the lower edge of the spectral display. When color is used, there may be peaks of color from the other end of the spectrum. A chirping sound may be heard as you angle through the stenotic area.

Explanation

The velocity is so high that the signal wraps around itself and peak velocities are displayed below the baseline (see Fig. 5-9). This problem arises because the selected PRF is too low to pick up the high velocities that are occurring.

CORRECTION TECHNIQUE

1. Place the baseline at its lowest site to allow the systolic peaks to be displayed.
2. Decrease the PRF, the velocity range. The smaller number of pulses transmitted per second will increase the measurable velocity range.
3. Some units allow the B-scan image to be frozen while the Doppler signal is obtained. This will also widen the measurable velocity range.
4. Increase the Doppler angle, but do not exceed 60 degrees.
5. Reduce the transducer frequency. Most units offer a choice of several Doppler frequencies for each transducer. Otherwise, change to a lower-frequency transducer.
6. Change to continuous wave.

Inadequate Venous Signal

Venous flow is difficult to detect even when the vessel is clearly demonstrated.

Explanation A

There may be little venous flow at rest.

CORRECTION TECHNIQUE. Respiration affects venous flow. With inspiration and the descent of the diaphragm, pressure increases in the abdomen but decreases in the extremities. Ask the patient to perform a Valsalva maneuver. (A Valsalva maneuver is performed by taking a deep breath, holding it, and tensing the abdomen.) As the breath is released, venous flow increases, and the venous signal will become more pronounced.

Explanation B

The vein may be compressed by patient position, for example extension of the leg.

CORRECTION TECHNIQUE. Ask the patient to flex the leg slightly and reevaluate. Utilize color flow in these instances to accentuate subtle flow.

Explanation C

The B-scan gain may be too low to demonstrate the clot within the vein.

CORRECTION TECHNIQUE. Increase the gain and apply gentle compression to see if the vein collapses.

Audible Signal but Vessel Not Seen

A venous signal can be heard, but a patent vessel cannot be visualized. The vein may be subtotally occluded or the presence of adjacent collaterals may cause the audible signal.

CORRECTION TECHNIQUE. Color flow will demonstrate the smaller collateral vessels as well as a small amount of residual flow in an almost-occluded vessel.

Spectral Broadening

Apparent spectral broadening may be caused by too much gain or by scanning too close to the vessel wall, picking up lower velocities.

CORRECTION TECHNIQUE. Make sure the supposed spectral broadening reflects true pathology, and is not just noise, by comparing it to an area known to be normal.

A Flickering Image

Sometimes it is difficult to evaluate the color flow of the image when obtaining a Doppler signal because the image flickers.

Explanation

A large amount of data is being processed to generate the image for each frame of information when obtaining the Doppler signal or color flow. Therefore, the frame rate is lowered and a flicker occurs.

CORRECTION TECHNIQUE. To reduce this flicker, evaluate one mode at a time (e.g., use color flow only) or reduce the size of the color flow box.

Color Misregistration Artifact (Color Flash)

If the transducer is rapidly moved, a flash of color may develop which is related to transducer movement and not to vascular flow.

CORRECTION TECHNIQUE. Use the filter to reduce noise and move the transducer slowly.

Tissue Vibration or Transmitted Pulsation

In the region of a highly pulsatile structure, such as an artery, neighboring structures may move, causing some color artifact in the surrounding tissues.

CORRECTION TECHNIQUE. Scan from a different axis, if possible.

Active Peristalsis

Active peristalsis may induce a color flow artifact.

Undue Color Gain

The outline of vessels may be misregistered owing to excessive gain, so the flow appears to fill in some of the surrounding tissues.

CORRECTION TECHNIQUE. Decrease gain so the color image corresponds to the vessel outline (Color Plate 5-3B).

SELECTED READING

Edelman, S. *Ultrasound Physics*. EST, Inc., 1994.

Kremkau, F. W. *Doppler Ultrasound Principles and Instrumentation* New York: Grune & Stratton, 1995.

MacSweeney, J. E., Cosgrove, D. O., and Arenson, J. Colour Doppler energy (power) mode ultrasound. *Clin Radiol* 51:387–390, 1996.

Polak, J. F. (Ed.). *Peripheral Vascular Sonography: A Practical Guide*. Baltimore, MD: Williams & Wilkins, 1992.

Zagzebski, J. *Essentials of Ultrasound Physics*, St. Louis: CV Mosby, 1996.

6

BASIC PRINCIPLES

NANCY SMITH MINER

SONOGRAM ABBREVIATIONS

Ao	Aorta
Du	Duodenum
F	Fibroid
GBL	Gallbladder
IVC	Inferior vena cava
K	Kidney
L	Liver
P	Pancreas
SMa	Superior mesenteric artery
Sp	Spleen
Spa	Splenic artery
Spv	Splenic vein
St	Stomach
Ut	Uterus

KEY WORDS

Acoustic Enhancement. Because sound traveling through a fluid-filled structure is barely attenuated, the structures distal to a cystic lesion appear to have more echoes than neighboring areas. Also referred to as *through transmission* (see below and Fig. 6-1).

Anechoic. Without internal echoes. Not necessarily cystic unless there is distal echo enhancement (good through transmission).

Complex. A structure that has both fluid-filled (echo-free) and solid (echogenic) areas.

Contralateral. On the other side of the body.

Cyst. Spherical, fluid-filled structure with well-defined walls that contains few or no internal echoes and exhibits good acoustic enhancement.

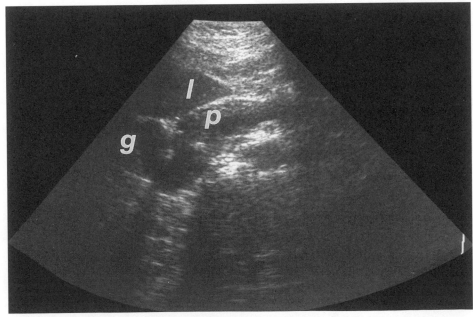

FIGURE 6-1. Transverse section of the upper abdomen showing the usual echogenicity of the organs in a young adult. Note that the pancreas (P) contains more echoes than the liver (L) and that the liver is slightly more echogenic than the kidneys (K). The gallbladder (GBl), a "cystic" (fluid-filled) structure, shows acoustic enhancement behind it, in the region of the duodenum (arrow). The spleen is slightly more echogenic than the liver.

Cystic. In ultrasonography, the word *cystic* does not necessarily refer to a cyst. The term is used (inaccurately) by some to describe any fluid-filled structure (e.g., urine-filled bladder or bile-filled gallbladder; see Fig. 6-1).

Distal. The extremity (limb) end of a body structure.

Echo-free. See *Anechoic*.

Echogenic. Describes a structure that produces echoes. Usually a relative term. For example, Figure 6-1 shows the normal texture of the liver and pancreas; the pancreas is slightly more echogenic. A change in the normal echogenicity signifies a pathologic condition.

Echogram. Term used by some to describe an ultrasonic examination, especially in cardiac work; an echocardiogram is frequently referred to as an "echo."

Echolucent. Without internal echoes; not necessarily cystic.

Echopenic. A few echoes within a structure; less echogenic. The normal kidney is echopenic relative to the liver (see Fig. 6-1).

Echo-poor. See *Echopenic*.

Echo-rich. See *Echogenic*.

Fluid-Fluid Level. Interface between two fluids with different acoustic characteristics. This interface has a horizontal level that varies with patient position.

Foot Print. Descriptive term for the amount of transducer face in contact with the patient (i.e., a small-head transducer has a small foot print).

Gain. The strength of the echoes throughout the image can be varied by changing the power output from the system.

Homogeneous. Of uniform composition. The normal texture of several parenchymal organs is homogeneous (e.g., liver, thyroid, and pancreas).

Hyperechoic. See *Echogenic*.

Hypoechoic. See *Echopenic*.

Interface. Strong echoes that delineate the boundary of organs and that are caused by the difference between the acoustic impedance of two adjacent structures. An interface is usually more pronounced when the transducer is perpendicular to it (Fig. 6-2).

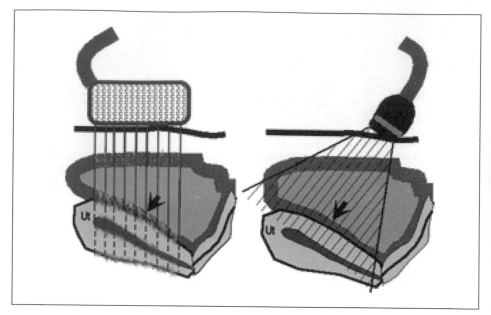

FIGURE 6-2. Interface (**A**) The "interface" between the bladder (black arrow) and the uterus (Ut) is poorly defined because the linear array beam is not perpendicular to the uterine wall. (**B**) The sector beam was angled perpendicular to the interface (black arrow) and is now well seen. The use of a small-headed scanner can bring out interfaces that are oblique to the linear array beam.

Ipsilateral. On the same side of the body.

Isoechoic. Of the same echogenicity as a neighboring area, but not necessarily of the same texture.

Noise. Artifactual echoes resulting from too much gain rather than from true anatomic structures.

Proximal. The trunk end of a limb or organ.

Reverberation. An artifact that results from a strong echo returning from a large acoustic interface to the transducer. This echo returns to the tissues again, causing additional echoes parallel to the first.

Ring Down. Extreme form of reverberation artifact that occurs when a long series of echoes, caused by a very strong acoustic interface and consequent reverberations, are seen.

Scan. Verb: to perform an ultrasound scan. Noun: a sonographic examination.

Shadowing. Failure of the sound beam to pass through an object. This blockage is caused by reflection or absorption of the sound and may be partial or complete. For example, air bubbles in the duodenum allow poor transmission of the sound beam because most of the sound is reflected. A calcified gallstone does not allow any sound to pass through, and shadowing is pronounced (Fig. 6-3). These degrees of acoustic shadowing may help in diagnosis.

Solid (Homogeneous). A mass or organ that contains uniform low-level echoes because the cellular tissues are acoustically very similar.

Sonodense. A structure that transmits sound poorly. A dense structure can attenuate sound so greatly that the back wall is poorly defined (Fig. 6-4). If it is very homogeneous, there may be few or no internal echoes, but the lack of acoustic enhancement and poor back wall help differentiate it from a cystic, echo-free structure.

Sonogenic. Handsome ultrasound image (like *photogenic*); for example, a good example of vascular anatomy.

Sonographer. A health professional who has learned how to perform quality sonography and can tailor the examination to individual patients.

Sonologist. A physician who specializes in ultrasonography and has appropriate training.

Sonolucent (Anechoic). Without echoes. Not necessarily cystic unless there is good through transmission.

Specular Reflector. Structure that creates a strong echo because it interfaces at right angles to the sound beam and has a significantly different acoustic impedance from a neighboring structure (e.g., diaphragm/liver or posterior bladder wall/bladder).

Static Scan. Not real-time. B scans produced with a fixed arm system. Obsolete technique.

Texture. The echo pattern within an organ; could be homogeneous or irregular.

Through Transmission. The amount of sound passing through a structure (see Fig. 6-1). Same as *acoustic enhancement* (see above).

Transonicity. Term used to indicate the amount of sound passing through a mass or cyst, usually qualified as good or poor. Same as *acoustic enhancement*.

Trendelenburg. A position in which a recumbent patient is tilted so that the feet are higher than the head.

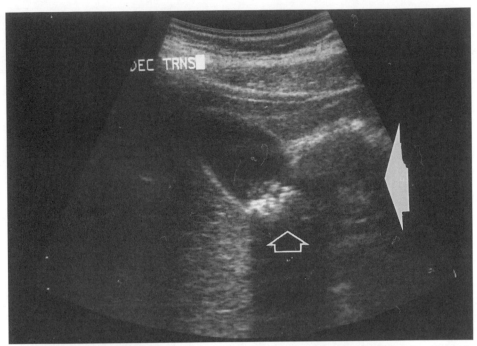

FIGURE 6-3. The acoustic shadowing from the stones in the gallbladder (GBl) is "sharp" (open arrow), whereas the shadowing from the bowel gas is "soft" (large arrow).

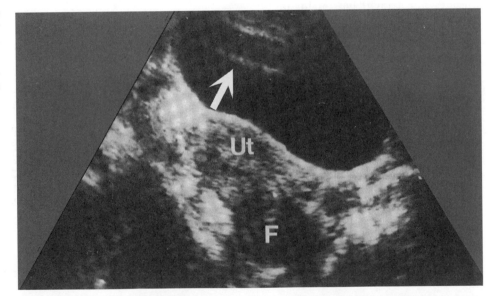

FIGURE 6-4. The fibroid (F) at the posterior aspect of the uterus is a solid homogenous mass with some internal echoes. Its density attenuates sound so the internal echogenicity diminishes near the backwall and there is poor through transmission. Note the reverberations in the anterior portion of the bladder (arrow).

TERMS RELATING TO ORIENTATION

Anatomic Terms

See Figures 6-5, 6-6, and 6-7.

Anterior or **Ventral.** Structure lying toward the front of the patient.

Distal. Away from the origin.

Inferior or **Caudal.** Terms denoting a structure closer to the patient's feet.

Lateral. Structure lying away from the midline.

Medial or **Mesial.** Structure lying toward the midline.

Posterior or **Dorsal.** Structure lying toward the back of the patient.

Prone. The patient lies on his or her stomach.

Proximal. Near.

Quadrant. The abdomen is divided into four quarters, each known as a quadrant.

Superior, Cranial, or **Cephalad.** Interchangeable terms denoting a structure closer to the patient's head.

Supine. The patient lies on his or her back.

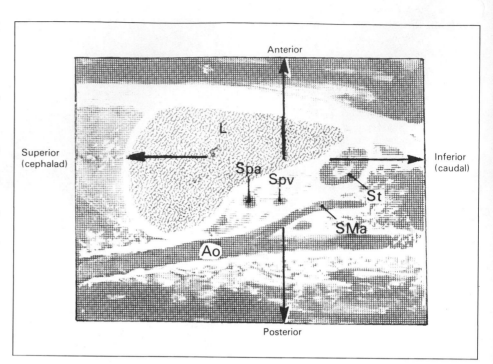

FIGURE 6-6. A longitudinal scan to the left of the midline showing normal strutures and orientation.

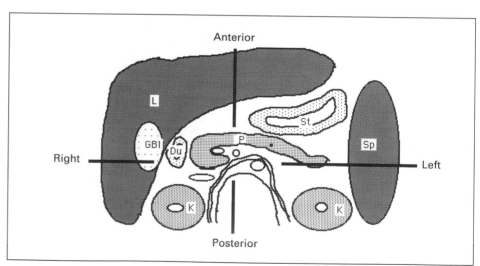

FIGURE 6-7. Transverse scan. The sonographic right and left are the opposite of the viewers right and left.

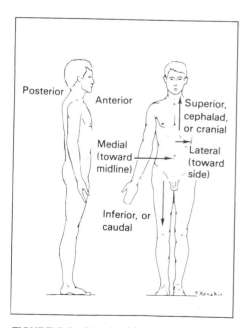

FIGURE 6-5. Standard labeling nomenclature used to show where structures lie in relation to each other.

TERMS RELATING TO LABELING

The American Institute of Ultrasound in Medicine (AIUM) has established standards for labeling studies so that a sonogram done in Columbus, Ohio, can be interpreted with no misunderstanding in Baltimore, Maryland. These standards are occasionally revised and are available on request from the AIUM.

One of the great features of real-time ultrasound is that structures can be visualized in their long axis, which may be oblique and not fall neatly into a sagittal or transverse plane. However, the basic principle of examining everything in at least two planes is a sound one, so suggestions for labeling an abdomen and a pelvis in longitudinal and transverse planes are discussed here.

Longitudinal (Sagittal) Scans

In the abdomen, the aorta and the inferior vena cava (IVC) may not follow an exact longitudinal plane, but should be imaged in their long axes if possible. Since these images also include other anatomy of interest—left lobe of liver, superior mesenteric artery, pancreas, and so forth—it suffices to label them "ML" (midline) unless you wish to draw the sonologist's attention to something in particular. For instance, if you get a nice look at the pancreatic head on your IVC image, you may want to label it "right ML, head of panc" or "ML, distal CBD" (common bile duct) if that appears in the head of the pancreas.

As you scan left, "left sag" will do unless, again, there is something of note. "Right sag" will suffice for the longitudinals on the right, although some sonologists may wish to know which images were obtained more coronally, so as you scan through the patient's ribs and come in through their side, "rt sag obl" is more precise. It is not generally necessary to label each organ; however, smaller organs or subtle structures such as the CBD, gallbladder, or pancreas are usually named (i.e., a section through the CBD will be labelled CBD).

Transverse Scans

Transversely, whether you are angling cephalad or not, on inspiration or not, "trans left," "trans right," "trans right obl," and "trans left obl" will cover most of the labeling needed in the abdomen. When a patient has pathology distorting the anatomy, or normal variants that you had to trace to their source to figure out, throw all those rules out the window and label copiously onscreen even at the risk of insulting your sonologist. Always remember that someone may pull that sonogram out of the jacket a month later, when you are not on hand to explain.

In the normal pelvis, the following labels do nicely, provided that you are certain that these are indeed the ovaries you are imaging:

ML

long. uterus

long. (or sag) right (or left) ovary

trans right (or left) ovary

trans C (cervix)

trans uterus or, perhaps, trans uterine
   fundus

Because patients often neglect to say things like "Oh yes, they removed my right ovary when they did my appendectomy 10 years ago," it is unwise to blithely label any lump of tissue in the adnexa "ovary." If unsure, stick to "right sag," "right trans," and "right adnexa."

Label all "endovag" images as such to avoid confusion. It is also important, on pelvic studies, to include the patient information on each image. Make sure the date of the last menstrual period (LMP) or last normal menstrual period (LNMP) is recorded, even if that date is "10 years ago." An otherwise unremarkable scan of a plump endometrial cavity takes on new meaning when it is made clear that the patient is postmenopausal or at an inappropriate stage of her cycle.

Decubitus (Figure 6-8)

These are scans taken with the patient lying on either side; following the traditional radiology standard, the label is for the side down (closest to the x-ray film). So, an image of the left kidney, taken with the patient on her right side, is labeled "right lateral decubitus." Frankly, this is confusing and is better labeled simply "left side up." The exception is the gallbladder, which is routinely examined with the right side up: "decub" will suffice, no matter what the plane.

Coronal

The term *coronal* implies a specific plane. The image is taken from the patient's side, whether the patient is decubitus or supine, if in the abdomen (see Fig. 6-8). In the neonatal head, coronal refers to images taken through the fontanelle, from side to side (see Chapter 50).

SCANNING TECHNIQUES AND CHOICES

General Principles

Regardless of the type of exam or transducer being employed, the following guidelines help ensure meaningful images.

1. *The beam should be as perpendicular as possible to the structure being imaged.* (Note: This is always true unless you are using Doppler—we'll discuss that later.)

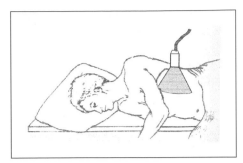

FIGURE 6-8. Left coronal, right decubitus, or left-side-up view.

2. *Scan through the best acoustic window possible*—this may be the liver, a mass, or the distended bladder. If no window is available, consider creating one by having the patient drink water to fill the bladder or filling the stomach with water.

3. *Get in the habit of demonstrating the long axis.* Ultrasound is flexible in scanning planes, unlike computed tomography, and any plane can be used as long as bone or gas does not interfere. The longest axis of the kidney, the aorta, or a tumor can be shown on real-time; then turn 90 degrees and demonstrate the short axis.

4. *Never carelessly photograph* an image that is suspicious for pathology when you think it is a scanning artifact, such as a pseudotumor caused by a rib shadow or the suggestion of gallstones created by artifact.

Transducers

Selection of the proper transducer is critical to the success of a scan. The wrong transducer shape or frequency can give you a passable scan in which the anatomy is demonstrated, but the pathology never shows up. Keep the following factors in mind, and *don't be lazy* about changing transducers from patient to patient or in the middle of a study.

Frequency

Use the highest frequency that will let you penetrate your object. Note, however, that you will defeat your purpose if the frequency is so high that your gain and time gain compensation settings are at their upper limits. Besides the absence of flexibility in changing controls, you've now put noise in your image that hides subtle changes.

Shape-Sector or Small Footprint Scanner

Advantages

- Useful for areas of small access: between ribs, through a urinary bladder, through a fontanelle.
- Good for angling up under or for wedging in between tight spots.

Disadvantages

- The wedge-shaped image gives you a limited near field of view (see Fig. 3-13C).

Curved Linear Array

Advantages

- Much bigger field of view, good for large structures and overviews.
- Near field is wider than sector (see Fig. 3-13D).
- Useful for second- and third-trimester obstetric patients, anywhere in abdomen that it will fit.

Disadvantages

- Larger transducer face than sector, may not fit in acoustic window.
- May get artifacts along sides of image due to poor contact.
- Near field is still more limited than linear array, but not by much, so it is becoming the most popular transducer design.

Linear Array

Advantages

- "Block" shape of image allows for large field of view in superficial areas; excellent for small parts, renal transplants, subfacial hematomas, and other superficial imaging (see Fig. 3-13A).
- Possible to hook up two images to form one very large field of view in cases where it is important not to extrapolate measurements (e.g., when measuring renal transplants or large masses undergoing radiation therapy, or when demonstrating hepatomegaly or polyhydramnios).

Disadvantages

- Can only be used where there is a large window, such as in the midline or in a pregnant uterus. Cannot get between ribs.
- Even where there are no ribs, the flat surface of the transducer makes it difficult to angle around pockets of gas or through small windows.

Endovaginal

Advantages

- No full bladder needed.
- Better resolution because decreased distance allows higher frequency.
- Good way to assess cervix without distortion caused by full bladder.
- Can see anatomy and fetal heart motion sooner than transabdominally (see Chapter 12).

Disadvantages

- Limited field of view (difficult to visualize a fibroid or large ovarian mass).
- Air in bowel can still interfere with seeing ovaries; may be easier through the bladder.
- More invasive; sometimes the patient may object. Note: The gender of the sonographer has to be considered here. Medico-legally, it is wise to have a female in the room during insertion and probably during the use of an endovaginal transducer.

There are many specialized transducers, including endorectal and intraoperative, that are described in other chapters. Most transducers, however, even small parts, generally fall into one of the above categories. Transesophageal and endoluminal transducers are not commonly used by sonographers or general sonologists so far and will not be considered further.

Color

The use of color is constantly being refined; currently, it is predominantly used to demonstrate fluid motion, and therefore flow, if the velocity is great enough. The color is coded to show the direction of the flow (see Color Plate 5-1).

Helpful

- Good as an adjunct to duplex Doppler scanning; maps out the vessels.
- Clarifies confusing Doppler values, such as those due to reversal of flow, etc.
- Establishes vascularity of an organ, as when questioning a torsed testicle.
- Establishes direction of flow at a glance, such as in the portal vein.

Not Helpful

- In instances of slow flow; if a tumor doesn't "light up" with color, it may still be a vascular tumor with low-velocity flow. A venous lake may contain blood, but the blood moves so slowly it does not light up with color (see Chapter 15).
- In precisely quantifying flow. Color gives an image of the actual flow in the lumen, but spectral analysis, which quantifies flow, is obtained from the traditional pulsed Doppler.

Cine Loop

Most machines offer this option to "rewind" the real-time images for several frames, a boon to those with a slow finger on the freeze button.

Helpful

- In catching a moving target, such as a four-chamber view of a fetal heart. Check back to make sure your frozen image is indeed the longest femur length, etc.
- When patients can't hold their breath, and the desired part flashes in and out of view.
- In fighting the "Was That a Real Lesion?" Syndrome. By all means, go back and look at it again, but remember, cine loop is . . .

Not Helpful

- When it causes you to violate one of the basic principles of scanning. If you can't duplicate a "lesion," maybe it was artifact in the first place. *Beware of creating pathology where it doesn't exist.*
- When students of scanning become too dependent on it. That stripped-down unit in Labor and Delivery probably won't offer it at 3:00 AM.

Contrast Media

So far, contrast media are not commonly available except in echocardiography, but they can be helpful in showing subtle intraluminal or intraparenchymal masses, enhancing color flow, and showing fallopian tube spill.

PATIENT PREPARATION

Gallbladder and Pancreas Scans

Patients scheduled for upper abdominal scans should ingest nothing that will make the gallbladder contract for at least 8 hours preceding the sonogram. Water is acceptable, but often the patient is scheduled for an upper gastrointestinal series the same day. This can be a problem if good visualization of the pancreas is required, since water in the stomach is often crucial to the ultrasound exam. In those cases requiring the ingestion of water, the GI series should be scheduled for the following day.

Pelvic Scans

The bladder should be distended to provide an acoustic window to the pelvic structures in patients undergoing a transabdominal pelvic scan. Outpatients should be instructed to drink enough fluid—at least 16 ounces—to make their bladder slightly uncomfortable at the time of exam. Since an endovaginal examination is very often used as a followup, we now recommend not emptying the bladder 2 hours before an exam rather than drinking water if a transvaginal exam is likely to be performed. Inpatients that are NPO (nothing by mouth) require alternative arrangements: an indwelling Foley can be clamped ahead of time, an IV flow rate can be increased, or permission can be obtained to insert a catheter so that the bladder can be filled in the ultrasound lab.

The endovaginal transducer has made bladder filling unnecessary in many situations. Remember that the bladder can be *too* full. An overdistended bladder can distort or displace pathology enough to hide it altogether. For rectal and endovaginal scanning, the bladder should be empty or only slightly filled for use as a landmark. Some prefer that patients undergoing a rectal scan be prepped with a Fleets enema, although it generally makes little difference.

Obstetric Scans

For early transabdominal obstetric scans, the bladder should be distended enough to visualize the lower uterine segments. After 20 weeks, the bladder should be empty to evaluate properly the cervix and its relationship to the placenta.

PATIENT–SONOGRAPHER INTERACTION

Talking to your patients will not only relieve anxiety, but also reassure them that you are interested in helping to diagnose their problem. Because sonography requires so much time and patient contact, a sonographer is in an excellent position to elicit pertinent information from the patient.

The information provided with outpatients is usually limited, so questions such as "What kind of trouble are you having?" or "Is this the first time you've been in the hospital?" can trigger a flood of information that can be relayed to the physician. With inpatients, it should be standard procedure to read the synopsis of a patient's chart. However, even with inpatients, conversation can yield information that helps focus a study: consider the case of a patient sent for a sonogram to rule out gallstones who casually mentions that pesky *renal* stone he passed 5 years ago.

Patients often ask the sonographer what the study shows. It is important to understand how much information the sonologist and the patient's clinician are willing to let the sonographer reveal. One way to answer questions without being too evasive is to explain that while sonographers are well-versed in anatomy, diagnosing pathology from the images is up to the doctors. Questions about bioeffects should never be evaded; the sonographer has a responsibility to keep up to date and answer the patient. At this time, no side effects from the levels of ultrasound used for diagnostic imaging have been documented, but the longest follow-up interval is about 10 years and power levels have been increasing.

SONOGRAPHER–SONOLOGIST INTERACTION

The sonographer and the sonologist should work together as a team. Once a preliminary scan is performed by the sonographer, both should discuss the findings, and the sonologist should rescan any confusing or unusual areas. Additional views can be made before the patient is removed from the table. The sonologist can benefit from watching the sonographer rescan a difficult area for which a specific scanning technique has been devised. If the sonologist is not available, it can be helpful to videotape confusing areas that are clarified by some dynamic process, for example, peristalsis in a very suspicious-looking "mass," or an alarming arrhythmia in a fetus where Doppler or M-mode is not available.

The physician should be informed about any problems encountered during scanning that may pertain to pathology—for instance, you may turn in a nice, homogeneous image of a liver, but to get that pretty picture you had to change to a much lower frequency transducer than you thought you'd need. This might bring fatty liver into question.

Perhaps one of the most significant contributions a sonographer can make to the diagnosis is to determine the source of a localized area of tenderness or of a palpable mass. The sonographer is in a unique position to see what lies directly beneath the patient's most tender spot. A good example is the patient with right upper quadrant pain in whom no gallstones are found. The presence of acute pain at the site of the gallbladder makes acute cholecystitis likely. The borders of a palpable mass can be defined on film by placing arrows where the edges are felt.

The value of this type of information is diminished if the films are read later in the day by a physician. Physician-to-patient contact may be essential to confirm such an important pathologic finding. A combined approach, using the expertise of both a sonographer and a sonologist, ensures that the best possible examination is made. As it becomes increasingly more common for the physician to see neither the patient nor the sonographer, it becomes increasingly important for the sonographer to leave an impression in writing for the sonologist.

SELECTED READING

Barnett, S. B. Ultrasound safety in obstetrics: What are the concerns? *Ultrasound Quart* 13:228–239, 1995.

INFERTILITY

For Ovulation Induction

ROGER C. SANDERS

SONOGRAM ABBREVIATIONS

Bl	Bladder
C	Cervix
CdS	Cul-de-sac
CE	Cervical endometrium
EC	Endometrial cavity
EV	Endovaginal probe study
FSH	Follicle stimulating hormone
GIFT	Gamete intrafollicular transfer
HCG	Human chorionic gonadotropin
Ip	Iliopsoas muscle
IVF	In vitro fertilization
L	Ligament
LH	Luteinizing hormone
OHS	Ovarian hyperstimulation syndrome
OI	Ovulation induction
Ov	Ovary
PCO	Polycystic ovary syndrome
PID	Pelvic inflammatory disease
Re	Rectum
St	Stroma
Sym	Symphysis
Ut	Uterus
V	Vagina
ZIFT	Zygote intrafollicular transfer

KEY WORDS

Adenomyosis. Deposition of endometrial tissue in the uterine myometrium. The endometrial tissue responds to hormonal stimulation and bleeds at the time of periods.

Amenorrhea. Absence of menstrual periods. If periods have never occurred, primary amenorrhea is present. If periods have occurred in the past, there is secondary amenorrhea.

Anovulation. Absence of ovulation. Menstruation and follicle development may still occur.

Ascherman's syndrome. Scarring of the endometrial cavity of the uterus, usually as a consequence of previous infection or surgery.

Chocolate Cyst. Blood-filled cyst associated with endometriosis.

Clomid. Hormone used to stimulate ovulation.

Corpus Albicans. Scar at the site of a previous corpus luteum.

Corpus Luteum (Lutein, alternative spelling). A cyst which produces progesterone that forms at the site of a burst dominant follicle; persists during the first trimester of pregnancy.

Cuff. After hysterectomy the blind end of the vagina is sutured and forms a fibrous mass, the cuff.

Estrogen. Hormone secreted by growing follicles that stimulates the uterine endometrium to regenerate.

Follicle. Fluid sac containing a developing ovum within the ovary. With each normal menstrual cycle follicles enlarge: the largest follicle is termed the dominant or graafian follicle. Ovulation takes place from this large follicle.

Fornix. The upper portion of the vagina surrounds the cervix. A vaginal pouch forms a recess around the cervix known as the fornix (see Fig. 7-2).

Gamete. Unfertilized egg.

Gamete Intrafollicular Transfer (GIFT). Technique whereby ova are removed, fertilized, and then placed within the fallopian tube.

Hirsutism. Excessively hairy.

Human Chorionic Gonadotropin (HCG). Hormone produced by the gestational sac trophoblastic tissue which increases with pregnancy. It can be measured in maternal blood.

In Vitro Fertilization. Technique for fertilizing eggs with sperm outside the body, in a culture dish.

Luteinizing Hormone. Hormone put out by the pituitary which stimulates ovulation.

Luteinized Unruptured Follicle Syndrome (LUFS). Term used for a type of infertility in which a normal follicle fails to rupture and ovulate and continues to grow on a repeated basis.

Nabothian Cyst. A cyst that forms in the cervix; it is a normal finding.

Nulliparous. A woman who has not been pregnant.

Ovarian Hyperstimulation Syndrome (OHS). Stimulation of ovulation by hormonal therapy.

Ovulation Induction (OI). Technique whereby ova are removed, fertilized, and placed within the uterine cavity.

Ovum (Ova, plural). An unfertilized egg within a follicle.

Parous. Previously pregnant woman.

Pergonal. Hormone that stimulates follicle growth.

Posterior Cul-de-sac. Pouch of Douglas space behind the uterus where fluid can collect.

Progesterone. Hormone secreted by the corpus luteum that prepares the endometrium to receive a fertilized egg.

Proliferative. Preovulatory phase of the menstrual cycle, at which time the endometrial cavity echoes form a single thin line (see Fig. 7-7).

Secretory. Postovulatory phase of the menstrual cycle, at which time the endometrial cavity echoes are thick (see Fig. 7-7).

Zygote. A fertilized egg.

 THE CLINICAL PROBLEM

Female infertility is a common problem, partly because many women defer pregnancy until a later age. If conception does not occur after a year or so of unprotected intercourse, couples seek advice from a reproductive endocrinologist. One of the first investigations performed is a sonogram. Both the ovaries and the uterus undergo ultrasonically obvious changes during ovulation and menstruation. Normally one out of several follicles becomes the dominant follicle; in midcycle this follicle bursts and releases an egg. Subsequently, a corpus luteum forms from the remnants of deflated follicle. In some instances, ultrasound can show that follicle production does not occur (anovulation) or the follicle continues to grow and does not release an egg (luteinized unruptured follicle [LUF]).

The causes of some types of ovulation failure can be determined only by biochemical assay, but ultrasound has a role in following follicular development so that hormonal intervention, intercourse, and follicular puncture can be performed when the follicle reaches an appropriate size. If the fallopian tube is blocked or absent, the ovum may be retrieved with a needle, fertilized outside the patient, and then placed back in the uterus, a technique known as in vitro fertilization. Ultrasound is generally used to guide ova retrieval. Replacement of the fertilized ova into the uterus or tube may be monitored with ultrasound. Placement of the fertilized ova into the fallopian tube is known as the GIFT (gamete intrafollicular transfer) or ZIFT (zygote intrafallopian transfer) technique. These techniques are not performed with ultrasonic aid.

At the time of the initial sonogram, the sonographer should also look for structural problems that prevent the process of conception. Look for these problems:

1. Congenital malformations such as a double uterus, bicornuate uterus, or hypoplastic uterus; uterine anomalies are associated with premature labor and spontaneous abortion
2. Blockage of the pathway of the sperm and ovum by adhesions or masses secondary to infection or endometriosis (e.g., hydrosalpinx and endometrioma)
3. Distortion of the endometrial cavity by fibroids or polyps

Menstrual Cycle Physiology

See Figure 7-1.

An average menstrual cycle lasts 28 days, but may vary between 25 and 35 days. Day 1 is the first day of bleeding. The hypothalamic-pituitary-ovarian axis regulates the normal menstrual cycle. Immediately following the onset of menses the hypothalamus prompts the pituitary gland to secrete follicle-stimulating hormone, which stimulates ovarian follicular growth. As the follicles grow, they produce estrogen, which induces endometrial regeneration. A dominant follicle (graafian follicle) develops, containing the egg (ovum). Follicles reach sizes of 1.5 to 2.5 cm. A large surge of the pituitary-secreted luteinizing hormone causes the graafian follicle to rupture, releasing the ovum. After ovulation the graafian follicle becomes a corpus luteum, producing progesterone, which prepares the uterine endometrium to receive a fertilized egg (zygote). If the egg is not fertilized, estrogen and progesterone levels fall, which causes bleeding (menses), and the cycle repeats itself. The corpus luteum degenerates into the corpus albicans, a small white scar on the ovary.

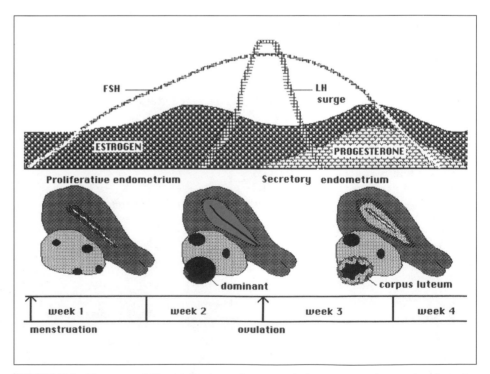

FIGURE 7-1. Diagram of the sequence of events during a normal menstrual cycle. The ovary contains several follicles; one (the dominant follicle) slowly increases in size until it ovulates. At the site where ovulation takes place, the corpus luteum develops. The developing follicle (a sonographic cyst) ovulates when it reaches a size of 15–25 mm. A degenerating corpus luteum has few internal echoes and a rather irregular border. The uterine endometrium thickens in the secretory phase prior to menstruation.

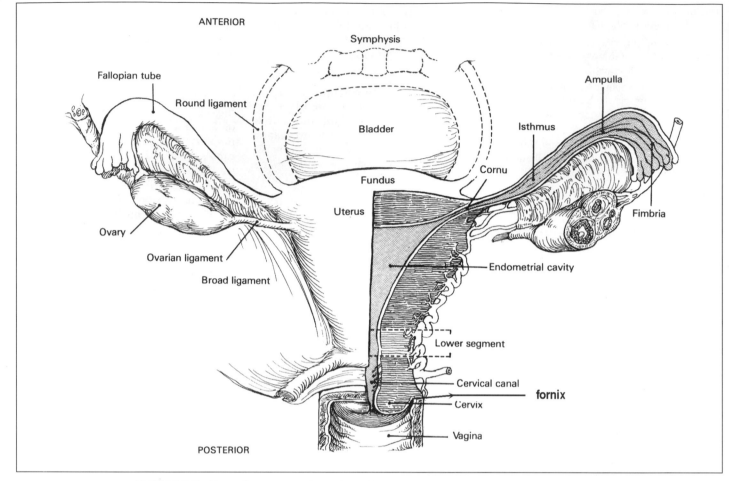

FIGURE 7-2. Normal uterus and ovaries. The ovaries are suspended from the broad ligament and lie adjacent to the ampullary end of the fallopian tube. The fallopian tube arises from the cornu of the uterus. The lumen is rarely visible.

Changes in the endometrium also occur. Shortly after menstruation, the endometrium is inactive and thin. As ovulation approaches, an echogenic rim develops on either side of the thin endometrium. After ovulation has occurred, the area between the echogenic rim and the central line fills in with echoes when the patient is in the secretory phase of the cycle (see Fig. 7-7).

ANATOMY

See Figure 7-2.

Vagina

See Figures 7-2 and 7-3.

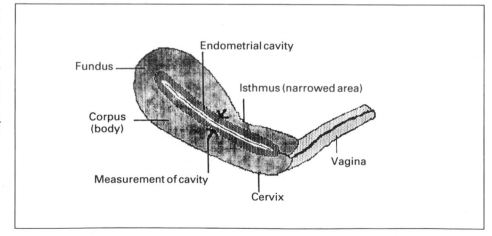

FIGURE 7-3. Uterus. Normal anteverted uterus with decidual reaction in the cavity. The anatomic components of the uterus—the cervix, corpus, fundus, and isthmus—are shown. The site for measuring the endometrial cavity echo is indicated.

A central bright linear echo represents the opposing inner vaginal walls. The surrounding muscular portion is more hypoechoic. After hysterectomy the blind end of the vagina is sutured to form a fibrous mass, the cuff. The cuff is variable in size but should not normally be more than 2.2 cm long.

Urethra

The posterior urethra forms a bulge in the posterior aspect of the female bladder, anterior to the vagina, that can be mistaken for a mass.

Uterus

The uterus is a thick-walled, pear-shaped, muscular organ lying posterior to the bladder and anterior to the rectum. A central echogenic line represents the endometrial cavity (Fig. 7-3). Small cysts in the cervical region are a common normal variant and are known as nabothian cysts. The uterus is composed of four parts: the fundus, the corpus (body), the isthmus, and the cervix (see Fig. 7-3).

Size

Normal uterine measurements in nulliparous menstruating women are 6 to 9 cm in length and up to 4 cm in anterior-posterior diameter and width. The uterus of parous women will have slightly larger dimensions. Before puberty the uterus is about 3 cm long and more or less tubular in shape (Fig. 7-4). After menopause the uterus shrinks in size but retains the shape it adopted with the onset of puberty.

Position

Usually the uterus is tilted anteriorly (anteversion; Fig. 7-5A), but may be normally tilted posteriorly (retroversion; Fig. 7-5B). An acute angulation in the midportion is known as an anteflexion (Fig. 7-5C) or retroflexion (Fig. 7-5D). Although usually in a midline position, the uterus may lie obliquely to the left or right.

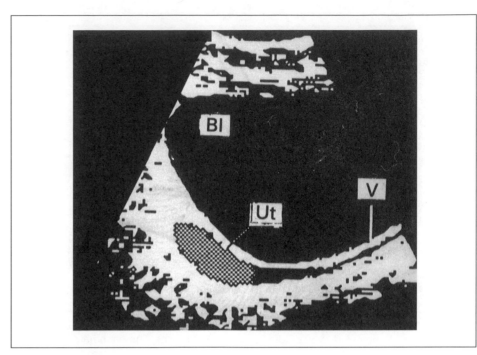

FIGURE 7-4. Prepubertal uterus. It will rapidly increase in size at puberty.

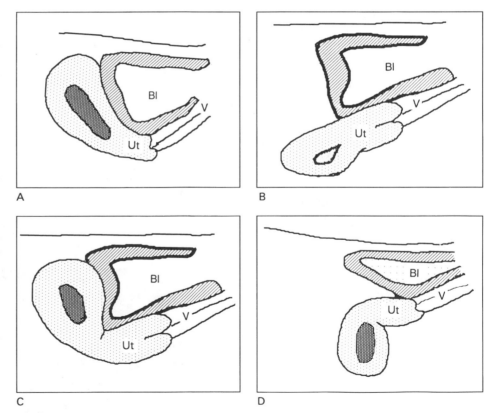

FIGURE 7-5. Various uterine positions. (**A**) Anteverted. (**B**) Retroverted. (**C**) Anteflexed. (**D**) Retroflexed. Note the septum where the uterus folds over on itself.

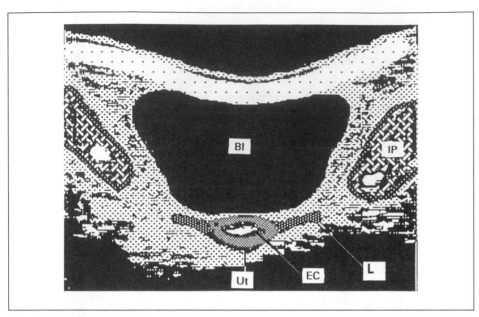

FIGURE 7-6. Transverse section through the fundus of the uterus (Ut), cornus, and proximal broad ligament (L); a decidual reaction is present. The endometrial cavity is shown (EC).

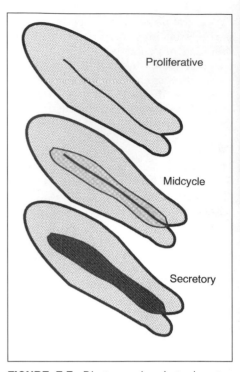

FIGURE 7-7. Diagram showing changes in the endometrial cavity over the menstrual cycle. The proliferative appearance is seen in the phase of the menstrual cycle leading up to ovulation. The endometrial cavity is less than 3mm thick. During this phase the dominant follicle is developing. Shortly before the time of ovulation the midcycle appearance is seen. Three echogenic lines are seen during this brief phase, which coincides with ovulation. The secretory phase (luteal phase) occurs after ovulation. At this time investigation of the endometrial cavity is limited because the endometrium is so thick and echogenic.

Shape

The menstruating uterus widens toward the fundus and the cornu, the bilateral, somewhat triangular regions where the fallopian tubes insert (Fig. 7-6). It is tubular in the part near the vagina known as the cervix.

Changes With Menstruation

The lining of the endometrial cavity is partially shed each month at menstruation, with consequent changes in cavity appearance during the course of the cycle (Fig. 7-7). During the preovulatory (proliferative) phase, the endometrial cavity echo is only about 3 mm thick and surrounded by an echopenic halo. Shortly before ovulation, two additional linear echoes outline the echopenic area (the "three line sign"). The echopenic area becomes more echogenic so that in the postovulatory (secretory or luteal) phase, the cavity echo becomes brighter and thicker (see Fig. 7-7). At this point, the width of the canal is between 9 mm and 1.3 cm thick.

Fallopian Tubes

The lumen of the normal fallopian tubes cannot be seen. The fallopian tubes lie within the broad ligament. They can often be traced from the uterine fundus to the ovaries on endovaginal views. This is especially easy if there is cul-de-sac fluid.

Ovaries

Location

The ovaries are usually found at the level of the uterine fundus where the uterus becomes triangular (the cornu) (Fig. 7-8; see also Figs. 7-2 and 7-6). Often the broad ligament can be traced laterally to the ovary. The ovaries often lie adjacent to the iliopsoas muscle, within which lies an echogenic focus that is due to the femoral nerve sheath (see Fig. 7-8). The iliac vessels usually lie lateral to the ovary.

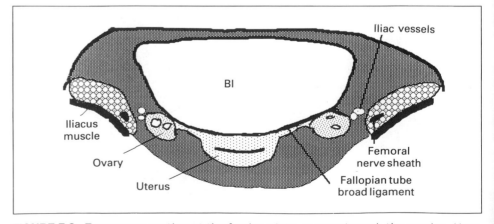

FIGURE 7-8. Transverse section at the fundus of the uterus through the ovaries. Note the iliacus muscle. The iliac vessels lie adjacent to the ovary. The ovaries normally lie close to the femoral nerve sheath.

Size

In a menstruating woman, ovaries normally measure approximately $2 \times 2.5 \times 3$ cm. There is variation, so $5 \times 2 \times 1.5$ cm or $4 \times 3 \times 1.5$ cm, for example, are measurements that may be within normal limits. The ovaries are about 1 cubic centimeter in young girls, gradually increasing in size as puberty approaches (see Appendix 24). In menopausal women the size of the ovary gradually decreases.

Menstrual Cycle Changes

Normally one follicle grows to a size of between 1.4 and 2.5 cm, alternating sides each menstrual cycle. Hormonal stimulation with drugs such as Pergonal or Clomid increases the number of dominant follicles, which may number as many as six or more in each ovary. Follicles are not seen in menopausal women, but are often seen in young girls before puberty. A dominant follicle normally bursts and disappears at midcycle. It is replaced by a corpus luteum. Typically, a corpus luteum has a thick, slightly echogenic, vascular rim (the rim of fire on color Doppler) and an echopenic center. The central echopenic area may be large if there is much bleeding at the time of ovulation.

The corpus luteum will usually disappear within a week or so.

Pelvic Muscles and Ligaments

Bands of muscle tissue play an important role in maintaining the position of the uterus and ovaries. The broad ligament extends from the lateral uterine walls to the pelvic sidewalls. The obturator internus muscles lie alongside the bony wall, lateral to the ovaries (Fig. 7-9). The iliopsoas muscles are lateral and anterior to the iliac crest; the femoral nerve sheath is seen as an echogenic area within the muscle (Fig. 7-10; also see Figs. 7-6 and 7-8). The levator ani, pyriformis, and coccygeus muscles make up the pelvic floor and are located posterior to the uterus, vagina, and rectum.

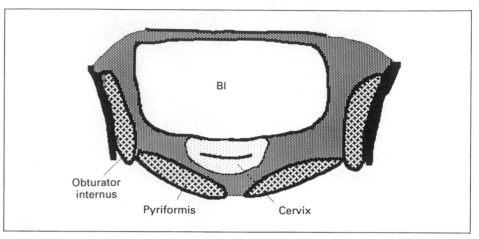

FIGURE 7-9. Transverse view at the level of the cervix showing the muscles that form the side walls of the pelvis.

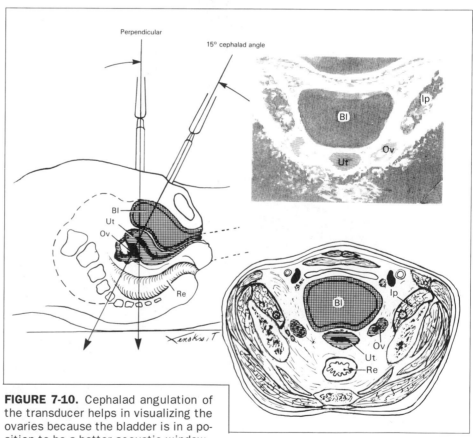

FIGURE 7-10. Cephalad angulation of the transducer helps in visualizing the ovaries because the bladder is in a position to be a better acoustic window.

Spaces Surrounding the Uterus

Small amounts of fluid may normally collect behind the uterus in the posterior cul-de-sac, also known as the pouch of Douglas (Fig. 7-11). The fluid may result from normal ovulation. The anterior cul-de-sac is anterior and superior to the uterine fundus.

▰ TECHNIQUE

Transabdominal Scanning

Distention of the urinary bladder is essential for a high-quality transabdominal pelvic sonogram. The full bladder displaces bowel and repositions the uterus in a more longitudinal fashion that allows the ultrasound beam to transect the uterus perpendicularly (see Fig. 7-10). The urinary bladder provides an acoustic window for better visualization of the pelvic structures. Overdistention or underdistention of the bladder can distort or obscure the view. A sufficiently full bladder will extend just over the uterine fundus. If the bladder is too full, encourage the patient to void into a paper cup so she does not empty her bladder completely.

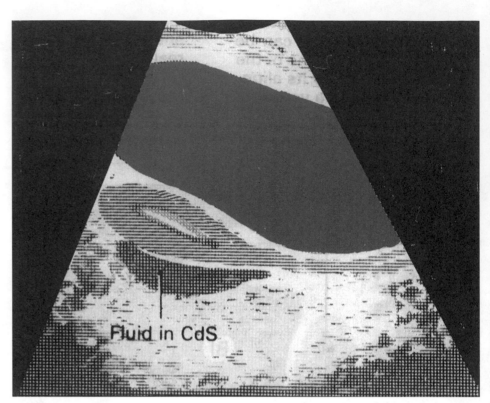

FIGURE 7-11. Fluid in the cul-de-sac. This amount of fluid may be seen in the course of the normal menstrual cycle following ovulation.

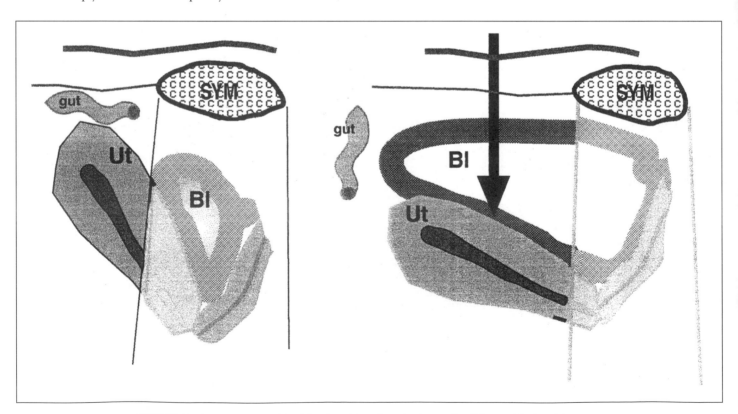

FIGURE 7-12. Filling the bladder to alter the uterine axis. When this bladder was filled (*right*), the uterus became less anteflexed. A retroverted uterus also usually adopts a more satisfactory position when the bladder is filled. Note the shadowing from the symphysis (Sym) obscuring the vagina and cervix unless the transducer is angled inferiorly.

1. The sonographic examination should begin in a longitudinal fashion by attempting to align the uterus with the vagina. The uterus can be recognized by the central line of the endometrial cavity and by its alignment with the vagina. The vagina is visualized as an echogenic line with relatively sonolucent walls.

    The uterus is normally located in the midline, but it may be deviated to either side in an oblique axis. Make sure that the bladder is full enough to show the fundus when the uterus is examined. An anteflexed or retroverted uterus may become more normal in position and shape if the bladder is filled (Fig. 7-12).

2. Scanning at right angles to the axis of the uterus should demonstrate the ovaries. The ovaries are usually close to the triangular cornual regions near the uterine fundus. Caudal angulation is helpful for visualizing the pelvic musculature and retroverted uteri. Cranial or caudal angulation may be necessary to see the ovaries.

3. A water enema can be helpful in the positive identification of bowel. Only a small amount of fluid need be run into the rectum through a small enema tube during observation with real-time. A flickering motion is visible when the water is running through the bowel. Do not mistake aortic pulsation or respiratory motion for peristalsis. This technique is rarely used now that endovaginal sonography is available (Fig. 7-13).

Endovaginal Scanning (Transvaginal Scanning, Vaginal Scanning)

Endovaginal (EV) scanning is becoming the dominant technique used for the examination of the female pelvic structures. Detail of the ovaries, endometrium, and myometrium is far superior to that obtained with the transabdominal approach. In addition, the vaginal probe can be used like an examining finger to decide the following:

1. Whether local tenderness is greatest in the ovaries, tubal region, or uterus
2. Whether the ovaries move freely; if the ovaries cannot be separated from the neighboring bowel or the adjacent uterus, adhesions are the likely cause

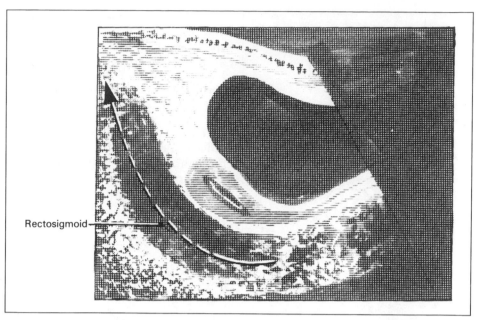

FIGURE 7-13. Water enema. A small amount of fluid is introduced through a tube into the rectum and watched under real-time as it fills the rectosigmoid colon.

Rectosigmoid

3. Whether a mass is intrauterine or extrauterine

Endovaginal scanning is essential whenever greater detail is required, for example in the following:

1. Ectopic pregnancy
2. Threatened abortion
3. Follicle monitoring and egg retrieval
4. A questionable adnexal mass
5. Intrauterine pathology (e.g., endometrial polyps or fibroids) and monitoring of endometrial thickness
6. Chorionic villi sampling
7. Early pregnancy

Endovaginal scanning is used following a transabdominal scan unless it is only follicles that are being monitored or it is suspected that the patient has an ectopic pregnancy and the bladder is empty. It is more convenient to perform the transabdominal study first since the bladder can easily be emptied, but takes at least 45 minutes to refill. The endovaginal pelvic examination cannot entirely replace the transabdominal pelvic sonogram for the following reasons:

1. It does not show the entire extent of large pelvic masses or midabdominal pathology.

2. It cannot be used in young girls or in some postmenopausal women—it may be too threatening for some sexually inexperienced women, and the older woman's vagina may not accommodate the probe.
3. Some ovaries are located at such a high level they can only be seen with transabdominal views.

Preparation

Since the endovaginal examination is similar to a pelvic examination, the male sonographer should have a chaperon. A clean transducer is covered with a condom after gel has been placed on the transducer tip. The bladder should be as empty as possible since urine in the bladder creates an artifact.

Instrumentation

The endovaginal transducer is a rod-shaped probe or wand approximately 6 to 12 inches in length with a handle at one end and the transducer crystal located in the tip at the opposite end. The ultrasound beam is transmitted from the tip parallel or at a slight angle to the probe shaft (Fig. 7-14).

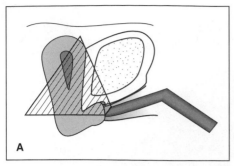

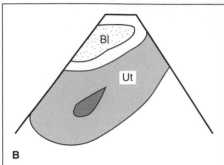

FIGURE 7-14. (**A**) View showing the segment of the uterus, cervix, and bladder that is visualized with a slightly off-axis vaginal sonogram. (**B**) The way the image will be presented on the TV screen. Note that the uterus appears to be back-to-front with the bladder to the left of the image.

SAGITTAL IMAGES. As the probe is advanced into the vagina, the cervix can be seen approaching the top of the screen with the uterus extending downward (see Fig. 7-14). By resting the monitor on its side one can see an orientation similar to that of a transabdominal pelvic scan.

CORONAL IMAGES. As the probe is advanced into the vagina a coronal slice through the cervix is obtained by angling the probe posteriorly and rotating the transducer head laterally (Fig. 7-15). With an anteverted uterus the

probe handle is angled posteriorly so the beam is perpendicular to the body and fundus. To obtain a coronal view the probe is rotated into a lateral position. A retroverted uterus requires anterior probe angulation.

When the probe is angled laterally the ovaries can usually be seen. If a transverse view through the fundus of the uterus is obtained, the broad ligament is usually found. In many women, tracing this structure laterally will lead to the ovary (Fig. 7-16).

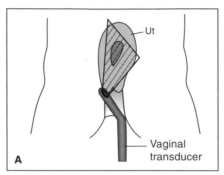
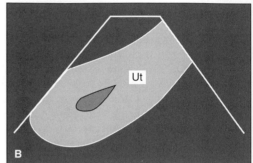

FIGURE 7-15. (**A**) Diagram showing the way in which a coronal view of the uterus obtained with an endovaginal approach can give a right-angle image to the sagittal view. (**B**) The resultant image as it appears on the screen.

Endovaginal Probe Technique

The probe is advanced approximately 3 to 4 inches into the vagina. The sonographer then directs the sound beam by rotating and angling the probe from anterior to posterior and sliding it in and out. If a gynecologic examination table with stirrups is not available, elevating the hip with a pillow may be necessary. This is particularly useful with an acutely anteverted uterus. The patient will let you know if she is experiencing discomfort; however, the vagina is very distensible, and angling the probe is usually pain-free unless the patient has a disease process such as pelvic infection.

Orientation

Sagittal and coronal images of the uterus and ovaries can be obtained transvaginally. Since the probe is inserted into the vagina with the ultrasound beam directed toward the uterus, the vagina itself is not normally visualized. The probe is partially withdrawn to visualize the cervix and distal vagina.

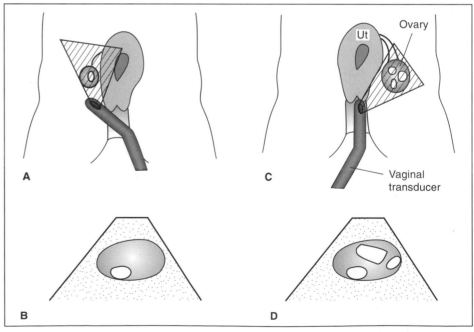

FIGURE 7-16. (**A**) Diagram showing the technique used to obtain a coronal view of the right ovary. (**B**) Image of the ovary seen on the screen. (**C**) Diagram showing the way in which a coronal view of the left ovary is obtained. (**D**) Image of the ovary seen on the screen.

◆ PATHOLOGY

Female infertility can be a result of the following:

1. Physiologic factors disrupting the hormonal control of ovulation.
2. Structural problems preventing fertilization.

Congenital Uterine Malformations

See Figure 7-17.

Uterine structural defects often cause repeated abortions rather than absence of pregnancy. One to two percent of the female population have some type of structural defect. The most common uterine anomalies are the following:

1. *Uterus didelphus:* Two adjacent cervices with two separate uterine bodies (Figs. 7-17 and 7-18).
2. *Septate uterus:* There is a partial lack of embryological fusion that results in a septated uterine body with two separate cavities within a single uterus (see Fig. 7-17).
3. *Bicornuate uterus:* The uterus has a single cavity in the cervix and lower uterine segment. The cavity splits in the fundus into two horns (see Fig. 7-17). Only one vagina is present. This is the most common structural defect.

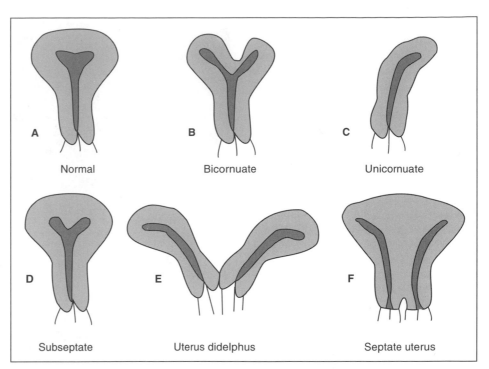

FIGURE 7-17. Congenital uterine anomalies. (**A**) Normal. (**B**) Bicornuate uterus. Note the V-shaped indentation in the fundus of the endometrial cavity. (**C**) Unicornuate uterus that has only one horn. No fallopian tube leads to the left ovary. (**D**) Uterus subseptate. There is no deformity of the uterine outline, but the two horns of the uterus are split. (**E**) Uterus didelphys. There are two uteri which are separate, two cervices, and two vaginas. (**F**) Septate uterus. Two completely separate uterine cavities are enclosed within a single uterine outline.

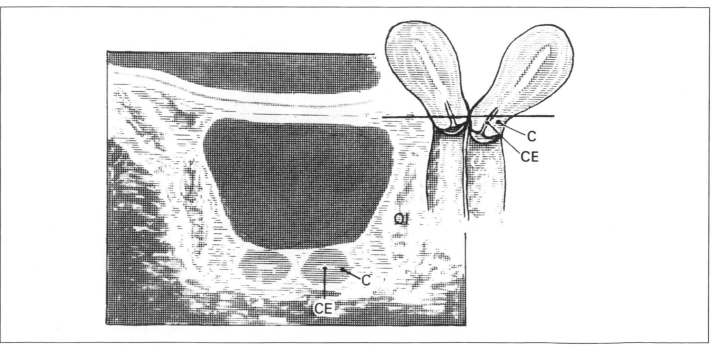

FIGURE 7-18. Diagram of one form of double uterus (uterus didelphus); there is complete separation of the uteri with two adjacent cervices. In another form, the two uteri are joined by a common midline septum.

4. *Uterus unicornis:* There is one uterine horn and cervix, and one vagina (see Fig. 7-17).
5. *Uterus subseptus:* The endometrial cavity bifurcates into two horns, but the uterine outline is unaltered.
6. *Hypoplastic uterus:* The uterus is normally formed, but is less than 4 cm long. Sometimes the patient can menstruate with a uterus this small.

Polycystic Ovaries (PCO)

See Figure 7-19.

Polycystic ovarian syndrome may cause only amenorrhea, but additional features sometimes seen are obesity and hirsutism. There is mild ovarian enlargement with numerous small cysts around the periphery of the ovary, best seen with the endovaginal transducer. The central cyst-free area is increased in size and is called stroma. Such sonographic appearances may be found in apparently normal women, so a diagnosis of polycystic ovaries is usually made in conjunction with biochemical tests.

Endometriosis

See Figure 7-20.

During the reproductive years, endometrial tissue may become implanted outside the uterine cavity, adhering to any structure, but particularly to the fallopian tubes, ovaries, and broad ligaments. The ectopic tissue undergoes cyclic changes with the menstrual cycle, and bleeding can occur, producing endometriomas, masses known as "chocolate cysts." Endometriosis is sometimes painful and is a very common cause of infertility.

Typical sonographic findings with endometriosis are fluid-filled circular or ovoid masses within or outside the ovary. These masses may

1. be echo-free.
2. contain low-level echoes.
3. look like a solid mass.
4. have echogenic areas or a septum within a fluid-filled mass.

One or more masses may be present. The abnormal endometrial tissue is not seen but there may be evidence of adhesions with an abnormal ovarian position (see Chapter 9).

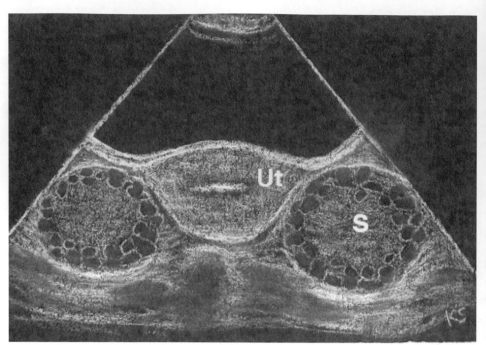

FIGURE 7-19. Polycystic ovaries are enlarged, round, and multiple small peripheral cysts. The central cyst-free area is called stroma (S). There is more stroma in an ovary with polycystic ovaries than in a normal ovary, so the ovary is enlarged overall.

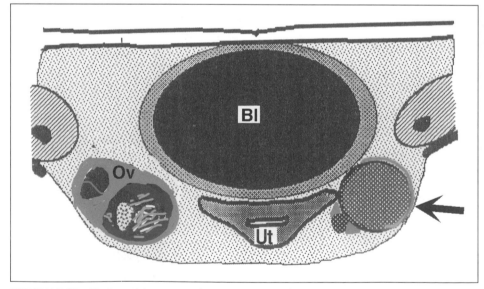

FIGURE 7-20. Endometrioma may have a variety of sonographic appearances. On the left (arrow), an endometrioma containing even lower level echoes with a small adjacent additional endometrioma is seen. On the right, two endometrioma can be seen within the right ovary. One contains many irregular echoes, consistent with blood clot. The other is an echo-free cyst with a septum. These are two of the other appearances that endometrioma may adopt.

If the condition involves the uterus it is known as adenomyosis. The uterus is enlarged. Ill-defined echopenic masses are seen in the myometrium adjacent to the endometrium. Occasionally cystic intramyometrial areas are seen. In most instances nothing can be seen on ultrasound, although adenomyosis is found at pathology.

Pelvic Inflammatory Disease (PID)

Pelvic inflammatory disease, when responsible for infertility, is characterized by tubo-ovarian abscesses and adhesions of the pelvic structures. Patency of the fallopian tubes is diminished secondary to scarring from infections, so bilateral hydrosalpinx may be seen. The sonographic findings of pelvic inflammatory disease are discussed in detail in Chapter 9. Previous pelvic surgery can also lead to adhesions and blocked fallopian tubes causing infertility due to hydrosalpinx. Tubal patency can be assessed using hysterosonosalpingography with the injection of fluid or ultrasonic contrast. This technique is described in Chapter 10.

Fibroids

Large uterine masses can hinder zygote implantation and cause premature labor or spontaneous abortion. Intracavitary fibroids are especially likely to prevent conception (see Chapters 8 and 10).

Uterine Synechiae

Previous intrauterine surgery, such as a dilatation and curettage, may result in fibrous strands across the uterine cavity, known as synechiae. These can prevent egg implantation. If many synechiae are present and the two walls of the endometrial cavity are gummed together, implantation cannot occur; this condition is known as Ascherman's syndrome. The endometrial cavity contents can be demonstrated by the use of the hysterosonogram (uterine infusion study) (see Chapter 10 for a description of this technique). Strands of fibrous tissue will be seen crossing the cavity. In the more severe form, the cavity will be obliterated and it will be impossible to get fluid into the cavity.

Anovulation

Anovulation is failure to ovulate characterized by poor ovarian follicular development or a dominant follicle that enlarges, but never bursts and ovulates (luteinized unruptured follicle syndrome). Serial sonograms during a cycle can reveal abnormal follicle development or even their absence. Unstimulated follicles normally burst when they reach a size of between 1.5 and 2.3 cm. The luteinized unruptured follicle syndrome (LUFS) is diagnosed when serial follow-up views show the follicle size continuing to increase beyond 2.3 cm. Eventually, the unruptured follicle will spontaneously disappear.

GUIDING THERAPY FOR INFERTILITY

Several approaches are used to assist infertile couples when anovulation is the problem. Most therapies involve using a pharmacologic agent, Clomid or Pergonal, to stimulate follicular growth. An HCG injection may then be used to initiate ovulation. Fertilization is planned by one of the following methods: intercourse, insemination, or in vitro fertilization. Lastly, some programs include implantation procedures (IVF and GIFT). An experienced sonographer is a necessary member of the team.

Serial Scanning for Follicles

1. A baseline study is performed shortly following the onset of menses to rule out any adnexal pathology or residual cysts from the previous cycle.
2. Serial sonograms are usually started 5 to 8 days following the onset of menses, preferably using the endovaginal route. Multiple small follicles under 1 cm in size should be visible at this time.
3. Follicles may be measured in three dimensions to produce a volume measurement using the formula length $\times$ height $\times$ width $\times$ 0.5233, or the largest dimension may be used for follow-up (Fig. 7-21). Be consistent in labeling so the growth of two different follicles is not confused.
4. As follicles increase in size, it can be confusing and time consuming to attempt to measure every follicle. We suggest noting the number of follicles over 8 mm in each ovary. Only the largest three are then measured.
5. As multiple follicles develop they may distort and compress adjacent follicles, which is why it is imperative to use all three measurements. An overdistended urinary bladder can also distort follicular size and shape.

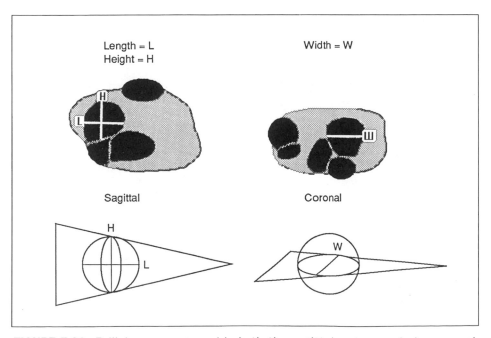

FIGURE 7-21. Follicles are measured in both the sagittal and coronal plane so volume can be calculated. It is very easy to be confused about which follicle you are measuring when you reexamine the patient on another day. Be consistent; start at 12:00 and label A, B, C clockwise on each ovary.

6. For consistent measurements, the same sonographer should examine a patient throughout the cycle.

7. Mature follicular size ranges from 1.4 to 2.3 cm. When stimulated, the follicles may reach a size of 3 cm. When a large size is reached and other biochemical indicators are appropriate, HCG is given to initiate ovulation.

8. A cumulus oophorus may occasionally be seen as a small septum or mass within a large follicle that is about to ovulate.

9. Endometrial changes have been used as an indicator of follicular maturity. When the endometrium develops three lines, ovulation is imminent (see Fig. 7-7).

10. Fluid in the posterior cul-de-sac may be a sign of follicular rupture (see Fig. 7-11).

11. When the follicle has ruptured, a corpus luteum forms where the follicle used to be. It is sonolucent with a thick, mildly echogenic border and some internal echoes. Color flow performed shortly after ovulation will show a rim of vessels around a corpus luteum (see Chapter 8).

12. A sonogram may be performed to prove that ovulation has occurred.

Hyperstimulation Syndrome

See Figure 7-22.

A dangerous side effect of inducing follicular development by hormone administration is the ovarian hyperstimulation syndrome (OHS). The features of OHS are the following:

1. Multiple, large, thin-walled cysts in both ovaries that are actually huge follicles; these are known as theca lutein cysts
2. Ascites
3. In severe cases, pleural effusions

If the patient fails to become pregnant, the cysts will usually resolve with the next cycle. If pregnancy occurs, the cysts will usually resolve within 6 to 8 weeks.

In Vitro Fertilization (IVF)

If the fallopian tubes are absent or blocked, conception cannot occur because the ova cannot reach the uterus. With in vitro fertilization, the mature follicles are aspirated to retrieve the eggs. The retrieval of the eggs is performed either at laparoscopy or under ultrasonic guidance. Ten to twenty-five percent of in vitro fertilization procedures will result in a pregnancy. Egg retrieval is generally guided with ultrasound.

Follicular Aspiration Under Ultrasonic Guidance

Three ultrasonic approaches have been used to aspirate follicles. All use an 18-gauge needle.

1. The needle is directed through the urinary bladder into the follicle through a guidance attachment to the transducer (Fig. 7-23). The needle path is monitored with ultrasound.
2. With the bladder full, the needle is pushed through the vaginal fornix into the ovary, being guided by real-time imaging through the bladder. Sometimes the needle traverses the bladder wall twice on its way to the ovary (Fig. 7-24).

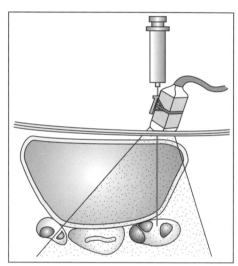

FIGURE 7-23. Diagram showing follicle puncture under transabdominal ultrasound guidance. The needle is passed through the bladder.

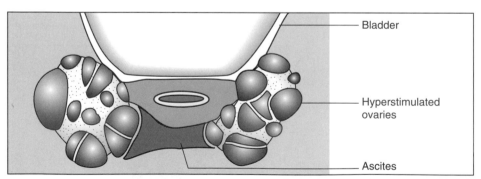

Bladder

Hyperstimulated ovaries

Ascites

FIGURE 7-22. Transverse scan. Hyperstimulation syndrome. Theca lutein cysts contain numerous septa, are frequently bilateral, and can be very large. They are associated with hydatidiform mole and the hyperstimulation syndrome. Ascites is often seen.

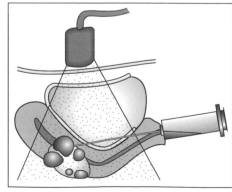

FIGURE 7-24. Follicle aspiration using the needle inserted through the vagina but with guidance performed with a transducer placed on the abdomen viewing the area through the bladder.

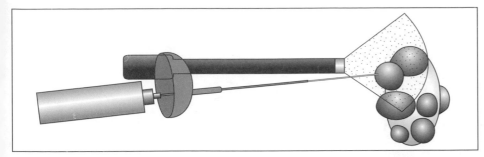

FIGURE 7-25. Follicle aspiration performed with transducer and the needle both inserted into the vagina.

3. The needle is inserted into the follicle alongside a vaginal transducer with the bladder empty (Fig. 7-25). This technique has proven to be the best and is almost universally used. Needle visualization is adequate, and with the bladder empty the ovary lies very close to the vaginal fornix so the possibility of damaging gut is reduced.

Gamete Intrafollicular Transfer (GIFT)

In the gamete intrafollicular transfer technique, follicles are removed from the ovary under sonographic control. They are then fertilized in a petri dish and a laparoscope is used to replace them within the fallopian tube.

PITFALLS

1. *Tampons in the vagina* can produce a mass-like effect or can cause shadowing if they do not contain blood.
2. *The degree of bladder distention* will affect the shape of pelvic structures. Overdistention will flatten and distort the ovaries and may make them undetectable, particularly with a vaginal probe. With underdistention, the ovaries may be obscured by gas on a transabdominal examination.
3. *The uterus is not always in the midline* and may lie on an oblique axis. Suspect adhesions if this is the case.
4. *Do not mistake rectum or sigmoid colon for a mass or fluid.* Watch for peristalsis or use a water enema to see movement (see Fig. 7-13).
5. *Failure to elevate the hips* during an endovaginal study may result in the ovaries not being seen and the urethra being mistaken for a mass.

6. *Nabothian cysts* can be mistaken for follicles if only a transvaginal approach is used.
7. *Compression of a follicle* can cause distortions in measurement. This is especially likely if only the longest dimension is used for comparison with previous studies. An overdistended bladder may compress follicles.
8. *The muscles of the pelvis*, in particular the pyriformis muscle, can be mistaken for ovaries. They lie more posteriorly, are ovoid in shape, and are symmetrical.
9. *Failure to empty the bladder* completely prior to an endovaginal study will lead to reverberation artifacts which may hide important structures.
10. *Difficulty in seeing the endometrial cavity.* Occasionally the endometrial cavity is difficult to see with the endovaginal probe because it is aligned in the same axis as the ultrasonic beam. Placing the patient in the knee elbow position and reinserting the endovaginal probe sometimes helps under these circumstances.

WHERE ELSE TO LOOK

1. *Uterine anomaly.* If a congenital uterine anomaly is present, such as a double uterus, be sure to check the kidneys since one may well be absent.
2. *Intrauterine pregnancy* with pain and bleeding in an infertile patient. Look for a heterotopic pregnancy—an ectopic pregnancy as well as an intrauterine pregnancy since infertility patients are at risk for ectopic.
3. *Hyperstimulation.* Check the abdomen for ascites and the chest for pleural effusions, which often occur with hyperstimulated ovaries.

SELECTED READING

Applebaum, M., and Parker, J. J. Endovaginal scanning in the "procto" position: An alternative approach. *Ultrasound Obstet Gynecol* 7:356–358, 1996.

Botchan, A., Yaron, Y., Lessing, J. B., Barak, Y., Yovel, I., David, M. P., Peyser, M. R., and Amit, A. When multiple gestational sacs are seen on ultrasound, "take-home baby" rate improves with in-vitro fertilization. *Human Reprod* 8: 710–713, 1993.

Botsis, D., Kassanos, D., Pyrgiotis, E., and Zourlas, P. A. Sonographic incidence of polycystic ovaries in a gynecological population. *Ultrasound Obstet Gynecol* 6:182–185, 1995.

Krysiewicz, S. Infertility in women: Diagnostic evaluation with hysterosalpingography and other imaging techniques. *AJR* 159:253–261, 1992.

Pache, T. D., Hop, W. C. J., Wladimiroff, J. W., Schipper, J., and Fauser, B. C. J. M. Transvaginal sonography and abnormal ovarian appearance in menstrual cycle disturbances. *Ultrasound Med & Biol* 17:589–593, 1991.

Pfeifer, D. G. The role of sonography in diagnosing and treating female infertility. *JDMS* 11:61–66, 1995.

Randall, J. M., and Templeton, A. Transvaginal sonographic assessment of follicular and endometrial growth in spontaneous and clomiphene citrate cycles. *Fertil Steril* 56: 208–212, 1991.

Sanders, R. C. Infertility diagnosis by ultrasound. *Urol Radiol* 13:41–47, 1991.

Shoham, Z., DiCarlo, C., Patel, A., Conway, G. S., and Jacobs, H. S. Is it possible to run a successful ovulation induction program based solely on ultrasound monitoring? The importance of endometrial measurements. *Fertil Steril* 56:836–841, 1991.

Zaidi, J., Campbell, S., Pittrof, R., and Tan, S. L. Endometrial thickness, morphology, vascular penetration and velocimetry in predicting implantation in an in vitro fertilization program. *Ultrasound Obstet Gynecol* 6:191–198, 1995.

RULE OUT PELVIC MASS

ROGER C. SANDERS, JOAN CAMPBELL

SONOGRAM ABBREVIATIONS

Bl	Bladder
C	Cervix
CdS	Cul-de-sac
CE	Cervical endometrium
Cy	Cyst
IC	Intracavitary
IM	Intramural
M	Mass
P	Pedunculated
SM	Submucosal
SS	Subserosal
Ut	Uterus

KEY WORDS

Adenomyosis. Generalized enlargement of the uterus due to endometrial tissue within the myometrium; condition similar to endometriosis.

Chocolate Cyst. Blood-filled cyst associated with endometriosis.

Corpus Luteum Cyst. Cyst developing in the second half of the menstrual cycle and in pregnancy that regresses spontaneously.

Cuff. After hysterectomy the blind end of the vagina is sutured and forms a fibrous mass, the cuff.

Dermoid. Form of teratoma that is benign and tends to occur in young women.

Endometrioma. Hematoma (*chocolate cyst*) caused by bleeding from abnormally implanted endometrial tissue.

Endometriosis. Deposits of endometrial tissue on the ovaries, the exterior of the uterus, and the intestines, among other places. They bleed at monthly intervals, causing development of hematomas and fibrosis.

Fibroid (Myoma). A benign tumor of the smooth muscle of the uterus. *Submucosal*—a fibroid bordering on the endometrial cavity. *Subserosal*—a fibroid bordering on the peritoneal cavity. *Myometrial*—fibroid within the wall of the uterus.

Follicle. Developing ovum within the ovary; can develop into a cyst.

Hematometrocolpos. Metra = uterus, culpa = vagina. Condition presenting at birth or at puberty due to an imperforate hymen. Blood or other fluid accumulates in the vagina and uterus.

Hydrosalpinx. Blocked fallopian tube that fills with sterile fluid as a consequence of adhesions from a previous infection.

Intramural. Term used to describe a lesion, such as a fibroid, that lies in the wall of the uterus.

Multiparous. A woman who has been pregnant more than once.

Myoma. See *Fibroid.*

Nulliparous. A woman who has not been pregnant.

Parous. A woman who has been pregnant.

Pedunculated. Term used particularly for fibroids describing a mass that is connected to its site of origin by only a short pedicle.

Polycystic Ovary Syndrome (PCO, Stein-Leventhal syndrome). Multiple cysts developing in both ovaries. The condition is traditionally associated with obesity and masculine distribution of body hair.

Progesterone. Hormone secreted by the corpus luteum that prepares the endometrium to receive a fertilized egg.

Pseudomyxoma Peritonei. Condition that occurs when an ovarian cystic tumor bursts and its contents spread through the abdomen, forming additional lesions.

Submucosal. Term used to describe a process, such as a fibroid, that is located adjacent to the uterine cavity within the uterus.

Subserosal. Term used to describe a lesion such as a fibroid that is on the surface of the uterus.

Teratoma. Tumor composed of the various body tissues including skin, teeth, hair, and bone, among others. May be malignant but is usually benign in the pelvic area.

Theca Lutein Cysts. Multiple cysts that develop in association with trophoblastic disease because of increased HCG levels. May also occur with multiple pregnancy and induced ovulation.

◆≫ THE CLINICAL PROBLEM

An ultrasound pelvic examination is often used as a supplement to the clinical pelvic examination. It may even replace an internal exam; cases in which a physical examination may be difficult to perform include (1) children—a pelvic exam is difficult or impossible; (2) obese females—the pelvic organs are difficult to palpate; and (3) patients with acute pelvic infection (pelvic inflammatory disease), in whom a pelvic examination is often painful.

A pelvic mass may come to light for a number of different reasons:

1. There may be pain on the side of the mass.
2. The mass may be found at a routine clinical examination.
3. Secondary obstruction of the genitourinary or gastrointestinal tract may occur.
4. An alternative imaging technique such as a CAT scan may show a mass.

The questions that need to be answered about a pelvic mass are the following:

1. Is a pathologic pelvic mass present or is the supposed mass a normal anatomic variant?
2. Is the mass uterine, adnexal, or neither?
3. Is the mass cystic, complex, or solid? If it is cystic, does it have septa?
4. Is there blood flow to the mass? Is the blood flow high or low resistance?
5. Is the mass involving or invading any other pelvic structure?
6. Are other associated findings such as ascites, metastases, or hydronephrosis present?

Using a combination of the clinical background and the sonographic appearance, a relatively specific diagnosis is usually possible. The sonographer needs the following information to perform a quality sonogram and to make sure that the sonogram is correctly interpreted:

1. What was the date of the first day of the last period (if the patient is still menstruating)?
2. Are menstrual cycles regular and how long do they last?
3. If the patient has had a hysterectomy, does she know when she ovulates?
4. How long ago did the patient stop menstruating (if she is menopausal)?
5. How many children has the patient had?
6. Has the patient had pelvic surgery? Have any pelvic structures been removed?
7. Has there been pain? If so, where is it located?
8. If the patient is postmenopausal, is she on hormone replacement therapy?

Pelvic mass assessment is helped by sonography in the following situations:

1. Ovarian masses in premenopausal women are usually followed for about 6 weeks to make sure the mass is not a physiological variant such as a corpus luteum. However, if the mass is greater than 10 cm in diameter or has typical dermoid appearances, or if there are sonographic features suggestive of malignancy, immediate surgery may be elected.
2. When fibroids are not treated surgically, they may be followed by serial sonography. Surgical planning for fibroid removal is aided by sonography.
3. Particularly in obese people, it may be difficult to be certain by pelvic examination whether a pelvic mass is present. Ultrasound can help by definitely showing a mass and determining whether it is uterine or ovarian.
4. Small cysts in postmenopausal women are common, and as long as they are echo-free, many cysts are followed with serial sonograms.
5. Screening for ovarian cancer in at-risk patients may be helpful in women over the age of 35 since this cancer has few signs and symptoms and usually presents when it has already metastasized. In women with a strong family history of ovarian cancer or of an associated cancer—colon, endometrium, and breast—annual sonograms for early cancer detection may be worthwhile.

ANATOMY

See Chapter 7.

▨ TECHNIQUE

See Chapter 7.

Investigation of masses in the female pelvis hinges on the identification of the ovaries and the uterus. The easiest structure to find is the uterus. Always note the patient's menstrual history on the film. The uterus is recognized

1. as a structure containing a linear echogenic structure—the endometrial cavity echoes.
2. by tracking the vagina to it; the uterus lies superior to the vagina. On some occasions, the uterus has an oblique axis.

Features to look for in a uterine mass include the following:

1. Cystic or solid
2. Location, e.g., fundal, cervical, lower segment, right or left, anterior or posterior
3. Relationship to endometrial cavity, e.g., intracavitary, submucosal, intramural, subserosal, or pedunculated
4. Secondary effects on the endometrial cavity, e.g., endometrial fluid above the level of the mass

The ovaries are recognized by:

1. their location at the end of the broad ligament.
2. the presence of follicles in women who are menstruating.
3. their proximity to the iliac vessels.

Features to look for in an adnexal mass include the following:

1. Is the mass cystic or solid? If the mass is cystic, does it contain septum or masses? Are the walls thin or fat? Are the walls smooth or irregular?
2. Is the mass inside or outside the ovary?
3. What is the size of the mass?
4. Is the mass round or some other shape, such as tubular?
5. Is there vascularity within the mass? Is the flow within the mass high or low resistance?

Maneuvers to Help in the Characterization of Masses

Endovaginal Transducer

The endovaginal transducer is helpful (1) to show mass detail—an extraovarian mass, for example, may turn out to have the shape of a dilated fallopian tube; (2) to distinguish the uterus from an ovarian mass; (3) to locate the site of local tenderness—the transducer is pushed toward the adnexa and the patient reports when and where there is a painful sensation; and (4) to see whether the ovary and neighboring gut move well. Polyps may be seen within the uterine cavity that cannot be seen from a transabdominal approach. The location of a fibroid in relation to the endometrial cavity can be determined.

Trendelenburg or Decubitus Position

Placing a patient in the Trendelenburg, or on their side (decubitus), should shift free fluid in the cul-de-sac out of the pelvis—but rarely does.

Doppler

Doppler analysis of pelvic cystic structures is worthwhile. Dilated veins in the region of the ovary can mimic ovarian cysts or hydrosalpinx. Malignant masses may show a low-resistance pattern. Doppler may be of assistance in determining whether an ectopic pregnancy is present, since a flow pattern with high diastolic flow (low resistance) is seen with ectopics and corpus luteum cysts. If a solid mass might be ovarian or a fibroid, use color flow to see whether vessels from the uterus enter and surround a fibroid.

◆ PATHOLOGY

Pelvic masses can be divided into four basic groups: (1) single cystic masses; (2) multiple cystic masses; (3) complex masses; and (4) solid masses. Unfortunately, many of these entities are not easy to distinguish from one another sonographically on a single examination. Using the clinical information and a follow-up examination, however, a relatively specific diagnosis can be made.

Cystic Masses

Cystic masses have well-defined smooth borders, show good through transmission, and are usually spherical.

Single Intraovarian Cysts

Cystic masses may originate in the ovary or may be separate from the ovary. The differential diagnosis is different depending on whether the cyst is within or outside the ovary. Intraovarian cysts are surrounded by a rim of ovarian tissue.

FOLLICULAR CYSTS (REPRODUCTIVE AGE GROUP). Follicular cysts (Fig. 8-1) are caused by continued hormonal stimulation of a follicle that does not rupture at ovulation. Cysts are considered worthy of follow-up when they are over 2.6 cm in diameter. Such cysts usually stay small, but can measure up to 10 cm in size. They disappear within a few weeks. Ovulation almost always takes place on alternate sides, so a repeat study after 3 to 4 weeks is desirable when a mass that could be a follicular cyst is found in a menstruating patient, to document its disappearance. Hemorrhage may occur within a follicular cyst and cause internal echoes, although such cysts are generally echo-free.

CORPUS LUTEUM CYSTS (REPRODUCTIVE AGE GROUP). Corpus luteum cysts are progesterone-producing cysts or masses that occur following ovulation or in the first 10 to 15 weeks of pregnancy. Their size is variable, and occasionally they become quite large (up to 10 cm). Although most often containing echoes, owing to hemorrhage, they may be echo-free. Characteristically there is a hyperechoic rim around the cyst. This rim is very vascular on color flow Doppler ("the ring of fire") shortly after ovulation.

SEROUS CYSTADENOMA (REPRODUCTIVE AND POSTMENARCHE AGE GROUPS). The most common benign tumors of the ovary, serous cystadenomas are large, thin-walled cysts that may have septa within them (Fig. 8-2). They occur most commonly in women between the ages of 20 and 50. These cysts may be small, but are usually large and may grow large enough to occupy most of the abdomen. About 30 percent are bilateral, but the contralateral cyst may be small. Color flow may show arterial flow in the septa which is typically high resistance.

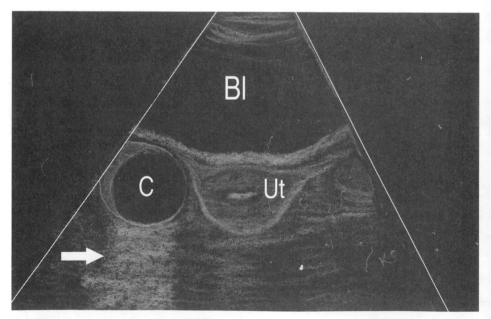

FIGURE 8-1. Cysts without internal structure in the adnexa are often follicular cysts that will disappear spontaneously. Note the rim of ovary surrounding the cyst (arrow).

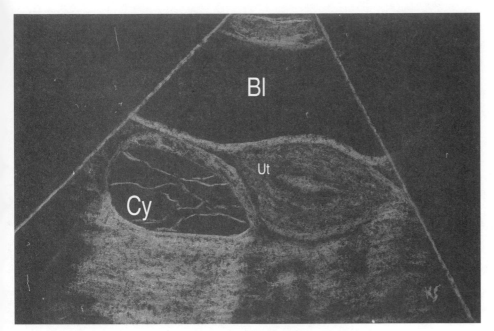

FIGURE 8-2. Serous cystadenoma are cysts that often contain thin septa.

POSTMENOPAUSAL CYSTS. Small cysts of up to 3 or 4 cm in diameter are commonly encountered in postmenopausal women. Many gynecologists now follow cysts of this type with serial ultrasound at 6-monthly to yearly intervals. The cyst must be shown by high-quality endovaginal ultrasound to be echo-free and without worrisome Doppler patterns in the wall. Many such cysts disappear spontaneously.

ENDOMETRIOMA. Endometrioma often occur within the ovary. (see Extraovarian Cystic Masses, later, for a detailed description of endometrioma.)

DERMOID. Although most dermoids contain echogenic structures or calcifications, some are entirely cystic.

CYSTADENOCARCINOMA. Although cystadenocarcinomas (Fig. 8-3) are practically never entirely cystic, they may be almost echo-free.

Extraovarian Cystic Masses

PARAOVARIAN CYST. Paraovarian cysts lie between the uterus and the ovary. Thought to represent embryonic remnants, they are ovoid and echo-free.

PERITONEAL INCLUSION CYST. Peritoneal inclusion cysts are a consequence of previous surgery or infection. The peritoneal surfaces become adhesed, and fluid slowly collects. These cysts may be of any shape and may contain septa and a few internal echoes.

ENDOMETRIOMA. An extraovarian fluid-filled mass that contains internal echoes in a patient without the clinical features of pelvic inflammatory disease probably represents an endometrioma. Not necessarily circular, they may be septated, and they are usually filled with homogeneously high-level echoes (see Chapter 7). Endometrioma are usually seen in the vicinity of the ovary but may occur anywhere in the pelvis including the abdominal wall at a surgical incision site. (see Multiple Cystic Masses.)

HYDROSALPINX. Hydrosalpinx are usually the sequelae of pelvic inflammatory disease (see Chapter 9) or, less often, of adhesive processes such as endometriosis involving the fallopian tube outlet. The pus in a pyosalpinx resorbs and is transformed into fluid. The sonographic findings may suggest hydrosalpinx when the tube folds over on itself and forms a funnel-shaped or kinked structure (see Chapter 9).

Single "Cystic" Masses Seen Within the Uterus

HYDROMETROCOLPOS (NEONATAL). In hydrometrocolpos, there is distention of the vagina and uterus with fluid. This is usually secondary to cervical or vaginal obstruction due to, for instance, an imperforate hymen. Usually the vagina is distended while the uterus is still small, however both uterus and vagina may be fluid filled. The fluid contents are usually anechoic.

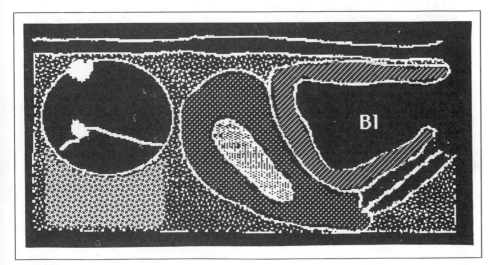

FIGURE 8-3. Cystadenocarcinoma. Note that the echogenic material within the cyst is eroding through the cyst wall, a sign of malignancy.

HEMATOMETROCOLPOS (PREMENARCHE). Hematometrocolpos occurs when the vagina and possibly the uterus are distended with blood at menarche, rather than the serous fluid of hydrometrocolpos. Internal echoes within the blood are usually seen (Fig. 8-4). Either the hymen is imperforate or there is a congenital narrowing of the vagina which only becomes apparent when menstruation starts. Hematometra, in which only the uterus is distended with blood, may be seen at menarche if there is a congenital stenosis of the vagina or the cervix. In older women it may result from cervical malignancy or postradiation cervical stenosis. As an acute problem it may be seen with an ectopic pregnancy or after uterine surgery.

PYOMETRA (REPRODUCTIVE OR POSTMENARCHE AGE GROUPS). Pyometra—distention of the uterus with pus—usually occurs secondary to a cervical obstruction of drainage of the normal uterine secretions, with subsequent superinfection. The patient is febrile and very sick. Low-level echoes are seen within the fluid in the endometrial canal.

FIBROIDS. Occasional fibroids appear cystic and are echopenic with acoustic through transmission.

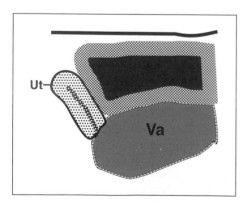

FIGURE 8-4. In hematocolpos the vagina is filled with blood because the hymen is imperforate. The uterus may or may not also be filled with blood. In this instance it is empty.

Extraovarian Multiple Cystic Masses

ENDOMETRIOSIS. A disease state that occurs during the reproductive years, endometriosis is caused by implantation of endometrial tissue in abnormal locations in the pelvis. This ectopic endometrial tissue responds to cyclic ovarian hormones and bleeds as if it were located within the uterus. Endometrial cysts (endometrioma) may develop in these areas of bleeding. Small cysts are termed blebs, whereas larger ones, because of their contents (blood) and color, are called chocolate cysts. This type of cyst may occur singly, but more than one are generally seen. Because these cysts contain blood, internal echoes may be present in the form of either many moderate-level echoes or a dense echogenic "blob" (see Fig. 7-20, Chapter 7).

TUBO-OVARIAN ABSCESSES. Tubo-ovarian abscesses are irregularly shaped, thick-walled, fluid-filled structures in the adnexa that may develop a few internal echoes and even an internal fluid-fluid level (see Fig. 9-2). Tubo-ovarian abscesses are usually bilateral. These abscesses are usually not an isolated finding; multiple abscesses are often noted elsewhere. They are very tender.

PYOSALPINX. Pyosalpinx are pus-filled fallopian tubes. Pyosalpinx have a tubular configuration that may be recognizable only when an endovaginal transducer is used. Internal echoes are generally present when the tube is pus filled (see Fig. 9-3). The tube walls are thickened and irregular. They are exquisitely tender when examined with the vaginal probe.

Intraovarian Cystic Masses: Complex

Complex masses in the ovary contain sonolucent and echogenic areas. The walls are generally smooth; the shape is usually spherical.

MUCINOUS CYSTADENOMA AND CYSTADENOCARCINOMA OF THE OVARY. These masses seen in the reproductive or postmenopausal age group are less common than the serous type of mass. They often have a characteristic sonographic appearance (see Fig. 8-3). A spherical cystic mass is present with many septa; there is some solid material (papillary fronds) arising from the septa. When benign, the margins are usually well defined. Malignancy is suggested by large amounts of solid tissue and ill-defined borders. Both benign and malignant mucinous tumors may be associated with free peritoneal fluid, but the presence of ascites favors malignancy. Color flow Doppler has been of some help in deciding whether a mass is malignant or benign. Malignant masses typically have a low impedance pattern with a resistive index of less than 4. Benign masses have a high-resistance Doppler flow pattern. Neither pattern is specific. Color flow is helpful in showing where to sample the small vessels that lie within the ovary. A tortuous course to the small vessels within the ovary suggests malignancy.

SEROUS CYSTADENOMA AND CYSTADENOCARCINOMA. These tumors (see Figs. 8-2 and 8-3) are similar to the mucinous form except that septa are thinner and papillary material is less common. Features that suggest malignancy are poorly defined walls, considerable amounts of solid tissue, and ascites. (see Mucinous Cystadenocarcinoma for details of Doppler use.)

CYSTIC TERATOMAS (DERMOIDS). Typically, although not exclusively, they occur in females aged between 10 and 30. Characteristically, dermoids are said to lie in a position anterior to the uterus or adjacent to the fundus. Cystic teratomas have a wide variety of sonographic appearances:

1. *Mainly cystic.* These often contain an echogenic area with acoustic shadowing due to calcium. Teeth may be seen on a radiograph.
2. *Complex internal structure.* There are echogenic areas from fat, hair, or bone, often with areas of shadowing.

3. *"Iceberg" appearance.* Dense echogenic material within a mass shadows the main bulk of the lesion, rendering much of the mass invisible. The use of the vaginal probe makes incomplete visualization of the mass much less common.

4. *Echogenic mass.* The echogenic mass may blend in with neighboring bowel, but the lesion's presence will be revealed by an indentation of the bladder or will be seen on endovaginal ultrasound (Fig. 8-5). The mass is ovoid and highly echogenic, with a well-defined border.

5. *Fluid-fluid level.* Dermoids may contain a fluid-fluid level (see Fig. 8-5). The echogenic material within the dermoid may lie either posteriorly or anteriorly. This latter finding is suggestive of a dermoid. Sometimes, there is a hairball floating on top of the posterior echogenic material; this appears as a mobile echogenic mass casting an acoustic shadow.

6. *Mucinous cystadenoma type.* Multiple thick septa are present within a round cyst. There may be echogenic masses attached to the septa.

OVARIAN CANCER. Ovarian cancer is one of the leading causes of death in women. An absolute diagnosis of malignancy cannot be made sonographically. However, several ultrasound features are strongly suggestive:

1. Poor definition of the lesion's borders due to tumor spread to adjacent organs
2. Multiple unconfined cystic areas containing irregularly shaped solid material
3. "Malignant" ascites—loculated fluid between fixed loops of bowel with peritoneal metastases (Fig. 8-6)
4. Solid ovarian masses (discussed later)
5. Bilateral nature
6. Low-resistance Doppler flow pattern from vessels within the mass. On color flow these vessels have a tortuous course.

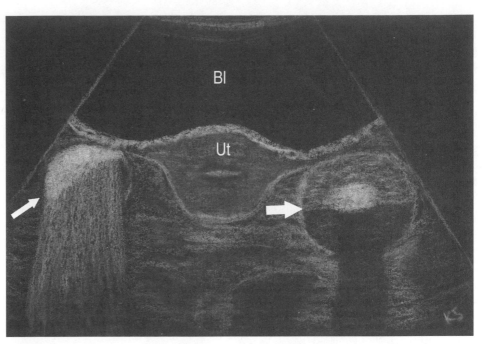

FIGURE 8-5. Dermoids or benign cystic teratomas have a number of sonographic patterns. In one of the most characteristic, echogenic material with acoustic shadowing occurs within a cystic lesion in association with a fluid-fluid level (on the left) [arrow]). In another characteristic appearance, a mass containing high-level echoes develops (on the right [smaller arrow]).

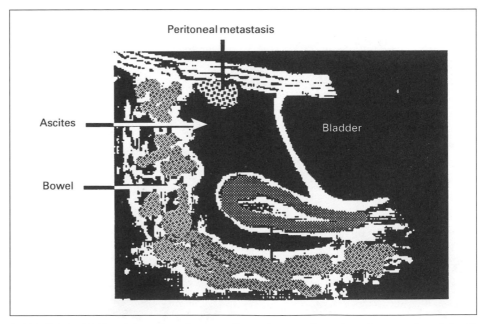

FIGURE 8-6. Malignant ascites. Loops of bowel are tethered to the anterior abdominal wall. Peritoneal metastatic lesions arise from the abdominal wall.

ENDOMETRIOMA. Endometrioma are frequently located within the ovary. A typical endometrioma is an apparently cystic mass which contains internal echoes. On high gain, the entire mass will be filled with relatively high-level echoes with an echogenic border. The appearances are typical for blood. The typical echogenicity is less than that seen with a dermoid but somewhat similar.

CORPUS LUTEUM HEMORRHAGE. A corpus luteum with hemorrhage looks somewhat similar to endometrioma. It also contains low-level echoes without quite the same evenness of texture. If the corpus luteum is examined shortly after ovulation, a ring of color Doppler will be seen, the so-called "ring of fire" which disappears after the corpus luteum hemorrhage has been there for awhile. The corpus luteum hemorrhage will be spontaneously resorbed after some weeks, so distinction between a corpus luteum with hemorrhage and endometrioma is made by performing a follow-up examination in approximately 6 weeks' time.

Complex Masses in the Uterus

PYOMETRA. A uterine cavity that contains echopenic fluid surrounded by myometrium may be caused by pyometra. Especially when significant debris or gas-forming organisms are present, echogenic areas with shadowing may occur.

FIBROIDS. Occasional fibroids that have degenerated have a complex appearance, with cystic areas in a predominantly solid mass.

Solid Masses

Solid masses contain only low-level echoes, show little or no through transmission, and have irregular or smooth walls.

Ovarian Masses

If a solid mass of the ovary is recognized sonographically, most often a specific diagnosis cannot be made. Nevertheless, the features of malignancy, as described previously, should be sought. Any solid ovarian mass in a postmenopausal woman carries a high probability of malignancy. In menstruating women an endometrioma should be considered.

FIBROMA. Fibromas are solid ovarian masses that affect menopausal and postmenopausal women. They tend to be large and have a similar sonographic appearance to fibroids. Basically echopenic, calcification can occur. Meigs' syndrome, in which there is associated ascites and pleural effusion, may be seen.

Uterine Masses

FIBROIDS (LEIOMYOMAS). Fibroids represent an overgrowth of uterine smooth muscle that forms a tumor. Leiomyoma is the benign form, and leiomyosarcoma the very rare malignant form. Fibroids are the most common tumors in women. They may grow progressively during the menstrual years but usually shrink after menopause. Common symptoms are heavy, prolonged periods; infertility; and pelvic pain. They may be intracavitary, submucosal, intramural, subserosal, or pedunculated. Sonographically, the features are as follows (Fig. 8-7):

1. An enlarged uterus, usually with a lobulated contour that may indent the bladder.

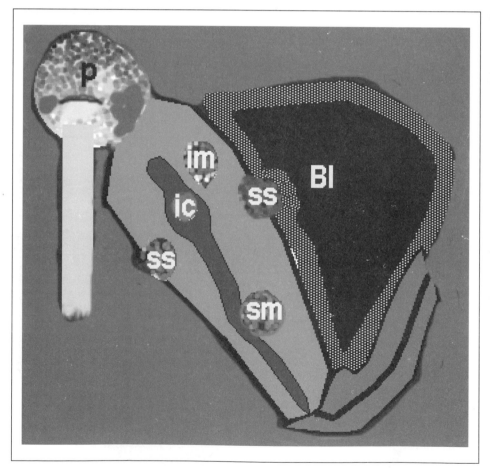

FIGURE 8-7. Fibroids may be located in several different sites. Subserosal (SS) fibroids lie on the edge of the uterus and may indent the bladder. They are usually asymptomatic. Intramural (IM) fibroids lie in the center of the myometrium (the muscular component of the uterus). If they do not secondarily distort the cavity, they are also usually asymptomatic. Submucosal (SM) fibroids lie on the edge of the endometrium. They often cause menstrual cramping and excessive menstrual bleeding. Intracavitary (IC) fibroids almost always cause cramping and bleeding. Pedunculated (P) fibroids are usually asymptomatic, but may twist on their stalk. They then become painful. This fibroid is calcified with shadowing, a common variety of fibroid degeneration.

2. Focal ovoid or circular masses within the uterus. These masses may have a similar echogenicity to the remainder of the uterus but tissue within is organized in a circular fashion.
3. The fibroid may be surrounded with a rim of calcification that can occasionally be so dense that the center cannot be seen with ultrasound.
4. The relationship of the fibroid to the endometrial cavity should be defined (see Fig. 8-7). Submucosal fibroids, that border on the endometrial cavity, often cause frequent lengthy periods with intramenstrual spotting and may cause infertility. Fibroids that lie within the cavity (intracavitary) are even more likely to cause such symptoms.
5. Fibroids that have a small neck and extend off the border of the uterus are termed *pedunculated*. They may be hard to distinguish from adnexal masses and may twist and infarct (torsion). This is very painful. It should be possible to track the myometrial arteries into the pedunculated fibroid with color flow.
6. If a fibroid is acutely tender, "red degeneration" may have occurred. The center of the fibroid looks somewhat cystic since a central bleed will have occurred.
7. Patients with fibroids may need serial ultrasound scans at intervals to rule out rapid growth; an abrupt change in size suggests malignancy. Malignant change is exceedingly rare.

CERVICAL CANCER. The most common genital tract malignancy in women is cervical cancer. The peak age for occurrence is in the fourth decade. Often the lesion is too small to be seen with ultrasound even if a Pap smear is suggestive or it can be seen with a speculum examination. Sonographically, the following may be seen:

1. Bulky cervix with an irregular outline, possibly extending into the vagina or peritoneum (Fig. 8-8).
2. A mass extending from the cervix to the pelvic sidewalls.
3. Obstruction of the ureters, producing hydronephrosis.
4. Invasion of the bladder, producing an irregular mass effect in the bladder wall.

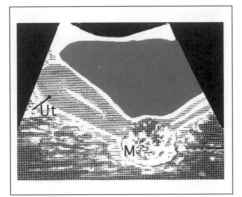

FIGURE 8-8. Cervical cancer causes a mass in the region of the cervix.

5. Para-aortic node formation and metastatic lesions in the liver.

✸PITFALLS

Endovaginal

1. *Gut vs. ovary.* When no follicles are seen in postmenopausal women, an indolent loop of feces containing bowel may be confused with an ovary. Watch for a considerable time for peristalsis. Look to see whether the supposed ovary lies close to the round ligament which can be seen leading from the lateral aspect of the fundus of the uterus, as an ovary should. Consider performing a water enema (see Fig. 7-13).
2. *Fibroid vs. ovarian mass.* If a mass lies adjacent to the ovary it can be very hard to distinguish between a fibroid and a solid intraovarian mass such as a fibroma. Push the vaginal probe between the mass and the uterus to see whether the two can be separated. A gap between the two structures needs to be seen at all sites for a mass to be definitely considered ovarian rather than a pedunculated fibroid. Use color flow to see whether there are vessels coming from the uterus to the mass.

3. *Endometrioma vs. corpus luteum.* A basically intraovarian mass with clumps of echogenic material within may represent a corpus luteum with hemorrhage, an endometrioma, or, much less likely, an ovarian neoplasm. Pulsed Doppler is not helpful since corpus luteum, neoplasm, and occasionally endometrioma may all show a low-resistance pattern. A repeat examination in the next proliferative phase of the cycle in about 6 weeks can help to distinguish between the lesions. A corpus luteum will alter configuration, whereas an endometrioma and a neoplasm will usually stay unchanged. At this point Doppler may be helpful since endometrioma are unlikely to have a low resistance pattern.
4. *Intracavitary masses in the secretory phase of the cycle.* The endometrial cavity echoes vary between .2- to .4-cm thick in the proliferative phase of the cycle and .8- to 1.3-cm thick in the secretory phase of the cycle. Small masses such as polyps or intracavitary fibroids can be concealed in the secretory phase. If possible, schedule patients with possible intracavitary masses for the proliferative phase of the cycle or repeat the study at that time.
5. *Pulsed Doppler sampling for signs of a neoplasm.* Pulsed Doppler sampling should be performed within or at the edge of a suspect ovarian mass. Sampling at other sites in the ovary can be misleading.
6. *Endovaginal scanning with a bladder containing some urine.* If the bladder is not completely empty, reverberation artifacts may obscure crucial structures and problem areas may be pushed too far away from the transducer.
7. *After hysterectomy.* The ovaries may be very hard to find since they may fall together in the center of the pelvis or be pulled laterally.

Transabdominal

1. *An empty bladder.* Lesions may be missed if the bladder is empty and an endovaginal sonogram is not possible. The bladder must always be adequately filled for transabdominal views. In filling the bladder, three techniques may be used: oral hydration, intravenous hydration, or catheterization of the patient.

2. An *overdistended bladder* will push adnexal structures, both normal and pathologic, to a high position where they are obscured by bowel. Free fluid may be missed owing to the compression of the posteriorly displaced organs.

3. *Excessive rapid oral hydration* may result in fluid in the small bowel that could be mistaken for a cystic lesion. Watch carefully for peristalsis.

4. *Foreign bodies in the vagina.* Tampons in the vagina cause an intravaginal mass. Usually there is acoustic shadowing since they generally contain air.

5. *Posthysterectomy changes.* A large vaginal cuff may mimic a recurrent mass.

6. The fundus of the *retroverted uterus* may be difficult to delineate if the beam lies at the same angle as the uterus. When acutely retroverted, the fundus may lie adjacent to the cervix and simulate a mass. Because a retroverted uterus is globular in shape, enlargement is hard to assess. A fibroid may be mistakenly diagnosed unless endovaginal views are obtained.

7. With *uterine anomalies* such as bicornuate and double uterus, the second horn may be mistaken for an adjacent mass. Careful longitudinal and oblique scanning should demonstrate an endometrial cavity in each (see Fig. 7-18). With a double uterus, two cervices and a vagina will be present.

8. By 1 week *postpartum* the uterus decreases in size to about one half its size at delivery. During the next 4 to 7 weeks the uterus gradually returns to normal size. If the history is unknown, the enlarged uterus may be misdiagnosed as fibroids or other uterine mass.

9. *Pelvic musculature* can be confusing. The iliopsoas and piriform muscles may be misinterpreted as pelvic masses. A solid knowledge of pelvic anatomy is essential.

10. *Bowel,* especially if distended with fluid, may mimic a cystic mass. Observation with real-time should show peristalsis in bowel. Alternatively, a water enema may confirm that this "cystic mass" represents fluid-filled colon (see Fig. 7-13).

11. *Fluid in the posterior cul-de-sac.* Ten to fifteen milliliters of fluid is normal in women in the reproductive years. A portion of this fluid is derived from follicular rupture.

12. Make sure the supposed pelvic mass is not a *pelvic kidney* (see Fig. 32-12). A pelvic kidney will have a central group of sinus echoes and a reniform shape.

13. An *ovarian cyst* located in the midline anterior to the uterus can be mistaken for the *bladder.* The cyst may compress the bladder, making the patient uncomfortable when the bladder is filled. The bladder will be seen as a small slit on the posterior-inferior aspect of such a cyst.

14. An *enlarged bladder* can be *confused with a cyst.* The patient voids incompletely and leaves a considerable amount of residual urine within the bladder. If you cannot see the bladder as well as a cyst, be cautious in diagnosing the presence of a cyst.

❓ WHERE ELSE TO LOOK

1. When performing a scan of a patient with a large pelvic mass of ovarian or uterine origin, the *kidneys* should also be examined to rule out *hydronephrosis* caused by pressure on the ureters.

2. If the patient is in the menopausal age group and the features of the pelvic mass suggest *malignancy*—large size, complex echoes, and ovarian origin—then a search for *metastatic lesions, nodes* and *ascites* should be carried out. The most common sites of metastatic lesions from pelvic masses are the peritoneum, para-aortic nodes, and liver.

3. If you suspect that a *pelvic kidney* is present, examine the normal sites where the kidney should lie, and make sure that two kidneys are not present in their usual location.

SELECTED READING

Atri, M., Nazarnia, S., Bret, P. M., Aldis, A. E., Kintzen, G., and Reinhold, C. Endovaginal sonographic appearance of benign ovarian masses. *Radiographics* 14:747–760, 1994.

Bourne, T. H. Transvaginal color Doppler in gynecology. *Ultrasound Obstet Gynecol* 1:359–373, 1991.

Caspi, B., Appelman, Z., Rabinerson, D., Elchalal, U., Zalel, Y., and Katz, Z. Pathognomonic echo patterns of benign cystic teratomas of the ovary: Classification, incidence and accuracy rate of sonographic diagnosis. *Ultrasound Obstet Gynecol* 7:275–279, 1996.

Cohen, L., and Sabbagha, R. Echo patterns of benign cystic teratomas by transvaginal ultrasound. *Ultrasound Obstet Gynecol* 3:120–123, 1993.

Fleischer, A. C., McKee, M. S., Gordon, A. N., Page, D. L., Kepple, D. M., Worrell, J. A., Jones III, H. W., Burnett, L. S., and James Jr., A. E. Transvaginal sonography of postmenopausal ovaries with pathologic correlation. *J Ultrasound Med* 9:637–644, 1990.

Fried, A. M., Kenney III, C. M., Stigers, K. B., Kacki, M. H., and Buckley, S. L. Benign pelvic masses: Sonographic spectrum. *Radiographics* 16:321–334, 1996.

Gross, B. H., and Callen, P. W. Ultrasound of the uterus. In P. W. Callen (Ed.). *Ultrasonography in Obstetrics and Gynecology.* Philadelphia: Saunders, 1991.

Huang, R. T., Chou, C. Y., Chang, C. H., Yu, C. H., Huang, S. C., and Yao, B. L. Differentiation between adenomyoma and leiomyoma with transvaginal ultrasonography. *Ultrasound Obstet Gynecol* 5:47–50, 1995.

Innocenti, P., Pulli, F., Savino, L., Nicolucci, A., Pandimiglio, A., Menchi, I., and Massi, G. Staging of cervical cancer: Reliability of transrectal US. *Radiology* 185:201–205, 1992.

Kurjak, A., Shalan, H., Matijevic, R., Predanic, M., and Kupesic-Urek, S. Stage I ovarian cancer by transvaginal color Doppler sonography: A report of 18 cases. *Ultrasound Obstet Gynecol* 3:195–198, 1993.

Laing, F. C. US analysis of adnexal masses: The art of making the correct diagnosis. *Radiology* 191:21–22, 1994.

Pellerito, J. S., Troiano, R. N., Quedens-Case, C., and Taylor, K. J. W. Common pitfalls of endovaginal color Doppler flow imaging. *Radiographics* 15:37–47, 1995.

Reinhold, C., McCarthy, S., Bret, P. M., Mehio, A., Atri, M., Zakarian, R., Glaude, Y., Liang, L., and Seymour, R. J. Diffuse adenomyosis: Comparison of endovaginal US and MR imaging with histopathologic correlation. *Radiology* 199:151–158, 1996.

Reuter, K. L., D'Orsi, C. J., Raptopoulous, V., and Evers, K. Imaging of questionable and unusual pelvic masses. *Br J Radiol* 59: 765–771, 1986.

Schincaglia, P., Brondelli, L., Cicognani, A., Buzzi, G., Orsini, L. F., Bovicelli, L., Jasonni, V. M., and Bucchi, L. A feasibility study of ovarian cancer screening: Does fine-needle aspiration improve ultrasound specificity? *Tumori* 80:181–187, 1994.

Van Nagell Jr., J. R. Editorial: Methods to improve the diagnostic accuracy of ultrasound in the detection of ovarian cancer. *Gynecol Oncol* 54:115–116, 1994.

Wu, A., and Siegel, M. J. Sonography of pelvic masses in children: Diagnostic predictability. *AJR* 148:1199–1202, 1987.

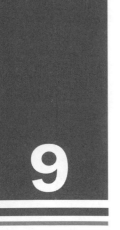

PELVIC PAIN

Without Positive Pregnancy Test

ROGER C. SANDERS

SONOGRAM ABBREVIATIONS

Ab   Abscess

Bl   Bladder

Ut   Uterus

KEY WORDS

Abscess. Localized collection of pus.

Adnexa. The regions of the ovaries, fallopian tubes, and broad ligaments.

Anteverted. The body of the uterus is tilted forward.

Corpus Luteum. Small structure that develops within the ovary in the second half of the menstrual cycle and secretes progesterone.

Crohn's Disease. Bowel inflammation which can affect any level of the bowel from stomach to anus. Fistula is a common complication.

Cul-de-sac. An area posterior to the uterus and anterior to the rectum where fluid often collects.

Dysmenorrhea. Difficult or painful menstruation.

Dyspareunia. Difficult or painful intercourse.

Endometrial Cavity, Canal. A potential space in the center of the uterus where blood or pus may collect.

Endometritis. Infection of the endometrial cavity.

Endometrium. Membrane lining of the uterus.

Follicle (Graafian Follicle). An intraovarian saclike structure in which the ovum matures prior to rupture at ovulation. The follicle is visualized as an ovoid cavity with fluid.

Hematocrit. The percentage of red blood cells in a given volume of blood.

Hydrosalpinx. Accumulation of watery fluid in the fallopian tube. The tube can be blocked at the peritoneal end by adhesions and fibrosis due to a prior infection.

Laparoscopy. Surgically invasive technique for viewing the pelvic anatomy in situ through a small tube using fiber-optics. The tube is inserted into the peritoneum through a small incision near the umbilicus.

Leukocyte Count. The number of circulating white blood cells. This count increases when an inflammatory process is present, as in PID (*pelvic inflammatory disease*), but remains normal in ectopic pregnancy and endometriosis.

Myometrium. Smooth muscle of the uterus.

Pelvic Inflammatory Disease (PID). Infection that spreads from the uterine tubes and ovaries throughout the pelvis; commonly due to gonorrhea.

Peritonitis. Inflammation of the peritoneum, which is the serous membrane lining the abdominal cavity.

Purulent. Containing pus.

Pyosalpinx. Accumulation of pus in the fallopian tube.

Retroverted Uterus. The long axis of the uterus points posteriorly toward the sacrum.

Salpinx. Fallopian tube.

Tubo-ovarian Abscess (TOA). An abscess involving the ovary and the fallopian tube.

Vulva. Region where the urethra and the vagina exit in the perineum.

◆》》 THE CLINICAL PROBLEM

One of the most common indications for a pelvic sonogram is pelvic pain. The differential diagnosis is narrowed by the duration of the pain. If the pain is acute and severe, obstetric disorders should be considered if the patient is of child-bearing age. In most parts of the world, rapid, reliable pregnancy tests are available and this possibility can usually soon be discarded. If the patient is pregnant, turn to Chapter 13. In the nonpregnant patient with acute pain of recent onset, pelvic inflammatory disease (PID), and ruptured or twisted ovarian cyst or ovary are the most likely diagnoses. If the pain is chronic and no mass can be felt the differential diagnosis is adhesions, endometriosis, hydrosalpinx, and peritoneal inclusion cyst.

Acute Pain

Pelvic Inflammatory Disease (PID)

Patients with PID are usually febrile and often have a purulent vaginal discharge. On clinical examination an adnexal mass may be felt, and the patient may have pain associated with movement of the cervix. Often physical examination is so painful that a thorough search cannot be completed. In these cases, a pelvic sonogram is needed as a supplemental examination, and at times it may replace the physical examination completely.

Acute or chronic PID is most commonly caused by gonorrhea or chlamydia. Pyogenic (*Escherichia coli*) and tuberculous infections are the other, more unusual causes. There is an association with the use of intrauterine contraceptive devices. PID due to gonorrhea and chlamydia spreads along the mucous membranes and travels from the vulva to the adnexa. However, the main site of localization is the fallopian tube. If left untreated, the course of tubal infection progresses as follows:

1. Endometritis (Fig. 9-1)
2. Acute salpingitis with cul-de-sac pus (see Fig. 9-1)
3. Chronic salpingitis
4. Pyosalpinx: A blockage of the peritoneal (fimbriated) end of the tube with an accumulation of pus (see Fig. 9-3)
5. Tubo-ovarian abscesses (TOA): Pus surrounded by tubal and ovarian tissue (Fig. 9-2)

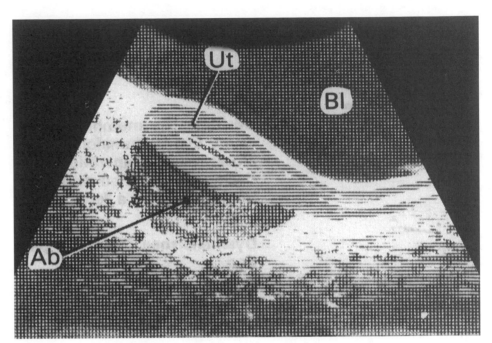

FIGURE 9-1. Pus in the cul-de-sac due to pelvic inflammatory disease. There is also a small amount of fluid in the endometrial cavity, a common finding with endometritis.

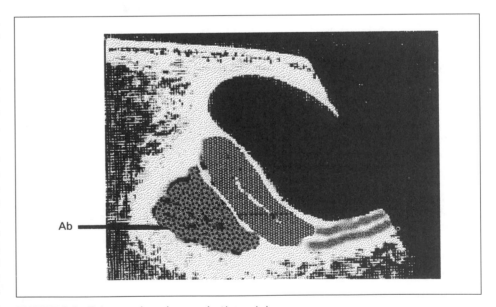

FIGURE 9-2. Tubo-ovarian abscess in the cul-de-sac.

6. Hydrosalpinx: The pus from a pyosalpinx resorbs and becomes sterile watery fluid (see Fig. 9-3)
7. Pelvic abscess: Abscesses outside of the tube in the region of the ovary or cul-de-sac (see Fig. 9-2)

The purulent contents of a TOA may escape the confines of the tube and ovary area and cause peritonitis or multiple pelvic abscesses.

The pelvic sonogram helps determine the extent of the disease, including the presence and size of adnexal masses. If large echo-free areas compatible with pus are present, surgical drainage rather than antibiotic therapy may be appropriate. If antibiotic therapy is given, the response to therapy can be followed by means of serial sonograms.

Cystic Masses

Rupture or bleeding of any pelvic mass causes acute pelvic pain similar to that seen in rupture of an ectopic pregnancy. Torsion (twisting of a cyst on a pedicle), hemorrhage, and rupture are the three complications that cause pain in cysts. Hemorrhage often results from torsion. In the absence of a pregnancy test, the sonographic findings of ovarian cyst rupture are confusingly similar to those of ectopic pregnancy, with free fluid present, and possibly an ill-defined mass in the adnexa. More specific changes are seen with hemorrhage (Fig. 9-4) and torsion, especially if there has been a previous sonogram showing a simple cyst.

Sonography helps (1) when clinical examination is not possible because of acute pain or obesity; (2) when accurate size estimation is necessary; (3) when it is unclear whether the mass is ovarian or uterine; and (4) in deciding whether a mass is cystic or solid.

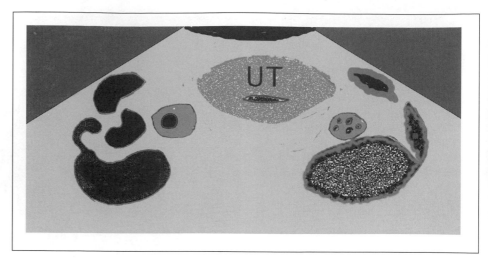

FIGURE 9-3. Transverse image. On the right the serpiginous fluid-filled structure with several smaller locules has the typical shape of a hydrosalpinx. It is larger posteriorly, smooth-walled, and rounded. The ovary is seen separately. On the left, the process is more acute and a pyosalpinx is present. Note that the walls are irregularly thickened and there are internal echoes within the fluid. This type of mass is exquisitely painful.

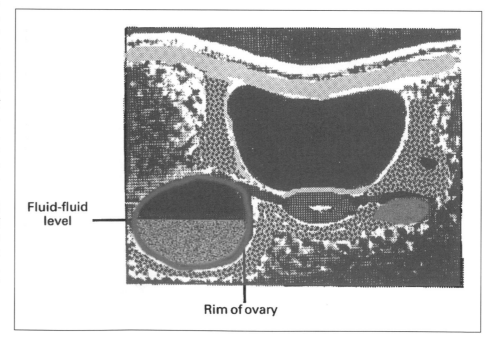

FIGURE 9-4. Hemorrhage into an ovarian cyst creates a fluid-fluid level, which changes position when the patient is shifted. Note the rim of ovary around the cyst.

Chronic Pain

Adhesions

The most common pelvic cause of chronic pain seen with ultrasound is adhesions. Most often this relates to underlying endometriosis, but other possible causes include previous surgery such as tubal ligation, cesarean section or appendectomy, and previous pelvic inflammatory disease. In some instances a nonpalpable endometrioma or hydrosalpinx will be found. Occasionally malignancy or radiation treatment for malignancy is the cause.

Chronic PID

Lingering chronic PID can cause chronic pain which is relieved by antibiotic treatment.

Masses

Many patients with masses have chronic pain and discomfort but since the mass can usually be palpated it becomes the principal indication for the sonogram.

Nonpelvic causes of pelvic pain such as gastrointestinal or genitourinary processes should be considered.

ANATOMY

See Chapter 7.

TECHNIQUE

See Chapters 7 and 8.

The endovaginal transducer is routinely used with patients with acute pelvic pain, either as a first approach or following an apparently normal transabdominal real-time study.

PATHOLOGY

Acute Pain

Acute Pelvic Inflammatory Disease

The sonogram is difficult to perform because the uterus and adnexa are so tender when the vaginal probe is inserted. The tenderness is maximal over the uterus and tubal region.

1. *Uterus.* On some occasions there is a thick-walled endometrial canal with fluid in the cavity (endometritis).

2. *Cul-de-sac.* Fluid often develops in the cul-de-sac (see Fig. 9-1). Such fluid almost always contains echoes and perhaps a fluid-fluid level when examined with the vaginal probe.

3. *Adnexa.* Bilateral cystic or complex masses located lateral, posterior, or superior to the uterus may be seen. These represent pyosalpinx or a closely related entity, tubo-ovarian abscess (TOA) (see Figs. 9-2 and 9-3). On endovaginal examination, the typical appearance of a pyosalpinx is a smooth-walled curving tubular structure with a club shape (see Fig. 9-3). The walls of the dilated tubes may be thickened and irregular if the acute infection has been present for awhile. The tubal contents may contain internal echoes. Unilateral pyosalpinx is uncommon since most relate to venereal diseases such as gonorrhea or chlamydia. Local inflammatory disease such as Crohn's disease or diverticulosis may cause a unilateral pyosalpinx. Although the ovaries may be surrounded by infected material they are practically never directly involved by PID.

Hemorrhagic Cysts

Hemorrhagic cysts are blood-filled cysts containing echoes that may form a fluid-fluid level (see Fig. 9-4) or a clumplike pattern due to clot. Severe pain develops when the bleeding into the cyst takes place. Bleeding into a cyst sometimes occurs at the time of ovulation with the formation of the corpus luteum. In some unlucky women, large hemorrhagic cysts, in association with ovulation, occur repeatedly. In other women, bleeding into a cyst occurs when a preexisting cyst, either a follicular cyst or a cystadenoma, twists and torts. In both situations, a cystic mass is seen in the ovary that contains either (1) a fluid-fluid level; (2) a crescent-shaped mass of low-level echogenicity; (3) clumps of echogenic material; (4) diffuse, even, echogenic material; or (5) diffuse low-level echoes.

Torted Ovary or Cyst

If the ovary twists on its mesenteric attachment, much pain develops. Usually some blood will be seen in the region of the ovary and the ovary will be very tender and enlarged on endovaginal examination. Color flow analysis of the blood supply to the ovary in torsion has been confusing since there is double arterial supply. If no flow can be demonstrated while flow to the other ovary can be seen, torsion is probable. However, evidence of normal flow does not rule out torsion since blood supply from the ovarian artery can continue while the uterine artery supply is occluded, or vice versa.

Cysts in the ovary may be associated with torsion. The cyst is very tender with the endovaginal probe and often contains a fluid-fluid level. A thick rim may surround the ovary.

Ruptured Cyst

Common features of a ruptured cyst include the following:

1. An adnexal mass with an irregular shape.
2. Cul-de-sac fluid.
3. Evidence of bleeding with development of a relatively echogenic mass of blood (hard to separate from the uterus), as in ruptured ectopic pregnancy (see Chapter 13).

Chronic Pain

Adhesions

Adhesions (1) occur as a consequence of previous infection or surgery (such as tubal ligation); (2) may be seen with endometriosis; and (3) occur very occasionally with malignancy. Adhesions represent the most common cause of chronic, nagging pelvic pain. Although the adhesions cannot be seen with ultrasound, there are several indirect signs:

1. Uterine deviation to left or right or extreme retroversion
2. An ovary positioned in a high or low lateral position
3. An ovary located adjacent to the uterus which cannot be moved with the vaginal probe and is locally tender. This is a very reliable sign.

4. An ovary which feels stiff when pushed with the transducer and which remains adjacent to a loop of bowel. Normally, the ovary can be pushed away from surrounding bowel with the transducer.

Chronic Pelvic Inflammatory Disease

In some instances pelvic inflammatory disease becomes chronic and longstanding. Typically, the patient has a chronic pelvic ache. The ovaries and uterus generally appear normal. Using the endovaginal probe, local tenderness is maximal over the tubes rather than the uterus or ovaries.

Endometriosis

It is not unusual for an endometrioma to be seen with ultrasound that cannot be felt (see Chapter 7 for detailed description).

PITFALLS

1. *Cul-de-sac fluid.* A small amount of normal fluid may appear in the region of the cul-de-sac during a normal menstrual period.
2. *Bowel.* Bowel may masquerade as an abnormal adnexal mass. This is such a common finding that any questionable complex mass must be proved to be truly pathologic. Real-time or a water enema allows the distinction to be made (see Fig. 7-13).
3. *Adhesion assessment.* If the uterus lies between the probe and the ovary one may not be able to determine whether or not the ovary moves or is locally tender.

? WHERE ELSE TO LOOK

1. *Appendicitis.* Some retrocecal cases of appendicitis lie low in the pelvis and can mimic an adnexal cause of acute pain. Sonographic appearances are described in Chapter 30. Some cases of appendicitis are best seen with the vaginal probe.
2. *Renal colic.* Pain referred into the adnexa can originate from a ureteric stone (see Chapters 24 and 33). The endovaginal probe is a good way of seeing renal calculi impacted at the ureterovesical junction (UVJ). Calculi have been seen with the endovaginal probe that are not visible from the standard abdominal approach.
3. *Gut lesions.* Gut problems located in the true pelvis can present with adnexal pain. Crohn's disease is particularly likely to involve the adnexa and can create fistulous connections to the fallopian tube. The typical appearances are described in Chapter 30.

SELECTED READING

Fedele, L., Bianchi, S., Dorta, M., and Vignali, M. Intrauterine adhesions: Detection with transvaginal US. *Radiology* 199:757–759, 1996.

10 VAGINAL BLEEDING WITH NEGATIVE PREGNANCY TEST

ROGER C. SANDERS

SONOGRAM ABBREVIATIONS

Ut Uterus

KEY WORDS

Adenomyosis. Endometrial tissue extends into the myometrium. Blood cysts develop with menstruation in the myometrium.

Bleeding Dyscrasia. Abnormality of the factors that control clotting and platelet function.

Dysmenorrhea. Painful periods with excessive bleeding.

Endometrial Cavity, Canal. A potential space in the center of the uterus where blood or pus may collect.

Endometritis. Infection of the endometrial cavity.

Endometrium. Membrane lining of the uterus.

French. A measure of catheter size.

Hematometrocolpos. Metra = uterus, culpa = vagina. Condition presenting at birth or at puberty due to an imperforate hymen. Blood or other fluid accumulates in the vagina and uterus.

Hysterosonogram. Procedure in which a catheter is placed in the cervical cavity and saline is infused into the endometrial cavity. Used to show intracavitary pathology.

Menorrhagia. Heavy bleeding with period.

Metromenorrhagia. Excessive bleeding occurring with or between periods.

Proliferative. Preovulatory phase of the menstrual cycle, at which time the endometrial cavity echoes form a single thin line.

Secretory. Postovulatory phase of the menstrual cycle, at which time the endometrial cavity echoes are thick.

Submucosal. Term used to describe a process, such as a fibroid, that is located adjacent to the endometrial cavity within the uterus.

Tamoxifen. Antiestrogenic drug used in patients with breast cancer to prevent a recurrence. It carries a risk of endometrial neoplasm and produces a reaction in the endometrium.

◆ ⟫ THE CLINICAL PROBLEM

Vaginal bleeding between periods or at any time in the premenstrual or postmenstrual nonpregnant patient is abnormal and is an indication for a sonogram. In the premenstrual patient, vaginal bleeding may be a sign of precocious puberty. Other clinical features which occur in the child with precocious puberty include large breasts (gynecomastia), excessive growth, and the development of an adult pubic hair distribution.

There are many possible reasons for intramenstrual bleeding. Conditions that may cause abnormal bleeding but do not distort the normal pelvic anatomy (e.g., bleeding dyscrasias) cannot be detected by sonography. Sonographically visible findings include the following:

1. *Retained products of conception.* If the patient has been pregnant in the recent past, a retained fragment of placenta may cause persistent bleeding. This is particularly likely after a termination.

2. *Fibroids that border on the endometrial cavity.* As mentioned in Chapter 8, fibroids can occur in a number of locations. Those that border on the cavity (submucosal) and those that lie within the cavity (intracavitary) are particularly likely to cause intramenstrual bleeding.

3. *Intracavitary masses.* Some intracavitary lesions such as polyps are usually well defined with ultrasound, whereas others, such as cancer of the endometrium (see Fig. 10-2) or endometrial hyperplasia, may merely cause an increased thickness to the endometrial cavity borders. These entities may also cause excessively heavy periods.

4. *Adnexal masses.* Occasionally, an ovarian mass, such as a hormone-secreting ovarian neoplasm or dermoid, may cause vaginal spotting.

Changes With Menstruation

The lining of the endometrial cavity is partially shed each month at menstruation, with consequent changes in cavity appearance during the course of the cycle. During the preovulatory (proliferative) phase, the endometrial cavity echo is only about 3-mm thick and surrounded by an echopenic halo. Shortly before ovulation, two additional linear echoes outline the echopenic area (the "three-line sign"). The echopenic area becomes more echogenic so that in the postovulatory (secretory or luteal) phase, the cavity echo becomes brighter and thicker (see Fig. 7-7). At this point, the width of the canal is approximately 9 mm.

Ascertain the following prior to starting a study for vaginal bleeding:

1. What was the first day of the last period?
2. Are menstrual cycles regular and how long do they last?
3. How long ago did the patient stop menstruating if menopausal?
4. If the patient is postmenopausal, is she on hormone replacement therapy? Hormone replacement therapy with estrogen or a combination of estrogen and progesterone thickens the endometrium. Unopposed estrogen (estrogen only) is particularly likely to thicken the endometrium. A postmenopausal endometrial cavity thickness of greater than 8 mm is a signal for further investigation such as endometrial sampling.
5. Is tamoxifen being administered? Tamoxifen, a commonly administered antiestrogenic chemotherapeutic drug, is given to women who have had breast cancer. Although it reduces breast cancer recurrence, there is a slight increase in the number of endometrial neoplasms. After 6 months to a year, 60% of women develop secondary changes in the endometrium.

ANATOMY

See Chapters 7, 8, and 9.

TECHNIQUE

Transvaginal

The endometrium can only be satisfactorily assessed with the vaginal probe. Detail is never satisfactory with the transabdominal approach.

Hysterosonogram

This technique is used for the further investigation of the cause of abnormal vaginal bleeding (Fig. 10-1). Informed consent is usually obtained since the procedure involves placing a catheter within the endometrial cavity, although the risks of infection and bleeding are minimal. In patients with a history of pelvic inflammatory disease, antibiotic prophylaxis with an antibiotic such as doxycycline is given. Pain and cramping occur if a balloon catheter is inserted, so if that is planned, an analgesic such as ibuprofen is given prior to the procedure. The procedure is performed as follows:

1. A speculum is inserted. A plastic translucent speculum with a built-in light is useful, since visualization of the cervix is important.

2. The cervix is cleansed with iodine.
3. A small catheter such as a 5 Fr Soules catheter is inserted into the cervix, using sponge forceps. If this catheter cannot be inserted or will not stay in place, a 7 Fr balloon catheter is inserted. The balloon is inflated with a fluid such as normal saline to prevent air within the balloon from causing a shadow that would make visualization of uterine pathology impossible. If the balloon is difficult to insert, a technique whereby the balloon is inflated, deflated, withdrawn, pushed in again, and then reinflated may be helpful in getting the catheter in place.

PATHOLOGY

Endometrial Cancer

Endometrial cancer, a tumor of the uterine endometrial lining, is most common after menopause and is associated with abnormal bleeding (Fig. 10-2). Typically, there is an echogenic mass in the endometrium. The management is changed and prognosis is worse if the echopenic area around the endometrium is penetrated by the tumor. Fluid in the endometrial cavity may occasionally be an indication of an underlying endometrial neoplasm.

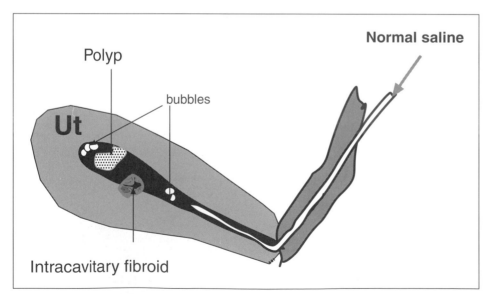

FIGURE 10-1. Hysterosonogram. A catheter is inserted into the endometrial cavity through which normal saline is infused. The catheter tip lies in the middle of the endometrial cavity and can be moved back or pushed forward under direct ultrasonic visualization. Normal saline causes bubbles which accumulate at the fundus if the uterus is anteverted and dissipate spontaneously if the uterus is retroverted. Polyps are typically on a stalk, mobile and echogenic with irregular borders. Fibroids indent into the myometrium and are usually evenly echopenic with a well-defined border.

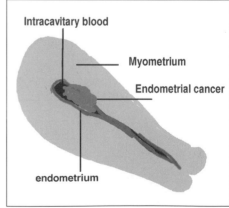

FIGURE 10-2. Endometrial cancer. A mass is seen arising from the endometrium which expands into the myometrium. Often, as in this case, there is secondary intracavitary blood due to the obstruction caused by the endometrial cancer.

Benign Endometrial Hyperplasia

The endometrium becomes irregularly thickened (over 8-mm thick) and echogenic. Small cysts lie within the echogenic area in the cavity border. This entity is usually seen after menopause.

Endometrial Polyp

Polyps within the endometrial cavity are common. Typically, they are round and echogenic. If the examination is performed in the secretory phase of the menstrual cycle, polyps may be concealed within the normal echogenic thickening that occurs at this phase of the cycle. Many are asymptomatic but some present with heavy periods or intramenstrual bleeding. If there is uncertainty regarding whether a polyp is present, a hysterosonogram is helpful. When outlined by fluid with a hysterosonogram, polyps are markedly echogenic, have an irregular border, and can be seen to move if they are on a stalk, as they often are (see Fig. 10-1).

Fibroids

Fibroids that abut on the endometrial cavity (submucosal) or that lie within the endometrial cavity (intracavitary) are a frequent cause of heavy periods, intramenstrual spotting, or postmenopausal bleeding. When outlined by fluid, during the performance of a hysterosonogram, they have a smooth, mildly echogenic border and less echogenic internal contents. They are immobile and they can be seen to extend beyond the confines of the endometrial cavity as a rule (see Fig. 10-1).

Retained Products of Conception

This cause of endovaginal bleeding only occurs after a patient has been recently pregnant. Endovaginal probe views will show echogenic material within the endometrial cavity, possibly with an area of acoustic shadowing related to a bony fragment. As a rule, the retained product is a portion of the placenta and will have typical placental texture. Blood and retained products can look very similar. A hysterosonogram can help differentiate blood from retained products since retained products will adhere to the endometrium, whereas blood will float around. If the endometrial cavity appears empty, this is helpful to the referring clinician since it means that any retained products are trivial.

Tamoxifen

Tamoxifen changes are of two types:

1. Cystic and echogenic areas reminiscent of benign endometrial hyperplasia (Fig. 10-3). These changes are due to subendometrial adenomyosis; a hysterosonogram or hysteroscopy shows nothing since the surface of the endometrium is uninvolved.
2. Multiple polyps, which may be very large, lie in the endometrium. These may develop into cancerous masses (Figs. 10-3 and 10-4).

✴ PITFALLS

1. *Intracavitary masses in the secretory phase of the cycle.* The endometrial cavity echoes vary between .2 to .4 cm thick in the proliferative phase of the cycle and .8 to 1.3 cm thick in the secretory phase of the cycle. Small masses such as polyps or intracavitary fibroids are often concealed in the secretory phase. If possible, schedule patients with possible intracavitary masses for the proliferative phase of the cycle or repeat the study.

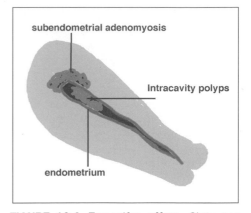

FIGURE 10-4. Tamoxifen effect. Sixty percent of women on long-term tamoxifen have secondary effects on the endometrial cavity. In subendometrial adenomyosis, the endometrial cavity appears to be widened by an echogenic process which is interspersed with cysts. If a hysterosonogram is performed, the endometrial cavity wall will be seen to be smooth and the entire process is beneath the endometrium. Intracavitary polyps are also commonly seen. Polyps associated with tamoxifen often contain small cysts. Sometimes secondary fluid builds up behind the polyp, outlining it. These are difficult to distinguish from endometrial cancer, which also occurs with greater frequency with tamoxifen. Endometrial cancers tend to burrow into the myometrium.

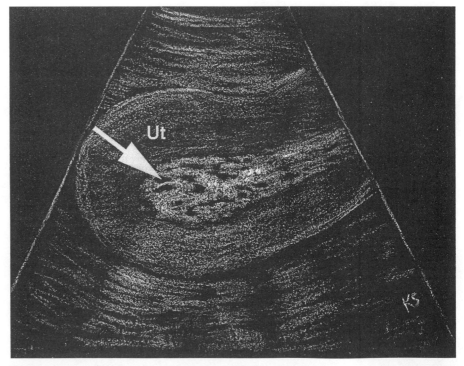

FIGURE 10-3. Typical appearances of tamoxifen effect on the endometrium are shown. The endometrium is markedly thickened and echogenic. Numerous small cysts are present within the area of thickening, which may represent either adenomyosis occurring deep to the endometrium, or cystic areas within polyps. A hysterosonogram is required to make this distinction.

2. *Blood clot vs. intracavitary mass.* In a patient with a history of intramenstrual bleeding or heavy periods an apparent intracavitary mass may represent a blood clot.
3. *Endovaginal scanning with a bladder containing some urine.* If the bladder is not completely empty, reverberation artifacts may obscure crucial structures and problem areas may be pushed far away from the transducer.
4. *Hysterosonogram in the secretory phase.* If a hysterosonogram is performed in the secretory phase, the endometrium is fragile. The catheter can push up the endometrium so it looks like a polyp. A polyp can be suspected when none is present since the borders of the cavity are often irregular in the secretory phase.
5. *Bubbles on hysterosonogram.* Air can accumulate at the fundus and conceal pathology if the uterus is anteverted.

SELECTED READING

Bourne, T. H., Lawton, F., Leather, A., Granberg, S., Campbell, S., and Collins, W. P. Use of intracavity saline instillation and transvaginal ultrasonography to detect tamoxifen-associated endometrial polyps. *Ultrasound Obstet Gynecol* 4:73–75, 1994.

Dubinsky, T. J., Parvey, H. R., Gromaz, G., Curtis, M., and Maklad, N. Transvaginal hysterosonography: Comparison with biopsy in the evaluation of postmenopausal bleeding. *J Ultrasound Med* 14:887–893, 1995.

Odom, L. D. Endometrial surveillance in tamoxifen-treated patients. *Contemp OB GYN* Mar:133–144, 1996.

Speroff, L. Tamoxifen: Special considerations for gynecologists. *Contemp OB GYN* 50–61, 1992.

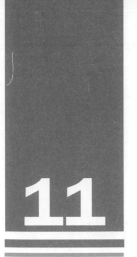

INTRAUTERINE CONTRACEPTIVE DEVICES

"Lost IUD"

PATRICIA MAY KAPLAN

SONOGRAM ABBREVIATIONS

IUD   Intrauterine device

KEY WORDS

Adnexa. Area of the broad ligament and ovaries.

Cul-de-sac. Area posterior to the uterus and anterior to the rectum, a common site for fluid collections.

Endometrial Cavity. Potential space in the center of the uterus where blood or pus may collect.

Myometrium. Uterine smooth muscle.

Os. *External*: The mouth of the uterus at the level of the cervix as it joins the vagina. *Internal*: Junction of the cervix and uterus proper.

Pelvic Inflammatory Disease (PID). Infection that spreads throughout the pelvis, often due to gonorrhea. If it is secondary to an IUD, other bacteria are usually found.

Retroverted. A uterus that points toward the sacrum.

 THE CLINICAL PROBLEM

Intrauterine contraceptive devices (IUDs, IUCDs) were, at one time, the second most popular means of birth control after oral contraceptives. Although many varieties of IUDs have been used, only the most commonly used devices will be discussed here.

Because pelvic inflammatory disease (PID) is a common side effect in women who use IUDs, only two IUDs are still being sold in the United States: the Progestasert and the Paragard. However, many other IUDs were inserted in the past and are still in place, and many others are used in other countries.

The proper location of an IUD, regardless of type, is in the endometrial cavity at the uterine fundus. The remainder of the device should be above the cervix. A nylon thread, which extends from the uterus into the vagina, is attached to the proximal end of all IUDs. This string should be palpable or visible on pelvic examination. If this string cannot be identified, the patient may be referred for evaluation of a "lost IUD."

Some patients have no complaint other than a lost string. Others, however, present with cramping, pain, or abnormal bleeding. In either case, the position of the IUD must be demonstrated. If the uterus is empty, the device has been expelled or has perforated the uterus. An IUD outside the uterus is usually not seen with ultrasound because it is surrounded by gut.

ANATOMY

Anatomy of the pelvic area is discussed in Chapter 7.

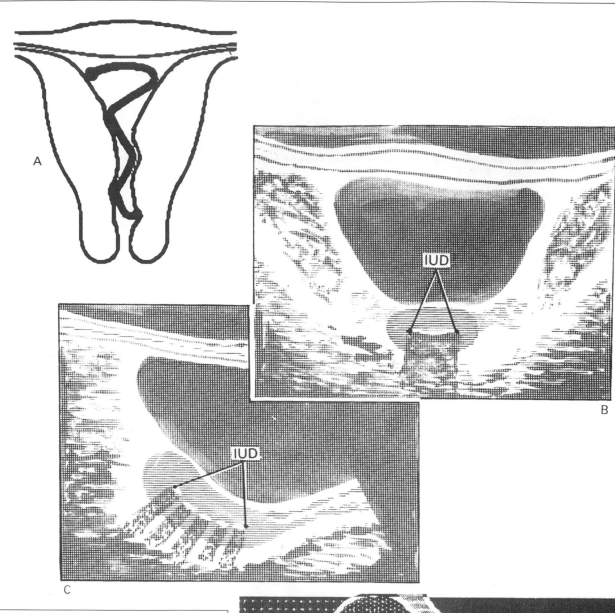

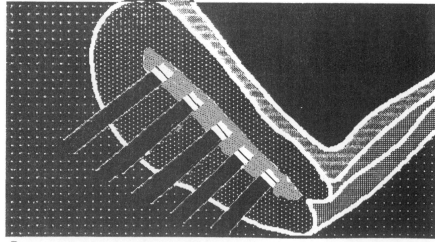

FIGURE 11-1. Lippes loop. (**A**) Lippes loop in the endometrial cavity. (**B**) Transverse view of one rung of the Lippes loop. (**C**) Longitudinal view of five rungs of the Lippes loop. (**D**) Diagram showing the Lippes loop within the uterus with entrance and exit echoes.

Types of Devices

Lippes Loop

The Lippes loop was the most widely used IUD and there are still some in use.

In a long-axis view, the loop has two to five echogenic components, depending on whether or not a true long-axis IUD view has been obtained (Fig. 11-1A and C). Transversely, the device is visualized as a single line (Fig. 11-1B).

Dalkon Shield

Insertion of the Dalkon shield was suspended some years ago because of a large number of associated infections. There are still a few women using the device. The Dalkon shield is the smallest of the IUDs. On both longitudinal and transverse scans, it appears as two echogenic foci (Fig. 11-2A and B).

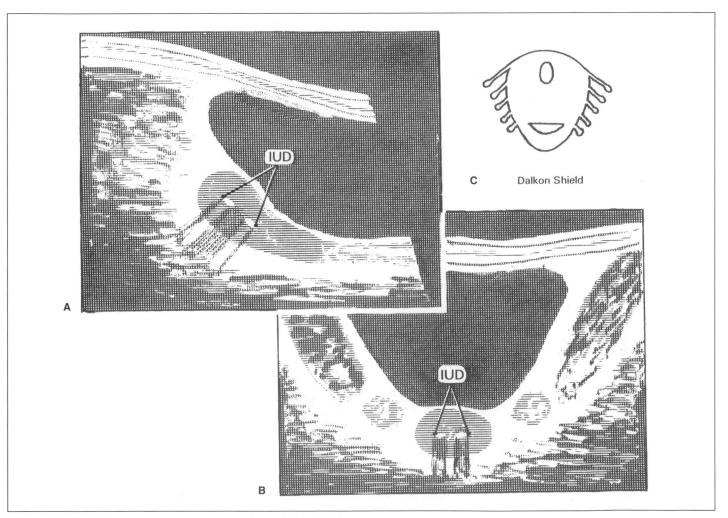

C   Dalkon Shield

FIGURE 11-2. (**A**) Longitudinal and (**B**) transverse views of a uterus containing a Dalkon shield. (**C**) Diagram of the device.

Copper 7 and Copper T, Progestasert and Paragard

The Copper 7 and Copper T IUDs differ from the others in that a band of copper is wound around one end. On long-axis views, both usually appear as a line with thickening at the upper end of the bend that forms the 7 or the T and at the lower end owing to the band of copper. Transversely, the devices will appears as a dot except at the upper end, where a short line can be seen owing to the 7 or T configuration (Fig. 11-3). The Progestasert and Paragard have an indistinguishable appearance.

 ## TECHNIQUE

IUD Position

The position of the IUD and its relationship to the uterus should be clearly shown. An IUD located in the lower uterine segment and extending into the vagina, or one that is too large for the uterine cavity, will probably be expelled.

Transabdominal Approach

Longitudinal and transverse scans of the uterus are necessary to demonstrate the position of an IUD properly. A full bladder is essential to visualize the pelvic structures and adequately demonstrate the uterine fundus. IUDs may be difficult to see when the uterus is retroverted. A full bladder can push the uterus into a more anteverted position.

Varying the gain may help to distinguish an IUD from an endometrial reaction. The IUD will remain visible when the decreased gain has eliminated most other signals.

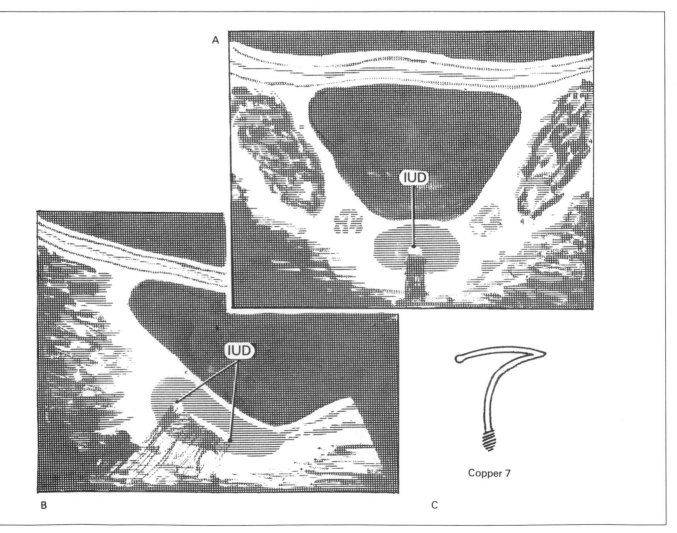

FIGURE 11-3. (**A**) Transverse view of a uterus containing a Copper 7 (Cu 7) IUD. Note shadowing behind the IUD. (**B**) Saggital view of Copper 7 (Cu 7 IUD). Note the separate echoes from the transverse and linear components of the device. Progestasert, Paragard, and Copper T would have similar appearances. (**C**) Diagram of the device.

Endovaginal Approach

The endovaginal probe has a number of advantages over a transabdominal approach:

1. Providing the IUD is in the uterus, it can be seen throughout its extent, whatever the uterine position.
2. The string can be seen as a thin longitudinal echo. If it is balled up into a clump, a small echogenic mass will be found near the inferior end of the IUD.
3. Should the IUD have perforated the myometrium, the site and amount of intramyometrial extension can be quantitated.
4. If the IUD is extrauterine, a small abscess or fluid collection may form around it and it may be visible from an endovaginal viewpoint, even when it cannot be seen on a transabdominal sonogram.

Remember that not all patients have a midline uterus. It may be necessary to scan obliquely in order to obtain a long-axis view of the uterus. Transverse scans are useful in demonstrating that the entire device is within the endometrial cavity and has not penetrated or perforated the myometrium.

There are two echoes associated with an IUD, known as the "entrance" and "exit" echoes. These subtle linear echoes are diagnostic of a foreign body (see Fig. 11-1D).

 PATHOLOGY

Perforation

Perforation of the uterus by an IUD may be complete or incomplete. If incomplete, a portion of the IUD may be demonstrated within the uterine wall. If a complete perforation has occurred, the IUD may be invisible because of overlying bowel gas.

It is important to show the relationship of the IUD to the endometrial cavity. If any portion of the device is in contact with the cavity, the IUD can be withdrawn, but if the IUD is entirely in the myometrium the uterus may have to be surgically removed (Fig. 11-4).

If the IUD cannot be seen with ultrasound it may have fallen out or it may be in the pelvis outside the uterus. A radiograph or CAT scan will show whether it is still inside the patient.

Pregnancy

Pregnancy can occasionally occur with IUDs. When an IUD with a coexisting pregnancy is discovered, one should determine the relationship of the device to the gestational sac (i.e., superior or inferior). This relationship is important in deciding whether an IUD can be safely removed. If it is left in place, a severe infection may occur. In the later stages of pregnancy, the location of the IUD is difficult to determine because of the large volume of the uterus occupied by the fetus.

Pelvic Inflammatory Disease

IUDs are associated with an increased incidence of PID. If a patient presents with pain or bleeding and the IUD is properly positioned, check the adnexal areas and the cul-de-sac for evidence of PID (as discussed in Chapter 9).

PITFALLS

Secretory Phase

The decidual reaction in the secretory phase of the endometrial cavity may obscure an IUD. Be sure to know the patient's menstrual history. IUD echoes are more readily reproducible, are associated with shadowing, and are generally stronger than decidual echoes. If the gain is decreased, IUD echoes will still be visible.

WHERE ELSE TO LOOK

If an IUD cannot be found with ultrasound despite a thorough search, and pregnancy has been ruled out, an abdominal radiograph or CAT scan will reveal the location of a migrated IUD or prove that the IUD has been expelled.

SELECTED READING

Callen, P. W. Ultrasonography in the detection of intrauterine contraceptive devices. In P. W. Callen (Ed.). *Ultrasonography in Obstetrics and Gynecology* (3rd ed.). Philadelphia: Saunders, 1994.

Nelson, A. Patient selection key to IUD success. *Contemp OB GYN* Oct:49–62, 1995.

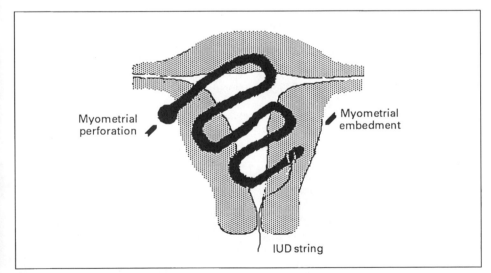

FIGURE 11-4. Diagram of an intramyometrial IUD. Portions of the IUD are outside the cavity within the myometrium or peritoneum.

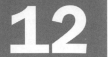

12 FIRST TRIMESTER BLEEDING

JOAN CAMPBELL, ROGER C. SANDERS

SONOGRAM ABBREVIATIONS

Bl Bladder

C   Cervix

F   Fetus
Fi Fibroid
FP Fetal pole

GS Gestational sac

Pl Placenta

RP Retained products

Ut Uterus

KEY WORDS

Abortion. Termination of pregnancy prior to 26 weeks; various types of abortion are discussed in the text.

Amniotic Membrane. Thin membrane sometimes visible in the first trimester sac. Fuses with chorionic membrane at 12 to 16 weeks.

Anembryonic. Gestation without development of a fetal pole (blighted ovum).

Bleeding Dyscrasia. An abnormality of the factors that control clotting and platelet function.

Blighted Ovum. See *Anembryonic*.

Chorionic Membrane. Membrane that surrounds the amniotic cavity and lies within the gestational sac. Not seen ultrasonically. Normally fuses with amniotic membrane at 12 to 16 weeks.

Decidual Cast (Reaction). If a pregnancy is located outside the endometrial cavity, hormonal stimulants cause the endometrium to thicken.

Dilatation and Curettage (D-and-C). Dilatation of the cervical canal and surgical removal of the uterine contents.

Double Decidual Sign. If a pregnancy is intrauterine and not ectopic, a decidual reaction occurs related to the gestational sac and a second reaction occurs due to reactive endometrial changes.

Embryo. See *Fetal Pole*.

Endocrine. Pertains to organs that secrete hormones directly into the bloodstream.

Endometrium. Membrane lining the cavity of the uterus.

Estrogen. Hormone secreted by the ovary and in pregnancy by the placenta.

Extracelomic Space. The area between the chorion and amnion.

Fetal Pole. The early developing fetus appears as a small collection of echoes within the gestational sac. More correctly termed an "embryo."

Gestational Sac. Sac-like structure that is normally within the uterus and that houses the early developing pregnancy.

Human Chorionic Gonadotropin (HCG) (Beta Subunit). Hormone that rises to very high levels in pregnancy. Assessed with a radioimmunoassay test, which is very sensitive and accurate when performed on a blood sample (serum). Pregnancy testing is almost as accurate with urine samples of HCG.

Hydatidiform Mole. Benign neoplasm that develops from the placenta of a missed abortion. High levels of HCG are produced by the tumor.

Macerated Fetus. The degenerative changes and eventual disintegration of a fetus retained in the uterus after fetal death.

Missed Abortion. A fetus which has died prior to approximately 13 weeks. Only macerated remnants may be seen.

Progesterone. Hormone produced by the corpus luteum in the second half of the menstrual cycle that modifies the endometrium in preparation for implantation of a fertilized ovum.

Septic. Pertaining to the presence of pathogenic bacteria and their products in blood or tissue; the patient becomes ill.

Spontaneous Abortion. An unplanned abortion (miscarriage) of the fetus and gestational sac before 23 weeks' gestation. After 23 weeks the spontaneous loss of pregnancy is termed premature delivery.

Triploidy. Chromosomal anomaly that often causes early pregnancy failure.

Trophoblast. Tissue that supports the developing pregnancy, for example, the gestational sac.

Vitelline Duct. A membrane supplying the yolk sac that is visible at approximately 6 weeks only.

Yolk Sac. Circular structure seen between 4 and 10 weeks that supplies nutrition to the fetal pole. It lies within the extracelomic space between the amnion and chorion.

◆>> THE CLINICAL PROBLEM

Vaginal bleeding in the first trimester is common and very worrisome to the patient. A sonogram can soothe maternal fears a lot by showing a normal, live fetus. Obstetric disorders that may cause abnormal bleeding include spontaneous abortion, ectopic pregnancy, premature separation of the placenta (abruption), placenta previa, and trophoblastic neoplastic conditions such as hydatidiform mole and choriocarcinoma.

Neoplasms (see Chapter 8) and second and third trimester bleeding problems such as placenta previa and abruptio placentae are discussed in Chapter 15. Therefore, this section will focus on spontaneous abortions. Ectopic pregnancy, which can also cause vaginal bleeding in the first trimester, is described in Chapter 13.

The majority of spontaneous abortions occur between the fifth and twelfth weeks of pregnancy; a patient may therefore consult her physician for abnormal bleeding without suspecting that she is pregnant. A pregnancy test is usually performed, but false-negative results may occur with an early pregnancy when a urine pregnancy test is used. Urine tests are, however, often waived in favor of blood tests, which are increasingly available and completely reliable. The physician may then send the patient for a sonogram to determine the viability and location of the pregnancy.

Follow-up with a combination of serum beta subunit (blood) pregnancy estimations and ultrasound studies is continued until it is evident whether the fetus is viable or dead.

Seven different types of spontaneous abortion can be distinguished sonographically:

1. Threatened abortion: a viable fetus with vaginal bleeding
2. Incomplete abortion: partial evacuation of the fetus and placenta
3. Complete abortion: No retained products
4. Missed abortion: retained dead fetus and placenta
5. Blighted ovum: anembryonic pregnancy
6. Inevitable abortion: abortion in progress
7. Septic abortion: infected dead fetus or retained products

Differentiation between a blighted ovum and an early pregnancy can be difficult to determine transabdominally; endovaginal ultrasonic analysis allows much earlier diagnosis of viable pregnancy at about 5½ weeks and is essential in early diagnosis. It does not harm the pregnancy.

Hydatidiform mole is a condition in which pregnancy develops abnormally into a form of neoplasm. The uterus is filled with grapelike structures (vesicles). This condition causes bleeding, vomiting, and an enlarged uterine size for dates. The human chorionic gonadotropin (HCG) titer is very high. Dilatation and curettage (D-and-C) is performed because the condition may develop into a neoplasm that spreads to other portions of the body.

ANATOMY
Gestational Sac

The uterus enlarges in relation to the length of pregnancy. A gestational sac is visible as a well-defined circle of echoes in the fundus of the uterus. The sac may be seen as early as 4 weeks (Fig. 12-1B), and by 6 weeks it can be demonstrated reliably on a transabdominal scan (Fig. 12-1C). At first, the sac should occupy less than one half of the total volume of the uterus and may appear echo-free because echoes from the fetal pole may not yet be visualized. Gestational sac visualization with the endovaginal probe is possible at 4 weeks. Fetal pole visualization is usually successful at about 4½ to 5 weeks (Appendixes 3, 4, and 5). A yolk sac is visible before the fetal pole can be seen.

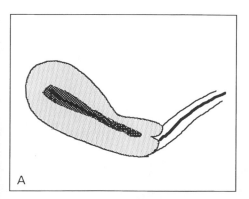 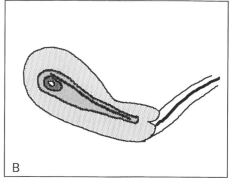 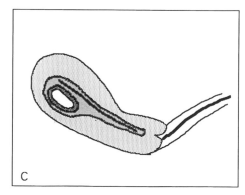

FIGURE 12-1. (**A**) Normal uterus. (**B**) Normal gestational sac at 4 weeks. (**C**) Normal gestational sac at 6 weeks. Note that the gestational sac is enclosed by the decidual reaction at this early stage.

The fetal pole (embryo) may lie between two small sacs, the yolk sac and the amniotic sac, at this very early stage (Fig. 12-2). The amniotic sac expands thereafter but is difficult to see. An additional linear structure, the vitelline duct, may be seen (Fig. 12-3). A gestational sac is surrounded by a decidual reaction between 4 and 7 weeks (see Fig. 12-1).

By 8 weeks, the sac should occupy approximately one half of the uterine volume, and by 10 weeks the entire uterine cavity should be encompassed (Fig. 12-4; Appendix 3). The gestational sac is encompassed by a ring of echoes (the decidual reaction), which should be well defined and of uniform thickness except at the site where the placenta will develop. At this implantation site, the ring is single and slightly thickened. Elsewhere it is double layered, although the second layer is sometimes subtle. The inner layer is composed of the chorion and the decidua capsularis. The outer layer is the decidua vera; together they are considered the double decidual sac (see Fig. 13-2) seen around true intrauterine gestations.

A sonolucent extra gestational sac space ("implantation bleed") is a relatively common feature of normal pregnancy between the sixth and tenth weeks (see Fig. 12-6). Sometimes an apparent implantation bleed contains venous flow on color flow Doppler.

Yolk Sac

The yolk sac can be seen slightly earlier than the fetal pole, at about 4 weeks transvaginally and 5½ weeks transabdominally. It disappears by 10 weeks (see Figs. 12-2 to 12-4).

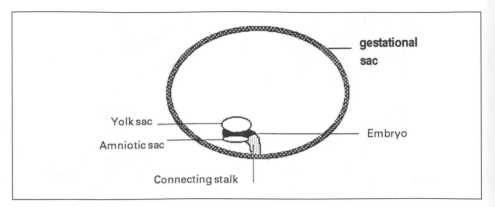

FIGURE 12-2. When the fetal pole is first seen, it lies between two small cysts, the yolk sac and the amniotic sac. Fetal heart motion can be seen at this 4 ½-week stage.

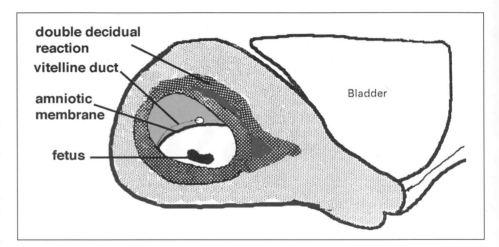

FIGURE 12-3. The yolk sac lies within the chorionic sac. The fetus lies within the amniotic sac. The vitelline duct may be seen supplying the yolk sac at 6 ½ weeks.

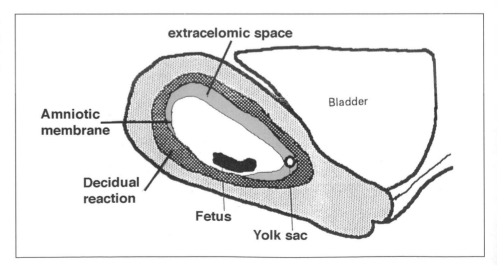

FIGURE 12-4. The amniotic membrane may be seen as a subtle line within the amniotic fluid at 7 ½ weeks.

Amniotic Membrane

The tiny crescentic line that constitutes the amniotic membrane can be seen within the gestational sac in the first trimester with high-quality ultrasound systems. It encloses the amniotic cavity. The yolk sac lies in the extracelomic cavity outside the amniotic membrane (see Figs. 12-3 and 12-4). At about 4 weeks the amniotic sac is about the same size as the yolk sac. Both lie within the chorion (see Fig. 12-2). A second membrane, the vitelline duct, may be seen leading to the yolk sac (see Fig. 12-3).

Fetal Pole (Embryo)

By 5 to 6 weeks with transvaginal ultrasound and by 7 weeks transabdominally, the fetus should be seen within the uterus as a small collection of echoes known as a fetal pole, or embryo (see Figs. 12-2 to 12-5). Measuring maximum fetal length (crown-rump length) is a very accurate method of dating between 5 and 12 weeks (see Appendixes 4 and 5). Almost as soon as the fetus is visible, the fetal head and body can be made out and facial structures can be seen. A mass may be seen at the cord insertion site, which is a physiologic omphalocele or midgut herniation. Such a physiologic omphalocele represents the normal gut rotation occurring outside the fetal trunk; this normal variant is present about half the time between 6 and 10 weeks.

Fetal heart motion is visible with good equipment almost as soon as the fetal pole is seen. It is always seen when the fetal pole is 4-mm long or greater.

The fetal heart is seen as a tiny fluttering structure within the fetal body. It beats at about double the maternal rate if the fetus is normal. If the fetus is sick the rate will be slow or irregular. The fetal pulse rate increases during the first trimester (Appendix 28).

◢ TECHNIQUE

Full-bladder Technique

The full-bladder technique should be used with the transabdominal approach. For details of this technique for identification of the uterus and ovaries, see Chapter 7. Overdistention can make the fetus difficult to see. If the bladder is full enough and if nothing can be seen, look transvaginally with the bladder emptied or ask the patient to half-void.

Measuring Gestational Sacs

The gestational sac measurement is an average of the width, length, and anteroposterior (A-P) dimensions of the sac. Measurements for width are taken at the transverse view demonstrating the widest portion of the sac, and measurements for the length are taken on the longest sagittal view. It is important to obtain the A-P diameter from a sagittal image as well, because the angle of the uterus can be taken into account (Fig. 12-5A). Sac shape can change owing to extrinsic factors, such as fibroids or bladder distention; all three dimensions should be measured on-screen within a few minutes of each other so that all of the measurements relate to each other. *Measure at the fluid-sac interface; do not include the decidua in your measurements.*

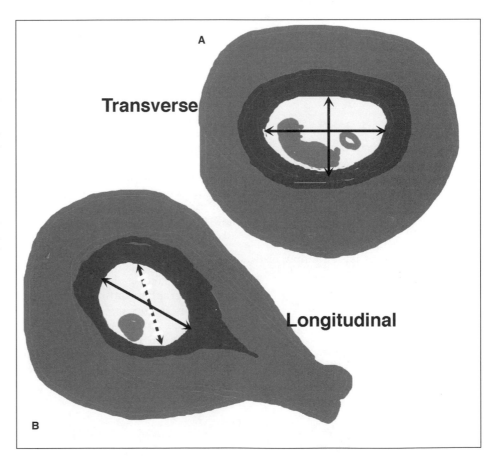

FIGURE 12-5. Longitudinal and transverse views of the uterus showing the views to measure a gestational sac. The width, length, and height diameters are obtained. The measurement is averaged. Take the longest length, rather than an oblique, shorter measurement as shown in the longitudinal diagram in dots.

Measuring Crown-Rump Length (CRL)

The dominant feature in a very early embryo is the pulsating heart in the center of a small lump of tissue—the crown and rump are the same size and virtually indistinguishable. At this stage it is easy to get an accurate measurement of the whole embryo.

Later, at about 9 weeks, it is possible to see the cranium as a separate entity from the fetal body. A crown-rump measurement is taken at the longest axis, which may require patience because the fetus curls and flexes at this stage (Fig. 12-6). It is worth taking a few measurements to determine whether the longest axis has indeed been recorded; however, it is not appropriate to average the shorter measurements—this decreases your accuracy. If your machine does this automatically, go into the OB program and remove the CRLs which are too short. The crown-rump length is still the dating method of choice until the intracranial anatomy is clear enough, at 12 weeks, to begin measuring biparietal diameters.

Endovaginal Technique

The endovaginal technique is a preferable technique for the examination of the first trimester pregnancy. It is particularly helpful in the following circumstances:

1. When it is uncertain whether there is a fetus or whether it is alive
2. When the patient has an empty bladder

3. To look for bleeds in or around the sac
4. If ectopic pregnancy is a possibility

◆ PATHOLOGY
Threatened Abortion

Threatened abortion is not visible sonographically. This diagnosis is made whenever vaginal bleeding occurs within the first 20 weeks of pregnancy with a closed cervix. The sonogram should demonstrate a pregnancy corresponding to the patient's dates.

Most such pregnancies will proceed to term, but because of the threat of abortion and increased risk of bleeding later in pregnancy, serial sonograms during the pregnancy may be requested.

A low fetal cardiac rate (less than 80) suggests impending fetal death.

Incomplete Abortion

If a threatened abortion progresses and some of the products of conception are passed as tissue with bleeding, the clinical diagnosis is an incomplete abortion. However, portions of the placenta and some fetal parts may remain within the uterus, resulting in continued bleeding. Sonographically, the uterus appears enlarged. With incomplete abortion, the sonographer may note an empty, ill-defined gestational sac within the uterus or a sac with internal echoes that are not clearly fetal. Occasionally, no sac at all can be identified, but large clumps of echoes in the center of the uterus may be seen. These echoes may represent parts of the fetus, placenta, or blood. This sonographic confirmation of diagnosis is useful because a D-and-C (dilatation and curettage) may be necessary to complete the process of abortion (Fig. 12-7). If the uterus appears normal by ultrasound many would not consider a D-and-C worthwhile.

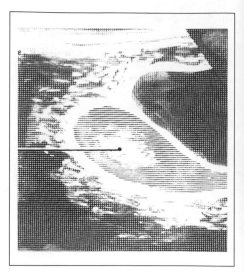

FIGURE 12-7. Incomplete abortion with retained product of conception. There is a featureless mass in the uterus.

Complete Abortion

With complete abortion, all products of conception pass. Sonographically, the uterus appears enlarged, but a gestational sac or fetus cannot be identified. However, a line of central echoes—a prominent thickening of the central cavity interface—within the uterus representing a decidual reaction may be present. The uterus may remain enlarged for up to 2 weeks after the abortion. After the initial passage of clots, bleeding is minimal, and the patient usually does not require any further treatment.

The sonographer's role is to confirm that the uterus is empty. Echoes within the cavity may represent blood rather than retained products of conception (Fig. 12-8).

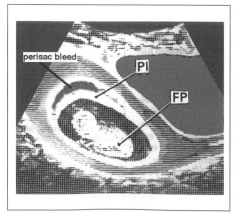

FIGURE 12-6. Normal fetal pole and gestational sac at 9 weeks. The placenta is beginning to be visible. A small implantation bleed is showing.

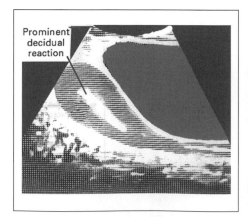

FIGURE 12-8. Pronounced decidual reaction due to some retained products of conception or blood.

Missed Abortion

When the fetus dies but is retained within the uterus, a missed abortion has occurred. Sonographically, the uterus is often too small for the expected dates. Most frequently, missed abortions occur between 6 and 14 weeks of gestation. In an early missed abortion, the gestational sac contains the fetal pole which shows no heart motion.

A diagnosis of a missed abortion can be made if a fetus measures 4 mm or more but no fetal heart motion is seen. If the fetal pole measures 3 mm and no fetal heart motion is seen, it is usually considered wise to rescan in a few days to confirm fetal death.

The fetal pole may assume an abnormal shape (Fig. 12-9). With later missed abortions, the placenta may become large, resembling a hydatidiform mole; these changes are termed hydropic changes.

Intrasac and Perisac Bleeds

Bleeds in or around the sac (Fig. 12-10) are common. Bleeds are seen (1) as a group of echoes within the amniotic sac adjacent to the fetus; (2) as low-level echoes in the space between the amniotic and chorionic membranes (extracelomic space); (3) as a group of echoes in a crescentic shape in a subchorionic location; or (4) between the gestational sac and the decidual reaction. In any location, as long as fetal heart motion is seen, management of the bleed should include a follow-up sonogram in 1 or 2 weeks.

Fetal survival is much more common than death if fetal heart motion is seen.

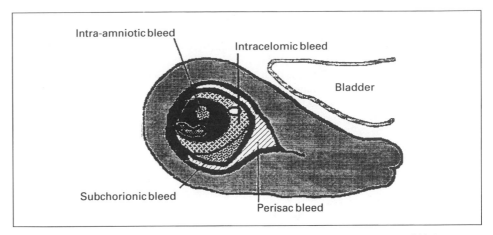

FIGURE 12-10. Perisac bleeding with threatened abortion may occur (1) between the gestational sac and the endometrial cavity, (2) in a subchorionic location, (3) within the chorionic sac, (4) within the amniotic sac.

Blighted Ovum

The definition of a blighted ovum is an anembryonic pregnancy. This means that the sac develops but the embryo does not. Clinically, the patient usually has slight vaginal bleeding. The pregnancy test may be positive even though no embryo is present because there is continued production of HCG by the trophoblasts in the sac. The growth of the sac will not increase as it would have in a normal pregnancy. Although eventually a blighted ovum will abort, the physician may intervene with a D-and-C before that occurs.

The main sonographic finding is a trophoblastic ring within the uterus. This ring may look like a gestational sac, although the borders are usually less regular and are ill defined (Fig. 12-11). No fetal pole is seen within the sac. If the mean sac diameter is 25 mm or more and on transabdominal examination no fetal pole is seen, or the mean sac diameter is 20 mm and no yolk sac is seen, a blighted ovum is considered to be present.

USING THE ENDOVAGINAL PROBE. A fetal pole should be seen when the gestational sac diameter is 17 mm or more. A yolk sac should be seen when the gestational sac has a mean diameter greater than 8 mm. Be cautious about using these measurements in the diagnosis of blighted ovum if there is a question of monoamniotic monochorionic twins.

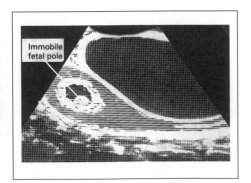

FIGURE 12-9. Gestational sac containing a macerated immobile fetus—a missed abortion.

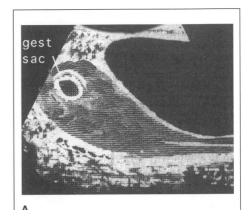

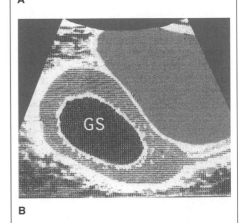

FIGURE 12-11. Blighted ovum. (**A**) A small sac with a thin irregular trophoblastic ring in a large uterus. (**B**) A large sac with a poorly defined border in a small uterus. Either an unduly large or small sac may occur with blighted ovum.

There may be a fluid-fluid level due to blood within the gestational sac; this is definitive evidence of fetal death.

The absence of a fetal pole is inconclusive evidence of blighted ovum if the gestational sac is small, because early normal gestational sacs with a diameter of less than 8 mm also appear to be without a fetal pole. To solve this dilemma the patient may be asked to return in a week or two for a repeat sonogram. Serial serum beta subunit pregnancy tests may be performed.

There may be a discrepancy between the size of the sac and the uterine size, with the sac being too large or too small for the uterus (see Fig. 12-11).

Inevitable Abortion

Pregnancies suffering an inevitable abortion are usually clinically obvious. The patient consults her physician because she is experiencing some bleeding. The physician examines her and discovers that her cervix is dilating and the pregnancy is doomed to be aborted. Sonographically, the area of the cervix may appear to be widened and fluid filled owing to blood and dilatation. A sonolucent space around the sac may be present where the sac has dissected away from the uterine wall. A fluid-fluid level may be present within the aborting sac. The gestational sac may lie at the level of the cervix and may be in the process of being aborted (Fig. 12-12).

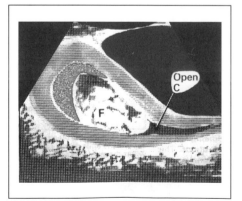

FIGURE 12-12. Incompetent cervix with inevitable abortion. One can see fluid in the cervix almost to the vagina. Note the irregular macerated fetus within the amniotic cavity. The fetus is in the process of being aborted.

Septic Abortion

In septic abortion there are infected products of conception in the uterus, perhaps as a result of surgical abortion with nonsterile devices. Alternatively, infection may occur in retained products after a spontaneous or induced abortion. Sonographically, the uterus is enlarged, and there are increased endometrial echoes. If the infection is caused by gas-forming organisms, areas of shadowing may be produced (Fig. 12-13). Shadowing may also be caused by retained bony fragments following an attempted abortion.

Hydatidiform Mole

Vaginal bleeding, excessive vomiting (hyperemesis gravidarum), and high blood pressure suggest the presence of a mole. The uterus will be filled with echoes interspersed with echo-free spaces (see Fig. 12-14).

Large echo-free spaces may occur within a mole, and the process may be confused with a missed abortion or a fibroid; however, the HCG titers will be markedly elevated. Large cysts may be seen in the ovaries. These theca lutein cysts represent follicles greatly stimulated by increased HCG.

Invasive Mole

Some hydatidiform moles recur after the performance of a curettage and invade the muscle of the uterus. Residual molar tissue is highly vascular and lights up using the color flow system. Without color flow, remaining invasive tissue may be overlooked.

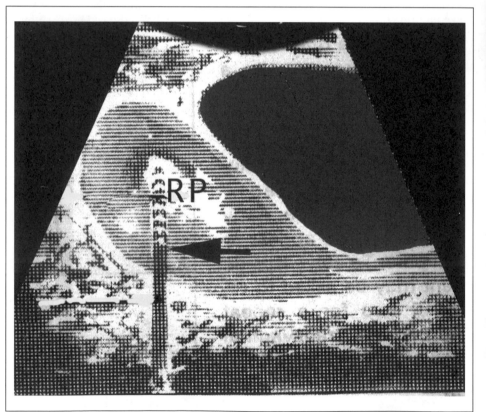

FIGURE 12-13. Retained products of conception with infection. Gas associated with retained products is responsible for some acoustic shadowing (arrow shows shadow).

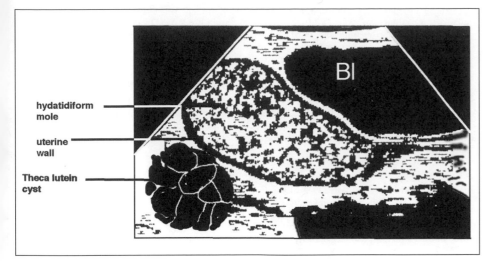

FIGURE 12-14. A hydatidiform mole fills the uterus with low-level echoes interspersed with echoic spaces. A theca lutein cyst is seen. Multiple follicles enlarge under the influence of HCG to form a multilocular ovarian mass.

Choriocarcinoma

Molar tissue has the potential to develop into an aggressive malignancy known as a choriocarcinoma. When seen in the uterus, this tumor has cystic centers with echogenic borders. Although easily treatable, it metastasizes early. When a patient with a positive pregnancy test is seen with a very high HCG, and masses with an irregular appearance and cystic center are present within the uterus, the liver should be examined for metastatic lesions, which are generally echopenic.

Partial Mole

When a mole and a fetus are present together it is possible (1) that there are twins and that one twin has become a mole or (2) that there is a "partial mole." A chromosomal anomaly, triploidy, causes placental changes that resemble a mole. The fetus is anomalous and almost always dies. Sometimes the fetus is hydropic (see Chapter 18).

PITFALLS

1. *Changes in sac shape* may be caused by external compression due to an overdistended bladder or bowel or to fibroids in the uterine wall (Fig. 12-15). Myometrial contractions may distort the sac shape in the first trimester.

2. *Other entities may mimic* the complex echo pattern seen in a molar pregnancy. These include degenerating fibroid, missed abortion, and necrotic placenta.

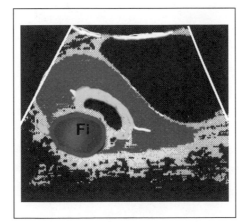

FIGURE 12-15. Fibroid distorting the uterus. This fibroid is more echogenic than the remainder of the uterus; other fibroids may be less echogenic.

3. *A sonolucent space around a portion of the gestational sac* may be seen between the sixth and eighth weeks of pregnancy as a normal variant. Subtle venous flow is usually visible within the area.

4. *A cervical pregnancy and an impending abortion* appear similar. If the pregnancy is aborting the sonographic findings will change rapidly and the patient will be bleeding.

5. *Underdistention and overdistention of the bladder* may prevent gestational sac visualization. The bladder should rise approximately 1 to 2 cm above the uterine fundus for satisfactory transabdominal evaluation.

6. Although *a gestational sac size of greater than 17 mm with no evidence of fetal pole or yolk sac* using an endovaginal probe suggests blighted ovum, monozygotic twins may still be present. The gestation is earlier than the sac makes it appear; rescan later if twins are suspected.

WHERE ELSE TO LOOK

Hydatidiform Mole

If a molelike appearance is seen in the uterus (see Fig. 12-14):

1. Look hard for evidence of an intrauterine fetus. Missed abortion with a macerated fetus can look like a mole.

2. Look for a theca lutein cyst, which is seen with 40 percent of moles.

3. Look for liver metastases, which are commonly seen with choriocarcinoma.

SELECTED READING

DuBose, T. J., Butschek, C. M., Hill, L. W., Dickey, D., Porter, L., and Poole, E. K. Fetal heart rates. *J Ultrasound Med* 8:407–408, 1989.

Frates, M. C., Benson, C. B., and Doubilet, P. M. Pregnancy outcome after a first trimester sonogram demonstrating fetal cardiac activity. *J Ultrasound Med* 12:383–386, 1993.

Horrow, M. M. Enlarged amniotic cavity: A new sonographic sign of early embryonic death. *AJR* 158:359–362, 1992.

Jaffe, R. Investigation of abnormal first-trimester gestations by color Doppler imaging. *J Clin Ultrasound* 21:521–526, 1993.

Jaffe, R., and Warsof, S. L. Color Doppler imaging in the assessment of uteroplacental blood flow in abnormal first trimester intrauterine pregnancies: An attempt to define etiologic mechanisms. *J Ultrasound Med* 11:41–44, 1992.

Kurtz, A. B., Needleman, L., Pennell, R. G., Baltarowich, O., Vilaro, M., and Goldberg, B. B. Can detection of the yolk sac in the first trimester be used to predict the outcome of pregnancy? A prospective sonographic study. *AJR* 158:843–847, 1992.

Laboda, L. A., Estroff, J. A., and Benacerraf, B. R. First trimester bradycardia. A sign of impending fetal loss. *J Ultrasound Med* 8:561–563, 1989.

Levi, C. S., Dashefsky, S. M., Holt, S. C., Lindsay, D. J., and Lyons, E. A. Ultrasound of the first trimester of pregnancy. *Ultrasound Quarterly* 11:95–124, 1993.

Lindsay, D. J., Lovett, I. S., Lyons, E. A., Levi, C. S., Zheng, X. H., Holt, S. C., and Dashefsky, S. M. Yolk sac diameter and shape at endovaginal US: Predictors of pregnancy outcome in the first trimester. *Radiology* 183:115–118, 1992.

McKenna, K. M., Feldstein, V. A., Goldstein, R. B., and Filly, R. A. The "empty amnion": A sign of early pregnancy failure. *J Ultrasound Med* 14:117–121, 1995.

Sohaey, R., Woodward, P., and Zwiebel, W. J. First-trimester ultrasound: The essentials. *Semin Ultrasound, CT and MRI* 17:2–14, 1996.

Wagner, B. J., Woodward, P. J., and Dickey, G. E. From the archives of the AFIP: Gestational trophoblastic disease: Radiologic-pathologic correlation. *Radiographics* 16:131–148, 1996.

13

PELVIC PAIN WITH POSITIVE PREGNANCY TEST

ROGER C. SANDERS

SONOGRAM ABBREVIATIONS

DR Decidual reaction

E Ectopic

F Fetus

Pl Placenta

Ut Uterus

YS Yolk sac

KEY WORDS

Abdominal Pregnancy. A pregnancy that occurs outside the fallopian tube or uterus and, therefore, expands without causing bleeding. Occasionally, abdominal pregnancies go to term.

Adnexal Ring. Extraovarian adnexal mass with thick echogenic border; this finding is suspicious for ectopic pregnancy.

Amenorrhea. Absence of menstruation. Can be primary if menstruation never occurs or secondary if menstruation occurred in the past.

Beta Subunit. Portion of human chorionic gonadotropin (HCG) measured to determine pregnancy status.

Cervical Pregnancy. Ectopic pregnancy located in the cervix. It is a dangerous site because there is heavy bleeding when the pregnancy is lost.

Cornual Pregnancy. Ectopic pregnancy located at the origin of the fallopian tubes from the endometrial cavity.

Ectopic Pregnancy. Pregnancy that is located in a site other than within the fundus of the uterine cavity.

Laparoscopy. A surgical procedure in which a tube is introduced into a small incision made, as a rule, adjacent to the umbilicus. Air is placed within the maternal abdomen. This allows visualization of pelvic structures through a small, movable tube.

Methotrexate. Chemotherapeutic drug which in a single dose can eliminate an ectopic pregnancy, leaving no scarring. It is now being used with increasing frequency with unruptured ectopic pregnancies.

THE CLINICAL PROBLEM

The most common cause of pelvic pain with a positive pregnancy test is ectopic pregnancy. This is a common diagnosis, now occurring in as many as 1 in 200 pregnancies. Pregnancies occurring outside the uterine cavity are termed ectopic pregnancies.

Ectopic pregnancies are most frequent in the following types of patients:

1. Patients with a history of pelvic inflammatory disease
2. Patients with a previous or current intrauterine device
3. Patients undergoing infertility treatment
4. Patients with a history of previous tubal surgery

After successful nonsurgical treatment of an infection, thickened and scarred fallopian tubes may remain. Although these injured tubes may not prevent the passage of sperm for fertilization of ova, the scarring may retard the return of a fertilized zygote to the uterine cavity. The zygote may begin to develop and grow in the fallopian tube, and eventually pain will result due to distention and rupture of the fallopian tube.

Ectopic pregnancy may occur at various sites, including the abdominal cavity, the fallopian tubes (as previously mentioned), the cornu of the uterus, and the cervix (Fig. 13-1). Pregnancies in the uterine cornu are the most difficult to diagnose because sonographically they appear at first to be partly in the uterine body. If misdiagnosed, they will progress to a more advanced stage before causing symptoms.

The clinical symptoms that suggest an ectopic pregnancy are as follows:

1. Acute pelvic pain (before or after rupture)
2. Vaginal bleeding (before or after rupture)
3. Amenorrhea (consistent with pregnancy)
4. Adnexal mass (before or after rupture)
5. Positive pregnancy test
6. Cervical tenderness (usually after rupture)
7. A drop in hematocrit (usually after rupture)
8. Shock (after rupture)

A feared complication of ectopic pregnancy is rupture of the ectopic sac. Rupture usually occurs at or before the eighth week of gestation. A ruptured ectopic pregnancy is an urgent surgical emergency. The diagnosis usually cannot be made on clinical grounds alone; pelvic sonography is helpful in making a more specific diagnosis. Unruptured ectopic pregnancy is much less of an emergency

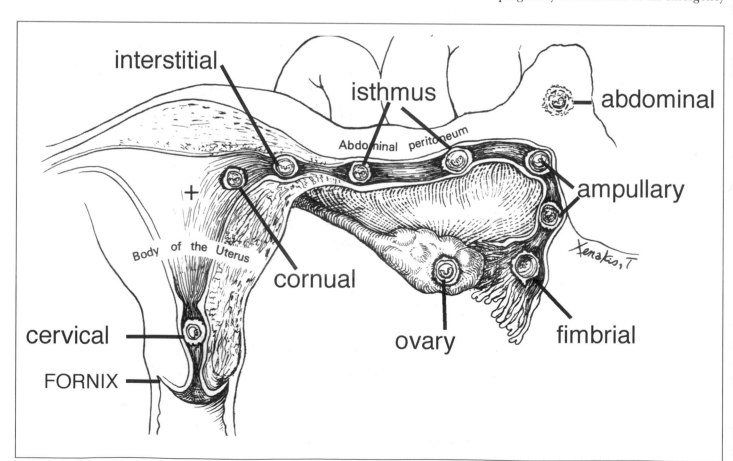

FIGURE 13-1. Possible sites for ectopic pregnancy. Note that the type of ectopic pregnancy is named after its site. The fornix is the structure in which the vaginal probe is normally placed. The fornices are very distensible, so the end of the vaginal probe can be at miduterine level.

and may be treated conservatively with methotrexate. Often sonography in a patient with the clinical features of ectopic pregnancy demonstrates an intrauterine pregnancy, thus precluding surgical intervention. Sometimes the sonographic picture of an ectopic pregnancy is so typical that the obstetrician can proceed straight to appropriate therapy (30 % of cases). In other cases, laparoscopy may be necessary to make a definitive diagnosis. Since serum pregnancy tests are so reliable, referral to the ultrasound unit should ideally wait until pregnancy test results are available.

Although unruptured ectopic pregnancies may be medically treated with methotrexate administration, the diagnosis is still one that requires an immediate call to the referring doctor.

Abdominal pregnancy outside the tube and uterus is rare. Although abdominal pregnancies can be carried to term, they are most often removed when diagnosed because they have a poor outcome and are associated with many complications. Clinically, in an advanced abdominal pregnancy the fetal parts are easily palpable.

The pregnancy test remains positive for up to 2 months after an abortion or an ectopic pregnancy has been removed. Quantitation of the beta subunit helps in the diagnosis of ectopic pregnancy. In normal pregnancy the level should double every other day. Once it reaches a level of about 1000 international units (depending on the test used), a normal gestational sac will be seen within the uterus. Falling levels may be due to complete or incomplete spontaneous abortion rather than dead ectopic pregnancy.

Cystic Masses

Rupture or bleeding of any pelvic mass in a pregnant patient causes acute pelvic pain similar to that seen in rupture of an ectopic pregnancy. Torsion (twisting of a cyst on a pedicle), hemorrhage, and rupture are the three complications that cause pain in cysts. Hemorrhage often results from torsion. The sonographic findings of ovarian cyst rupture are confusingly similar to those of ectopic pregnancy, but more specific changes are seen with hemorrhage and torsion, especially if there has been a previous sonogram showing a simple cyst.

ANATOMY

Approximately 95 percent of ectopic pregnancies occur in the fallopian tubes; it is increasingly easy to visualize tubes with endovaginal sonography. There are four subdivisions: the mouth of the fallopian tube into the endometrial cavity termed the cornix; the short interstitial portion, which is intramural and surrounded by the wall of the uterus; the long tubal segment termed isthmus; then the ampulla, which is open to the abdominal cavity and which receives the ovulated egg into the tube at the fimbria (see Fig. 13-1). The normal tube is about 10-cm long and is suspended by the broad ligament.

▦ TECHNIQUE

See Chapter 7.

Go ahead and use the endovaginal probe. It is not dangerous and is an invaluable diagnostic tool in this emergency clinical situation. Endovaginal views are usually obtained first since the patient is often NPO in preparation for surgery. If nothing is seen in or outside of the uterus on endovaginal views and the pregnancy test is positive, than it may be appropriate to fill the bladder with a foley catheter and perform transabdominal views for those ectopic pregnancies that lie high in the abdomen.

PATHOLOGY

Ectopic Pregnancy

The ultrasonic features of ectopic pregnancy are as follows:

1. A *gestational sac in the adnexa containing a fetal pole with heart motion and a yolk sac* is a diagnostic finding (see Figs. 13-3 and 13-4). This used to be a rare finding, but is not uncommon when an endovaginal transducer is used. Endovaginal visualization of the fetus is possible as early as 4 weeks and 3 days after menstruation. A yolk sac has such a distinct shape that a diagnosis of ectopic pregnancy can also be made when only a yolk sac is seen in an adnexal sac (see Fig. 13-3).

   Fetal heart motion may be seen with high-quality equipment when the fetal pole itself is not seen and the gestational sac is very small.

2. *Uterine enlargement or a decidual reaction in the endometrium without a gestational sac.* A decidual reaction has a single outline, whereas an early gestational sac has a double decidual reaction. Low-level echoes due to blood often occur in a decidual reaction (Fig. 13-2).

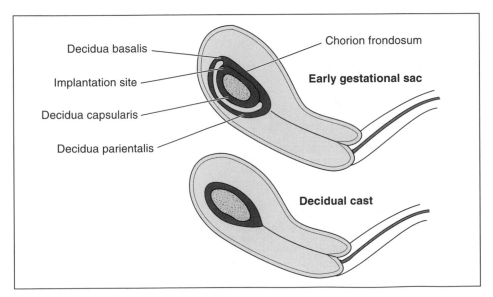

FIGURE 13-2. Decidual reaction compared with early gestational sac. Note the double outline in a normal pregnancy. The decidual cast is filled with blood.

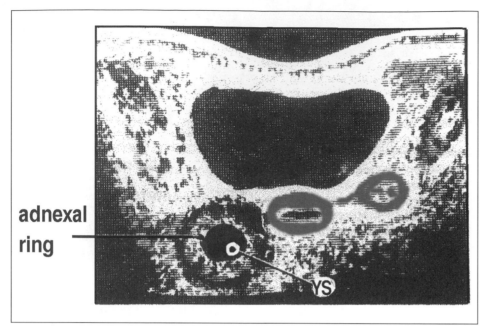

FIGURE 13-3. Ectopic pregnancy. A mass in the cul-de-sac has the configuration termed an adnexal ring. There is some fluid forming a decidual reaction within the endometrial cavity. The decidual reaction may not be this prominent. The yolk sac (YS) can be seen within the adnexal ring—definitive evidence of an ectopic pregnancy.

3. An *adnexal mass*, which may be echo filled or hypoechoic (Fig. 13-4 and see Fig. 13-5). The use of color flow Doppler may be helpful here since a low-resistance pattern in the center of a nonspecific extraovarian mass is typical of ectopic. However, this pattern is also seen in association with corpus luteum cysts.
4. A gestational sac with a thick rind in the adnexa without an identifiable fetal pole (Fig. 13-4). When this lesion is less well defined, the term *adnexal ring* is used.
5. *Cul-de-sac fluid.* If there are many adhesions, *free intraperitoneal fluid* will not pool in the cul-de-sac but will be seen in the *subhepatic space* or the *paracolic gutters.* Those areas should be examined whenever pelvic findings are negative and ectopic pregnancy is suspected.

The presence of free fluid suggests a ruptured ectopic pregnancy, especially if internal echoes are visible within the free fluid. This represents a dangerous situation and an immediate call should be made to the referring physician.

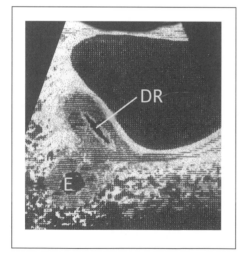

FIGURE 13-4. Diagram showing an adnexal ring posterior to the uterus (E). A thick ring of echogenic material surrounds some fluid, but no fetal pole or yolk sac is seen.

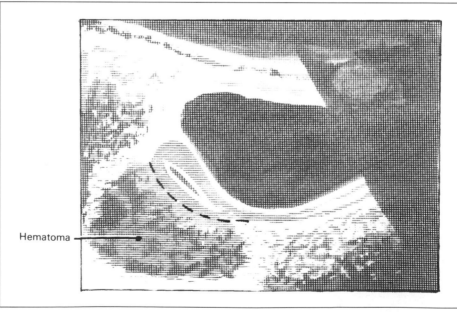

FIGURE 13-5. Ectopic pregnancy after rupture. A hematoma obscures the uterine outline.

6. *Empty uterus with a positive pregnancy test.* If the pregnancy test is positive, but nothing is seen in the pelvis, an ectopic pregnancy is possible. However, a more likely diagnosis is early pregnancy (before the gestational sac can be seen) or complete spontaneous abortion (if the patient has vaginal bleeding). An ectopic pregnancy becomes almost certain on endovaginal examination if:
   a. There is no intrauterine pregnancy.
   b. The patient has had no vaginal bleeding.
   c. The beta subunit is more than 1000 international units.

With Bleed (After Rupture)

If bleeding has occurred, there is a loss of uterine outline due to hematoma. Blood may surround the uterus, giving a "pseudouterus" effect (Fig. 13-5); the presence of blood may not be obvious because the complex mass can look like the uterus.

Interstitial Pregnancy

When the fertilized egg implants in the intrauterine portion of the tube (intramural), it is termed an interstitial pregnancy (Fig. 13-6). Interstitial pregnancies are difficult to diagnose because the gestational sac appears to be within the uterus, although there is a relative absence of surrounding myometrium. An interstitial pregnancy usually presents at a later date than an ectopic pregnancy (8–10 weeks) with catastrophic bleeding. The pregnancy may look as if it is in the edge of the myometrium or may lie very close to the uterus.

Cornual Pregnancy

This type of ectopic pregnancy is located in the mouth of the tube as it passes through the wall of the uterus (Fig 13-7, and see Figs. 13-1 and 13-6). This is a very confusing location because a normal gestational sac may not lie in the center at the fundus of the uterus. In addition to a variant of normal, two other common causes of lateral gestational sac location exist:

1. Fibroids at the fundus. The gestational sac is displaced to one side by a fibroid. The texture of the fibroid is usually distorted and easily distinguished from the normal uterus.

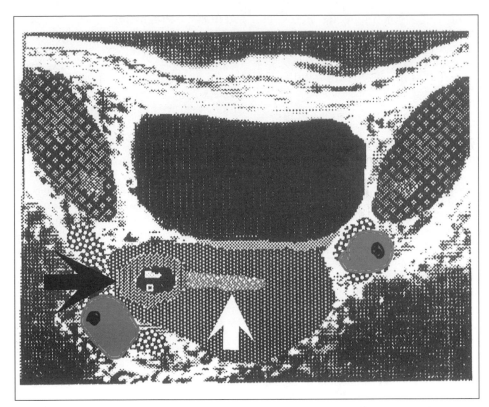

FIGURE 13-6. In an interstitial pregnancy the myometrium around the sac is barely visible (black arrow). The decidual reaction can be seen in the center of the uterus (white arrow).

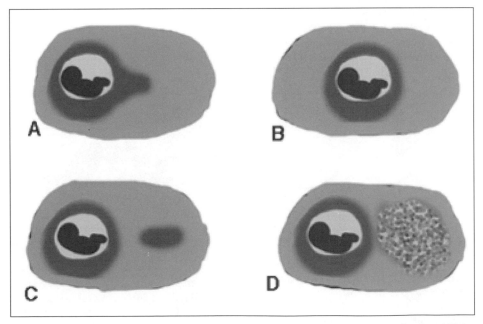

FIGURE 13-7. Possible explanations for eccentrically placed gestational sacs. (**A**) Interstitial pregnancy. Note that the endometrial cavity echoes are still seen next door to the sac. (**B**) A normal pregnancy. (**C**) A septated uterus with second decidual reaction. Note the echoes on the opposite side of the uterus. (**D**) Fibroid displacing the sac to the right. The fibroid can be seen as a mottled pattern on the left.

2. Bicornuate or subseptate uterus. The pregnancy develops in one horn and is, therefore, eccentrically located. A second well-defined decidual reaction should also be seen on the other side of the uterus.

If neither of these entities are present and the gestational sac is eccentrically located, reexamine with a different degree of bladder filling. The sac may then appear in the midline. Management of gestational sacs in this location is very difficult because so many turn out to be normal variants. On reexamination at another time, the gestational sac may adopt a normal location. If the myometrium is very thin over the lateral side of the gestational sac, the diagnosis becomes more likely, but even then a later examination may be normal.

Cervical Pregnancy

Another rare ectopic location where a pregnancy can implant is the cervix (Fig. 13-8). The gestational sac will be in a low position with little or no myometrium surrounding its inferior aspect. Cervical pregnancies present at a later date than ectopic pregnancies (8–10 weeks), often with severe bleeding. An intra-amniotic injection of methotrexate, a new chemotherapeutic drug, under ultrasound control, has been performed as a therapeutic maneuver. Such pregnancies are now usually treated with oral methotrexate.

Abdominal Pregnancy

Abdominal pregnancy (Fig. 13-9) is rare. The pregnancy develops outside the tubes within the peritoneal cavity. These pregnancies may grow to a large size, since they are not surrounded by the fallopian tube, and can present at term with unsuccessful labor. Three sonographic findings suggest an abdominal pregnancy:

1. The fetus, placenta, and amniotic fluid are superior to the uterus. The uterus may lie between the bladder and the pregnancy; the endometrial cavity is the giveaway finding. Less commonly, the uterus may lie posterior to the pregnancy, in which case the diagnosis is often missed.
2. The surrounding membrane around an abdominal pregnancy will be very thin since there is no myometrium.
3. The pregnancy lies close to the abdominal wall.

Often abdominal pregnancies fail before term. During the surgical removal of an abdominal pregnancy the placenta may be left in place because it is too dangerous to remove. If it is attached to the intestines it slowly regresses over the ensuing months under the influence of the chemotherapeutic agent methotrexate.

Corpus Luteum Problems

1. *Hemorrhage.* Corpus luteum cysts may become filled with blood and form a painful mass. This can be mistaken for an ectopic pregnancy. The corpus luteum will lie within the ovary, whereas an ectopic pregnancy as a rule lies outside the ovary. A search for the normal ovary should enable one to differentiate between ectopic pregnancy and a corpus luteum with hemorrhage.
2. *Rupture of Corpus Luteum.* The common features of a ruptured corpus luteum include the following:
   a. An adnexal mass with an irregular shape
   b. Cul-de-sac fluid
   c. Evidence of bleeding with development of a relatively echogenic mass of blood (hard to separate from the uterus)

   The ovary will lie in the center of this mass. This pattern may be indistinguishable from ruptured ectopic pregnancy. In both, a low-resistance Doppler pattern is seen within the mass.
3. *Ovarian Torsion.* If the ovary twists, it causes a great deal of pain. Usually there is some blood in the region of the ovary, and the ovary will be very tender and enlarged on endovaginal examination. If a cyst is present, it may well develop blood clot within.

⭐ PITFALLS

1. A *cervical pregnancy* and an *impending abortion* appear similar. If the pregnancy is aborting the sonographic findings will change rapidly and the patient will be bleeding.
2. *Pelvic adhesions.* Check in the upper abdomen if nothing is seen in the pelvis. If many adhesions are present in the pelvis, free fluid may only be seen in the lateral paracolic "gutters" or in the subhepatic space.
3. *Abdominal pregnancies.* Abdominal pregnancies are easily missed unless the empty uterus is recognized lying between the bladder and the pregnancy. Always look for myometrium surrounding the fluid and placenta in any pregnancy.

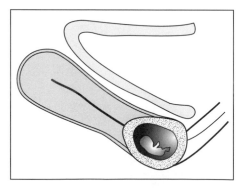

FIGURE 13-8. Cervical pregnancy. The gestational sac lies within the cervix. An impending abortion could have a similar appearance but would be in this site for a very short time, and the cervix would likely be open.

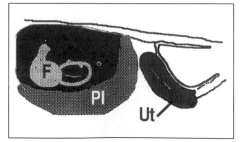

FIGURE 13-9. Abdominal pregnancy. The placenta, amniotic fluid, and fetus lie superior to the uterus which can be seen separately. The uterus is often very small and difficult to see.

4. *Decidual cast (reaction) versus gestational sac.* Many decidual casts have been mistaken for intrauterine pregnancies. The clue to the diagnosis of decidual cast is the absence of a double outline that is normally seen in an early intrauterine gestational sac.

5. *Cornual ectopic vs. eccentrically located normal pregnancy.* It is hard to distinguish these two entities since the normal gestational sac may be eccentrically located. A fibroid may displace the sac to one side. With a bicornuate uterus there will be an eccentric gestational sac position, but a second decidual reaction will be seen.

6. *Color flow Doppler.* Low-resistance Doppler flow can be found both with a corpus luteum with hemorrhage and with ectopic pregnancy. This finding is only helpful if the normal ovary has been located, a separate mass is seen, and flow is found within the mass.

？ WHERE ELSE TO LOOK

Empty Uterus With Positive Pregnancy Test

If the uterus appears normal but the pregnancy test is positive, look in the cul-de-sac and the adnexa for evidence of ectopic. If there is nothing to see the possibilities are (1) early pregnancy; (2) complete spontaneous abortion; or (3) ectopic pregnancy. Profuse vaginal bleeding favors complete spontaneous abortion.

SELECTED READING

Atri, M., Leduc, C., Gillett, P., Bret, P. M., Reinhold, C., Kintzen, G., Aldis, A., and Thibodeau, M. Role of endovaginal sonography in the diagnosis and management of ectopic pregnancy. *Radiographics* 16:755–774, 1996.

Brumsted, J. B. Managing ectopic pregnancy nonsurgically. *Contemp OB GYN* Mar:43–56, 1996.

Filly, R. A. Ectopic pregnancy: The role of sonography. *Radiology* 162:661–668, 1987.

Fleisher, A., et al. Ectopic pregnancy: Features at transvaginal sonography. *Radiology* 174:375–378, 1990.

Frates, M. C., and Laing, F. C. Sonographic evaluation of ectopic pregnancy: An update. *AJR* 165:251–259, 1995.

UNCERTAIN DATES

Elective Cesarean Section, Late Registration

ROGER C. SANDERS, NANCY SMITH MINER

14

SONOGRAM ABBREVIATIONS

Ce Cerebellum
CP Choroid plexus
CSP Cavum septi pellucidi

FH Frontal horns

GB Gallbladder

H Heart

K Kidneys

L Liver
LV Lateral ventricles

OH Occipital horns

P Peduncles (cerebellar)
PV Portal vein

St Stomach

Th Thalamus
TV Third ventricle

UV Umbilical vein

KEY WORDS

Amniocentesis. Procedure involving the insertion of a small needle into the amniotic cavity to obtain fluid for cytogenic or biochemical analysis.

Brachycephaly. Short, wide fetal head—a third-trimester normal variant.

Breech Presentation. The fetal head is situated at the fundus of the uterus (see Fig. 14-11).

Cephalic Presentation. The fetal head is the presenting part in the cervical area; also known as a vertex presentation (see Fig. 14-11).

DeLee's Test. The first time the fetal heart can be heard with the fetal stethoscope, usually at about 16 weeks' gestation.

Dolichocephaly. Long, flattened fetal head—a normal variant.

Ductus Venosus. Fetal vein that connects the umbilical vein to the inferior vena cava and runs at an oblique axis through the liver.

Face Presentation. The fetal face is the presenting part. This suboptimal position is more likely in a fetus that is lying on its back.

Gestational Age. As used with ultrasound studies, this term refers to the pregnancy age since the first day of the last menstrual period.

Gravid. Pregnant.

High-Risk Pregnancy (HRP). Pregnancy at high risk for an abnormal outcome. Typical examples of high-risk pregnancies are those that involve (1) maternal disease (e.g., kidney or heart disease); (2) maternal drug ingestion (e.g., alcohol or cigarettes); (3) a previous pregnancy with a small fetus; and (4) a family history of congenital malformations.

Hydrocephalus. Enlargement of the cerebral ventricles; can be associated with spina bifida.

Late Registration. A pregnant woman who first attends the obstetric clinic when she is 20 or more weeks pregnant is termed a late registrant. At this stage of pregnancy, clinical dating is difficult because several important dating landmarks have passed (e.g., quickening and the DeLee's test).

Menstrual Age. Age of the pregnancy calculated from the last menstrual period.

Microcephaly. Unduly small skull and brain. Associated with mental deficiency.

Para. Term used to describe how many pregnancies a woman has undergone and their outcome. The first number represents the total number of pregnancies. The second number represents the number of abortions. The third number indicates the total number of premature births. The fourth number shows the number of full-term pregnancies. For example, para 4112 represents four pregnancies, one abortion, one premature birth, and two full-term deliveries.

Quickening. The time when the mother first feels the baby move—about 16 to 18 weeks.

Shoulder Presentation. The fetal shoulder is the presenting part (see Fig. 14-11).

Transverse Lie. A fetus that is lying transversely so that head and trunk are at approximately the same level (see Fig. 14-11).

Umbilical Vein and Arteries. Vessels within the cord. There are two arteries and one vein.

Ventricular Outflow Tracts. Term used for a view showing the chambers of the heart and the aorta and a second view showing the pulmonary artery as it leaves the main chambers of the heart.

Vertex Presentation. The fetal head is the presenting part. This is the usual presentation; it can be face first or brow first (see Fig. 14-11).

 THE CLINICAL PROBLEM

Uncertain Dates

Pregnant women are often referred to ultrasound to confirm gestational age. One of the common reasons for referral is uncertainty about when the mother became pregnant. The mother (1) may be uncertain whether her last menstrual period was a genuine period; (2) may have a history of infrequent periods; or (3) may be a late registrant, first attending the clinic after dating landmarks such as the DeLee's test, quickening, and findings on the first trimester physical examination have already passed. A sonogram is also usually recommended to confirm the maternal dates when a woman has had a previous cesarean section. Another cesarean section is often performed with any subsequent pregnancy, and in such patients the gestational age must be accurately determined so that a cesarean section will not be performed too early, possibly resulting in a child with immature lungs.

Dating by ultrasound should take place before 28 weeks, because at a later stage in pregnancy, the biparietal diameter may vary within a 4-week range of possible dates. Ideally, a dating sonogram should be performed between 16 and 20 weeks so that the timely diagnosis of twins, fetal anomalies, or placenta previa can be made.

If an earlier sonogram is available, continue to date by those measurements. If dating is being performed for the first time after 28 weeks, be sure to issue a report that gives a range of possible dates (and weights) for a given measurement. Reporting by computer saves a lot of time because a date and a range of possible dates can be generated effortlessly without the tedium and possible inaccuracy associated with gathering the information from tables (see Appendixes).

Fetal Presentation

It can be difficult for the clinician to tell which part of the baby is going to be delivered first. Most babies are delivered head first (cephalic or vertex presentation). Others are delivered foot or bottom first (breech presentation). The latter is a much more dangerous mode of delivery and generally requires cesarean section. Other dangerous fetal positions are shoulder presentation and transverse lie. The sonographer should therefore make a point of mentioning the fetal position if a preliminary report is being issued.

If the fetus is lying on its back with the head presenting, this is known as a dorsoposterior fetal position. It is worthwhile mentioning that a fetus is in this position because there is a greater chance that this fetus will be difficult to deliver because the face is the presenting part.

The sonographer's preliminary report on an obstetric sonogram should include (1) fetal position; (2) number of fetuses; (3) placental position; (4) measurements of the biparietal diameter, femoral length, and abdominal and head circumference (after 16 weeks); and (5) whether evidence of fetal movement or fetal heart movement was observed. It is wise to document images that correspond with those suggested by ACR/AIUM/SOGU guidelines (see Appendix 35 and Fig. 14-1).

ANATOMY

The anatomy described in this chapter is limited to that required for a basic obstetric ultrasound exam.

In a basic exam, a series of transverse views of the fetus are obtained (see Fig. 14-1).

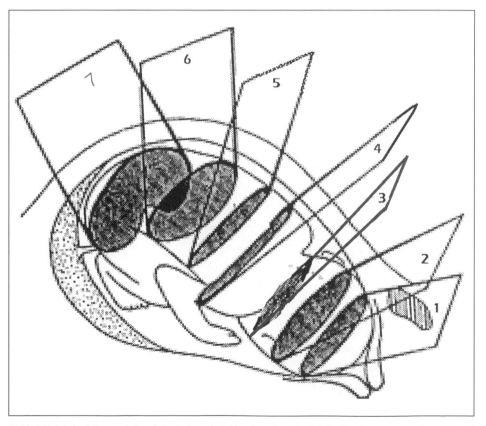

FIGURE 14-1. View of the fetus showing the levels at which the transverse images of the fetus are obtained to satisfy the ACR/AIUM/SOGU guidelines. Level 1 is obtained at the level of the lateral ventricles; level 2 at the level of the biparietal diameter; level 3 at the level of the cerebellum; level 4 at the level of the fetal heart; level 5 at the trunk circumference level; level 6 at the level of the fetal kidneys; and level 7 at the level of the lumbar spine and bladder.

Fetal Head

Cross-sectional anatomy of the fetal head should be defined at varying levels, starting at the level of the lateral ventricles (Fig. 14-2) and moving inferiorly (Figs. 14-3 and 14-4). Structures that should be routinely identified are the thalamus (see Fig. 14-3), the lateral ventricles (see Fig. 14-2), the third ventricle (see Fig. 14-3), the cavum septi pellucidi (see Fig. 14-3), the sylvian fissures (see Fig. 14-3), the cerebellar hemispheres (see Fig. 14-2), the vermis of the cerebellum, and the cisterna magna.

Abnormalities in the posterior fossa structures or enlargement of the ventricles raise suspicion of spinal abnormalities.

Fetal Chest

On either side of the heart one can see the fetal lungs, which are evenly echogenic but have a slightly different texture from the liver. The diaphragm can be seen as an interface between the liver and the lung (see Fig. 14-4). Fetal breathing with movement of the diaphragm is commonly present at approximately 24 weeks. The ribs cast acoustic shadows across the chest.

Fetal Heart

On this transverse section, a normal heart will occupy about one third of the chest, predominantly on the left side.

The four chambers of the fetal heart should be routinely identified on a four-chamber view (see Fig. 20-3).

The right and left ventricular outflow tract views (RVOT and LVOT) (Figs. 20-3 and 20-4) are useful additional views. If normal four-chamber and outflow tract views of the heart are obtained, most cardiac malformations can be excluded. A brief look to see whether the rhythm is regular and the rate normal is desirable.

Fetal Abdomen, Liver, Gallbladder, and Spleen

On a high transverse section of the fetal abdomen the liver, umbilical and left portal veins, stomach, aorta, adrenal glands, and spine should be visible (see Fig. 14-4).

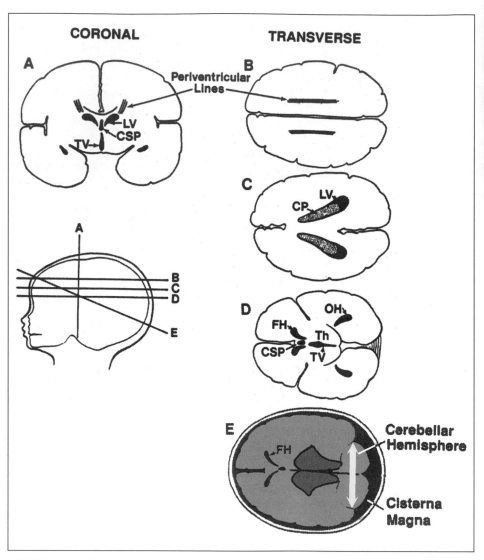

FIGURE 14-2. Series of normal transverse sections and coronal sections. On the coronal view A note the lateral ventricles (LV) with the cavi septi pellucidi (CSP) between them. The third ventricle (TV) is immediately inferior. The transverse B shows the periventricular lines that can be seen on the coronal view. These periventricular lines were for a time mistaken for the lateral ventricles. They actually represent a series of blood vessels which lie superior to the lateral ventricles. C is a section taken at the level of the lateral ventricles (LV). A choroid plexus (CP) can be seen within the lateral ventricles. Section D is taken at the level normally used for a biparietal diameter. One can see the cavum septi pellucidi (CSP), the frontal horns (FH), and the occipital horns (OH). The thalamus (Th) surrounds the third ventricle (TV). Section E, which is more oblique, is a section through the cerebellum and the front horns (FH). This is the section used to measure skin thickness, cerebellar width, and cisterna magna size (reprinted with permission by D. Nyberg).

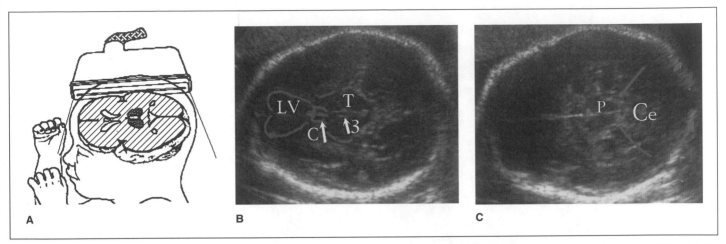

FIGURE 14-3. (A) Diagram showing the axial approach to obtaining views of the thalami (which is level D on the inset of Fig. 14-2). (B) Sonographic appearances: The thalamus (T) should have a diamond shape, and the third ventricle should be seen between them. The cavum septi pellucidi (C) is visible. Too much of the cerebellar vermis should not be visible for acceptable head circumference views. The occipito-frontal diameter is obtained at this level. The biparietal diameter should be taken from the near-side echoes to the inner aspect of the far-side echo (arrows)(LV = lateral ventricle). (C) Diagram C is taken at the level of the cerebellar peduncles (P). The cerebellum (Ce) is shown at the same level. This level gives an erroneous biparietal diameter.

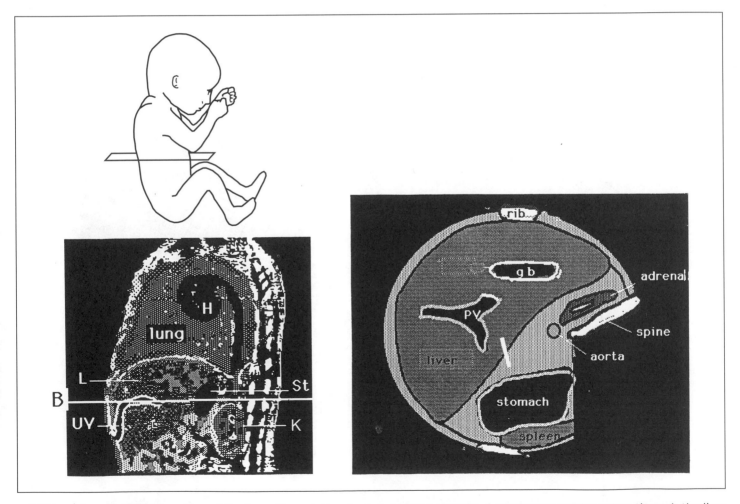

FIGURE 14-4. Longitudinal section of the fetus through the chest and abdomen (left). A transverse section taken through the liver (L) shows the aorta, stomach, and portal vein. Inset diagram (top) shows the level at which the trunk circumference is obtained. Trunk circumference view (right) shows the gallbladder (gb) the portal vein (PV), the adrenal gland, the aorta, and stomach, and symmetrically placed ribs if the view is of good quality. Shadowing behind the spine obliterates part of the abdominal outline.

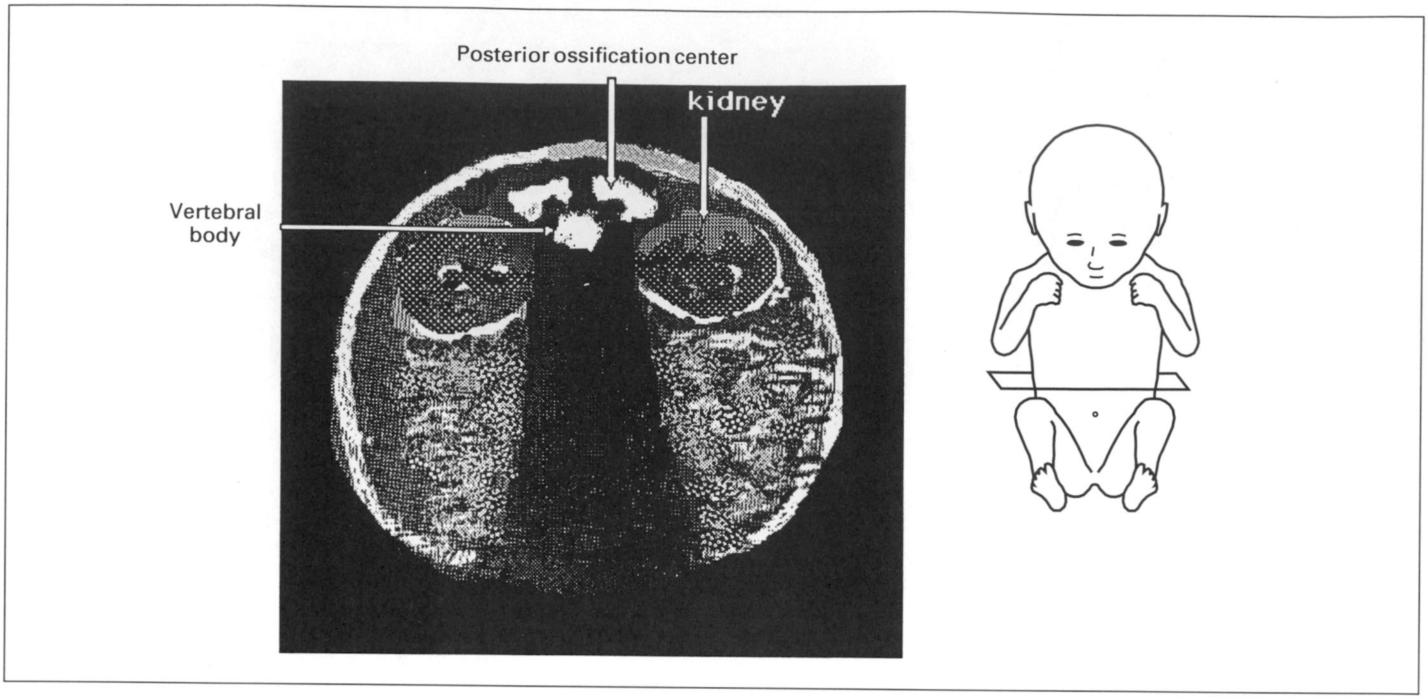

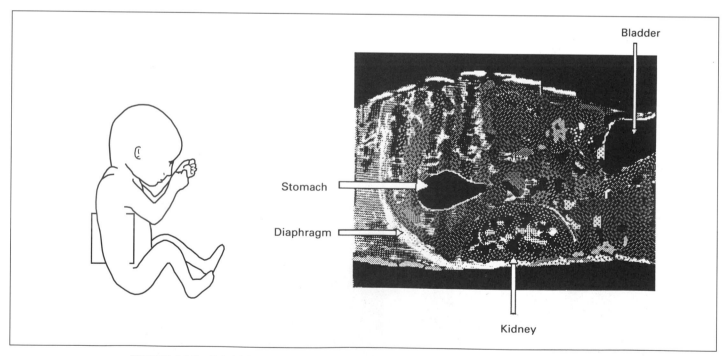

FIGURE 14-5. Transverse section through the kidneys showing the fetal spine.

FIGURE 14-6. Fetal kidneys. Long section of the fetus showing the fetal kidneys (arrow). The diaphragm, stomach, and bladder can also be seen.

The gallbladder can often be seen within the liver contour and may be confused with the umbilical vein. A fetal liver has the same homogeneous appearance as an adult liver. The liver edge can usually be delineated adjacent to fetal bowel.

The spleen may be visible on the side of the abdomen opposite the liver. The pancreas is hard to distinguish from the liver (see Fig. 14-4); often the vascular anatomy is the best clue to finding the fetal pancreas.

Kidney and Bladder

On lower transverse sections, the fetal kidneys can be seen (Fig. 14-5). They are paraspinous (see Fig. 14-6) and have a configuration similar to that of adult kidneys. A small degree of dilatation of the central sinus echoes is permissible as a normal variant. The dilatation is accepted as a normal variant if it is less than 5 mm and probably normal if it is between 5 and 10 mm.

At a still lower section, the fetal bladder should be recognizable (Fig. 14-7; see also Fig. 14-6). It empties and fills over the course of about an hour and is rarely completely empty.

While small bowel is echogenic, large bowel contains meconium, which can look echopenic or echogenic in the third trimester.

A fetal long-axis section that demonstrates the bladder, stomach, and heart is desirable (see Fig. 14-6).

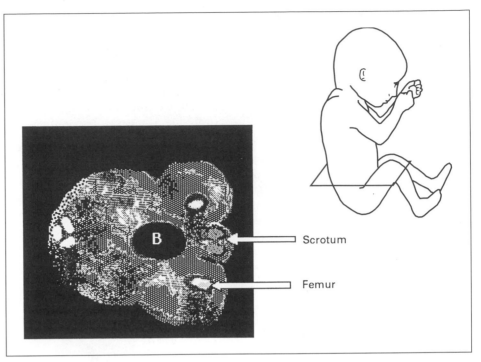

FIGURE 14-7. Transverse section through the level of the fetal bladder showing the scrotum and hips.

Genitalia

From 16 to 20 weeks on, the penis and scrotum can be made out (Fig. 14-8A and B). The testicles normally descend into the scrotum at 28 weeks. Females can be recognized by the labia with a linear echo from the vagina in between (Fig. 14-8C).

Most patients are anxious to know the fetal sex. We inform the parents of the fetal gender but say that there is a chance that we are wrong (even if we are certain).

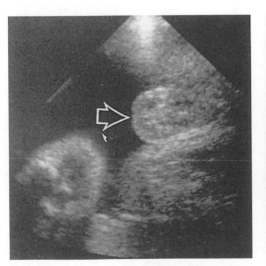
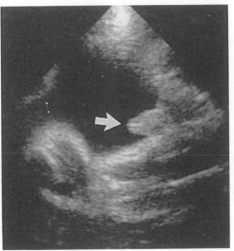
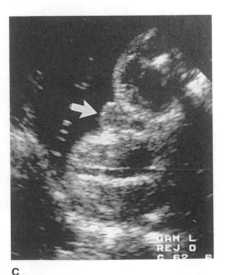

FIGURE 14-8. (A) View of the scrotum with two testicles present (arrow). **(B)** View of the penis (arrow). **(C)** View of the labia. The similarity between the labia and the scrotum can be seen (arrow); at times the labia are even more pronounced, owing to maternal hormonal stimulation.

The gender of the fetus can be important information from an obstetric point of view; there may be sex-linked chromosomal anomalies or a need to determine the type of twin. The fetal sex is often important to the parents, and not only from a planning point of view. Studies have shown that parents who see their baby on ultrasound undergo a sort of prenatal bonding experience, which can result in greater compliance with prenatal care. Problems that interfere with gender identification, such as swollen labia from maternal hormones or difficult fetal lie, should be carefully explained to the parents to temper their expectations.

Bones

The upper arm and thigh (femur), which contain single bones, generate only a single linear echo, whereas the distal limbs generate two parallel linear echoes. Bones are seen as echogenic lines with acoustic shadowing (Fig. 14-9).

Individual digits can be counted reliably from about 16 weeks' gestational age, earlier in ideal patients. Soft tissues can be seen around the bones, and some epiphyses can be seen. Cartilaginous structures such as the femoral head are visible (Fig. 14-10).

Visualization of the distal femoral epiphysis, the proximal humeral epiphysis, and the proximal tibial epiphysis is used to aid dating (see Fig. 14-10 and Appendix 21).

Fetal Spine

Although a comprehensive examination is not required by the ACR/AIUM/SOGU guidelines, it is imperative to take a good look at the spine. To rule out spina bifida, serial transverse views must be obtained of the entire spine. On a transverse view of the fetal spine, three echogenic structures that form a complete ring can be seen. These are the posterior elements and the posterior ossification center of the vertebrae. On long-axis views, two of the three ossification centers, the posterior ossification center of the vertebrae, and the posterior elements are seen. On a coronal view, both posterior elements can be seen by 12 weeks. The posterior elements are composed partly of the pedicles and partly of the lamina. The bony ring formed by these ossification centers contains the spinal canal. The spinal cord may be seen within the spinal canal and can be traced to about the level of L2. It is more echopenic than the other contents of the spinal canal. The normal spine has a gentle curve forward in the thoracic area and a posterior bend in the sacral region on the longitudinal view. The fetal spine widens slightly in the cervical and lumbar areas.

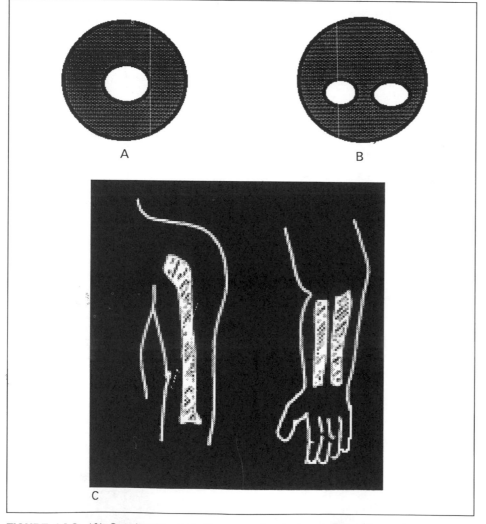

FIGURE 14-9. (**A**) Section through the arm showing a single echogenic area from bone. (**B**) Section through a distal arm showing two echogenic areas. (**C**) On the left, a single bone limb, the humerus, is shown, and on the right, a two-boned limb, the forearm (the radius and ulna), is shown.

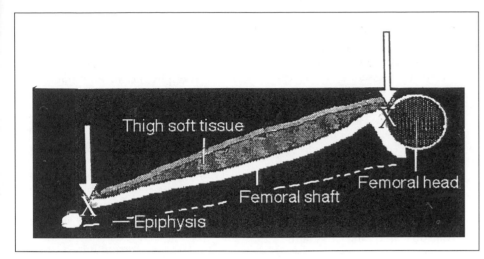

FIGURE 14-10. View of the femur. The femoral length is measured along the shaft from X to X (arrows). The cartilagenous femoral head can be seen. The hook at the proximal end of the femur is now considered to represent the undersurface of the femoral head rather than the greater trochanter. Note the epiphysis at the distal end of the femur (white dot). This structure first appears at 22 weeks. The soft tissue on the underside of the femur is dotted in. It is normally shadowed out by the femoral bone.

Amniotic Fluid

The amount of amniotic fluid varies with the gestational age, so no single measurement can be used throughout pregnancy. The amniotic fluid index (AFI) is a crude method of quantifying amniotic fluid. The uterine cavity is divided into quadrants and the vertical depth of the largest fluid pocket is measured. Values between 10 and 20 are considered normal—the normal values vary with gestational age, however (see Appendix 26 and Chapter 19). There should be a lot of fluid in the second trimester and a steadily lessening amount in the third trimester, so not much is present at term.

If the only fluid present is a pocket of less than 2 cm, this is abnormal at any stage of pregnancy. A pocket of more than 8 cm indicates polyhydramnios.

Placenta

The placenta is discussed in Chapter 15. The placental site should be mentioned, but prior to 20 weeks it may appear to cover the cervix. The placental position changes as the pregnancy proceeds, and most such pregnancies are normal. We therefore use the phrase "covers the cervix" rather than "placenta previa" in a preliminary report before 20 weeks so we do not cause needless alarm.

If the placenta is covering the cervix prior to 20 weeks, we recommend a further sonogram at 24 to 26 weeks to make sure it has shifted position.

 TECHNIQUE

Bonding

A sonogram is a powerful experience for a pregnant woman and should, if possible, be shared with the father. The mother and the father appreciate, often for the first time, that a little person lies within. Once it is determined that the fetus is sonographically normal, the maternal feelings induced by the sonogram should be reinforced by showing the mother the heart, limbs, genitalia, and other structures. If an abortion is planned, we do not recommend that the patient view the fetal anatomy unless the patient insists. If an anomaly is found, we do not show the mother the details of the abnormality until we are as clear as possible about the diagnosis and have contacted the referring physician.

Giving the Patient a Picture

Most patients request a picture of the fetus. We believe the psychological benefit in giving them an image of the profile, the genitalia, or the hand far outweighs any legal hazard.

Allowing the patient to watch the realtime as the sonogram is being performed enhances the bonding process.

Videotaping

Many patients request that a videotape of the obstetric sonogram be made. Some institutions do not permit videotaping because they fear that the videotape will be used as evidence, were there to be a malpractice suit. Our practice is to perform a standard obstetric study first. If the sonogram is normal the *doctor* videotapes selected areas at the end of the study. If the sonogram is abnormal and termination or still birth is a possibility, we do not provide a videotape because we feel that repeated viewing of the tape may exacerbate the grieving process.

Endovaginal Approach

A complete fetal survey can be performed with the vaginal probe with a pregnancy that is less than 15 weeks; this is particularly helpful in obese patients.

We prefer to use the endovaginal approach as a primary imaging technique in fetuses that are less than 14 weeks in age.

While such exams are increasingly commonplace, they are sometimes unexpectedly invasive for the patient, and she may be ill at ease. It is appropriate (if sometimes inconvenient) to have a female in the room, at least during insertion of the probe.

Gel is placed on the transducer, then a sterile condom is placed over it and fastened on with a rubber band. Further instructions for ensuring sterile technique are discussed in Chapter 56.

The patient should be instructed to empty her bladder *before* she gets on the table. Because so much manipulation of the transducer is necessary to see all of the anatomy, these exams are much more easily accomplished on a lithotomy table. If one is not available, it is usually necessary to build up the patient's hips with pillows or towels; this creates enough space to angle the transducer up or down as needed. The patient's knees are also dropped to allow movement from side to side, visualizing the adnexae. To demonstrate the cervix, the transducer is pulled out until it comes into view.

Linear Versus Sector Transducer

Linear arrays that allow one to place two images alongside each other are helpful for obstetric work. A composite long view of the fetus can be created. Sector scans are less desirable because the pie-shaped image cuts off the near field, and there may be some distortion of measurements. Curved linear views combine the virtues of both approaches.

Patient Preparation

It is not necessary to have the bladder full prior to starting a study unless the pregnancy is under 20 weeks. A sector scan taken on a patient with a full bladder may make you suspect a placenta previa when none is present. However, the bladder may need to be filled if an important fetal structure such as the head is low in the pelvis and not seen well. The patient's bladder should be empty or only slightly full before an endovaginal exam.

Routine Approach

The following is the suggested routine when examining women with an apparently normal pregnancy. Bear in mind, however, that when a sonogenic view of the spine rolls by, or the fetus waves at you—affording a lovely view of five normal fingers and a photo-op for mom—*freeze it and photograph it.* You may not get another chance. Conversely, don't waste time sticking to a routine if the fetus refuses to cooperate. Come back later.

1. Sweep first. A quick scan through the uterus to check for gross pathology and fetal viability allows you to set the tone for how much to share the exam with the patient and family.

2. Lower uterine segment. Do it early, before the bladder fills, potentially distorting the cervical length or its relationship to the placental margin. Include the presenting fetal part.
3. Long-axis and transverse views of the spine, if the fetus is in a convenient position. This localizes the fetus for the axial views to follow.
4. The head (it may not be as easy to view later in the exam).
5. Transverse views of the chest to show a four-chamber view.
6. The trunk circumference view, making sure to include the stomach.
7. Transverse and long views of the kidneys.
8. Views of the cord insertion.
9. Bladder views (long view to include the stomach, heart, and diaphragm).
10. Femur views and evidence that all four extremities are present.
11. A sweep through the entire fetus and an informal biophysical profile.
12. Views of the placental site and amniotic fluid volume.

Fetal Lie

Demonstrate the fetal position by taking a view that shows the fetal head and the maternal bladder if there is a vertex (head first) position. The term *cephalic presentation* may be preferable because it doesn't imply whether the face or the back of the head is coming first. If the fetus is foot or bottom first (breech) or in an oblique position, take a view that shows the lower uterine segment and the presenting fetal structures (Fig. 14-11).

Lower Uterine Segment

Sector scan views of the lower uterine segment in the midline are helpful. If the maternal bladder is empty, the relationship of a low-lying placenta to the cervix can be shown and the presence of a placenta previa established.

A post-void view of the normal cervix and vagina should be obtained. The normal cervical length is 3.5 cm or more. Translabial or endovaginal views of the cervix are now routinely performed in many institutions since they give a superior view of the placenta/cervix relationship and show whether or not cervical incompetence is present (Figs. 15-4–15-6).

Spine

Localize the spine next. Many views such as those of the kidneys and the truck circumference require knowledge of how the spine lies for orientation.

1. It may be impossible to get the entire spine on a single cut if the fetus is curled. Dual or "long" linear array views may be used for the long axis.
2. The iliac crests may conceal the sacrum. Views from a more dorsal approach are needed for this area. Inclusion of the iliac crests on the transverse view is evidence that the scan was obtained in the lumbosacral region.
3. If possible, get prone long-axis views of the fetus that show the skin covering over the spine—this is a good way to show subtle myelomeningoceles. The skin over the lumbar spine must be demonstrated from a sagittal posterior aspect for this approach to be useful. This image must be pursued if an abnormal cerebellum suggests spinal pathology.
4. Transverse views showing the relationships of the posterior elements to the vertebral body should be obtained at several sites in the lumbosacral area and at several sites in the abdomen and chest. Show some other anatomy, such as the iliac crest or kidneys, so the level can be recognized later (see Figs. 14-5 and 14-6).
5. Coronal views obtained in a long axis, from the side of the fetus, are an excellent way of showing widening of the spinal canal. This view is especially valuable if the fetus is in a supine position. Check to make sure there is an equal amount of soft tissue on either side of the spine to ensure that you are in the best plane.

Four-Chamber View

Once the spine is localized, turn the transducer 90 degrees at the level of the heart and record an image documenting four chambers and the interventricular septum. The septum between the atria doesn't always look intact on still images because the foramen ovale is flipping in and out of the left atrium; watch this on real-time. The cine loop option is very helpful in finding the optimal image on this view.

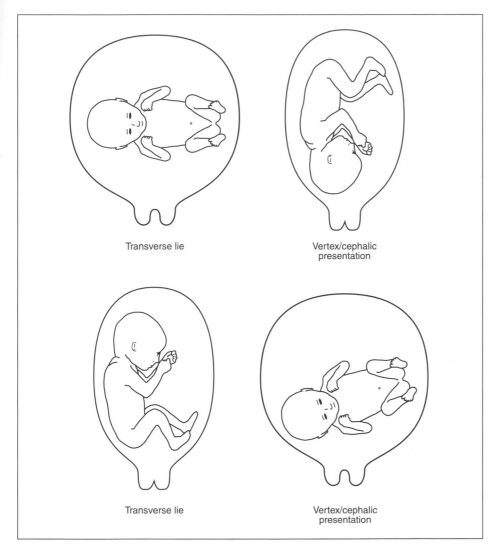

Transverse lie

Vertex/cephalic presentation

Transverse lie

Vertex/cephalic presentation

FIGURE 14-11. Diagram of different fetal positions. A fetus in breech position can have its legs extended or flexed. This information is helpful to the referring obstetrician. To determine the situs of the fetal organs, use the following rule: If the fetal head is down and fetal back is to the left, the left side of the fetus (stomach, heart) is down. Conversely, if the fetal head is up (breech) and the fetal back is to the mother's right, the right side of the fetus is up. If the fetal head is up and the fetal back is to the left, the left side is up.

Limbs

Once the proximal femur is found below the iliac crest, rotate the transducer so the rest of the bone is lined up. Use the same technique for other bones. In a dating series, all that is required are images that show there are four extremities. If possible, demonstrate both feet and hands.

Always start from a known landmark in the trunk and work outward through the femur or humerus. The lower leg can easily be mistaken for the forearm.

Amniotic Fluid

Document the largest pocket of amniotic fluid by taking two views of it at right angles. Look for evidence of internal echoes or septa within the amniotic fluid. Views across the short axis of the fetus and the fluid pocket in true transverse and longitudinal planes show the fluid amount. Oblique views may be misleading. A view that shows all four limbs extending into the amniotic fluid is useful evidence that all four limbs exist and that the fluid quantity is normal or increased.

Placenta

Document the placental site, size, and texture by taking views at right angles that show its maximal extent. A long-axis view of the lower segment of the uterus and cervix shows placental maturation and placental relationship to the cervix.

If the placenta appears to obscure the cervix, repeat this view with an empty bladder. If it is still unclear whether the placenta relates to the cervix, place a probe on the labia and examine the cervix through the vagina (see Chapter 15).

Cord

Take a short-axis view of the cord that shows whether there are two or three vessels (Color Plate 14-1). If the cord is very twisted, it may be difficult to decide whether there are one or two arteries present. Look with color flow for pulsating arteries on either side of the bladder within the fetus. If the cord is uncoiled, take an image. A noncoiled cord is a nonspecific indicator that the fetus is at increased risk for perinatal morbidity and mortality. If amniocentesis is being performed, show the cord's entrance site into the placenta.

Take a view of the cord insertion.

Truncal Views

Once the spine has been plotted out, it is easy to take transverse views at the level of the stomach, kidneys, bladder (see Fig. 14-7), heart, and trunk circumference (see Figs. 14-4 through 14-7). If the stomach is not seen, come back and try later. Some fluid should be visualized in a normal fetal stomach during the course of an exam. When the kidney view is taken, try to slide the transducer to a position where the spine's shadow does not obscure the second kidney. Turn the transducer at right angles and take a longitudinal view that shows the diaphragm, stomach, and bladder, if possible, on a single view (see Fig. 14-6).

Gut extending through the fetal anterior abdominal wall, a normal finding until about 11 weeks, can confuse the long-axis image. In early pregnancy, the fetal anatomy is poorly seen. One should measure the longest length on a view that shows the fetal heart. Don't include the yolk sac in the measurement. Very small fetuses may lie adjacent to the yolk sac. Always do more than one measurement to find the longest one, and use the system's electronic calipers.

Measurements to Perform

Critical obstetric management decisions hinge on accurate measurements, so be certain that the system is properly calibrated.

Crown-Rump Length

In a dating examination performed in the first trimester, the crown-rump length is the optimal method of establishing fetal age (Fig. 14-12).

This measurement is performed using a real-time system by finding the longest axis of the rapidly moving fetus. This value can be obtained between approximately 5 and 12 weeks quite easily. (See Appendixes 4 and 5.)

Cerebellar View (Posterior Fossa)

An inferiorly angled view to show the cerebellar hemispheres (useful in excluding spina bifida) will also, if obtained at 18 weeks, show the skin thickening around the neck that is seen in Down syndrome (Fig. 14-13).

Now required by the guidelines, this is an essential screening view. Be sure to include the shape of the cerebellar lobes, and try to demonstrate the cisterna magna.

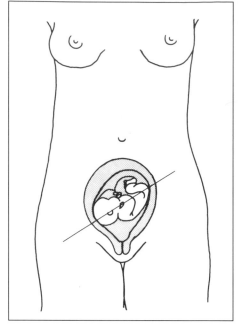

FIGURE 14-12. Diagram showing the way in which the crown-rump length is measured with real time.

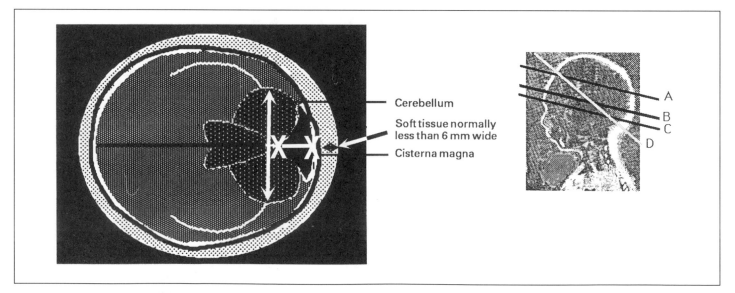

Cerebellum

Soft tissue normally less than 6 mm wide

Cisterna magna

FIGURE 14-13. Angled view of the cerebellum (level D) showing the cerebellar hemispheres. The thickness of the soft tissue at the back of the neck should not be greater than 6 mm. If it is over 6 mm, one should be concerned about Down syndrome. Note the cisterna magna adjacent to the cerebellar hemispheres, which must be seen as a fluid-filled structure to be considered normal. The cisterna magna should not measure more than 9 mm (white X's). The transcerebellar distance (white arrow) in millimeters is equivalent to a gestational age in weeks, up to about 26 weeks.

The transcerebellar diameter can be used as a dating technique. The diameter in millimeters corresponds to the gestational age throughout the first 26 weeks of pregnancy.

This image is easy to obtain once the transducer is positioned for a biparietal diameter by angling the posterior aspect of the transducer inferiorly on the fetal head. The cisterna magna should be photographed on this view. It should not measure more than 9 mm.

Dating Measurements

Biparietal Diameter

For dating after 12 weeks, the biparietal diameter is used (see Appendix 9). Find the cervical spine as it enters the head at its widest point. Place the transducer at right angles to this axis and adjust the angulation of the transducer so that it is at a right angle to the midline echo. Take images at the level of the thalami (see Figs. 14-2 and 14-3), which are recognizable as hypoechoic, blunted, diamond-shaped structures in the center of the brain. Structures visible at the desirable level include the thalamus, the third ventricle, and the cavum septi pellucidi (see Fig. 14-3). Do not take a biparietal measurement at the level of the two lines parallel to the midline (see Fig. 14-2A and B), which were formerly thought to represent the lateral ventricles and which have now been shown to represent venous structures. Make sure to obtain the ovoid shape that is desirable. Measurements are made from the outer side of the near skull to the inner side of the distal skull echoes.

Accuracy with this technique is ±1 week prior to 20 weeks and ±10 days until about 28 weeks. Beyond this point, accuracy diminishes to ±2 to 4 weeks; therefore, dating by biparietal diameter measurement alone is undesirable after about 28 weeks (see Appendix 9).

A ratio of the biparietal diameter to the longest distance from the front of the head to the back of the head (occipitofrontal diameters; see Fig. 14-3) is useful in the diagnosis of dolichocephaly. This normal variant—a long, flattened fetal head in the third trimester—produces erroneous biparietal diameters. The normal ratio is 0.74 ± 0.08 (see Appendix 10).

An unduly wide head (brachycephaly) is less frequently seen and is also usually of little significance.

Head Circumference

The head circumference is obtained from a good biparietal image that shows the thalamus, third ventricle, and falx and does not show the cerebellum (see Appendixes 7 and 8). If the vermis of the cerebellum or the cerebellar hemispheres are visible, the section is too steeply angled (see Figs. 14-2 and 14-3). If the fetal head is deep in the pelvis or if the face is looking in the direction of the transducer, it may be difficult or impossible to obtain a head circumference, although a biparietal diameter is usually possible.

Changing the maternal position may allow visualization. Use of the endovaginal probe approach is helpful with a vertex presentation.

Measure around the perimeter of the skull, including the bone but *not* fetal hair and scalp. Use the electronic ellipse or track ball if possible; always move the posterior caliper from the inside of the cranium to the outside before taking circumference measurements. If the system only allows for diameter measurements, measure the diameter from outside to outside and then move to a right-angle position and repeat the measurement. Average the two measurements and use this with the formula πD.

Femoral Length

The femoral length is an additional method of estimating gestational age. Overall, it is a slightly more accurate predictor of age than the biparietal diameter. Tables of normal values are available (see Appendix 11). The lateral and medial aspects of the femur have different appearances. The lateral aspect is straight, whereas the medial aspect is curved. If a femur length is obtained from the medial surface, the femur may be thought to be bowed.

To ensure that one has the longest femoral length, measurements should be taken along an axis that shows both the round, echopenic, cartilaginous femoral head and the femoral condyles (see Fig. 14-10). A portion of the femoral condyle may be ossified as the distal femoral epiphysis. Angle to show the entire femoral shaft. It is easy to underestimate length, so take more than one measurement. Measure the straight lateral surface rather than the bowed medial surface. Noting the date of first appearance of condyles can be used as a dating technique (see Appendix 21). The distal femoral epiphyses are visible after 32 weeks. The proximal tibial epiphysis becomes visible at around 35 weeks and can also be used for dating purposes.

The proximal humeral epiphysis appears so late that its appearance has a good correlation with fetal lung maturity.

Abdominal Circumferences (or Diameter)

The abdominal circumference (see Fig. 14-4) is usually used for detecting intrauterine growth retardation (IUGR) (see Chapter 16), as well as for dating the fetus (see Appendixes 12 through 14).

For further details, see Chapter 16.

Femoral Length/Abdominal Circumference Ratio

The femoral length/abdominal circumference ratio is 22 and is constant from 22 weeks on. It may be of help in the diagnosis of fetuses with the long, lean type of IUGR.

Dating With Other Measurements

Tables exist that allow one to obtain the gestational age from the size of numerous other parts of the body, such as the orbits, foot, and clavicle. These measurements are useful if only a small segment of the fetus can be seen or much of the fetus is abnormal (see Appendixes 2 and 17 through 20).

✳ PITFALLS

1. An inaccurate *biparietal diameter* is obtained if
   a. the biparietal diameter is not taken at the level of the thalamus and cavum septi pellucidi.
   b. the head is round (brachycephalic) or flattened (dolichocephalic) rather than ovoid.
   c. the head measurement is taken at a point where the distance between one side of the skull and the midline is not the same as the other side and is asymmetrical.
   d. the measurement is first obtained in the third trimester when there is a wide variation of dates for any given measurement.
   e. the measurement is taken inferior to the thalamus at the level of the cerebellar peduncles and cerebellar hemispheres (see Figs. 14-2 and 14-3).
2. The *crown-rump length* is inaccurate if
   a. it is obtained after 12 weeks.
   b. no persistent effort is made to find the longest length by varying the transducer axis.
   c. the yolk sac is included in the length measurement.
3. The *femoral length* may be erroneous if
   a. it is really the humerus that is being measured.
   b. only one length is obtained.
   c. a sector scanner is used at an oblique axis or with the femur in the far field.
   d. the measurement is faulty because the calipers were put at the wrong site.
   e. too much gain is used or abnormal ossification occurs at the distal end of the femur.
4. The *head circumference* will be underestimated if
   a. too steep an axis is used so that the cerebellum is prominent.
   b. the measurement line does not follow the external borders of the head outline.
5. The *biparietal diameter in the third trimester is less than caliper measurements at birth* because of the measurement site used and because the assumed speed of sound is slightly slower than it really is—1540 m/sec versus 1610 m/sec.
6. Failure to check the *calibration system* may lead to incorrect measurements. Wrong measurements can have serious clinical and legal consequences. Fortunately, modern digital systems rarely vary.
7. By *not using the calipers* on screen that were incorporated into the system, it is easy to mismeasure the image by 1 cm.
8. Using the *wrong nomogram* for the measurement technique employed will yield erroneous dates. The technique used in the creation of the measurement tables for dating must be used. For example, different biparietal diameter measurement sites, such as outer table to outer table of the skull, have been used in different tables.

❓ WHERE ELSE TO LOOK

1. If the biparietal diameter and femoral length do not indicate the same fetal age, perform the measurements suggested for IUGR (see Chapter 16).
2. If the biparietal diameter is less than expected, consider the possibility of microcephalus by looking at the head circumference/abdominal circumference ratio. Check the intraorbital distance and look for ventriculomegaly.
3. If the biparietal diameter is more than expected, make sure that hydrocephalus is not present (see Chapter 18) and look for evidence of IUGR (see Chapter 16).
4. If the femoral length is too short, consider the possibility of dwarfism (see Chapter 18):
   a. Check the length of the humerus, tibia, fibula, radius, and ulna.
   b. Count the number of digits, and look at the hand and feet position.
   c. Look at the ratio of abdomen to chest size; it should be greater than .87.
   d. Examine the head and spine for the appearances described in Chapter 18.
5. If the femur is too long or too short, check the size of the mother and father to see whether they are short or tall.
6. If the abdominal circumference is unusually large relative to other measurements later in pregnancy, consider diabetes mellitus. Look for scalp edema and skin thickening, and ask the patient whether she is diabetic or there is a family history of diabetes.
7. If no fetal movement or fetal breathing is seen, do a biophysical profile (see Chapter 19).
8. If the fetal head is unduly large relative to other measurements and dates and there is no hydrocephalus, perform views of the orbits, hands, and feet. There may be a chromosomal anomaly present. Hand, foot, and face problems are common with chromosomal anomalies. Check the maternal and paternal head size. Familial large head is common.
9. If the measurement data are less than expected, perform a biophysical profile and use the protocol suggested for IUGR (see Chapter 16).

SELECTED READING

Bowerman, R. A., and DiPietro, M. A. Erroneous sonographic identification of fetal lateral ventricles: Relationship to the echogenic periventricular "blush." *AJNR* 8:661–664, 1987.

Callen, P. W. (Ed.). *Ultrasonography in Obstetrics and Gynecology* (2nd ed.). Philadelphia: Saunders, 1994.

Chinn, D. H., Callen, P. W., and Filly, R. A. The lateral cerebral ventricle in early second trimester. *Radiology* 148:529–531, 1983.

Craig, M. Family-centered sonography. *Journal of Diagnostic Medical Ultrasound* 2:96–103, 1986.

Gardberg, M., and Tuppurainen, M. Dorsoposterior fetal position near term—a sonographic finding worth noting? *Acta Obstet Gynecol Scan* 74:402–403, 1995.

Hearn-Stebbins, B. Normal fetal growth assessment: A review of literature and current practice. *JDMS* 11:176–187, 1995.

Lea, J. H. Psychosocial progression through normal pregnancy. *J Diag Med Sonography* 1:55–58, 1985.

Shepard, M., and Filly R. A. A standardized plane for biparietal diameter measurement. *J Ultrasound Med* 1:145–150, 1982.

Strong, T. H., Elliott, J. P., and Rudin, T. S. Noncoiled umbilical blood vessels. A new marker for the fetus at risk. *Obstet Gynecol* 81:409–411, 1993.

15

SECOND AND THIRD TRIMESTER BLEEDING

ROGER C. SANDERS

SONOGRAM ABBREVIATIONS

Bl   Bladder

FH   Fetal head
FT   Fetal trunk

M   Myometrium

Pl   Placenta

Re   Rectum

T   Transducer
Tu   Tumor

V   Vagina

KEY WORDS

Abruptio Placentae (Accidental Hemorrhage). Bleeding that occurs when the placenta separates from the uterine wall. A serious condition that threatens the life of the fetus and the mother. It is usually seen by the sonographer only when it is relatively mild; other cases go straight to the operating room.

Amnion. The membrane that lines the fluid cavity (amniotic cavity) within the uterus in pregnancy.

Amniotic Sac Membrane. This membrane surrounds the amniotic fluid. It is not normally seen sonographically after the first trimester, except when the separation between two amniotic sacs is visualized in a multiple pregnancy.

Cervix. Most inferior segment of the uterus. It is more than 3.5 cm long during a normal pregnancy, but decreases (effaces) in length during labor (see Fig. 15-1).

Cesarean Section (C-section). Operation performed to deliver a fetus. An incision is made transversely in the lower anterior wall of the uterus. In a "classic" cesarean section, the incision is made vertically at the fundus of the uterus.

Chorionic Plate. Term used to describe the interface between the amniotic fluid and the placenta.

Circumvallate Placenta. A rim develops around the placental edge. This condition is thought to be associated with bleeding at delivery.

Double Set-Up. Examination performed by an obstetrician on a patient with a suspected placenta previa. Owing to the risk of placental rupture, the examination is performed in the operating room so that a cesarean section can be done immediately if necessary.

Effaced. The cervix becomes shortened towards the end of labor. When it is very thinned out and there is a lot of fluid within the internal os, it is known as effaced.

Infarct of the Placenta. Loss of tissue blood supply due to arterial occlusion.

Low-Lying Placenta. The inferior edge of the placenta is close to but does not cover the inner aspect of the cervical os.

Marginal Placenta Previa. The edge of the placenta is at the margin of the internal os.

Migration. Term used to describe the apparent shift in position of the placenta from the cervical to the fundal area that often occurs during the course of pregnancy.

Myometrium. The muscle that forms the wall of the uterus.

Oligohydramnios. Too little amniotic fluid for a given pregnancy stage.

Os. Term used to describe the upper (internal) and lower (external) entrances to the cervical canal (see Fig. 15-1).

Partial Placenta Previa. The internal os is just covered by the placenta.

Placenta Percreta. In placenta percreta the placenta extends through the myometrium. The placenta burrows into the myometrium, causing an unduly firm attachment that bleeds at delivery since it does not separate normally.

Placenta Previa (Total). The placenta completely covers the internal os.

Polyhydramnios. Too much amniotic fluid for a given pregnancy stage.

Ripening. As the cervix softens and the internal and external os dilate close to the end of pregnancy, the cervix is said to be ripening.

Succenturiate Lobe. Anomaly in which the placenta is divided into two segments that are connected by blood vessels. The second lobe may be so small that it is overlooked sonographically. This anomaly occurs in less than 1% of cases.

Vasa Previa. The umbilical cord vessels as they enter the placenta are the presenting part of the internal os.

Velamentous Insertion. The cord bifurcates before reaching the placenta and lies within a membrane. Especially common in twins.

◆>> **THE CLINICAL PROBLEM**

Vaginal bleeding in the second or third trimester is an ominous clinical sign. Although such bleeding may be due to unimportant conditions such as cervical erosions or vaginal piles, it may signify placenta previa or abruptio placentae.

Placenta Previa

In placenta previa the placenta covers the internal os of the cervix and bleeds because the placenta has separated from the myometrium. When the placenta covers the cervix (total placenta previa), cesarean section is necessary because vaginal delivery would endanger the fetus. Unless a double set-up has been prepared, a pelvic examination is avoided because it may provoke bleeding. With lesser degrees of placenta previa vaginal delivery may be attempted. Ultrasound is the best noninvasive method of establishing a diagnosis of placenta previa (Color Plate 15-1).

Abruptio Placentae

Although abruptio placentae is about as common in clinical practice as placenta previa, ultrasonic examinations may not be performed because many patients with abruptio placentae are taken straight to the operating room as a clinical emergency. The primary event is a bleed between the placenta and the uterine wall, but blood also frequently enters the amniotic cavity, where it can be visualized sonographically. Abruptio may be present, yet not visualized sonographically.

ANATOMY

Placenta

In the second trimester the placenta is evenly echogenic with a smooth, well-defined border marginated by the chorionic plate. An irregular border and textural changes often occur in the third trimester (see Placental Maturation in Chapter 16).

Echopenic areas in the placenta in a subchorionic location are a normal finding. Venous lakes, which are echo-free areas, may show flow with real-time. Alternatively, echopenic areas may represent deposits of a material known as Wharton's jelly, of no pathologic significance.

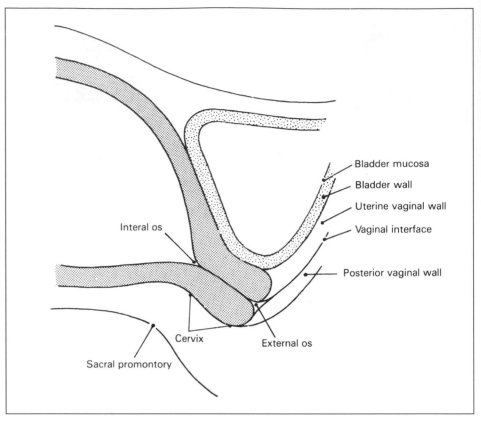

FIGURE 15-1. Diagram showing the cervix and surrounding structures.

Vagina and Cervix

The vagina can be seen transabdominally as an echogenic line with echo-free walls. It ends at the cervix. The internal os, external os, and cervical canal can be seen within the cervix (Fig. 15-1).

These structures are best examined with the endovaginal probe, but may often be well seen using the translabial approach. Occasionally, they can be seen adequately on a postvoid transabdominal view.

Cord

The cord normally comprises three vessels—two small arteries and one large vein (see Color Plate 14-1). About 2% of the time there are only two vessels, with one of the arteries missing. There is an increased incidence of fetal abnormalities when there are only two vessels.

Amniotic Fluid

Amniotic fluid is produced by the mother until between 15 and 18 weeks. After that it is produced by the fetus. The fetus swallows the fluid, absorbs it, and excretes it through the kidneys. If the fetus cannot swallow, polyhydramnios develops. If the fetus cannot urinate, oligohydramnios occurs. There is a steady reduction in amniotic volume as the pregnancy proceeds. Fluid volume is maximal between 20 and 30 weeks. In the third trimester, small particles known as vernix can be seen in the normal amniotic fluid.

◾ **TECHNIQUE**

Filled Bladder and Uterus

Between 16 and 20 weeks, pregnant women are optimally examined with the maternal bladder full. Beyond 20 weeks, the fetus usually lies at a sufficiently high level that a full bladder is unnecessary. Prior to approximately 13 to 14 weeks, the fetal examination is best performed using the endovaginal approach, which requires an empty bladder.

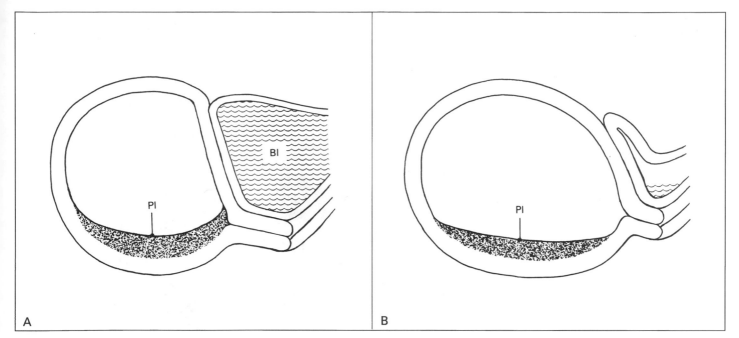

FIGURE 15-2. Overdistended bladder and placenta previa. (**A**) An overdistended bladder may compress the anterior wall of the uterus against the posterior wall, causing an appearance resembling a placenta previa. (**B**) With the bladder empty, the true length of the cervix is seen; the placenta ends above the cervix.

If the placenta extends into the lower uterine segment, demonstrate the vagina and cervix with the bladder empty (Fig. 15-2) because there may be a placenta previa. Only with the bladder empty can you be sure the cervix is not artificially lengthened from being squashed by the distended bladder (see Fig. 15-2). The axis of the vagina and cervix may not be longitudinal, and oblique sections may be required to show this critical relationship. If the placenta appears to lie adjacent to the cervix, scan transversely at right angles to see whether the placenta is centrally located or whether it lies to one side of the cervix and lower uterine segment (Fig. 15-3). This relationship is easy to determine if the fetus is breech, but more difficult with a cephalic (vertex) presentation.

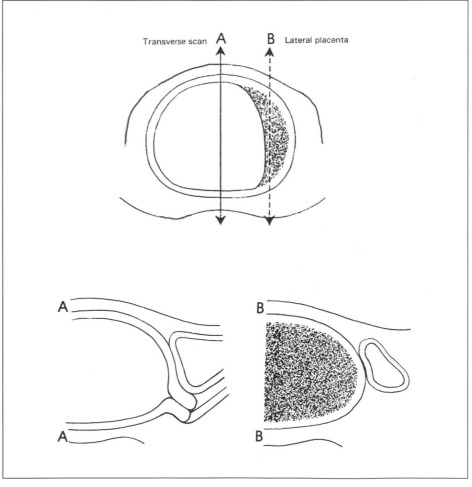

FIGURE 15-3. A longitudinal section at level A in the midlines through the vagina shows no placenta covering the cervix. Longitudinal section at level B gives the impression of a placenta previa, but the placenta is off to the left.

Maneuvers to Show Placenta Previa

1. Make sure that the bladder is empty before trying any of the following maneuvers. When the bladder is filled, the anterior wall of the uterus may be compressed against the placenta, giving a false impression of placenta previa (see Fig. 15-2). If the fetal head is more than 2 cm from the sacrum, the possibility of placenta previa exists, and certain maneuvers can be performed to show the area behind the fetal head.

2. Push the transducer into the maternal abdomen just superior to the pubic symphysis, and while scanning, arch it longitudinally toward the patient's feet.

3. Have a physician move and hold the fetal head out of the pelvis with an abdominal rather than a vaginal approach and scan the lower uterine segment.

   These techniques have, for the most part, been replaced by the transvaginal and transperineal (translabial) approaches.

4. *Transperineal (translabial)*. Place a covered curved linear array probe (5 MHz) against the labia and optimize settings so that the bladder can be seen (Fig. 15-4). The vagina will be seen as an apparently vertically placed echopenic area and the cervix will be visualized at right angles, at the lower end of the vagina. The fetal head or fetal parts will be seen posterior to the bladder, which should be almost empty. The cervix will be somewhere between 2.9 and 5 cm long. It should be closed. If there is a V-shaped opening at the fetal end of the cervix, this is indicative of cervical incompetence (Fig. 15-5). The cervix is an active structure and may be closed at times and open at others. To provoke it to open, press gently but firmly on the maternal abdomen at the fundus to increase pressure at the internal os, the proximal end of the cervix. Occasionally, the entire cervix is then filled with fluid and the membranes balloon out of the external os. This is an emergency situation and an obstetrician needs to be called immediately.

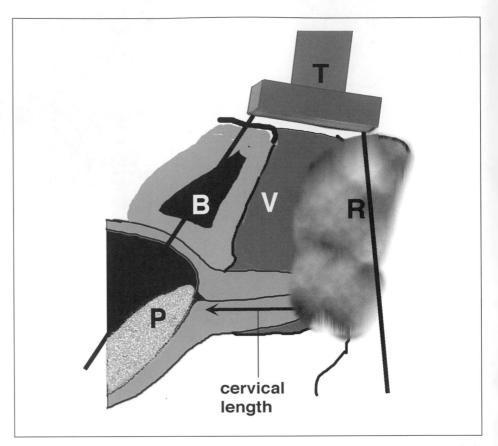

FIGURE 15-4. Diagram of a translabial view of the cervix displayed in the way it is seen on the monitor. The transducer (T) is placed against the labia with the patient with legs flexed and wide apart. The transducer is covered with gel and plastic wrap to prevent infection. The vagina (V) is an echopenic vertical structure which leads directly down to the cervix. The bladder lies superiorly as does the fetus. The cervix is almost always "horizontal" to the vagina, although it may be oblique or even angulated towards the bladder (B). The rectum (R) may interfere with the image and prevent the inferior end of the cervix from being seen. In this case the entire placental length cannot be examined and the external os cannot be seen. If rectal gas interferes, an endovaginal probe view will be required. In this example, the placenta (P) covers the cervix and is a marginal previa.

Gas in the rectum sometimes obscures the external os when using a transperineal approach, so the entire cervical length cannot be measured. The patient may then be placed in the left-side-down decubitus position. If this maneuver fails, an endovaginal examination of the cervix shows the entire cervical length.

5. *Endovaginal*. The endovaginal probe is cautiously introduced, viewing the cervix as one puts it in place. After only a short distance, the cervix will be seen. Since the cervix is usually at right angles to the vagina, the procedure is not dangerous providing that the cervix is watched as the probe is introduced. In addition to allowing a beautiful look at the entire cervix, one can gently probe the cervical firmness with the endovaginal probe. If it is soft this indicates that the cervix is ripening and becoming effaced. Again, press on the fundus to provoke dilatation of the internal os.

   Using either technique, the relationship of the placenta to the internal os will be seen well (Figs. 15-4 to 15-6).

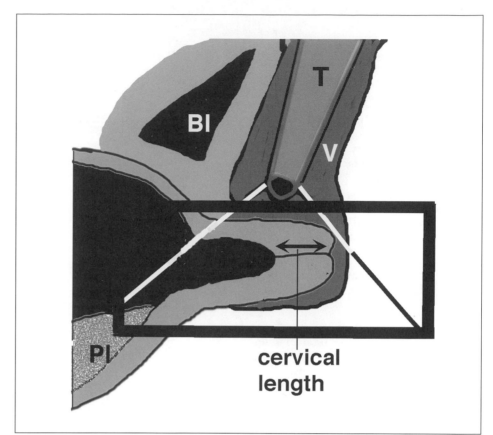

FIGURE 15-5. Endovaginal view of the cervix. Note that the vaginal probe (T) is located directly adjacent to the cervix, so an excellent view is obtained. Cervical incompetence is present. Cervical length can be accurately measured and the cervix can be gently prodded with the end of the transducer to see if it is soft. When the cervix is partly effaced as in this case, the remaining cervical length is measured (arrow). The placenta (P) is low-lying but is not a placenta previa. Box shows area seen on the monitor.

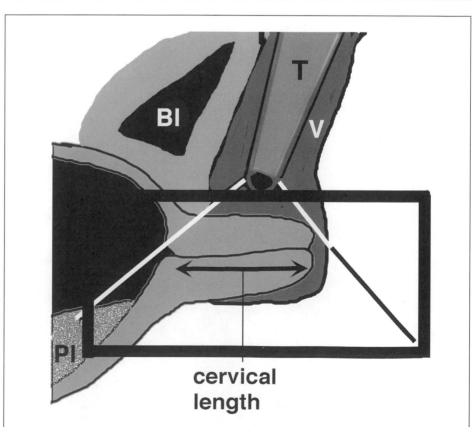

FIGURE 15-6. View of normal cervix using the endovaginal probe showing measurements (arrow). Area enclosed in the box is seen on the TV monitor.

◆ PATHOLOGY

Placenta Previa

Placenta previa is present whenever the placenta can be shown to lie adjacent to the internal cervical os. There are four low placental positions (Fig. 15-7):

1. *Low-lying* when the placenta is close to the os but not overlying it. This is not a placenta previa.
2. *Partial* when the placenta extends to the internal os, but does not cross it.
3. *Marginal* when the placental margin extends just over the cervix.
4. *Complete* or *total* when it completely overlies the internal os.

An apparent placenta previa in the second trimester usually ceases to be a placenta previa in the third trimester. Possible explanations include the following:

1. Overdistention of the fetal bladder (see Fig. 15-2).
2. Myometrial contractions giving the impression of a placenta previa (see Fig. 15-15).
3. A placenta that lies adjacent to the cervix but is not attached to the placental wall at that site.

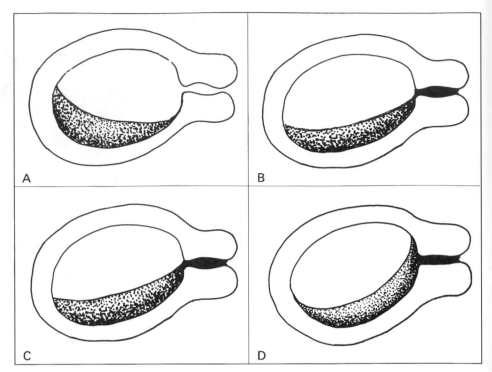

FIGURE 15-7. The types of placenta previa. (**A**) Low-lying—abutting on the internal os but not covering it. (**B**) Partial—extending to the internal os. (**C**) Marginal—just covering the internal os. (**D**) Total—completely covering the internal os.

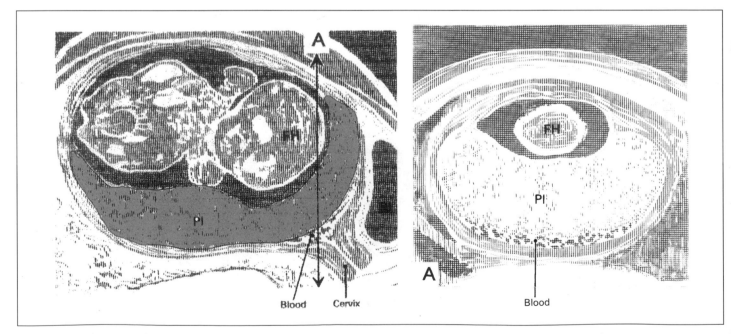

FIGURE 15-8. Total posterior placenta previa. Note the blood between the cervix and the placenta. The scan plane was taken at the level marked "A."

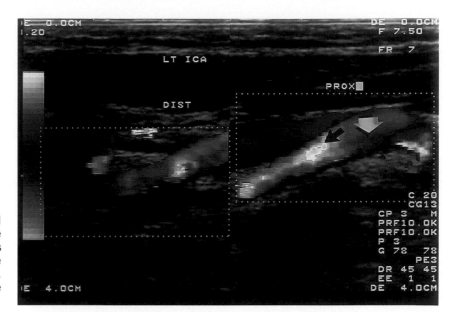

COLOR PLATE 5-1. Color flow of the left internal carotid artery is shown. Flow is away from the transducer, hence the color blue. Faster velocities are assigned brighter colors (small arrow) while slower velocities are darker colors (large arrow). When the vessel runs an oblique course to the probe, color entirely fills the vessel.

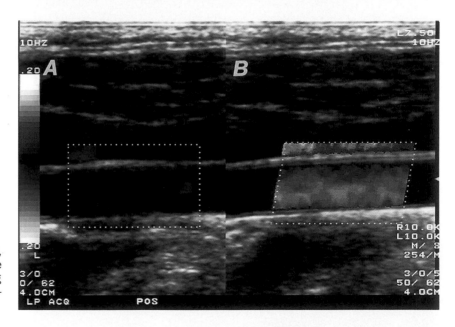

COLOR PLATE 5-2. (**A**) Color flow, like Doppler, will not receive the returning signals when the probe is 90 degrees to the vessel. (**B**) Obliquing the probe will generate the angle needed to receive the returning signals and display color.

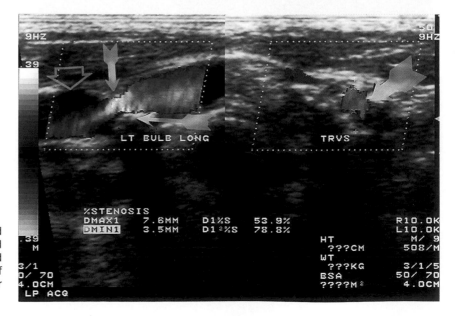

COLOR PLATE 5-3. (**A**) Soft plaque is outlined well with color flow (open arrow). An area of hard plaque with internal echoes is also seen (closed arrows). (**B**) Calculating the diameter stenosis of the residual lumen is easier when utilizing color flow (large arrow).

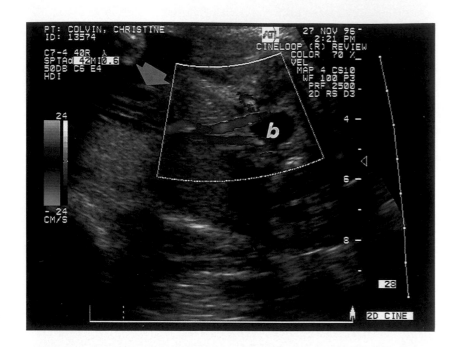

COLOR PLATE 14-1. Color flow image showing the two umbilical arteries alongside the bladder (b). This proves there is a three-vessel cord present. The cord outside the fetal abdomen is imaged (arrow); it is unclear whether there are two or three vessels present.

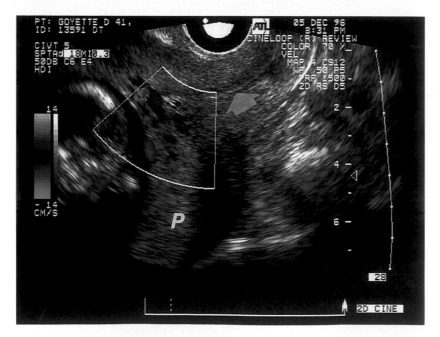

COLOR PLATE 15-1. Color flow view of the cervix showing a placenta previa. The cervical canal is shown (arrow). A posterior placenta ends at the internal os. Large vessels shown in color, lie at the internal os.

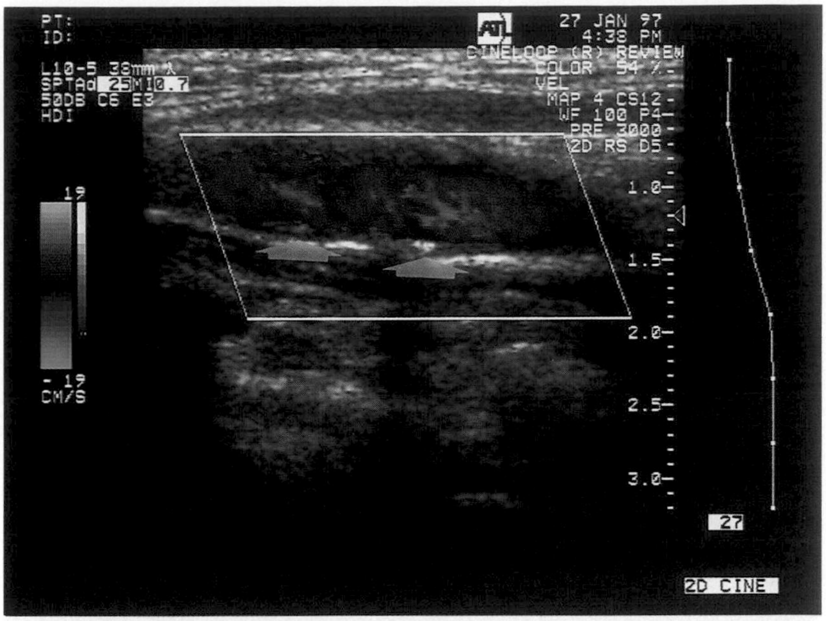

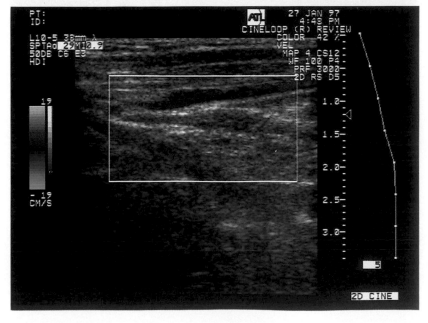

COLOR PLATE 53-1. Color flow within a vessel outlining a plaque (arrows).

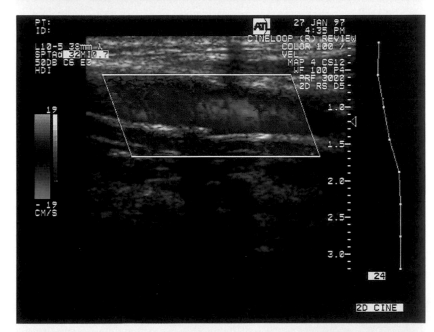

COLOR PLATE 53-2. Same patient. Excessive color flow gain has been used so that the plaque is obliterated by the color flow within the vessel.

COLOR PLATE 53-3. View of a peripheral vessel showing relatively insignificant color flow with the beam angled at right angles to the vessel.

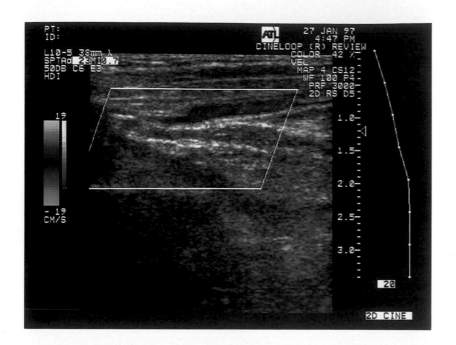

COLOR PLATE 53-4. After angling the beam obliquely and with the color gain unchanged, the amount of color flow within the vessel increases substantially.

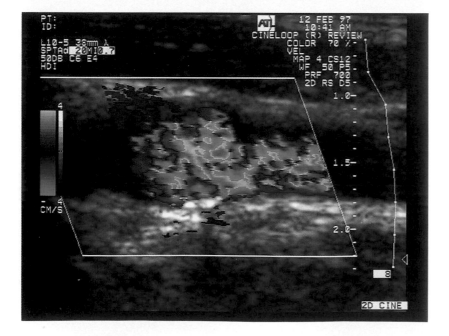

COLOR PLATE 53-5. Color flow image of a carotid artery. Within the normal red signals, from the flow within the artery, are interspersed areas of blue related to aliasing.

4. Placental atrophy. It is thought that the placenta atrophies at sites where there is poor blood supply such as in the cervical region.

A placenta previa is a type of abruptio with separation of the internal os tissues from the placenta as the cervix becomes effaced. When the placenta previa is symptomatic, it is sometimes possible to discern blood between the internal os and the placenta (Fig. 15-8).

In our practice serial ultrasonic examinations are obtained when placenta previa is discovered, with the hope that the placenta will change position during the course of pregnancy. At term, it frequently lies at the fundus, whereas previously it was close to the cervix (Fig. 15-9). In asymptomatic patients, the placenta often covers the cervical os early in the second trimester.

Occasionally the placenta is split into two segments. The smaller satellite segment is called a succenturiate lobe.

Vascular Connections Between a Succenturiate Lobe and the Placenta

If a succenturiate lobe is found in the inferior portion of the uterus and the placenta is located anteriorly, it is possible that the vessels that communicate between the two portions of the placenta run across the cervix.

Should the fetus break these vessels, as it delivers, the blood loss could be disastrous.

The only way to discover this very unusual finding is to look at the cervical region with color flow. Prominent vessels will be seen running across the cervix.

Vasa Previa

If the placenta is located in a low position and the cord insertion into the placenta is at the rim of the placenta, there is a possibility of vasa previa. With a velamentous insertion, the three vessels that make up the cord become separated and lie in a membrane as they reach the placenta. If this membrane lies across the cervix, it can act in the same way as a placenta previa and cause even more serious blood loss.

A velamentous insertion can only easily be recognized with color flow and should be looked for whenever the placenta is low lying and vaginal bleeding occurs. Velamentous insertions occur much more commonly with twin pregnancies than with singleton pregnancies.

Incompetent Cervix

A cervix that starts to dilate prematurely in the absence of labor contractions is known as an incompetent cervix (see Fig. 15-5). The mucous plug that fills the cervix can be lost at the time that this dilatation takes place. This causes a brief episode of vaginal bleeding.

Whenever a patient presents with vaginal bleeding in the second or third trimester, cautiously examine the cervix with the vaginal probe. The probe can be inserted about 2 cm to see whether there is any evidence of cervical incompetence. There will be a V-shaped indentation at the internal os if incompetence is present.

If none is seen, the vaginal probe can be moved onto the cervix to look for placenta previa, vasa previa, or crossing vessels. Cautious pressure is applied to the cervix with the vaginal probe to see whether it has softened. Put pressure on the maternal abdomen to see whether the internal os opens. If there is evidence of fluid in the cervical canal, these maneuvers are not performed. Be especially cautious if there is evidence of fluid throughout the canal with "ballooning" membranes prolapsing out of the external os into the vagina.

Cord Prolapse

Prolapse of the umbilical cord into the endocervical canal occurs at delivery in .5% of cases. There is a high chance of fetal loss secondary to cord compression if the cord is in this location. This rare problem occurs most often with polyhydramnios, a nonvertex presentation, and multiple gestation. If the cord is found with color flow to be the presenting structure at term or if the patient is in labor, then the obstetrician should be called.

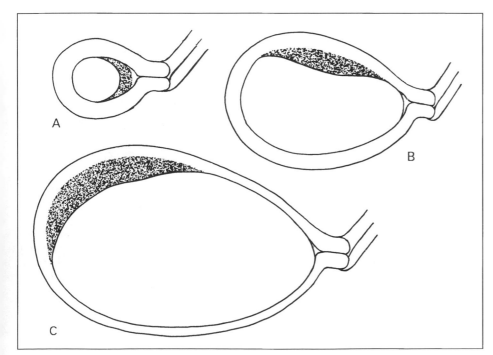

FIGURE 15-9. Placental "migration." (**A**) Early in pregnancy the placenta overlies the internal os. (**B**) With selective growth of the lower uterine segment the placenta moves to an anterior site. (**C**) Late in pregnancy the placenta typically lies at the fundus of the uterus.

Abruptio Placentae (Accidental Hemorrhage)

Bleeding from the placenta in any of a number of sites is known as abruptio placentae. The condition has several sonographic manifestations (Fig. 15-10).

A Gap Between the Myometrium and the Placenta

The collection of blood between the myometrium and the placenta may be completely sonolucent, or it may contain low-level internal echoes due to the blood. The border of the placenta will be displaced away from the myometrium. The textures of the blood clot and of the placenta can be similar. This type has the worst prognosis. Using color flow helps in showing that myometrium is present rather than clot since vessels will be seen.

Echoes Within the Amniotic Fluid Due to Blood

Echoes within the amniotic fluid due to blood may be focal and present in small clumps or they may be evenly echogenic and extensive, resembling vernix, and even form a fluid-fluid level.

Bleeding in a Subchorionic or Subamniotic Location

The blood within the subchorionic or subamniotic space may be relatively similar in texture to that of the placenta, but it will eventually become sonolucent.

Subchorionic blood in front of the placenta is considered particularly dangerous because it may compress the cord.

Marginal Bleed

The amniotic or chorionic sac membrane is displaced away from the placenta in a marginal location (see Fig. 15-10). This is the most common form of abruptio. In most instances, the collection develops at the edge of the placenta (a marginal bleed).

With normal gain settings the only sign of this type of abruption may be a membrane within the amniotic fluid adjacent to one end of the placenta. If gain is increased the blood within this area becomes more echogenic than neighboring amniotic fluid because it has a more-proteinaceous composition.

The prognosis with this type of bleed is good.

Intraplacental Bleed

An echopenic or echogenic area within the placenta can represent an intraplacental bleed or infarct (see Fig. 15-10). Areas of infarction, while initially echopenic, may eventually calcify. Intraplacental bleeds or infarcts may be locally tender, allowing distinction from Wharton's jelly deposition.

Flow will be seen on real-time in an echopenic area due to vascular lakes, although the flow is usually too slow to be detected with Doppler.

Chorioangioma

A benign tumor arising from the amniotic surface of the placenta, chorioangioma is highly vascular. Profuse blood flow can be seen within it. Chorioangiomas are quite common and almost always of no consequence.

Extremely rarely, so much blood goes to the mass that the fetus becomes anemic and shows evidence of hydrops.

Chorioangioma of a size greater than 5 to 6 cm needs careful follow-up (Fig. 15-11).

Intra-amniotic Membranes

Membranes within the amniotic cavity may have a number of possible causes (Fig. 15-12).

1. *Abruptio.* See above.
2. *Amniotic sheets.* These membranes, which do not enclose a space, are double and have a small circular echopenic area in the portion adjacent to the amniotic cavity.

   Vascular flow can often be seen at the tip of the amniotic sheet where it widens. This is thought to represent a site where the amnion and chorion surround subamniotic adhesions (synechiae) present before the pregnancy occurred.
3. *Amniotic sac membrane.* In a proportion of twin pregnancies, one twin dies. The sac membrane enclosing amniotic fluid may persist when the fetus has disappeared, or resorbed.

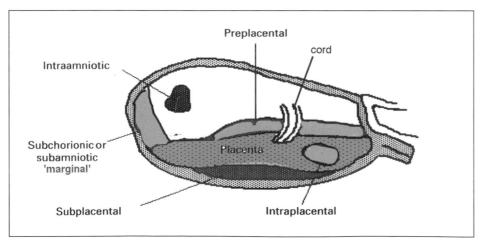

FIGURE 15-10. The various appearances of abruptio placentae: (1) Blood between the placenta and myometrium (subplacental). (2) Blood within the amniotic fluid (intra-amniotic). (3) Blood between the amniotic sac membrane and chorionic membrane (subchorionic or subamniotic). Usually the blood is adjacent to the placenta. If it is in a preplacental location the cord may be compressed. (4) Intraplacental blood.

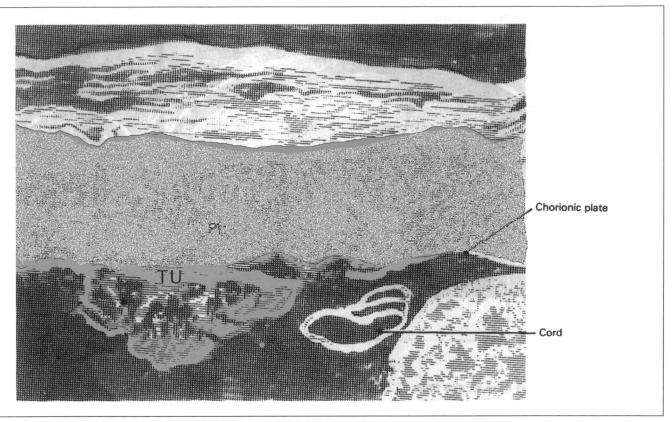

FIGURE 15-11. A placental tumor (TU) arises from the placenta. It has a slightly different texture and shows pulsation on real-time.

4. *Amniotic bands.* The amniotic membranes can break and curl up in amniotic fluid so the chorionic membrane is exposed to the amniotic fluid and the fetus. Portions of fetal limbs may be truncated if amniotic bands are present, perhaps because the fetus becomes attached to the chorion, which is not smooth and slippery like the amnion. Amniotic bands do not enclose amniotic fluid.

5. *Unfused amnion.* The amnion usually fuses with the chorion at about 14 to 16 weeks. Occasionally, fusion is delayed, which is of little clinical consequence. Following amniocentesis, blood may enter the extracelomic space between the amnion and chorion and prevent fusion. If this takes place, premature delivery may occur. Low-level echoes will be seen between the amnion and chorion, representing blood.

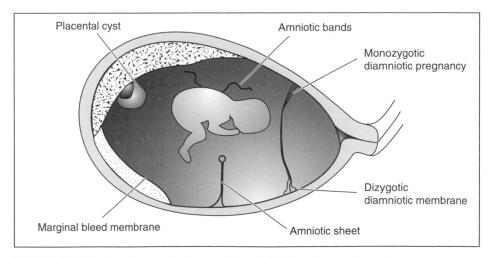

FIGURE 15-12. Membranes in the amniotic fluid. Four types of membranes are seen: (1) Membranes related to subamniotic blood. Increasing the gain shows low-level echoes within the enclosed space. (2) Amniotic sheets. There is a double membrane with a cystic area. (3) Amniotic bands adhering to the fetus. These are rare. (4) Placental cysts. (5) Membranes related to a twin pregnancy that has reabsorbed.

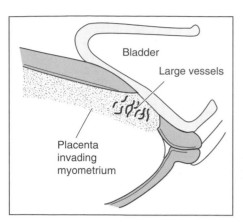

FIGURE 15-13. Placenta percreta. At the cesarean section incision site, the placenta invades the myometrium and bladder wall. Large vessels can be seen within the placental invasion site.

6. *Placental cysts.* Cysts may form on the amniotic surface of the placenta. They enclose a small tumor mass and much fluid. The cysts have no pathologic significance, but the membrane around the cyst may be confused with an amniotic band or other structures (see Fig. 15-12).

Placenta Percreta

If the placenta implants onto a previous cesarean section incision, placental tissue may invade the myometrium at the cesarean section site (Fig. 15-13). The invasion may be slight (acreta), into the myometrium (increta), or through the muscle wall (percreta). This is a rare but very dangerous condition with a high mortality rate. At the time of delivery, a large bleed occurs as the placenta and myometrium attempt to separate.

The sonographer can detect placenta percreta by concentrating on a previous cesarean section site and seeing the absence of myometrium. Many prominent arterial vessels will be seen flowing at right angles to the placental interface with the myometrium. Vessels will be seen on the bladder surface if a placenta increta is present.

★ PITFALLS

1. *Placental and uterine vessels.* Sometimes the blood vessels that supply the placenta are large and form spaces in the myometrium adjacent to the placenta (Fig. 15-14) that may be mistaken for abruptio placentae. Real-time visualization will document venous flow in these sinuses.
2. *Overdistended bladder.* An overdistended bladder may cause an appearance that suggests a placenta previa because the anterior wall of the uterus is compressed against the posterior wall (see Fig. 15-2). Postvoid films resolve this false-positive finding.
3. *Myometrium.* Mistaking the myometrium (uterine wall) for abruptio is possible. The normal sonolucent space around the placenta should be symmetrical at all sites, although this space is particularly obvious at the fundus of the uterus. An increase in gain will cause echoes in this area and not in adjacent amniotic fluid. Flow will be seen in uterine vessels with color flow Doppler.

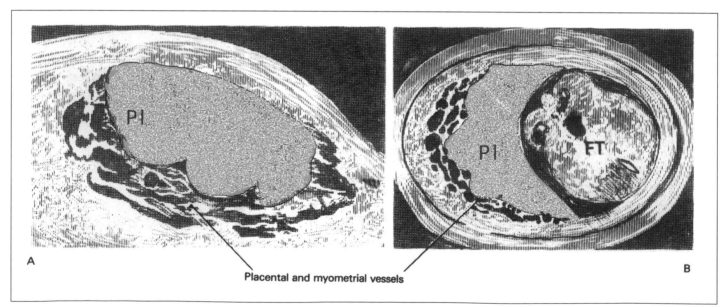

FIGURE 15-14. Pronounced placental and myometrial vessels may be seen as a normal variant. These vessels may be confused with abruptio placentae.

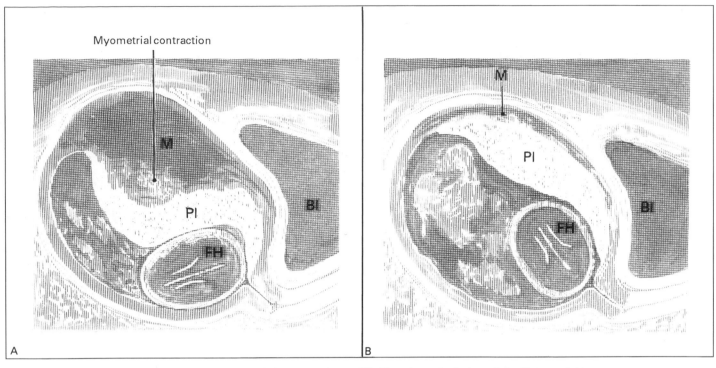

FIGURE 15-15. Myometrial contractions. (**A**) The placenta bulges into the amniotic cavity. A myometrial contraction is responsible. (**B**) After a wait of approximately 30 minutes, such contractions disappear. Fibroids do not have the regular texture of thickened myometrium.

4. *Myometrial contraction.* A myometrial contraction can temporarily displace the placenta and simulate a placenta previa when the contraction occurs in the lower uterine segment (Fig. 15-15). If the placenta appears to be visible at two separate sites, rescan after 30 minutes. One of the possible placentas will usually turn out to be a myometrial contraction. These are painless contractions of the uterine wall of no pathologic significance.

5. *Succenturiate lobe.* Succenturiate lobe is a rare variant of placenta occurring in approximately 1% of cases. The placenta is split into two parts. If the second part is small and located adjacent to the cervix, sonographic detection may be difficult.

6. *Subchorionic echopenic areas.* Sonolucent areas may be seen adjacent to the chorionic plate within the placenta. These represent either fibrin deposition or large placental vessels and are of no pathologic significance (Fig. 15-16).

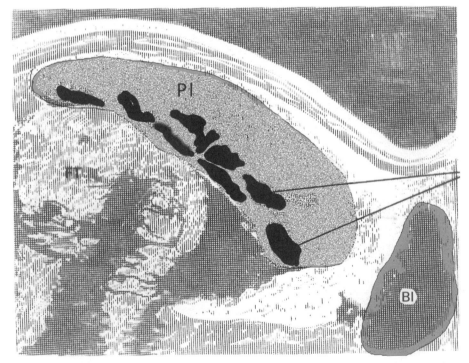

FIGURE 15-16. Sonolucent areas within the chorionic aspect of the placenta due to fibrin deposition or prominent vessels. These are a normal variant.

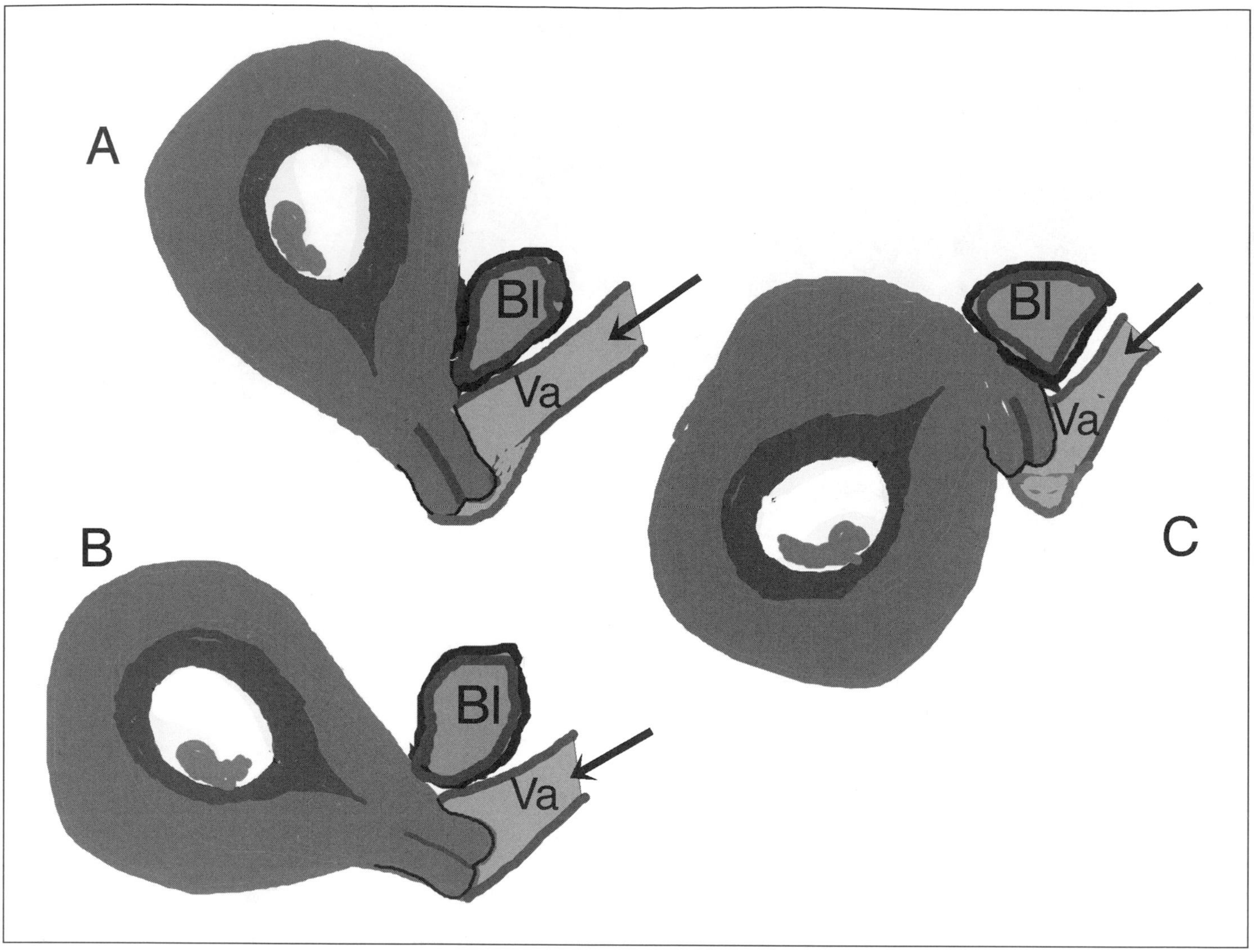

FIGURE 15-17. (**A**) This is the normal position for the cervix. The black arrow indicates the transducer or beam axis. (**B**) The cervix is at an oblique axis to the transducer. (**C**) The cervix is anteverted, but retroflexed. Note that most of the cervix is not readily seen through the vagina because it is more anteriorly located than usual. This type of cervix can easily be missed completely.

7. *Thinned myometrium at cesarean section site.* The myometrium can be markedly thinned at the cesarean section site. Although this is worth commenting on in a report, it is rarely of clinical significance. The myometrium can be so thin at the time of cesarean section that the fetus is visible within.

8. A *circumvallate placenta.* The placenta can burrow into the myometrium. An echogenic rim forms around the border of the placenta. This circumvallate appearance is worth noting. The placenta is more difficult to deliver if this abnormality is present.

9. *Low lateral placenta mimicking a placenta previa.* If the placenta lies lateral to the cervix but in the region of the lower segment, casual scanning may give the impression of a placenta previa (see Fig. 15-3). Make sure that a section is taken through the cervix and lower uterine segment simultaneously to be confident that a placenta previa is present.

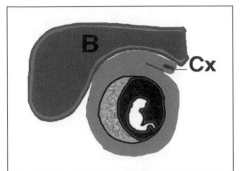

FIGURE 15-18. Retroverted uterus with anteverted, but retroflexed cervix with incarceration of the uterus. The pregnant uterus is expanding posteriorly and anteriorly rather than superiorly. Adhesions may be tethering the fundus of the uterus in the posterior position. The uterus is, therefore, indenting the bladder and causing retention.

10. *Intra-amniotic bleed versus fetal mass.* Maternal blood can collect in the amniotic fluid and create a mass that may look as if it arises from the fetus. It will change appearance if reexamined in a few days. If the maternal abdomen is jogged, the blood clot will move separately from the fetus.

11. *Placental lakes.* Echopenic areas within the placenta known as vascular lakes are common. Real-time will show vascular flow in these areas (see Fig. 15-16).

12. *Nuchal cord.* In about 20% of second and third trimester pregnancies, the cord is wrapped around the fetal neck. As a rule, this is an unimportant normal variant, but if the cord is wrapped around twice or the cord appears to be straightened and under tension, the obstetrician should be informed because fetal death could occur at the time of delivery.

13. *Unusual axes to the cervical canal.* When the cervix is examined, either with a translabial or endovaginal approach, the cervical canal is usually at a horizontal axis to the probe (Fig. 15-17A). On some occasions, the axis of the cervical canal is oblique to the vagina (Fig. 15-17B). A rare variant occurs when the uterus is retroverted and the cervix flips anteriorly (Fig. 15-17C). This type of cervix can be difficult to see because the cervix is displaced antero-superiorly. When the uterus is retroverted with an anteverted and retroflexed cervix, there is a danger of uterine incarceration (Fig. 15-18). In this condition, as the uterus expands, it compresses the bladder and eventually causes urinary retention.

SELECTED READING

Bromley, B., Pitcher, B. L., Klapholz, H., Lichter, E., and Benacerraf, B. R. Sonographic appearance of uterine scar dehiscence. *Internat J Gynecol Obstet* 51:53–56, 1995.

Callen, P. W. (Ed.). *Ultrasonography in Obstetrics and Gynecology.* Philadelphia: Saunders, 1994.

Cook, C. M., and Ellwood, D. A. A longitudinal study of the cervix in pregnancy using transvaginal ultrasound. *Br J Obstet Gynecol* 103:16–18, 1996.

Dudiak, C. M., Salomon, C. G., Posniak, H. V., Olson, M. C., and Flisak, M. E. Sonography of the umbilical cord. *Radiographics* 15:1035–1050, 1995.

Farine, D., Fox, H. E., Jakobson, S., and Timor-Tritsch, I. Vaginal ultrasound for diagnosis of placenta previa. *Am J Obstet Gynecol* 159:566–569, 1988.

Fleischer, A. E., et al. (Eds.). *The Principles and Practice of Ultrasonography in Obstetrics and Gynecology* (6th ed.). Englewood Cliffs, NJ: Appleton-Century-Crofts, 1991.

Harris, R. D., Cho, C., and Wells, W. A. Sonography of the placenta with emphasis on pathological correlation. *Semin Ultrasound, CT and MRI* 17:66–89, 1996.

Heinonen, S., Ryynanen, M., Kirkinen, P., and Saarikoski, S. Perinatal diagnostic evaluation of velamentous umbilical cord insertion: Clinical, Doppler and ultrasonic findings. *Obstet Gynecol* 87:112–117, 1996.

Huntington, D. K., and Sanders, R. C. Ultrasound of the placenta and membranes. *Ultrasound Quarterly* 12:45–64, 1994.

McCarthy, J., Thurmond, A. S., Jones, M. K., Sistrom, C., Scanlan, R. M., Jackobson, S. L., and Lowensohn, R. Circumvallate placenta: Sonographic diagnosis. *J Ultrasound Med* 14:21–26, 1995.

Nyberg, D. A., et al. Placental abruption and placental hemorrhage: Correlation of sonographic findings with fetal outcome. *Radiology* 164:357–361, 1987.

Reuter, K. L., Davidoff, A., and Hunter, T. Vasa previa. *J Clin Ultrasound* 16:356–348, 1988.

Sauerbrei, E. E., and Pham, D. H. Placental abruption and subchorionic hemorrhage in the first half of pregnancy: US appearance and clinical outcome. *Radiology* 160:109–112, 1986.

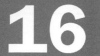

SMALL FOR DATES

ROGER C. SANDERS

KEY WORDS

Amenorrhea. Absence of menstruation.

Eclampsia. High blood pressure with urinary protein loss occurring in pregnancy. In its most severe form it is associated with epileptic seizure. It is a very serious condition that causes intrauterine growth restriction and often leads to fetal death.

Hyaline Membrane Disease (Respiratory Distress Syndrome). Respiratory condition occurring in the neonate as a consequence of delivery when the fetal lungs are still immature.

Intrauterine Growth Restriction (Intrauterine Growth Retardation) (IUGR). A fetus is suffering from IUGR when it is below the 10th percentile for weight at a given gestational age or weighs less than 2500 g at 36 weeks' gestational age.

Oligohydramnios. Too little amniotic fluid. No fluid or only small pockets of fluid are present.

Pre-eclamptic Toxemia. High blood pressure and proteinuria that precedes eclampsia.

Premature Rupture of Membranes (PROM). Leakage of fluid from the amniotic cavity occurring before the patient goes into labor. Most often results in premature delivery.

Trimester. Pregnancy is divided into three periods of 13 weeks each, known as trimesters. Obstetric problems are conveniently related to a given trimester.

 THE CLINICAL PROBLEM

Three possibilities should be considered when a fetus is small for dates.

1. The *mother's dates are wrong*, and the fetus is actually younger than indicated by her dates.
2. *Palpation is misleading* because of obesity or unusual uterine lie.
3. A small uterus with *oligohydramnios* is present owing to:
   a. Premature rupture of membranes (PROM)
   b. Intrauterine growth restriction (IUGR) with a small fetus and placenta and diminished amniotic fluid
   c. Fetal renal anomaly (see Chapter 18) with diminished fluid

Premature Rupture of Membranes

The rupture of membranes (a "show") early in pregnancy is an obstetric management problem. If the fetus is too small to survive outside the uterus, no efforts are made to salvage it. If the fetus is large enough to survive, the mother is put on bed rest and treated with antibiotics to stop infection of the uterine contents. Ultrasound is valuable in the following ways:

1. Showing how large the fetus is
2. Giving an idea of the mother's true dates
3. Excluding a fetal anomaly associated with polyhydramnios that might have caused premature rupture of membranes

This is an obstetric emergency study.

Intrauterine Growth Restriction

In IUGR, insufficient nutrition is supplied to the fetus. Fetuses are at risk if the mother is chronically ill (e.g., chronic heart disease), takes drugs (e.g., alcohol or cigarettes), does not eat well, is under 17 or over 35, or has had previous pregnancies in which there was poor fetal growth.

IUGR can exhibit an asymmetric, a symmetric, or a femur-sparing pattern. In asymmetric IUGR the fetal trunk is small but the skull is more or less normal in size. This type of IUGR is thought to be associated with placental problems that result in defective transfer of nutrients from the mother to the fetus. When the onset of fetal nutritional insufficiency is abrupt, the fetal brain is relatively spared, but the liver is severely affected, leading to an asymmetric growth pattern.

In symmetric IUGR the entire fetus is smaller than normal. This type of IUGR is thought to relate to a continued insult such as chronic maternal illness or drug intake.

In the femur-sparing type of IUGR all measurements apart from the femur length are small. The femur-sparing type of IUGR is relatively common. So far no specific clinical features have been recognized.

Diagnosis of symmetric IUGR requires accurate dating at an early stage. Most obstetricians feel that a routine biparietal diameter measurement at 17 to 20 weeks' gestation is desirable in mothers who are at risk for IUGR so that accurate dates are known.

IUGR is usually diagnosed by ultrasound when growth is less than expected in the third trimester. Establishing the diagnosis is crucial because of increased risk of difficult delivery and of stunted stature and intellect at a later age if the condition is not detected and remedied in utero. The fetal condition may be improved by maternal bed rest and other maneuvers such as eliminating cigarette smoking. The ultrasonic diagnosis depends on comparing the sizes of different structures in the fetal body, such as the overall size of the abdomen with the head size, and correlating these measurements with those expected according to standard experience for a given obstetric date.

If a fetus is first examined in the late second or third trimester and the trunk is too small or the femur is too long for other measurements, think of IUGR.

ANATOMY

For the standard approach to the fetal anatomy, see Chapter 14.

 TECHNIQUE

See the techniques described in Chapter 14.

 PATHOLOGY

Renal Anomalies

Eliminate the possibility of a renal anomaly by finding the kidneys and looking for the fetal bladder (see Chapter 14). If a normal-size bladder is present, the possibility of agenesis (absence) of the kidneys can be discarded. The bladder normally fills and partially empties over the course of about an hour. Slower rates of filling are associated with IUGR.

Premature Rupture of Membranes

In evaluating premature rupture of membranes (PROM) the obstetrician needs to know the following:

1. How much amniotic fluid there is
2. Whether there is a fetal anomaly that might cause polyhydramnios and thus induce premature rupture of membranes
3. The gestational age and size of the fetus

If there is uncertainty as to whether or not premature rupture of membranes has occurred, the cervix should be examined (see Chapter 15).

Intrauterine Growth Restriction

Measurements

IUGR is diagnosed by obtaining the following measurements.

BIPARIETAL DIAMETER. Normal growth charts of the biparietal diameter according to week of pregnancy are available. If the mother has accurate dates or has been dated by an earlier biparietal diameter measurement before 26 weeks, a diagnosis of IUGR can be made if a subsequent sonogram shows unduly small growth for the stage of pregnancy (see Appendix 9 and Chapter 14).

TRUNK CIRCUMFERENCE. The trunk or abdominal circumference is measured at the level of the portal sinus and the liver (Fig. 16-1). Adequate abdominal circumference measurements can be made using a small foot print transducer if the fetal trunk is not too large for the field of view. However, a curved linear array system is more appropriate.

Make sure that the trunk is more or less round at the point of measurement and that the umbilical vein, aorta, adrenal gland, stomach, and spine are visible. If the kidneys are present, the section is too low or angled improperly.

To measure a trunk circumference either find the circumference with the caliper-based system built into the ultrasound machine or measure the trunk diameter. The two approaches are comparable in accuracy. Two trunk diameters (D) at right angles are measured, and their averages calculated to yield an average trunk diameter (see Appendix 12). The circumference can be derived from the diameter by using the formula πD. Weight can then be estimated by measuring the biparietal diameter and the trunk circumference or diameter and using Appendix 13 to make the calculation.

Other tables use the head size, femur length, and abdominal circumference to compute weight (see Appendix 13). The abdominal circumference (transverse trunk diameter + anterior-posterior diameter $\times$ 1.57 = abdominal circumference) also represents another method of dating the fetus (see Appendix 6).

HEAD CIRCUMFERENCE. The measurement of the head circumference is valuable because the head-to-trunk ratio will allow the diagnosis of asymmetric IUGR. The head circumference should be obtained at a level that shows the thalami, the cavum septi pellucidi, the intrahemispheric fissure, and the third ventricle, as for calculating a biparietal diameter. Dating tables based on the head circumference are available (see Appendixes 7 and 8).

HEAD/TRUNK CIRCUMFERENCE RATIO. Finding the head/trunk circumference ratio and comparing it with normal tables (see Appendix 15) allows the recognition of asymmetric IUGR when the liver is unusually small (see Fig. 16-1) even if dates are unknown, providing intracranial structures appear normal.

If there is an abnormal head/trunk circumference ratio, consider the possibility that the fetus has hydrocephalus, which will give similar measurement findings. A low head/trunk circumference ratio suggests the possibility of microcephalus or a large fetus with macrosomia.

FEMORAL LENGTH. The femoral length measurement is described in Chapter 14. It is valuable in diagnosing IUGR because it represents another method of determining whether adequate fetal growth has occurred (see Appendixes 2 and 11). The femur is often spared by IUGR when the head and trunk are small.

FEMORAL LENGTH/BIPARIETAL DIAMETER RATIO. The femoral length/biparietal diameter ratio may reveal one type of IUGR in which the fetus is long but skinny. The femoral length/biparietal diameter ratio should be 0.79 ± 0.06.

CEREBELLAR WIDTH. The cerebellar width in millimeters is equivalent to the age in weeks. This measurement is less affected by excessive growth or IUGR than other measurements such as the abdominal circumference or head measurements. If a patient presents with no early sonogram or accurate last menstrual period, measurement of the cerebellar width may be valuable.

Fetal Anatomy

The fetal anatomy should be examined in considerable detail, because approximately 10% of IUGR cases are due to a congenital fetal anomaly (see Chapter 18). The kidneys and bladder should be examined in detail to exclude renal anomalies (see Chapter 18).

Biophysical Profile

If a fetus is found to have IUGR, perform a biophysical profile (see Chapter 19) and an umbilical artery Doppler study.

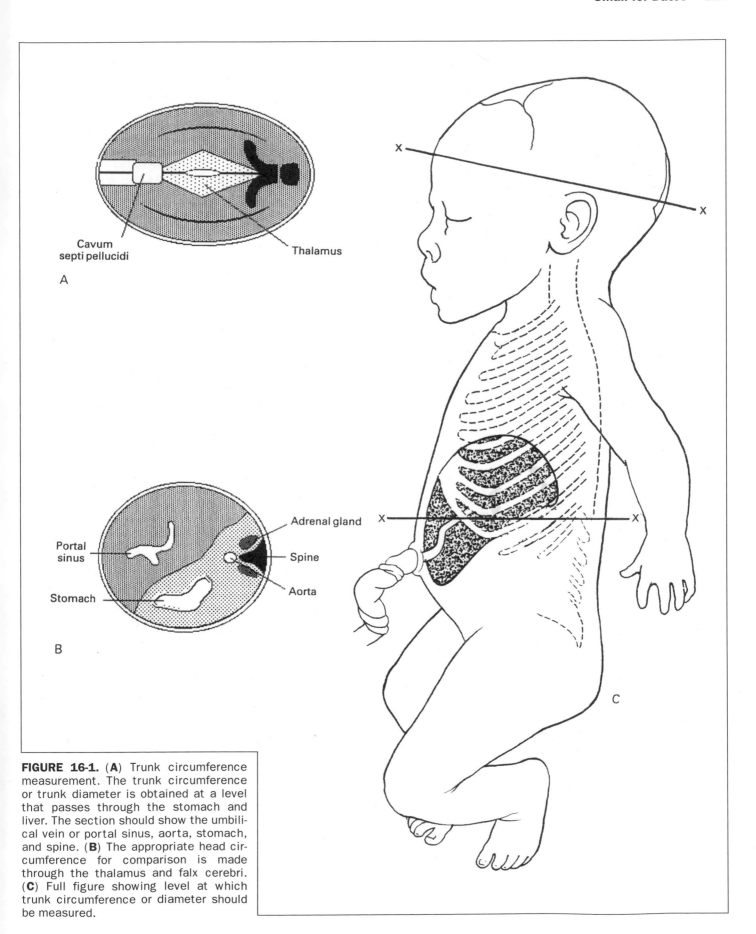

FIGURE 16-1. (**A**) Trunk circumference measurement. The trunk circumference or trunk diameter is obtained at a level that passes through the stomach and liver. The section should show the umbilical vein or portal sinus, aorta, stomach, and spine. (**B**) The appropriate head circumference for comparison is made through the thalamus and falx cerebri. (**C**) Full figure showing level at which trunk circumference or diameter should be measured.

Placental Maturation

The placenta is likely to be small with IUGR. Signs of premature placental aging (early calcification deposition) prior to 36 weeks suggest IUGR (Fig. 16-2). Grade III placental changes usually indicate that the fetal lungs are mature.

Amount of Amniotic Fluid

The amount of amniotic fluid is low in most cases of IUGR (oligohydramnios). Reduced amounts of amniotic fluid are normally seen in the third trimester.

Measurements of the largest pocket that is less than 2 cm in size is one method of quantifying oligohydramnios with IUGR, but if the fluid has diminished to this tiny quantity the situation is grave. Recognition of lesser amounts of oligohydramnios requires experience and comparison with gestational age.

The amniotic fluid index is a measure of amniotic fluid volume. Calculating the index allows one to follow changes in the amniotic fluid volume. The uterine contents are divided into four sections. The greatest depth of amniotic fluid is measured in each quadrant. The four measurements are then totaled and compared with the values in a standard graph (see Chapter 19 and Appendix 26).

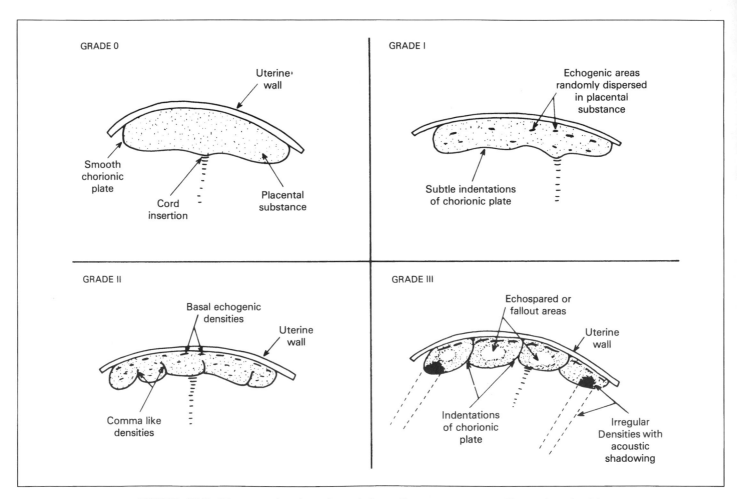

FIGURE 16-2. Diagram showing placental grading appearances. (Reproduced with permission from Grannum, P., Berkowitz, R., and Hobbins, J. The ultrasonic changes in the maturing placenta and their relation to fetal pulmonic maturity. *Am J Obstet Gynecol* 133:915–922, 1979.)

PITFALLS

1. *IUGR vs. hydrocephalus.* Remember that an abnormal head-to-trunk ratio may occur not only with IUGR, but also with hydrocephalus. Examine the ventricles carefully if you find an abnormally high head-to-trunk ratio.
2. *Inaccurate trunk circumference.* The trunk circumference will be inaccurate if:
   a. Too much umbilical vein is visible.
   b. The kidneys are visible.
   c. The view is oblique, showing ribs on only one side.
   d. Too much compression by the transducer has flattened the trunk shape so it is ovoid.
   e. The circumference is not measured along the outside border of the abdominal image.
   f. The measured outline does not correspond to the real outline. Place the tracing at the edge of the trunk outline. (Some machines have calipers that wander from the trunk outline. If you have such a cumbersome system, use the averaged diameter approach.)
   g. The fetus is prone, so the umbilical vein cannot be found. Results are still reasonably satisfactory if the kidneys and chest are not on the view.

WHERE ELSE TO LOOK

1. If IUGR is present, make a particular effort to look for signs of a chromosomal anomaly.
2. If apparent symmetric IUGR occurs at 30 weeks or more, look at the parents to see if they are small or of Asian origin. The fetal small size may be normal if the parents are also small.

SELECTED READING

Bronshtein, M. and Blumenfeld, Z. First- and early second-trimester oligohydramnios—a predictor of poor fetal outcome except in iatrogenic oligohydramnios post chorionic villus biopsy. *Ultrasound Obstet Gynecol* 1:245–249, 1991.

Callen, P. W. (Ed.). *Ultrasonography in Obstetrics and Gynecology* (2nd ed.). Philadelphia: Saunders, 1994.

Devoe, L. D., and Ware, D. J. Oligohydramnios: Definition and diagnosis. *Contemp OBGYN* Sept:31–40, 1994.

Doubilet, P. M., and Benson, C. B. Sonographic evaluation of intrauterine growth retardation. *AJR* 164:709–717, 1995.

Fleischer, A. E., et al. (Eds.). *Principles and Practice of Ultrasonography in Obstetrics and Gynecology* (6th ed.). Englewood Cliffs, N. J.: Appleton-Century-Crofts, 1991.

Gardosi, J. Ethnic differences in fetal growth. *Ultrasound Obstet Gynecol* 6:73–74, 1995.

Goldstein, I., and Reece, E. A. Cerebellar growth in normal and growth-restricted fetuses of multiple gestations. *Am J Obstet Gynecol* 173:1343–1348, 1995.

Lin, C. C., Sheikh, Z., and Lopata, R. The association between oligohydramnios and intrauterine growth retardation. *Obstet Gynecol* 76:1100–1104, 1990.

Moore, T. R., Longo, J., Leopold, G. R., Casola, G., and Gosink, B. B. The reliability and predictive value of an amniotic fluid scoring system in severe second-trimester oligohydramnios. *Obstet Gynecol* 73:739–742, 1989.

17 LARGE FOR DATES

ROGER C. SANDERS

KEY WORDS

Acardiac Acephalic Twin. One twin is malformed. No heart is present and circulation is pumped from the second twin. Either partial or complete absence of the head with cystic hygroma.

Conjoined (Siamese) Twins. Twins that are joined at some point in their bodies.

Corpus Luteum Cyst. A cyst developing as a response to human chorionic gonadotropin (HCG) in the first few weeks of pregnancy. Such cysts usually disappear by 14 to 16 weeks after the last menstrual period.

Cytomegalic Inclusion Disease (CMV). Viral disease characterized in utero by fetal ascites, intrauterine growth restriction, intrafetal calcification, and cardiac anomalies. The placenta is often enlarged.

Dizygotic Dichorionic. Twin pregnancies in which there are two nonidentical fetuses and two placentas.

Erythroblastosis Fetalis (Rh Incompatibility). A form of fetal anemia in which the fetal red cells are destroyed by contact with a maternal antibody produced in response to a previous fetus. Severe fetal heart failure results.

Fifth Disease. See *Parvovirus.*

Fraternal Twins. Dizygotic dichorionic nonidentical twins (see Fig. 17-2).

Gestational Diabetes. A form of diabetes mellitus that manifests itself only in pregnancy. Discovered by performing a glucose tolerance test, and associated with large babies.

Hydrops Fetalis. The fetal abdomen contains ascites and the skin is thickened by excess fluid. This condition has a variety of causes, of which the most well known is Rh (rhesus) incompatibility. Other causes are associated with what is known as nonimmune hydrops (see Chapter 18).

Locking Twins. Because the twins are not separated by an amniotic sac membrane, they become entangled and are consequently difficult to deliver.

Macrosomia. Exceptionally large infant with fat deposition in the subcutaneous tissues; seen in fetuses of diabetic mothers.

Monochorionic Diamniotic. Identical twins in two amniotic cavities.

Monochorionic Monoamniotic. Identical twins in a single cavity.

Monozygotic Monochorionic. Twin pregnancies in which the fetuses are identical; usually an amniotic sac membrane divides the two amniotic cavities, but it may be absent.

Multiple Pregnancy. More than a singleton fetus (e.g., twins, triplets, or quadruplets).

Myometrial Contraction. Localized slow, asymptomatic contraction of the uterine wall. Reexamination after 20 to 30 minutes will show it to have disappeared.

Nonimmune Hydrops. Not related to underlying immunologic problems. There are many different causes. A cardiac origin is the most common.

Parvovirus. Viral disease characterized by severe fetal anemia. It may result in hydrops. It usually occurs in child care providers.

Polyhydramnios. Excessive amniotic fluid. Defined as more than 2 liters at term.

Rubella. Viral disease occurring in utero with a number of associated fetal anomalies including congenital heart disease.

Stuck Twin. Massive polyhydramnios around one twin and severe oligohydramnios around the second. Almost always a fatal condition unless some of the amniotic fluid is withdrawn.

Toxoplasmosis. Parasitic disease affecting the fetus in utero, often resulting in intracranial calcification.

Twin-to-Twin Transfusion Syndrome. When monozygotic twins share a placenta, most of the blood from the placenta may be appropriated by one fetus at the expense of the other. One twin becomes excessively large, and the other unduly small.

VACTERL. Combination of findings seen mostly in diabetics. There are *v*ertebral, *a*nal, *c*ongenital heart, *t*racheoesophageal, *r*enal and *l*imb findings. The acronym is derived from the first initial of the components.

THE CLINICAL PROBLEM

If the pregnancy appears clinically more advanced than predicted by dates, several detectable causes should be considered by the sonographer. Most commonly the mother is wrong about her dates. Other possible causes of a uterus that is too large for dates include (1) polyhydramnios; (2) multiple pregnancy; (3) a large fetus; (4) a mass in addition to the uterus; and (5) a large placenta.

Hydramnios (Polyhydramnios)

In polyhydramnios there is excess amniotic fluid; consequently, the limbs stand out, separated by large echo-free areas devoid of any fetal structures. Detailed sonographic visualization of the fetal gastrointestinal tract and the skeletal and central nervous systems is required because anomalies in these areas are associated with polyhydramnios (see Chapter 18). Other causes of polyhydramnios include maternal diabetes mellitus, multiple pregnancy, and hydrops. Isolated mild to moderate polyhydramnios at 20 to 30 weeks is common and often precedes macrosomia.

Twins

It is important to establish whether there is a multiple pregnancy in a uterus that appears large for dates. Twins are at risk for a number of problems during pregnancy and have to be followed with serial sonograms to see that growth is adequate, that death has not occurred, and that one twin is not growing at the expense of the other. Careful sonographic examination of multiple pregnancy is necessary because the fetuses often adopt an unusual fetal lie. Additional fetuses, as in quintuplets, can easily be missed if careful scanning is not performed.

Macrosomia

Unduly large fetuses (over 4000 g at birth) pose management dilemmas for the obstetrician because they are difficult for the mother to deliver. They are often the fetuses of diabetic or obese mothers. Weight estimation is important here because the obstetrician must decide whether to perform a cesarean section and must be alert to the delivery problems that occur with the fetuses of diabetic mothers.

Mass and Fetus

Additional masses may give the impression that the uterus is larger than it really is, as with fibroids or ovarian cysts. Such problems are particularly important if an abortion is being considered because the clinician may incorrectly estimate the dates as being beyond the legal limits for abortion. Fibroids cause a number of problems during pregnancy, such as spontaneous abortion and difficulty in delivery, so that size estimation and location of fibroids are important.

Hydatidiform Mole

Hydatidiform mole causes uterine enlargement in the first and early second trimester. This condition is described in detail in Chapter 12.

ANATOMY

The following are important concepts to keep in mind regarding twins:

Amnionicity—the number of sacs

Chorionicity—the number of placentas

Monozygotic—single zygote that divides to form identical twins

Dizygotic—two zygotes that form fraternal twins

Amnionicity

Each sac is surrounded by an amniotic membrane and each placenta gives rise to a chorionic membrane. So, in a dichorionic pregnancy—that is, one with two placentas—it is possible to see four "leaves" of the membranes that separate the fetuses (possible, but, unfortunately, unlikely). Because these layers are difficult to separate, a subjective evaluation of the thickness is done; if only the amnions are present, the membrane is quite thin and may be difficult to see. No measurement of amniotic membrane thickness is used because the apparent thickness varies depending on the membrane angle to the ultrasonic beam. It is thickest at right angles to the beam. When there are two sacs and two placentas (diamniotic dichorionic), placental tissue often grows into the gap between the amniotic cavities, creating the "twin peak" sign (Fig. 17-1).

Chorionicity

The most common type of twins is dichorionic diamniotic (about two thirds of them). In monochorionic diamniotic pregnancy there is a shared placenta, but there are two separate cord insertions, each in its own sac. Monochorionic monoamniotic looks the same, with no sac membrane visible.

In dichorionic pregnancies, there may be adjacent placentas or two separate placentas. It can be difficult or impossible to tell a fused from an adjacent placenta, but is important to try and make this distinction (Fig. 17-2).

◼ TECHNIQUE

When a patient is large for dates owing to a multiple gestation, the scanning routine changes. The first rule of finding twins is: *Look for the third*. Woe be to the sonographer who gets caught up in the excitement of discovering twins, and neglects to hook that femur up to trunk number three.

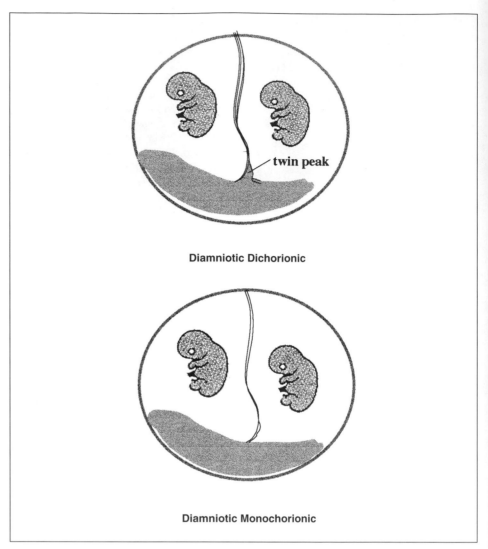

Diamniotic Dichorionic

Diamniotic Monochorionic

FIGURE 17-1. Diagram showing the two types of diamniotic pregnancies. In a dichorionic diamniotic pregnancy, four separate components make up the intervening membrane between the two cavities. There are separate amniotic and chorionic membranes from each pregnancy. In a dichorionic diamniotic pregnancy the placenta grows into the gap between the two amniotic cavities forming the twin peak sign. The presence of a twin peak sign supported by visualization of at least three membranes is reliable evidence of a diamniotic dichorionic pregnancy. In a monochorionic diamniotic pregnancy only two amniotic membranes make up the intervening membrane, so the membrane is thinner and has only two components. No twin peak sign will be seen in a monochorionic diamniotic pregnancy.

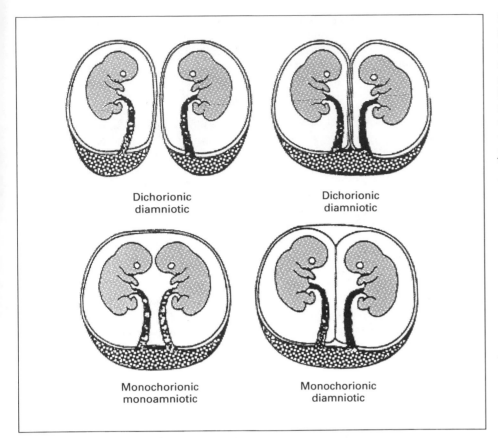

Dichorionic
diamniotic

Dichorionic
diamniotic

Monochorionic
monoamniotic

Monochorionic
diamniotic

FIGURE 17-2. Diagram showing the different types of twins. Dichorionic diamniotic twins may have a shared or adjacent placenta.

Counting and Assigning Position

So, the first order of business is to do a sweep through the uterus and count heads. Establish that each fetus has a beating heart, because there is a higher incidence of fetal death in multiple gestations, then assign a number or letter to each head, traditionally starting with the first to present. This does *not* mean the lowest head, necessarily. If both twins, for example, are cephalic, and twin A on the right is clearly lower, it still must be labeled as "A, right side," because on the subsequent exam it may be breech. With twins this is easy; with more than two, follow the membranes and placentas and draw a map to assign the letters, so anyone can perform the follow-up work and be sure to give the right set of measurements to each fetus.

When, and how, you tell the parents during this process depends on the rules of your department (some obstetricians like to break any unusual news, but that can be impossible to pull off in these circumstances) and your subjective evaluation of how they'll take it. It's a nice touch to be sure the father is seated first.

Determining Amnionicity and Chorionicity

Usually, multiple gestational patients are clinically large for dates early enough that it is not too crowded, and it is relatively easy to count placentas and look for membranes. Monochorionic membranes can be so hard to see that a higher frequency may help; don't just give up if you don't find the membrane easily, because a monochorionic monoamniotic pregnancy is a worrisome diagnosis. Use a high magnification and look for the twin peak sign (see Fig. 17-1) and at least three membranes to diagnose diamniotic dichorionic twins. Try squeezing the uterus up and down gently with the transducer while you watch the membrane to see if you can get the leaves to separate. Cine loop may be helpful in documenting temporarily splayed membranes. Look for cord insertions to help match placentas with fetuses.

Keeping Measurements Straight

Since most equipment has computer-generated computations, it's necessary to enter measurements for each fetus separately; sometimes it's necessary to trick the machine into thinking it is a different patient by erasing the mother's name, then re-entering "Nancy Smith—B" for the next one.

Before *every* measurement, start at the proper head and follow the spine to your destination. Healthy twins interact a lot in utero; arms and legs get surprisingly entangled.

Gender Determination

Establishing the fetal sex becomes important clinically in twins. If two genders are present it proves that they are dizygotic and rules out monochorionicity even if no membrane is found. Fetuses of the same sex, with one placenta and thin membranes, are monochorionic diamniotic; if amniocentesis is necessary, the greatest care should be taken to be sure there is a sample from each sac (see Chapter 52). If they are the same sex with no membranes (monoamniotic monochorionic), they are at risk for various problems, such as entangled cords and acardiac acephalic twins.

Special Views

Although measurements are done separately, some views should show the fetuses together. A view with both heads is definitive proof of twins. A split screen with a good abdominal circumference from each baby shows comparable growth at a glance and can document the position of both fetuses. How is baby B relative to baby A? or C? Don't forget to label whose part is presenting on the cervical evaluation views. These composite views are especially important when pathology is present, and the growth of one or more fetus is affected.

PATHOLOGY
◆ Large Fetus (Macrosomia)

Exceptionally large fetuses cause discrepancies between estimated dates and examination findings. Sometimes these fetuses are normally large infants. Often the mother has mild diabetes mellitus and the fetus is macrosomic. Polyhydramnios is commonly seen with macrosomia and often develops before the fetus enlarges.

When a large fetus is found, the following procedures are in order:

1. Measure the biparietal diameter.
2. Measure the trunk circumference. The normal head-to-trunk ratios are inappropriate in such babies, but the fetal weight can still be estimated. If the weight estimate is above the 90th percentile, the fetus is considered "macrosomic." If all measurements are normal, but the abdominal circumference is above the 90th percentile, this finding in itself is very suspicious for macrosomia, even though the overall weight is still less than the 90th percentile.
3. Search for evidence of scalp or trunk edema, which will be apparent as a second line running around the skull or trunk. This is a common finding in infants of diabetic mothers and is due to subcutaneous deposition of fat. The fetal cheeks are especially prominent.
4. Examine the placenta. The placenta is often increased in size in diabetic mothers.

5. Fetal anomalies related to the genitourinary tract, central nervous system, and cardiovascular system are more common in diabetic pregnancies than in others. Make sure that these areas are examined in detail. This constellation of anomalies is known as the VACTERL syndrome (vertebral, anal, cardiovascular, tracheoesophageal, renal, and limb).

Multiple Pregnancy

As mentioned in the Technique section, it is essential to determine whether there is a monochorionic or dichorionic pregnancy and whether an intersac membrane exists, because complications such as stuck twin and twin-twin transfusion only occur if there is a monochorionic pregnancy.

The membrane is absent in about 10 percent of monochorionic pregnancies. Absence of the membrane is associated with various abnormalities (e.g., conjoined twins, locking twins, polyhydramnios, asymmetric growth, and tangled cords).

Cord Problems

If there appears to be only one amniotic cavity, try to follow each cord and see whether they are entangled. The two cords are twisted around each other and may have as many as twelve twists.

Acardiac Acephalic Twins

An unusual variant of a twin pregnancy with no amniotic membrane present is an acardiac acephalic monster. A twin is seen with no heart, yet it may show movement. There is massive skin thickening of the trunk with cystic hygroma. The legs are spared. The head may be absent or partially present.

Conjoined Twins

Conjoined and locking twins should be ruled out by noting position changes. The body components of both fetuses move together if they are conjoined. If conjoined twins are found, make sure that there are two heads and trunks and eight limbs.

Death

Make sure all fetuses are alive—there is an increased incidence of fetal death in multiple pregnancy.

Twin-to-Twin Transfusion Syndrome

Identical twins share a common placental circulation. One twin may grow at the expense of the other (twin-to-twin transfusion syndrome), receiving some of the blood that should have reached the second. One twin becomes plethoric (too much blood), the second anemic. Polyhydramnios may be present.

If one twin is bigger than the other and the twin-to-twin transfusion syndrome seems possible, look for ascites in the larger twin, an early indication of heart failure. The other, smaller twin will have features of intrauterine growth restriction (IUGR) (see Chapter 16). IUGR of one twin also occurs with greater frequency than in singletons in the absence of twin-to-twin transfusion syndrome and may be seen in dizygotic pregnancies.

If the twin-to-twin transfusion syndrome is severe there will also be pleural and pericardial effusions and skin thickening in the larger twin. Look for IUGR or asymmetric growth. On follow-up examinations, measure the biparietal diameter, trunk circumference, and head/abdomen ratio on both twins every time. These measurements may be difficult, because multiple pregnancies often result in an unusual fetal lie.

Stuck Twin

The "stuck twin" syndrome is usually fatal unless recognized by ultrasound (Fig. 17-3). There is severe polyhydramnios around one twin and oligohydramnios around the second twin. It may be difficult to see the membrane around the stuck twin. The stuck twin will not move and may appear to be adhering to the anterior or lateral aspect of the uterus. Magnified views will show the membrane alongside the fetus. Aspirating large amounts of fluid from the polyhydramniotic sac may allow survival of the stuck twin. Fluid may then return within the sac that previously showed severe oligohydramnios. In most instances, this syndrome is related to the twin-to-twin transfusion syndrome.

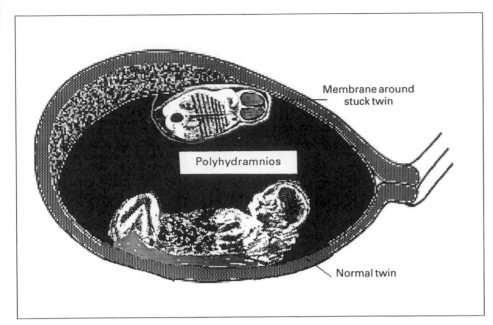

FIGURE 17-3. Stuck twin. There is polyhydramnios surrounding the normal twin. The smaller fetus is apparently attached to the anterior abdominal wall. The amniotic membrane can just be seen around the stuck twin.

Fetal Hydrops

A large-for-dates fetus may be the first indication of fetal hydrops with poly-hydramnios. Until a few years ago this condition was almost always due to Rh incompatibility (erythroblastosis fetalis). Hydrops due to Rh incompatibility is known as immune hydrops. This condition is now uncommon and is considered further in Chapter 18. Nowadays hydrops is more commonly due to certain congenital fetal anomalies and infections, in which case it is known as nonimmune hydrops. Nonimmune hydrops has particular sonographic findings.

The presence of any two of the following features allows a diagnosis of hydrops:

1. *Fetal edema.* The fetus may show evidence of scalp and skin edema as a double outline around the fetal parts (Fig. 17-4).
2. *Placental enlargement.* The placenta is often markedly enlarged with fetal hydrops and has an abnormal, homogeneous, echogenic texture. A large placenta is most likely to occur with Rh incompatibility, placental tumors, and fetal cardiac problems.
3. *Polyhydramnios.* Polyhydramnios is usually present and is responsible for the enlarged uterus.

4. *Ascites.* Fluid can be seen surrounding the bowel or liver and outlining the greater omentum, which is seen as a membrane.
5. *Pleural effusion.* Fluid outlines the lungs and diaphragm.
6. *Pericardial effusion.* Fluid surrounds the heart.

Underlying Causes

Nonimmune hydrops is a consequence of a number of different conditions, some of which can be detected ultrasonically.

PLACENTAL TUMORS. Placental tumors siphon off the blood destined for the fetus, and the fetus becomes anemic. A mass is seen adjacent to the placenta or within it (see Fig. 15-11). Almost all placental tumors are chorioangiomas. These tumors are very vascular and show visible real-time flow or flow on Doppler. Fetal ascites is a sign that the fetus is in danger and has heart failure due to anemia.

CARDIAC AND CHEST ANOMALIES AND FETAL TUMORS. Cardiac and chest anomalies and fetal tumors are considered in Chapter 18. All may cause hydrops.

VIRAL DISEASES. Diseases such as toxoplasmosis, cytomegalic inclusion disease, fifth disease (parvovirus), and toxoplasmosis are causes of fetal hydrops. Cytomegalic inclusion disease and toxoplasmosis may be associated with intracranial calcification and acoustic shadowing within the brain. Fetal hepatosplenomegaly is common. Large placentas may be seen with these conditions.

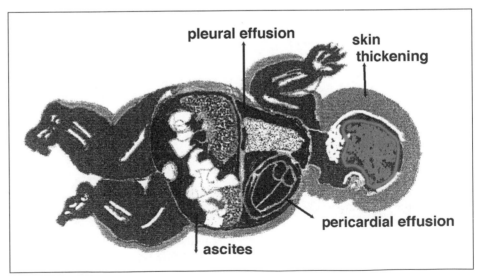

FIGURE 17-4. Sonographic findings in hydrops. Note the marked skin thickening, fluid surrounding the lung, the pericardial effusion, and fluid in the abdomen surrounding the small bowel loops.

Parvovirus infection causes fetal anemia and thus hydrops. Treatment with intracord blood transfusion is possible.

CHROMOSOMAL ANOMALIES. Some chromosomal anomalies are associated with hydrops (see Chapter 18). Discovery of hydrops is followed by:

1. Chromosomal analysis
2. Fetal echocardiogram
3. Tests for toxoplasmosis and cytomegalic inclusion disease

Additional Masses

The uterus may appear large for dates because of a mass. Either an ovarian cyst or mass or a uterine mass may be present in addition to pregnancy.

Fibroids

Fibroids (leiomyomas) are a common cause of apparent uterine enlargement. Fibroids may be confused with the placenta because they have a somewhat similar acoustic texture, but the texture of a fibroid is usually more disorganized and tends to bulge beyond the outline of the uterus. The uterine outline is distorted by a fibroid, but not by a myometrial contraction or placental process (Fig. 17-5). Fibroids located in the lower uterine segment near the cervix are clinically important because they can interfere with delivery. As fibroids are followed through pregnancy, they may change in texture, becoming less echogenic because of cystic degeneration. Most fibroids become difficult to find in the third trimester, but are visible again after delivery. Rarely there may be bleeding into a fibroid (red degeneration). A fibroid undergoing red degeneration is very tender and larger than on a previous study.

Ovarian Cysts

Physiologic ovarian cysts, known as corpus luteum cysts, are common in pregnancy. In the first few weeks of pregnancy, the increased amount of human chorionic gonadotropin stimulates the development of such cysts. They may achieve a large size (up to 10 cm), but involute spontaneously as pregnancy continues and usually disappear by 16 weeks. They are echo-free, apart from an occasional septum, unless bleeding has occurred within them.

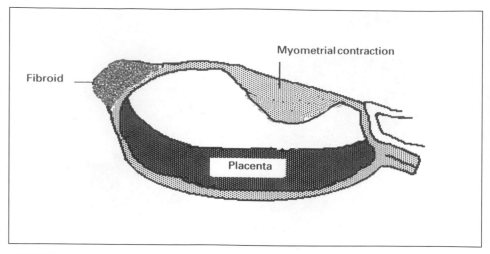

FIGURE 17-5. Fibroid versus myometrial contraction. The fibroid distorts the outline of the uterus. The myometrial contraction has uterine texture, is smoothly contoured, and expands toward the fetus.

Other types of cysts may occur in the ovaries, notably dermoids and serous cystadenomas. These cysts often contain internal structures such as calcifications or septa and do not decrease in size on follow-up sonograms. Cysts arising from the kidney or liver may appear on palpation to be associated with the uterus.

Occasionally a cyst or ovary may twist on itself. The cyst or ovary is locally tender, and may contain internal echoes due to hemorrhage. There may be blood around the cyst.

Abscess Formation

Abscess formation due to a ruptured appendix or pelvic inflammatory disease may occur at the same time as pregnancy. An abscess has a complicated internal texture, as described in Chapter 30, and is usually locally tender.

✴ PITFALLS

1. *Fibroids vs. myometrial contraction.* Uterine contractions occur throughout pregnancy and are known as myometrial contractions (see Fig. 17-5). They last for up to a half hour and may simulate a fibroid or placenta while in progress, although the internal texture is more even than that of a fibroid and different from placenta. To differentiate a myometrial contraction from a fibroid, reexamine the patient after approximately half an hour, or document a change in shape and size at the end of the exam. Most machines document the time onscreen.

2. *Cysts vs. bladder.* Cysts located anterior to the uterus have been mistaken for the bladder. The normal bladder should have a typical shape. Ovarian cysts are generally spherical. Asking the patient to void or fill the bladder will make the distinction apparent.

3. *Overlooking a triplet or twin.* A thorough search of the entire uterine cavity is the only way to avoid this disaster.

4. *Pseudoascites.* When the fetus appears to have ascites in a nondependent area think of pseudoascites. In this condition the sonolucent space is related to the paraspinous muscles and not to fluid.

5. *Fetal ascites vs. polyhydramnios.* If the fetus has massive fetal ascites mainly due to renal obstruction, the vast amount of fluid in the abdomen may be mistaken for polyhydramnios, since fetal renal ascites is associated with very severe oligohydramnios. Close inspection will show that the fetal bowel is floating in the ascites.

6. *Succenturiate lobe.* Even though there are two apparent placentas, there still can be a monochorionic diamniotic pregnancy if one of the apparent two placentas is actually a succenturiate lobe. Unless the twin peak sign is present or the fetuses are of different gender, continue to look for complications of twin pregnancies such as twin-twin transfusion syndrome and stuck twin syndrome.

❓ WHERE ELSE TO LOOK

1. *Cystic masses* should be followed sonographically because most, but not all, will go away. Those that do not disappear, or even grow, may be surgically removed.
2. *Polyhydramnios* necessitates a detailed anomaly search and extra growth parameters, such as limb lengths.

SELECTED READING

Abramowicz, J. S., Sherer, D. M., and Woods Jr., J. R. Ultrasonographic measurement of cheek-to-cheek diameter in fetal growth disturbances. *Am J Obstet Gynecol* 169:405–408, 1993.

Benson, C. B., and Doubilet, P. M. Ultrasound of multiple gestations. *Semin Roentgenol* 26:50–62, 1991.

Brown, D. L., Benson, C. B., Driscoll, S. G., and Doubilet, P. M. Twin-twin transfusion syndrome: Sonographic findings. *Radiology* 170:61–63, 1989.

Brown, D. L., Polger, M., Clark, P. K., Bromley, B. S., and Doubilet, P. M. Very echogenic amniotic fluid: Ultrasonography-amniocentesis correlation. *J Ultrasound Med* 13:95–97, 1994.

Callen, P. W. (Ed.). *Ultrasonography in Obstetrics and Gynecology* (3rd ed.). Philadelphia: Saunders, 1994.

Divon, M. Y., and Weiner, Z. Ultrasound in twin pregnancy. *Semin Perinatol* 19:404–412, 1995.

Elliott, J. P., Urig, M. A., and Clewell, W. H. Aggressive therapeutic amniocentesis for treatment of twin-twin transfusion syndrome. *Obstet Gynecol* 77:537–540, 1991.

Finberg, H. J. The "twin peak" sign: Reliable evidence of dichorionic twinning. *J Ultrasound Med* 11:571–577, 1992.

Monteagudo, A., Timor-Tritsch, I. E., and Sharma, S. Early and simple determination of chorionic and amniotic type in multifetal gestations in the first fourteen weeks by high-frequency transvaginal ultrasonography. *Am J Obstet Gynecol* 170:824–829, 1994.

Nicolaides, K. H., Fontanarosa, M., Gabbe, S. G., and Rodeck, C. H. Failure of ultrasonographic parameters to predict the severity of fetal anemia in rhesus isoimmunization. *Am J Obstet Gynecol* 158:920–926, 1988.

Reisner, D. P., Mahony, B. S., Petty, C. N., Nyberg, D. A., Porter, T. F., Zingheim, R. W., Williams, M. A., and Luthy, D. A. Stuck twin syndrome: Outcome in thirty-seven consecutive cases. *Am J Obstet Gynecol* 169:991–995, 1993.

Rosati, P., Exacoustos, C., Caruso, A., and Mancuso, S. Ultrasound diagnosis of fetal macrosomia. *Ultrasound Obstet Gynecol* 2:23–29, 1992.

Sahakian, V., Syrop, C., and Turner, D. Endometrial carcinoma: Transvaginal ultrasonography prediction of depth of myometrial invasion. *Gynecol Oncol* 43:217–219, 1991.

Sanders, R. C. (Ed.). *Structural Fetal Abnormalities: The Total Picture*. St. Louis: Mosby-Year Book, 1996.

Sohaey, R., Nyberg, D. A., Sickler, G. K., and Williams, M. A. Idiopathic polyhydramnios: Association with fetal macrosomia. *Radiology* 190:393–396, 1994.

Stoll, C. G., Alembik, Y., and Dott, B. Study of 156 cases of polyhydramnios and congenital malformations in a series of 118,265 consecutive births. *Am J Obstet Gynecol* 165:586–590, 1991.

Weiner, C. P. Challenge of twin-twin transfusion syndrome. *Contemp OB GYN* May:83–104, 1992.

18 POSSIBLE FETAL ANOMALIES

ROGER C. SANDERS

SONOGRAM ABBREVIATIONS

AH	Anterior horn
B,Bl	Bladder
BS	Brainstem
Ce	Cerebellum
Ch	Choroid
CV	Cavum vergi
D	Diaphragm
F	Falx
FH	Fetal head
FS	Fetal spine
H	Heart
He	Hematoma
L	Liver
LV	Lateral ventricle
M	Cisterna magna
N	Nose
Pe	Peduncle
Pl	Placenta
S, St	Stomach
T,Th	Thalamus
UPJ	Uteropelvic junction
V	Draining vein
VG	Vein of Galen aneurysm
3, 3rd	Third ventricle

KEY WORDS

Acetylcholinesterase. An enzyme found in the amniotic fluid when a neural crest anomaly is present. It may be found in trace amounts if an abdominal wall defect, such as omphalocele, is present.

Achondrogenesis. A lethal type of dwarfism similar to thanatophoric dwarfism.

Achondroplasia. A type of dwarfism characterized by a bulging forehead and short limbs.

Alpha-Fetoprotein (AFP). An enzyme found in maternal blood and amniotic fluid that is elevated in the presence of neural crest anomalies, some gastrointestinal anomalies, fetal death, twins, wrong estimation of dates, fetal masses such as sacrococcygeal teratoma and cystic hygroma, and maternal liver problems. Low levels of AFP are associated with Down syndrome.

Amniotic Band Syndrome. Bands within the amniotic fluid adhere to the fetus and amputate portions of limbs. In its most severe form it causes the limb/body wall complex.

Anal Atresia. Intestinal obstruction at the anal level due to failure to form the rectum; usually without sonographic features.

Anencephaly. Most common fetal intracranial anomaly. The base of the brain and face are the only things present in the head; the cranium is absent.

Anhydramnios. No amniotic fluid.

Arnold-Chiari Malformation (Type II). Low position of the cerebellum in the upper cervical spinal canal due to cord tethering. Associated with "lemon" skull shape, banana-shaped cerebellum, and hydrocephalus.

Banana Sign. Change in the shape of the cerebellum (it becomes curved) that occurs in the presence of spina bifida.

Cisterna Magna. Fluid-filled space at the back of the head that lies between the cerebellum and the skull.

Cleft Palate. Congenital gap in the midface that involves the palate, maxilla, and possibly the lip.

Cloaca. Fluid-filled bag into which ureters, rectum, and vagina enter; seen with certain developmental anomalies.

Closed Neural Defects. Neural defects in which the spinal cord and brain are not in contact with the amniotic fluid and thus are not associated with an elevated alpha-fetoprotein level.

Clubfoot. The foot is acutely angled. This abnormal foot position may be a sign of chromosomal anomaly.

Cyclops. A single eye is present. Associated with holoprosencephaly.

Cyllosoma (Limb/Body Wall Complex). Lethal abnormality thought to be due to amniotic bands. Features are gastroschisis, spina bifida, kyphoscoliosis, and absent limbs.

Cystic Adenomatoid Malformation. Anomaly in which a part of the lung is replaced by cysts.

Cystic Hygroma. Large fluid-containing sac filled with lymph, usually located in the region of the neck. May be part of a generalized fatal condition—lymphangiectasia—or a benign focal process. Associated with Turner's and Down syndrome.

Cytomegalic Inclusion Disease (CMV). Fetal viral disease sometimes resulting in intracranial calcification, microcephaly, and mental deficiency.

Dandy-Walker Syndrome. Brain anomaly with a dilated fourth ventricle and possible secondary dilation of the rest of the ventricles of the brain. A small cerebellum is the cardinal feature.

Diaphragmatic Hernia. A portion of one diaphragm is missing, and the bowel or liver lies in the chest.

Diastematomyelia. Bony spur in the center of the spinal canal, splitting the cord.

Double Bubble Sign. Sign of duodenal atresia in which two circular, fluid-filled structures, representing the stomach and duodenum, are seen in the upper abdomen.

Down Syndrome (Mongolism). Syndrome seen predominantly in the fetuses of women who are over 35 years old; recognizable at amniotic fluid analysis or chorionic villus sampling by the presence of an abnormal chromosome. It is associated with congenital heart disease and duodenal atresia.

Duodenal Atresia. Intestinal obstruction at a duodenal level with subsequent distention of the duodenum and stomach by fluid. Associated with polyhydramnios and Down syndrome.

Duplication Cyst. Congenital anomaly. A portion of the gastrointestinal tract, usually the stomach, is reduplicated. If a cystic mass can be seen with ultrasound, there is generally not a patent connection between the gut and the cyst.

Dysplasia. See *Multicystic (Dysplastic) Kidney*.

Ectopia Cordis. The heart partially lies outside and anterior to the chest. Associated with *omphalocele* and the *pentalogy of Cantrell*.

Ellis-van Creveld Syndrome (Six-Fingered Dwarfism). Type of dwarfism in which there are extra digits.

Encephalocele. Herniation of the coverings of the brain through defect in the skull. Brain tissue is contained within the herniation, although usually most of the contents of the sac are fluid.

Exencephaly. Variant of anencephaly in which some cortical brain remains.

Finnish Nephropathy. A cause of renal failure and increased AFP. The kidneys are often normal but may be large and echogenic.

Gastroschisis. Condition similar to *omphalocele* except that no membrane covers the herniated material. Gut floats freely in the amniotic fluid. The wall defect is in the right lower part of the abdomen.

Holoprosencephaly. Intracranial anomaly. A horseshoe-shaped ventricle replaces the two lateral ventricles. Usually fatal or causes severe mental retardation. Associated with trisomy 13 and facial defects such as cleft lip, palate, and hypotelorism, and in extreme cases, cyclopia and proboscis.

Holt-Oram Syndrome. Congenital syndrome consisting of a combination of heart disease and absence of a digit or the radius in the arm.

Hydranencephaly. Absence of the cortical brain. Portions of the midbrain and brainstem are present. Not compatible with life.

Hydrocephalus. Marked enlargement of the cerebral ventricles. Implies ventricular obstruction. A better term is ventriculomegaly or nonspecific ventricular enlargement.

Hydronephrosis. An obstructed kidney with a dilated collecting system.

Hydrops Fetalis. The fetal abdomen contains ascites and the skin is thickened by excess fluid. This condition has a variety of causes, of which the most well known is rhesus incompatibility (Rh disease). Other causes are grouped as nonimmune hydrops.

Hypoplastic Left Heart Syndrome. Congenital abnormality in which the aorta and left side of the heart are too small. This condition is often fatal after birth, even with surgery.

Hypotelorism. Condition in which the orbits are too close together.

Ileal Atresia. Intestinal obstruction at a midgut level. Filling of small bowel loops with fluid; associated with polyhydramnios.

Infantile Polycystic Kidney. A congenital condition in which large kidneys are filled with tiny cysts.

Iniencephaly. Defect consisting of an encephalocele that involves the posterior aspects of the skull and the cervical vertebrae; some vertebrae may be missing.

Karyotype. Process of performing chromosomal analysis on a fetus.

Kleebattschadel Deformity. Skull deformity in which there is a large bony bulge off the superior aspect of the head.

Kyphoscoliosis. Spine that is bent sideways and unduly flexed.

Lamina. Lateral bridge of bone covering the posterior spinal canal.

Lemon Sign. Deformity of the skull in which it assumes a shape similar to a lemon. The frontal areas become flattened. This type of anomaly is seen when spina bifida is present.

Limb/Body Wall Syndrome. See *Cyllosoma*.

Lymphangioma. See *Cystic Hygroma*.

Meckel's Syndrome (Meckel-Gruber Syndrome). A lethal syndrome consisting of infantile polycystic kidney, encephalocele, and extra digits (polydactyly).

Meconium. Contents of the fetal bowel.

Meconium Peritonitis. Bowel rupture in utero, which leads to meconium spillage with consequent calcification. There is usually bowel obstruction.

Megacystis Microcolon Syndrome. Rare anomaly with huge bladder, dilated ureters and calyces, and minute large bowel. Only the bladder is visible with ultrasound. Most patients are female, and there is often polyhydramnios.

Meningocele. Spinal bone defect with cerebrospinal fluid pouch.

Microcephaly. Unduly small skull and brain; associated with mental deficiency.

Micrognathia. Small or absent jaw. A feature of a number of rare syndromes.

Multicystic (Dysplastic) Kidney. Developmental abnormality of the kidney in which the normal renal parenchyma is totally replaced by cysts of varying sizes. If bilateral, it is not compatible with survival.

Myelocele. Spinal bone defect with spinal cord protrusion, but no cerebrospinal fluid pouch.

Myelomeningocele. Bone defect associated with tethering and distortion of the spinal cord and a fluid-containing cavity at the level of the abnormality.

Mutation. Spontaneous change in the chromosomal make-up of a cell.

Neural Crest Anomaly. A brain/spinal defect in which there is no skin covering on the spine or brain, and therefore contact between some portion of the central nervous system and the amniotic fluid occurs. This combination gives rise to a raised alpha-fetoprotein level. Anencephaly, encephalocele, and spina bifida are examples of neural crest anomalies.

Omphalocele. Herniation of some of the gut, including the liver, out of the abdomen through an umbilical opening (see *Gastroschisis*). A membrane covers the herniated contents. Associated with other congenital anomalies.

Osteogenesis Imperfecta. Congenital anomaly in which bone fractures occur.

Pentalogy of Cantrell. Combination of partial diaphragmatic absence, ectopia cordis, omphalocele, sternal abnormality, and pericardial deficiency.

Phocomelia. Most of the arms or legs are absent so that flippers originate from the trunk. Used to be seen following thalidomide administration.

(continues)

Posterior Urethral Valves. Valves situated in the posterior urethras cause partial or complete obstruction of the bladders, ureters, and kidneys. Occurs only in males.

Potter's Syndrome. Fetus with bilateral renal abnormalities, which may consist of absent kidneys, bilateral hydronephrosis, bilateral multicystic dysplastic kidneys, or infantile polycystic kidney. Anhydramnios may accompany this syndrome. The consequences of absent amniotic fluid—unusual face, deformed limbs, and hypoplastic lungs—will be seen at birth. Most such fetuses are stillborn.

Proboscis. Instead of a nose, this soft tissue tubular structure may be seen above the eyes in holoprosencephaly.

Prune Belly (Eagle-Barrett) Syndrome (Agenesis of the Abdominal Muscles). Congenital condition in which there are weakened or absent abdominal wall muscles, markedly distended ureters with tiny or hydronephrotic kidneys, and a large bladder.

Pulmonary Hypoplasia. Condition associated with oligohydramnios and extrinsic pressure on the chest, due to fluid or masses, in which the lungs never function adequately after birth.

Rachischisis. The bone and soft tissues that cover the posterior aspects of the spinal canal are unfused so the spinal cord is exposed.

Reflux (Vesicourethral). In the normal fetus, the ureter enters the bladder through a long tunnel which allows urine to pass into the bladder, but not to go back to the kidney. If this tunnel is short, urine can pass in either direction. Reversal of urine flow back to the kidney is known as reflux.

Rhesus (Rh) Incompatibility (Erythroblastosis Fetalis). The fetal blood possesses a different Rh group from the maternal blood. When maternal blood cells leak into the fetal circulation, they interact, forming antibodies. In the next pregnancy there is hemolysis, and the fetus is left anemic with hydrops.

Rockerbottom Foot. Abnormal foot with very prominent heel. May be an indication of a chromosomal anomaly.

Rubella. Viral disease that is associated with a number of fetal anomalies, including congenital heart disease, when occurring in utero.

Sequestration. Anomaly in which a segment of the lung does not connect with the trachea and has its own blood supply. Sometimes the abnormal segment of the lung develops below the diaphragm.

Spina Bifida. Bony spinal defect over the spinal canal. Nearly always accompanied by some form of myelomeningocele, sometimes with hydrocephalus.

Teratoma. Tumor composed of multiple different tissues that may arise anywhere in the body, but usually in the sacrum.

Tethering. The lower end of the cord normally ascends from the sacrum to level L2 in utero. With anomalies such as spina bifida and lipoma, it does not ascend, but terminates at a lower level, e.g., L5.

Thanatophoric Dwarf. Form of dwarfism that affects not only the limbs but also the chest, which is too small. Invariably fatal.

TORCH. Group of congenital infectious diseases with similar features: toxoplasmosis, rubella, cytomegalic inclusion disease, and herpes.

Toxoplasmosis. Parasitic disease affecting the fetus in utero and causing intracranial calcification.

Tracheoesophageal Fistula. Obstruction of the esophagus usually associated with a fistula to the trachea. Sometimes there is also a connection to the stomach through the trachea. In the most severe form no fluid reaches the stomach.

Triploidy. There are one and one half times as many chromosomes as there should be. Causes fetal death and a large, abnormal placenta that may look like a mole.

Triradiate. The fingers in thanatophoric dwarfism are separated and short, forming a triradiate shape.

Trisomy. Abnormal chromosomes are present; three are present where a specific pair should be. The most common types are 13, 18, and 21 (hence trisomy).

Turner's Syndrome. One sex chromosome is absent. Associated with cystic hygroma, a webbed neck, and mental deficiency.

Vein of Galen Aneurysm. A large arteriovenous fistula seen as a sizable cyst in the posterior aspect of the brain, above the tentorium.

Ventriculomegaly. Enlargement of the intracranial ventricles, not necessarily associated with obstruction.

 THE CLINICAL PROBLEM

Fetal anomalies as small as an extra digit or an abnormal little finger can be discovered by an accomplished sonographer. To distinguish normal from pathologic, all sonographers should have a detailed knowledge of normal fetal anatomy.

Anomalies should, if possible, be discovered before the fetus is 23 to 24 weeks old. If the fetus has a condition not compatible with normal life, therapeutic abortion may be desirable, but in many states it cannot be legally performed after 6 months gestational age. A practical limit of 23 weeks is often used, because beyond this age a fetus may be viable.

Nevertheless, discovery of an anomaly at a later stage of pregnancy is of practical importance because the optimal fashion and time of delivery can be arranged, and the patient can, if necessary, be transferred to a hospital that has neonatal care and pediatric surgical facilities. Fetuses with anomalies that may rupture at the time of delivery (such as an encephalocele) may be best delivered by cesarean section. If the fetal prognosis is very poor, those with a fluid-distended abdomen or head may be decompressed under ultrasound control prior to delivery in order to avoid a needless cesarean section.

Some clues to the presence of a fetal anomaly are discussed in the following sections.

Elevated Alpha-Fetoprotein Levels

Elevated alpha-fetoprotein (AFP) levels are associated with a number of anomalies, among which are:

1. Neural crest problems: anencephaly, spina bifida, and encephalocele
2. Abdominal wall problems: omphalocele and gastroschisis

For a detailed list see pathology section.

AFP can be measured in the mother's blood (serum AFP; evaluates AFP produced by both mother and fetus) and in the amniotic fluid at amniocentesis (evaluates only AFP produced by the fetus). Levels increase with gestational age. Acetylcholinesterase, found in the amniotic fluid, is increased only with anomalies.

Family History

Most hereditary anomalies are dominant, in which case there is a one in two chance of recurrence, or recessive, when the chance of recurrence is one in four. Usually there is a family history of an affected sibling, parent, or cousin, but the condition can be seen for the first time if a spontaneous mutation occurs. Examples of genetic conditions are adult polycystic kidney (dominant), infantile polycystic kidney (recessive), and osteogenesis imperfecta (dominant and recessive types). Usually the mother is referred for an ultrasound study because her family history is suspicious. On other occasions the family history is elicited only when an anomaly is seen and the patient is questioned.

Maternal Age

The risk of chromosomal anomalies increases as the mother ages. Amniocentesis for Down syndrome is recommended for pregnant women aged 35 or more. The risk of other chromosomal defects is also increased (Table 18-1).

Triple Screen

Maternal blood screening for AFP, estriol, and HCG is widely used between 16 and 22 weeks. Down syndrome and trisomy 18 result in changes in the level of these three substances in the mother's blood and reflect changes in the fetus. Levels of all three substances are increased with Down syndrome, whereas with trisomy 18, the level of all three substances is decreased from the normal maternal blood screening level. Increased alpha-fetoprotein is suspicious for a neural crest anomaly or an abdominal wall defect, as stated earlier.

TABLE 18-1. Incidence of Down Syndrome and Chromosomal Abnormalities According to Maternal Age

Maternal Age	Down Syndrome	Chromosomal Abnormalites
20	1/1923	1/526
21	1/1695	1/526
22	1/1538	1/500
23	1/1408	1/500
24	1/1299	1/476
25	1/1205	1/476
26	1/1124	1/476
27	1/1053	1/455
28	1/990	1/453
29	1/935	1/417
30	1/885	1/384
31	1/826	1/384
32	1/725	1/322
33	1/592	1/285
34	1/465	1/243
35	1/365	1/178
36	1/287	1/149
37	1/225	1/123
38	1/177	1/105
39	1/139	1/80
40	1/109	1/63
41	1/85	1/48
42	1/67	1/39
43	1/53	1/31
44	1/41	1/24
45	1/32	1/18
46	1/25	1/15
47	1/20	1/11
48	1/16	1/8
49	1/12	1/7

Teratogenic Drugs

Many drugs are said to have been responsible for fetal anomalies. Appendix 25 gives a list of drugs with an alleged risk. The only one that seems important in practice is the relationship between antiepileptic drugs and facial/spinal deformities. A dangerous nonprescription drug that causes intrauterine growth retardation is nicotine.

Polyhydramnios

Polyhydramnios is a clue to the presence of fetal anomalies that interfere with the intake and absorption of amniotic fluid. For a detailed list of the causes see the pathology section.

Small for Dates With Oligohydramnios

Look for a genitourinary problem when the fetus is small for dates and there is oligohydramnios. Very severe intrauterine growth retardation with oligohydramnios occurring before 28 weeks has a strong chance of being related to a chromosomal anomaly.

Lack of Fetal Mobility

Fetal activity is often absent or slowed with anomalies. Take a very good look around if the fetus is unduly still.

ANATOMY

The relevant anatomy is described in Chapter 14.

◢ TECHNIQUE

See Chapter 14 for appropriate technique in routine scanning of pregnant women. Additional areas that need examining when an anomaly search is being performed are the following.

The Hands

Anatomy

The hands are usually mildly flexed with all fingers and thumbs aligned. They should flex and extend frequently. After 15 to 16 weeks, the number of fetal digits (fingers and toes) can be counted.

Technique

To find the hands start scanning at the trunk. Find the humerus and continue out to the radius and ulna until you see the hands. When you have found the knuckles, angle the transducer slightly until you can see all fingers and the thumb simultaneously (Fig. 18-1). If the fetus is moving, snap an image of the hands as they fly by or use cine loop. Obtain a view that shows four or five digits simultaneously and see if any digit is out of alignment.

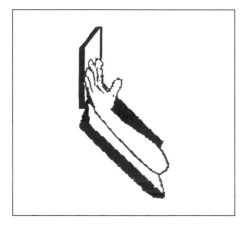

FIGURE 18-1. View showing the angle at which the hand and arm should be imaged to show the lower arm and hand position.

Pathology

If the fourth finger is overlapped by the third and fifth finger a chromosomal anomaly may be present. Unusual thumb positions may be a clue to a chromosomal anomaly or particular type of dwarfism (e.g., Hitchhiker thumb in diastrophic dwarfism). Count the number of digits, especially when investigating syndromes in which extra digits are present (e.g., Meckel's syndrome and Ellis-van Creveld syndrome) or in which a digit is missing (e.g., Holt-Oram syndrome). A small, incurved fifth finger (klinodactyly) with a short middle phalanx is seen with Down syndrome.

The Feet

Technique

Showing the feet and legs simultaneously is difficult. Inspect the toes like you inspect the fingers, for number, alignment, and position. Find the feet by tracing the hips to the femur to the fibula and tibia. It is not difficult to obtain a view that shows the bones of the foot and the toes. The trick is to line up the lower leg and foot together so you can determine whether there is an abnormal angle (Fig. 18-2). This requires patience and subtle angulation of the transducer.

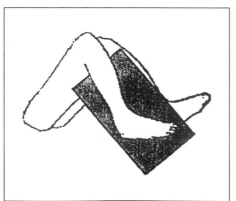

FIGURE 18-2. View showing the angle at which the foot and leg should be imaged to show relative position and exclude clubfeet.

Pathology

There should not be too large or small an angle between the foot and the lower leg. Acute or extended angulation of the foot is a feature of clubfoot. In addition the foot is inverted so the long axis of the foot and both long bones can be seen at the same time. Strange foot position is often seen with chromosomal anomalies (Fig. 18-3). A gap between the big toe and the remaining toes suggests Down syndrome. Excessive heel tissue suggests a rockerbottom foot (see Fig. 18-3).

The Limbs

Technique

In addition to the femur (see Chapter 14), the tibia and fibula, radius and ulna, and humerus should all be imaged and measured in an anomaly search. Be systematic about the measurements of long bones. Start with the femur or the humerus and work out to the tibia and fibula or radius and ulna so as not to confuse the arms and legs. In distal limbs, photograph one long bone after the other and label as you go. Bowing is a clue to some anomalies. Absent limbs are seen in some syndromes (e.g., limb/body wall complex).

If the femur length is short by more than two standard deviations, all long bones should be measured. Normal length tables for all bones are available (see Appendix 2).

Pathology

Grossly short (less than the fifth percentile), barely visible long bones are associated with polyhydramnios. Unduly short or large limbs may indicate fetal anomalies. However, if a long bone such as the humerus or femur is short and the condition is symmetrical and localized there may be familial focal limb shortening.

To diagnose specific lethal defects described later in this chapter, look at the following:

1. Chest/abdomen ratio
2. Amount of soft tissue around the limbs
3. Amount of ossification of the spine
4. Shape of the head

Look for angulation and fractures in the long bones if the bones appear poorly ossified. With less-marked limb shortening, look for asymmetry, epiphyseal changes, bowing, increased digit number, or angulation with a fracture.

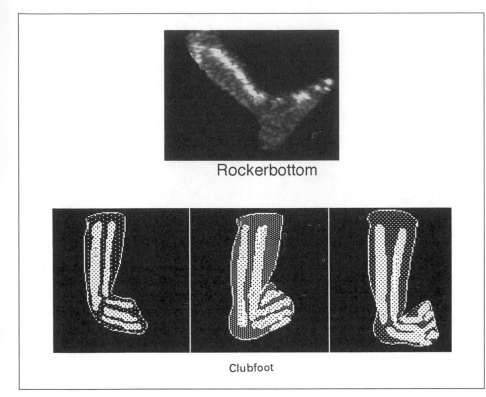

Rockerbottom

Clubfoot

FIGURE 18-3. In clubfoot there is an abnormally small or large angle between the lower leg and the foot, and the foot does not align with the leg normally and appears twisted. The lateral aspect of the foot and both long bones of the leg can be seen on a single view. Normally only a single long bone is seen on a view that shows the lateral foot. With rockerbottom foot (see inset) the heel is unduly prominent. Both are common with chromosomal anomalies.

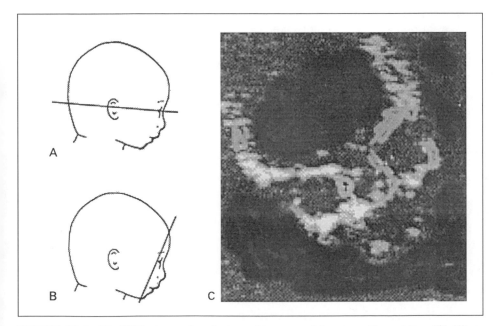

FIGURE 18-4. (**A, B**)Diagram showing positions used to show the orbits. (**C**) Ultrasonic view of the orbits. Technique A is more likely to be accurate than technique B since it is harder to be off axis.

The Brain

In addition to visualizing the cerebellum, note should be made of the cisterna magna, which is a cystic space between the occipital bone and the cerebellum. The cisterna magna should be no more than 10 mm in diameter (see Fig. 14-13) as measured on a cerebellum view. In Dandy-Walker syndrome, the cisterna magna will be larger than 10 mm, whereas in spina bifida, the cisterna magna will not be seen. The entire cerebellum may not be visualized in cases of severe spina bifida because the cerebellum partially lies in the upper spine. The cavum septi pellucidi is absent in holoprosencephaly and related conditions. The lateral ventricular width should be measured at the atrium (see Fig. 18-26). Its normal width is 10 mm or less. Demonstrate that the cisterna magna, cavum septi pellucidi, and atrium of the lateral ventricle are normal. If all are present and normal, this is a quick screening technique that demonstrates that the brain as a whole is normal.

The Orbit

To find the orbit, obtain the standard axial view, as for the biparietal diameter, and then change to a right-angle axis. Continually change the axis until you have determined where the orbits appear largest and the intraorbital distance is greatest (Fig. 18-4). A small intraorbital distance is associated with cranial problems, particularly holoprosencephaly. Measurements of the orbits represent another method of estimating gestational age (Fig. 18-5; see Appendix 18).

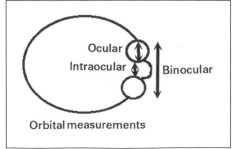

Orbital measurements

FIGURE 18-5. Sites for taking orbital measurements.

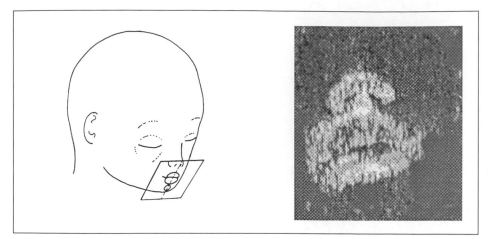

FIGURE 18-6. Views required to show the nose, lips, and palate with ultrasonic images.

The Face

Views of the maxilla and lips are essential to exclude cleft palate. Angle inferiorly to display the maxilla, the lips, and the mandible (Fig. 18-6). To see a gap in the upper lip and maxilla beneath the nose, as in cleft lip and palate, obtain a transverse view through the face and orbits, and then shift anteriorly to the maxilla and upper lip, which lie just beneath the nose (Fig. 18-7).

The Profile

Place the transducer at right angles to the views that show the maxilla to see the profile. Ensure that the profile view does not include the orbits and includes the chin (Fig. 18-8). It is easy to take a profile view that is slightly oblique and create a diagnosis of micrognathia.

The Ears

Make an attempt to show the position of the ears in relation to the cervical spine on a single view. A low position of the ears is seen with anomalies, but deciding whether the ears are too low is very difficult. Abnormally small or misshapen ears indicate a chromosomal anomaly.

The Nose

When taking views of the maxilla, take a view through the nose to ensure that two nostrils are present (see Fig. 18-6). A single nostril suggests holoprosencephaly.

The Spine

Take transverse views at many levels at right angles to the long axis view of the spine to show the relationship of the posterior elements to the vertebral bodies and to exclude spina bifida (see Figs. 18-43 and 18-44). This is especially difficult in the lumbosacral region where the spine changes direction. Obtain a prone sagittal view of the distal spine that will show the skin posterior to the spine. This will bring out a subtle meningocele. The coronal view, which shows both posterior ossification centers simultaneously, is also valuable (Fig. 18-9). This view will help to exclude diastematomyelia.

The Diaphragm

Find the diaphragm bilaterally to exclude diaphragmatic hernia. When the fetus is breathing, visualization of the diaphragm on longitudinal views is easier.

The Cord Insertion

Make sure the cord inserts into the abdominal wall normally. Small omphaloceles might be overlooked, and this view gives you an opportunity to count the three vessels in the cord. If only one artery is present, an anomaly is more likely.

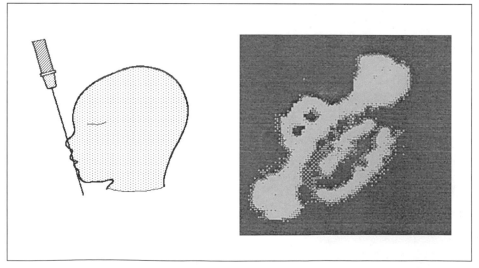

FIGURE 18-7. Diagram showing the axis at which the transducer should be placed to obtain adequate views of the upper lip to exclude cleft palate and lip.

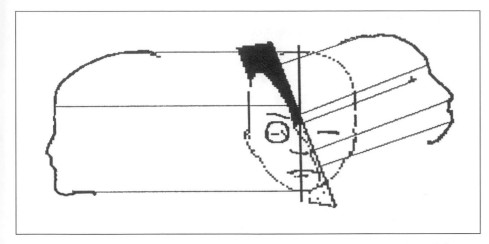

FIGURE 18-8. Diagram showing the technique used to obtain a straight view of the profile (on the left). The oblique view (on the right) will show the orbits and a small chin.

The Neck

Look at the cervical spine area of the neck to exclude small cystic hygromas and to check for small encephaloceles.

The Liver and Spleen

Try to visualize the liver length at right angles to the diaphragm. There are normal size standards (see Appendix 20). Also make an effort to see the spleen lateral to the stomach (see Fig. 17-4). There are normal standards for spleen size when its length is measured on a coronal view.

Mass Arising From the Head or Neck

Most masses arising from the head or neck are cystic. First establish whether the mass arises from the head or neck by carefully showing landmarks such as the jaw and shoulder. If a cystic mass arises from the head, whether anterior or posterior, look for a bony defect in the skull, which is seen with encephalocele. Look for brain tissue within the mass and secondary intracranial ventricular dilation.

If the cystic mass arises in the neck, see whether it is bilateral and in a posterolateral location. This favors cystic hygroma. Septations are seen in most cystic hygroma and skin thickening with hydropic changes is common. If the cystic mass is posterior, look for spinal defects as with iniencephaly or a low encephalocele; also look for secondary hydrocephalus.

Mass Arising From the Trunk

If the mass is anterior, determine whether the mass is cord or bowel loops. Cord will show flow on Doppler and light up with color flow. Slightly dilated bowel loops can look like cord. If the mass is enclosed in a membrane, as seen in omphalocele, see whether there is liver or gut within the mass.

If the mass is posterior, see whether the spine is intact and look at the head for evidence of Arnold-Chiari malformation. Also see whether the bladder and kidneys are obstructed and look for evidence of hydrops.

When investigating omphalocele, define the extent of the defect on transverse and longitudinal views. Also take a view that shows the cord insertion, the omphalocele, and the spine simultaneously, if possible.

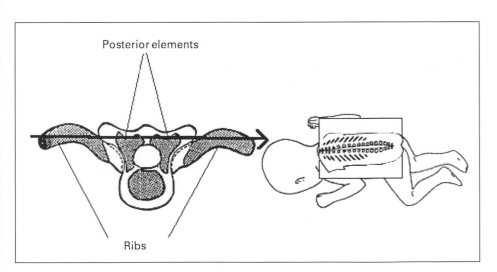

FIGURE 18-9. Diagram showing the technique used for obtaining a coronal view of the spine.

◆ PATHOLOGY

Most fetal anomalies are unsuspected prior to the sonogram. If there is a family history or a risk factor such as maternal drug intake, then the examination is much simplified because a specific anomaly can be sought. Three important nonspecific clues channel the way the fetus is examined because they are associated with defined groups of anomalies.

1. *Polyhydramnios.* The followings anomalies are associated with polyhydramnios:
   a. Gut anomalies
      duodenal atresia
      omphalocele
      gastroschisis
      diaphragmatic hernia
      esophageal atresia and tracheoesophageal fistula
      small bowel atresia
   b. Swallowing problems
      cleft palate
      tracheoesophageal fistula
      small lower jaw (micrognathia)
   c. Central nervous system anomalies (if the swallowing center is impaired)
      anencephaly
      hydrocephalus
      encephalocele
   d. Neck problems
      goiter
      cystic hygroma
      cervical teratoma
   e. Short-limbed dwarfism with small chest (presumably compressing the esophagus)
      thanatophoric dwarfism
      achondrogenesis
      osteogenesis imperfecta
   f. Lung problems (with esophageal compression)
      cystic adenomatoid malformation
      isolated pleural effusion
   g. Nonimmune or immune hydrops
   h. Renal problems with too much urine production or renal enlargement compressing gut as with ureteropelvic junction obstruction

2. *Oligohydramnios.* Too little urine output causes less amniotic fluid or no amniotic fluid at all.
   a. Renal anomalies
      renal agenesis
      infantile polycystic kidney
      bilateral dysplastic kidney
      posterior urethral valves
      prune belly syndrome
   b. Others
      limb/body wall syndrome (amniotic bands)
      some spina bifida
      some cranial problems
   c. Intrauterine growth retardation (IUGR)

3. *Increased alpha-fetoprotein*
   a. Open neural crest defects
      spina bifida variants
      encephalocele
      anencephaly
      iniencephaly
   b. Abdominal wall defects
      omphalocele
      gastroschisis
      limb/body wall syndrome (amniotic bands)
   c. Tumorous lesions
      cystic hygroma
      sacrococcygeal teratoma
   d. Renal problems (rarely)
      renal agenesis
      posterior urethral valves
      hydronephrosis
      Finnish nephropathy
   e. Placental problems (e.g., triploidy)
   f. Rudimentary or dead twin

Most fetal anomalies, however, are unexpectedly discovered during a sonographic study. This section is therefore organized by the presenting sonographic finding, in the following order:

Cyst in the abdomen
Cysts and masses in the chest
Cyst in the head
Head and brain malformations
Mass arising from the head or neck
Limb shortening
Blood tests or maternal age suspicious for Down syndrome
Mass arising from the trunk
Stomach not seen
Fetal ascites
Skin thickening
Bilateral large echogenic kidneys
Absent or small kidneys
Masses in the region of the kidneys

Cyst in the Abdomen

Three normal cystic structures lie in the abdomen: the stomach in the left upper quadrant, the gallbladder, and the bladder. Abnormal cystic processes occur in three locations between the diaphragm and the genitalia: those related to the kidney, those related to the gastrointestinal tract, and intraperitoneal and pelvic cystic processes.

Kidney (Renal) Cystic Processes

Cystic structures of renal origin normally occur in a paraspinal location. Provided the kidneys are present, gastrointestinal processes do not extend to contact the spine or into the paraspinal area. Establish whether one or more cysts are present and whether the cysts interconnect and connect with the renal pelvis. (The cysts in a dysplastic multicystic kidney may not connect, will vary in size, and are laterally placed.) If kidney parenchyma can be seen around the suspect lesion, the process is most likely related to hydronephrosis.

Look for a dilated ureter or ureters. Look at the bladder to see whether it is enlarged. Note whether the kidney process is bilateral. Horseshoe and pelvic kidneys may lie at a low level in front of the spine in the midline. If these anomalies are present, no kidneys will be seen in the normal location. Dysplastic changes are more common in pelvic kidneys.

Renal Obstruction

Some renal cysts are related to obstruction, either unilateral or bilateral hydronephrosis. These conditions can be detected and explored sonographically. Renal pelvicalyceal distention suggestive of hydronephrosis has been subclassified depending on whether there is calyceal as well as pelvic distention.

Type 0: no pelvic distention
Type 1: pelvic distention only
Type 2: pelvic and calyceal distention
Type 3: pelvicalyceal distention with parenchymal narrowing

Technique

1. Measurements of renal pelvic dilation are made in an anteroposterior direction at the level of the renal pelvis (Fig. 18-10).

2. A longitudinal coronal view angled so that the bladder is also seen shows the full extent of the pelvicalyceal system well. This view may show the ureter passing towards the bladder. (The ureter can be confused with the fetal psoas muscle and the iliac artery. Color flow can help with this. Also, try to demonstrate the ureter emerging from the renal pelvis.)

3. Watch the dilated renal pelvis for several minutes. If the renal pelvic size varies over the course of the examination, reflux should be considered. Alternatively, the renal pelvic dilation may be a response to fetal bladder dilation and may disappear when the fetus voids. Reexamine the renal pelvis after the fetus voids if possible.

4. Examine the renal parenchyma. If it is markedly echogenic, dysplasia should be suspected. The earliest definitive sign of renal dysplasia is the presence of tiny peripherally placed cysts which enlarge as the condition becomes more severe.

Mild Pelvic Enlargement

See Figure 18-10.

1. Pelvic distention to 4 mm or greater associated with increased risk of Down syndrome.

2. If there is no calyceal distention and the renal pelvic distention is less than 10 mm, long-term follow-up is not advised. If there is calyceal distention, serial sonograms are arranged which vary in frequency depending on the severity of the pelvic distention.

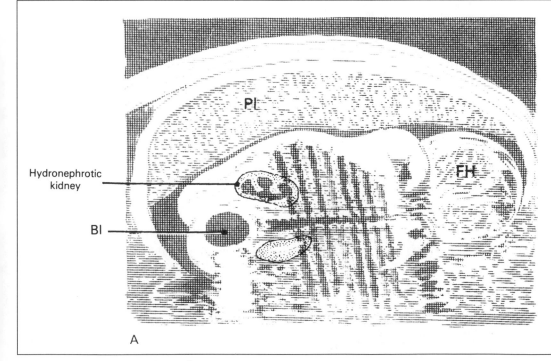
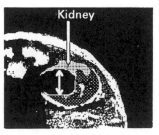

FIGURE 18-10. (A) Kidney showing evidence of mild hydronephrosis. With this degree of hydronephrosis the finding may be transitory and disappear after delivery. **(B)** Transverse view showing the site at the renal pelvis where renal measurements for hydronephrosis are made.

Ureteropelvic Junction Obstruction (UPJ)

1. If the renal pelvis is large and rounded, the diagnosis is likely to be ureteropelvic junction obstruction. Generalized calyceal distention is seen with a large renal pelvis having a rounded shape.
2. Echogenic parenchyma due to dysplasia is very uncommon with UPJ.
3. Sometimes the renal pelvis is very large with or without calyceal distention; it may appear to be a cyst in the midabdomen (Fig. 18-11).

4. Both renal pelves may have a UPJ configuration. As a rule, the degree of renal pelvic dilation is asymmetrical with one renal pelvis being larger than the other. If the hydronephrosis is severe there may be decreased amniotic fluid (oligohydramnios).
5. With severe unilateral or bilateral renal pelvic enlargement, there can be polyhydramnios.

UNILATERAL HYDRONEPHROSIS. There will be a normal amount of amniotic fluid with unilateral hydronephrosis.

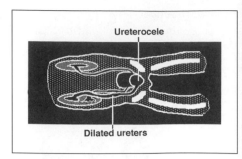

FIGURE 18-12. Ureterocele is a small sac at the base of the bladder. The distal ureter balloons out into a cobra head–shaped deformity. Most ureteroceles occur in a double collecting system. The upper half of the kidney is connected by a dilated ureter to the ureterocele. The second ureter that connects to the lower pole of the kidney is dilated due to reflux. Note that the ureter from the lower pole is inserted into the bladder in an ectopic location, compared to the normal insertion site which is seen on the opposite kidney.

1. *Ureteropelvic junction obstruction.* Generalized calyceal distention is seen with a large renal pelvis with a rounded shape. This condition is common (see Fig. 18-11). There can be polyhydramnios, thought to be due to gut compression by the dilated renal pelvis.
2. *Hydronephrosis due to ureterocele.* A tortuous dilated ureter can be traced from the renal pelvis to the bladder. The dilated ureter can be so redundant with multiple dilated loops that it looks like many centrally placed cysts and seems to be of gut origin. A small spherical membrane, the wall of the ureterocele, can be seen within the bladder. If a ureterocele is very large it can obstruct the ureter draining the other kidney. Many ureteroceles are found in kidneys with double collecting systems. The ureterocele may be draining only the upper half of the kidney, and the lower half of the kidney may not be hydronephrotic if it is a double collecting system (Fig. 18-12). Alternatively, the lower pole may be dilated related to reflux. With the similar entity ectopic ureteric insertion, the dilated urethra inserts low and can be traced to a site at the inferolateral aspect of the bladder. Both ureterocele and ectopic ureter can occur in single kidneys.

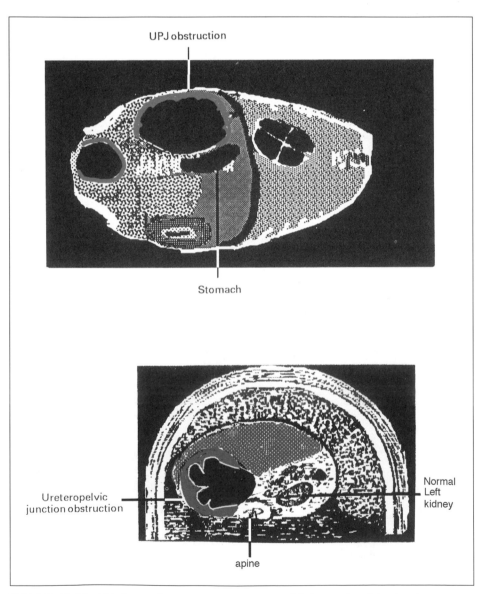

FIGURE 18-11. (A) Coronal view showing a dilated left renal pelvis due to ureteropelvic junction obstruction (UPJ) compressing the stomach. **(B)** Transverse view of UPJ. Note that the kidney lies alongside the spine.

VESICO URETERIC REFLUX. Reflux is a condition in which some urine returns from the bladder to the kidney when the fetus voids. The one-way valve at the junction between the ureter and the bladder may not be fully formed in utero; this valve may leak so some urine flows back to the kidney from the bladder when the bladder contracts. Ultrasonic signs are (1) dilated pelvicalyceal system; (2) dilated ureter which shows much peristalsis; and (3) distention of the renal pelvis as the bladder empties. Often, the bladder is large but thin walled since it never empties well. This condition is much more common in males than females in utero and the reverse of the situation in small children, when reflux is much more common in girls than in boys. Usually, reflux seen in utero resolves over the course of the pregnancy or in the first few months of life.

BILATERAL HYDRONEPHROSIS. If the hydronephrosis severely compromises renal function, there will be decreased amniotic fluid (oligohydramnios).

1. *Bilateral ureteropelvic junction obstruction.* Renal function is rarely impaired, but with severe obstruction the dilated kidney compresses intestines and polyhydramnios may result. Oligohydramnios is rare. The degree of hydronephrosis is usually asymmetrical. The renal pelves are large in comparison with the calyces.

2. *Posterior urethral valves (PUV).* Valves in the posterior urethra of males may obstruct the urethra.

   An obstruction in the posterior urethra causes the bladder to dilate.
   Oligohydramnios is usual.
   The bladder has a V-shaped area known as a "keyhole" arising from its inferior end—the dilated posterior urethra (Fig. 18-13).
   The kidneys often show evidence of renal dysplasia.

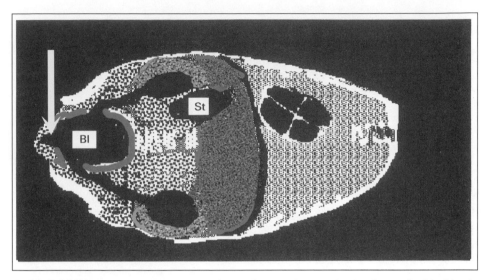

FIGURE 18-13. In the most common form of posterior urethral valves, the bladder is large with a V-shaped inferior extension (white arrow), the posterior urethra is dilated, and the ureters and kidneys are dilated.

Several appearances can be seen:

a. The bladder may be enormously distended without the kidneys showing hydronephrosis. The kidneys are often densely echogenic since they are dysplastic. Confusion with a large pelvic cyst can occur. This form of PUV is always fatal. There will be no amniotic fluid if this form is seen after 18 weeks because complete urethral obstruction is present.

b. The bladder may be quite large with both kidneys hydronephrotic. Dilated tortuous ureters are seen.

c. Severe fetal ascites can be seen without the skin thickening, pleural effusions, or placentomegaly of hydrops. The bladder, ureters, and kidneys are distended. This variant of PUV is thought to result in the prune belly anomaly (Eagle-Barrett syndrome) (Fig. 18-14).

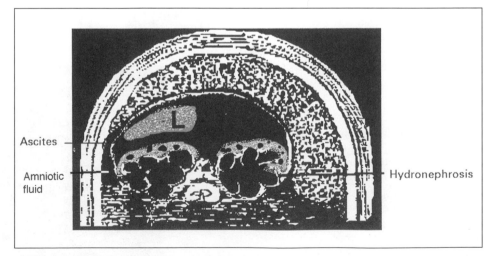

FIGURE 18-14. Bilateral hydronephrosis, fetal ascites, and oligohydramnios. Note the absence of skin thickening. It is easy to confuse the picture of ascites with no amniotic fluid with the picture of polyhydramnios. Both kidneys show evidence of renal dysplasia with several small cysts in echogenic parenchyma.

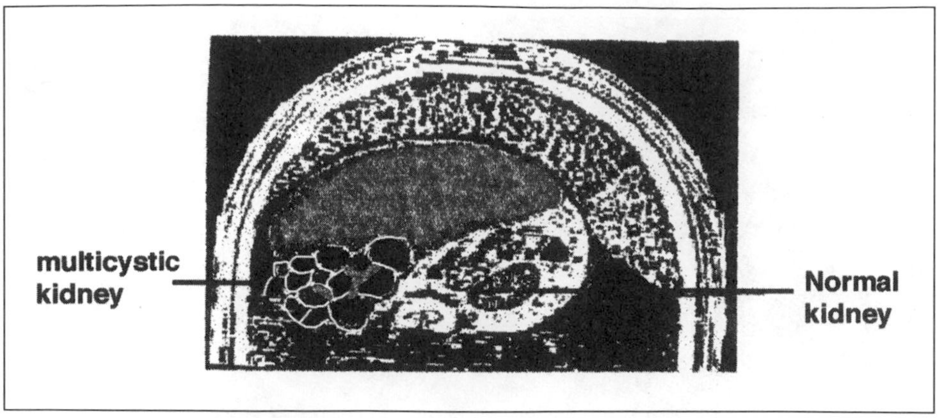

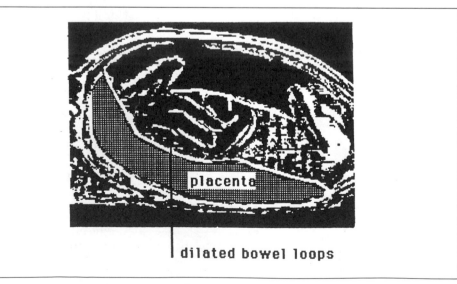

FIGURE 18-15. Multicystic kidney in utero. In contrast with the normal kidney, which has an echogenic center and an even renal parenchyma, a multicystic kidney contains cysts that vary in size and shape.

Fetuses with PUV may be considered for in utero drainage. Before a procedure is performed the diagnosis must be well established and the following problems excluded:

a. Chromosomal abnormality. Before a drainage procedure is used, karyotyping is performed since there is an association with chromosomal abnormalities, particularly trisomy 21.
b. Dysplasia. The fetal kidneys are inspected carefully to ensure that dysplasia is not present. If the kidneys are echogenic with peripherally placed cysts, one can be sure that dysplasia is present. Often the kidneys are echogenic but no cysts can be seen, so a diagnosis of dysplasia can be suspected but not definitively made (discussed later).
c. Amniotic fluid. Most groups only perform drainage procedures when amniotic fluid is still present but is decreasing in amount.

The fetal bladder is punctured under ultrasound control and a double pigtail catheter is pushed through a wide metal catheter so that one pigtail end lies in the bladder and the other in the amniotic fluid. A special introducer is used which has a pigtail catheter and a pusher on a single needle. This technique is difficult and should only be performed in specialized units.

3. *Ureterovesicle junction obstruction (UVJ).* In this rare condition both ureters are dilated and there may be pelvicalyceal dilation. The bladder may be small or normal in size since the partial obstruction is at the level of the insertions of the ureters into the bladder.
4. *Idiopathic megaureter.* The ureters are dilated and there may be some dilation of the renal pelvis. There is no urethral obstruction. The distal portions of the ureters do not function normally. It is hard to distinguish this condition from reflux which may also occur in utero. Watch for changes in size of the kidneys and ureters after fetal voiding.

Multicystic Dysplastic Kidney

If renal obstruction occurs early in pregnancy, before approximately 15 weeks, permanent damage to the kidneys termed dysplasia may occur (see Figs. 18-14 and 18-15). When dysplastic changes are present the kidneys become more echogenic and develop parenchymal cysts. The cysts vary in size and do not generally communicate. If the cysts are large, the condition is known as multicystic kidney rather than dysplasia. If dysplasia is generalized with visible cysts, the kidneys do not function. Dysplasia may result from ureteropelvic, distal urethral, or ureteric obstruction; both kidneys are involved if the urethra is obstructed, and fetuses with this condition do not usually survive.

Gastrointestinal Cystic Processes

With the exception of duplication, proximal gastrointestinal processes associated with gut obstruction cause polyhydramnios. Distal gut atresias such as anal or colonic atresia are not associated with polyhydramnios.

If the obstruction is below the level of the stomach there will be several cyst-like structures that are really dilated loops of small bowel (Fig. 18-16).

SMALL BOWEL ATRESIA. The most common cause of obstruction is gut atresia, when a loop of bowel does not form or atrophies due to inadequate blood supply.

FIGURE 18-16. With intestinal obstruction, fluid-filled tubes are seen within the fetal abdomen.

1. Obstruction occurs either in the jejunum, when both stomach and small bowel are dilated, or in the ileum, when the stomach is usually not enlarged. Both processes cause polyhydramnios. Multiple fluid-filled tubular structures are seen in the abdomen (see Fig. 18-16). Occasionally, peristalsis may be visible.

2. Malrotation with an unusual axis to the stomach and duodenum may be seen. Sometimes the obstruction is due to volvulus; a single, very distended loop of bowel will be seen with other, less dilated loops.

3. Distal gut atresias such as anal or colonic atresia are not associated with polyhydramnios. Dilated large bowel is occasionally seen with these abnormalities. Usually intestinal appearances are normal because the colon does very little in utero. An echogenic spot seen on a transverse view which includes the genitalia is normally present and represents the anus. It is absent with anal atresia (imperforate anus) (Fig. 18-17).

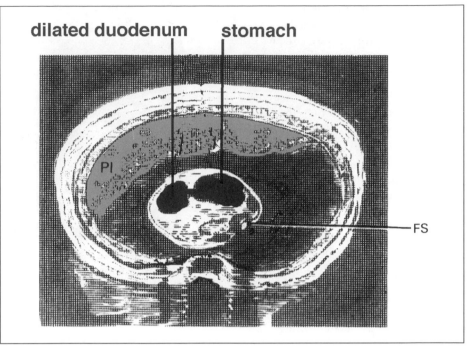

FIGURE 18-18. In duodenal atresia there are two large, round, upper-abdominal fluid-filled cavities that can be shown to communicate.

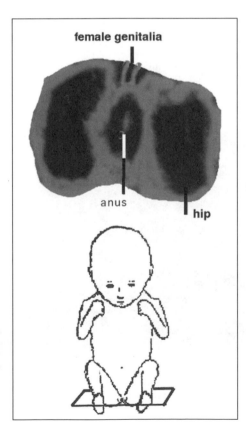

FIGURE 18-17. View of the anus in a female patient. The anal orifice is a small echogenic area surrounded by the echopenic anal muscles.

DUODENAL ATRESIA. Two large sonolucent spaces (the double bubble sign) are visible within the upper abdomen in duodenal atresia.

1. Demonstrate the connection between the distended fluid-filled stomach and the duodenum which form the two spaces (Fig. 18-18).

2. Between 30 and 50% of duodenal atresia cases are associated with Down syndrome and cardiac anomalies.

3. Severe polyhydramnios is always present.

4. With duodenal atresia, obstruction may not develop until as late as 24 weeks, so an 18-week sonogram may appear normal.

Intraperitoneal Cystic Processes

This category includes cystic processes that lie outside the kidney and the gut in the midabdomen at a distance from the spine.

MECONIUM CYST AND PERITONITIS. Spillage of fetal intestinal contents (the meconium) results in calcification, usually in a ringlike shape, in the fetal abdomen.

1. This condition may be associated with bowel obstruction.
2. Initially, a cyst with irregular echogenic walls is seen. Over time the cyst often disappears and calcification develops at the cyst site (see Fig. 18-19).
3. Linear groups of calcification, typically superior to the liver, are considered to represent the remnants of similar episodes that were not seen with ultrasound. Extraintestinal calcifications not associated with gut dilation have no long-term clinical significance.

MESENTERIC CYST AND DUPLICATION. Mesenteric cysts and duplication are extremely rare echo-free cysts. They are indistinguishable from an ovarian cyst except they may occur in males.

CHOLEDOCHAL CYST. Choledochal cysts are bile filled and occur only adjacent to the liver. A dilated bile duct may be seen entering the cyst. The gallbladder should be seen as well as the cyst. These are also very rare.

OVARIAN CYSTS. In the late second and third trimester, the mother's hormones affect the fetus, occasionally causing the formation of breasts in male and female fetuses (gynecomastia). In the female fetus the hormones affect the ovary and cause ovarian cyst formation. A cyst may be round and echo-free or contain echoes that are due to bleeding following twisting (torsion) (Fig. 18-20). Echoes may be seen throughout the cyst or form a curved area to one side thought to represent retracting clot. The cysts lie in the anterior part of the abdomen but are often close to the liver rather than in the pelvis.

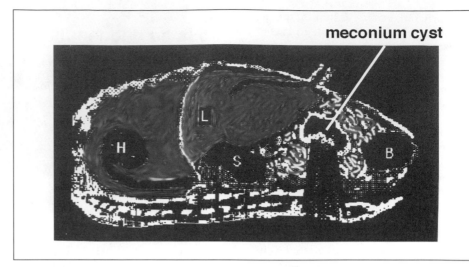

FIGURE 18-19. Meconium cysts have an irregular shape and lie in the center of the abdomen. Their walls are often calcified and ascites may be present.

Pelvic Cystic Processes

BLADDER. The bladder must be visualized in the pelvis on every obstetric scan. When there is renal obstruction without hydronephrosis the bladder may be very large and may be confused with an ovarian cyst. The bladder may contain a septum when a ureterocele is present.

The bladder may be large as a normal variant. Examine the fetus over a 2-hour period to see whether the bladder contracts. The bladder normally empties partially within an hour.

RECTUM AND COLON. Normal meconium-filled large bowel can appear cystic in the third trimester. The rectum may be mistaken for a cyst.

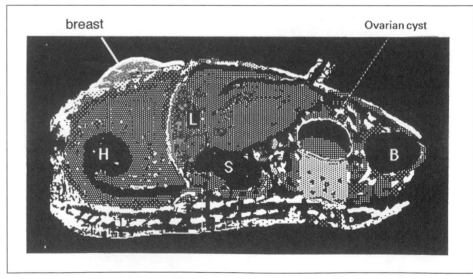

FIGURE 18-20. Most ovarian cysts are echo-free. Some have an area of echoes (clot) within that assume a half-moon shape. This indicates torsion. Note the acoustic transmission distal to the cyst.

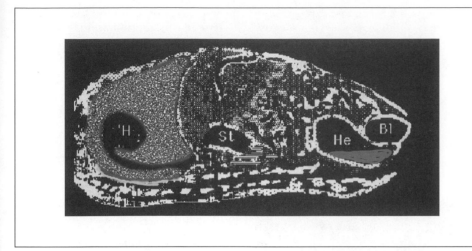

FIGURE 18-21. Hydrometrocolpos. A cystic structure (He) that may contain some internal echoes arises from the pelvis posterior and slightly inferior to the bladder (Bl).

Cysts and Masses in the Chest
Pleural Effusion

Pleural effusions can be recognized surrounding the lungs at the level of the heart or above it (Fig. 18-22). They may be unilateral or bilateral. Although pleural effusions are usually associated with the changes of hydrops, they may be an isolated finding. Isolated pleural effusions are usually composed of lymph. As a rule, they are small and do not push the diaphragm down (diaphragmatic eversion) or displace the heart. Small pleural effusions often disappear over the course of the pregnancy. Large pleural effusions with these findings may cause secondary hydrops. Catheter drainage in utero has been advocated for this type of effusion. Some have performed needle aspiration shortly before birth for large effusions. Aspiration after birth is usually rapidly curative.

HYDROMETROCOLPOS. In the female fetus, a cystic structure posterior to the bladder extending out of the pelvis is likely to be an obstructed vagina due to an imperforate hymen. The uterus is usually not dilated or seen. The bladder and kidneys may also be obstructed (Fig 18-21). A cloaca, a combined bladder and vagina, may be present.

MEGACYSTIS MICROCOLON SYNDROME. If the bladder is overdistended but there is polyhydramnios, consider the megacystis microcolon syndrome. The ureters and kidneys may or may not be dilated. The bowel is small, malformed, and obstructed, but not seen as such, and there is a normal or excessive amount of amniotic fluid. The fetus is almost always female with this very rare syndrome.

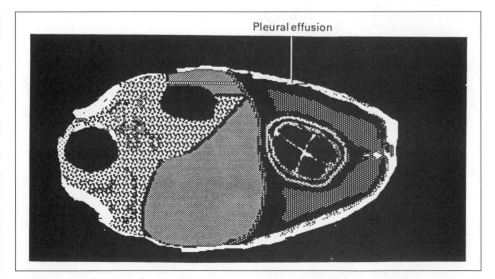

Pleural effusion

FIGURE 18-22. Pleural effusions have a typical shape as they surround the lung. There is a small pericardial effusion present within the pericardium surrounding the heart.

Cystadenomatoid Malformation of the Lung

1. In the type 1 and 2 forms of cysta-denomatoid malformation of the lung, there are multiple cysts with echogenic areas in between. The heart is displaced and the entire chest or a portion of the chest appears filled with cysts. The cysts are large in type 1 (Fig. 18-23) and smaller, but visible, in type 2.

2. In the type 3 form, cysts are present but too small to be seen as cysts. There are echogenic areas in the lung (see Fig. 18-23).

3. Polyhydramnios and nonimmune hydrops are often present with any of the three types. Usually hydrops results in stillbirth.

4. All three types may regress in utero and the lung may be normal at birth.

5. Sequestration can look the same as a type 3 cystadenomatoid malformation of the lung, however, a large supplying artery may be visible on color flow.

High Left Diaphragm

The diaphragm may be difficult to see. The left diaphragm is often a little higher than the right. On a casual look, a high subphrenic stomach may appear to lie above the diaphragm. Intra-abdominal processes may herniate into the chest, but they may just appear to lie in the chest if the diaphragm is high.

Left-side Diaphragmatic Hernia

Left-side diaphragmatic hernia is a difficult condition to recognize because the small bowel in the chest resembles lung.

1. The stomach is not seen in the abdomen but lies alongside the heart in the chest; the heart is shifted to the right (Fig. 18-24). No left hemidiaphragm is visible.

2. The texture of the left lung will be slightly different from that of the right lung. Since there are multiple loops of small bowel in the chest, fluid-filled loops may be seen, but empty gut and lung can look amazingly similar.

3. The liver will be displaced to the left and often lies partially in the chest. It is the presence of the liver in the chest that makes in utero surgery very difficult and almost always unsuccessful. Sonographic clues to the presence of the liver in the chest are the distortion and posterior position of the liver vessels and the position of the stomach in the chest.

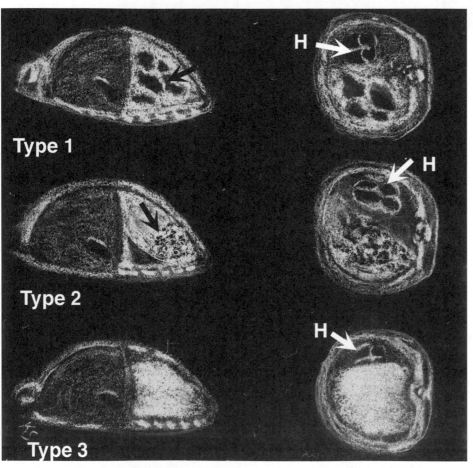

FIGURE 18-23. The three types of cystadenomatoid malformation of the lung are seen. At the top is type 1. Large cysts (black arrow) are visible within the cystadenomatoid malformation. Note the echogenic area of lung around it. Type 2, in the middle section, smaller cysts are visible (black arrow). Notice that the heart is displaced to the right. Again, there is echogenic tissue surrounding the small cysts. Type 3, although cysts are present, they are so small they are only seen as echoes. This type tends to displace the heart more and has a greater association with hydrops. On some occasions, however, it has been seen to regress and disappear over the course of the pregnancy.

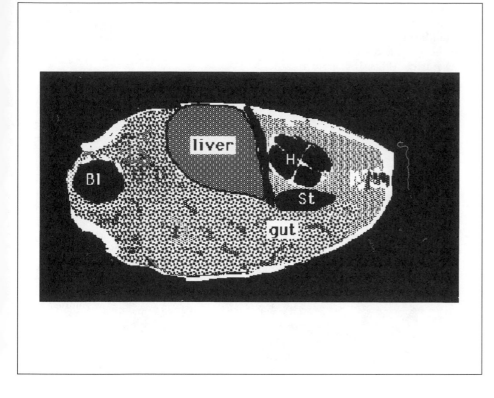

FIGURE 18-24. Diaphragmatic hernia. The stomach is seen alongside the heart. The gut in the chest apart from the stomach has almost the same acoustic appearance as the lung.

Right-side Diaphragmatic Hernia

A right-side diaphragmatic hernia is ever more difficult to diagnose because the herniated liver looks so similar to the lung.

1. The stomach will not be seen or will be deviated to the right.
2. The apparent lung on the right will have visible portal veins within that can be tracked to the liver with color flow.
3. The heart will be displaced to the left.
4. Right-side hernia is much less common than left-side hernia. Both types of hernias are associated with other anomalies such as hemivertebrae and hydronephrosis.

Bronchogenic Cyst and Neuroenteric Cyst

Bronchogenic and neuroenteric cysts are rare. A single cyst is seen in the posterior midline portion of the lung near the spine. As a rule they are echo-free. They are associated with vertebral anomalies.

Cyst in the Head
Technique

1. Most cystic lesions in the head represent dilation of two or more ventricles, so it is first necessary to identify the ventricles and the choroid plexus. Lateral ventricles can be recognized by the presence of the choroid plexus even when very distorted.
2. Reverberations from the skull obscure the ventricle closest to the transducer on axial views; apparent asymmetrical dilation of the down-sided ventricle is often a technical artifact because the superficial ventricle cannot be well seen.
   a. Try to scan the head from a coronal axis when side-to-side comparisons are made (see Chapter 50).
   b. It is usually possible to see the hidden lateral ventricle if the probe is placed in a good position to see the down ventricle on an axial view and then angled inferiorly.
   c. If the fetus is in a cephalic presentation, try an endovaginal probe to visualize the ventricular system in a fashion similar to neonatal head imaging (see Chapter 50).
3. Bananas and lemons. Be sure your images demonstrate the entire shape of the skull and the posterior fossa; both are abnormally shaped in the Arnold-Chiari malformation (see discussion later and Fig. 18-28).

The Lateral Ventricles

1. ***Normal lateral ventricular size.*** The lateral ventricles and choroid plexus do not change size during the second and third trimesters. At any stage of pregnancy beyond 12 weeks the lateral ventricular width toward the posterior aspect of the ventricle (atrium) should be no more than 10 mm, and the choroid plexus should fill most of the ventricle (Figs. 18-25 and 18-26).

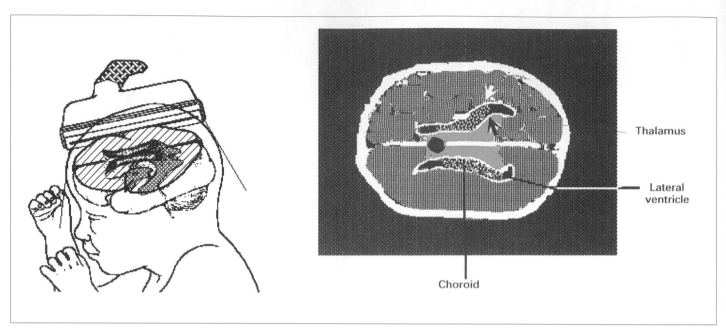

FIGURE 18-25. Axial view showing the way the lateral ventricles are imaged. The normal choroid should fill the lateral ventricle. The lateral ventricle width, measured at the atria, should be less than 10 mm.

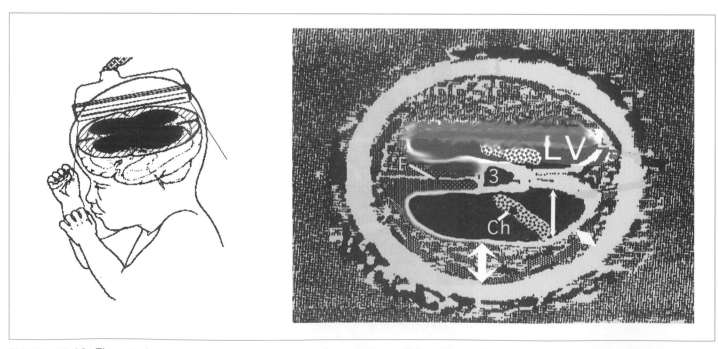

FIGURE 18-26. The usual type of hydrocephalus. Much of the skull is filled with two large structures obstructed by the lateral ventricles. The cortical mantle thickness is the term used to describe the width of the remaining brain. Details of the dilated lateral ventricle on the side of the brain near the transducer are usually poor because of the reverberations. Note the choroid plexus within the dilated ventricle, assuming an angle of greater than 75 degrees (dangling choroid). The arrow is placed at the site in the atrium of the lateral ventricle, just behind the choroid, where measurements of lateral ventricular width are made.

2. *Mild ventriculomegaly.* There should be a gap of no greater than 3 mm between the choroid plexuses and the walls of the lateral ventricles. The choroid plexuses are compressed in hydrocephalus. Noting the discrepancy between the choroid plexus and ventricle sizes allows a diagnosis of mild ventriculomegaly when the ventricular size is still within normal limits (see Fig. 18-26). (The ventriculohemispheric ratio of midline-to-lateral-ventricular-wall distance to hemispheric distance is no longer considered helpful because the normal ratio changes over the course of pregnancy.)

3. *Hanging choroid sign.* The choroid plexuses are gravity dependent. In the normal ventricle they are angled at less than 25 degrees from vertical. In hydrocephalus the angle is greater, and the choroid plexuses "dangle" (see Fig. 18-26). An angle of 75 degrees or more is pathologic, even if the choroid plexuses are in contact with the lateral ventricular wall.

4. *Mantle thickness.* It is important to obtain a good view of the amount of cortex (the "mantle") around the ventricle, because the width of the mantle has some relationship to whether or not the fetus will have diminished mental capacity. Measurement of the mantle should be made. Measuring the thickest and thinnest points may be helpful in follow-up (see Fig. 18-26).

5. *Establishing the level of obstruction.* If hydrocephalus is present and lateral ventricles are symmetrical, try to visualize the third and fourth ventricles to establish the level of obstruction. Selective dilation of the lateral ventricle without third and fourth ventricle involvement is unusual and suggests hydranencephaly or holoprosencephaly.

6. *Look elsewhere.* Most cases of ventricular dilation are associated with an anomaly elsewhere. The spine, orbits, face, feet, and hands may be affected.

Hydrocephalus

If the fourth ventricle is not dilated, consider the following possibilities:

AQUEDUCTAL STENOSIS. A common form of ventriculomegaly known as aqueduct stenosis results from narrowing of the aqueduct of Sylvius, which connects the third and fourth ventricles (Fig. 18-27). The sonographic features are as follows:

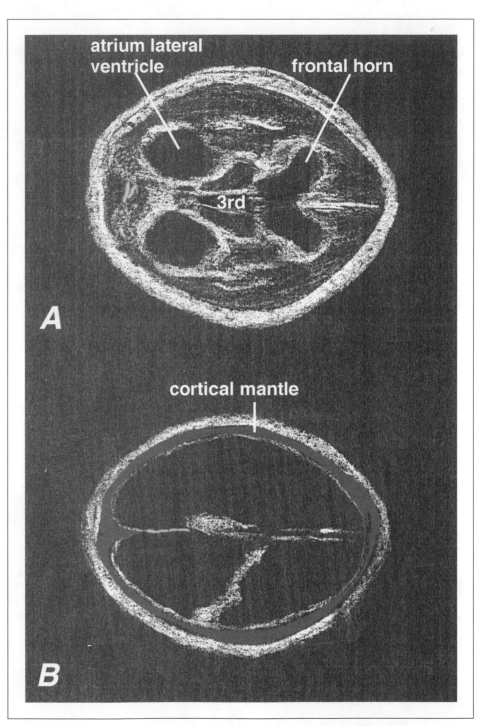

FIGURE 18-27. Aqueduct stenosis. (**A**) Note the dilation of the lateral and third ventricles, but the fourth ventricle is not affected. (**B**) The lateral ventricles only are visualized. A hanging choroid is seen. The cortical mantle is markedly thinned.

1. Symmetrical dilation of both lateral ventricles with intact intrahemispheric fissure. Usually the degree of dilation is relatively mild with considerable preserved brain mantle.
2. Dilated third ventricle without dilation of the fourth ventricle.
3. Dilated aqueduct. This structure may be seen as a small tube extending toward the tentorium on a sagittal midline view.
4. The cerebellum and cisterna magna will be normal.

Mild ventriculomegaly with similar features is associated with Down syndrome. The prognosis with aqueduct stenosis diagnosed in utero is poor; the outcome for almost all children is severe retardation or death.

ARNOLD-CHIARI MALFORMATION. The Arnold-Chiari malformation (type II), a common type of hydrocephalus, is usually, but not necessarily, associated with spina bifida (Fig. 18-28). Long-term intellectual capacity can be good, even when the cortical mantle width is very narrow. With spina bifida the spinal cord ends at a lower level than L2 owing to tethering, so a portion of the cerebellum lies below the skull and is compressed as it is pulled through the cisterna magna. The sonographic features are as follows:

1. Dilation of the lateral ventricles, usually asymmetrical and often severe.
2. Partial absence of the septum pellucidum.
3. Dilation of the third ventricle and aqueduct.
4. "Banana" shape to the cerebellum instead of the usual bilateral "apple" shape. The cerebellum may not be seen if it is in the upper cervical spine.
5. Usually a "lemon" shape to the skull with a more narrow anterior portion.
6. Overall small cranial size. In general, small head size associated with ventricular dilation suggests atrophy, but in a case of Arnold-Chiari malformation, considerable ventriculomegaly can be present although the overall head size is smaller than expected.

HYDRANENCEPHALY. Hydranencephaly is an uncommon anomaly and is lethal (Fig. 18-29). It is due to an infarct of the cortex of the brain. The sonographic features are as follows:

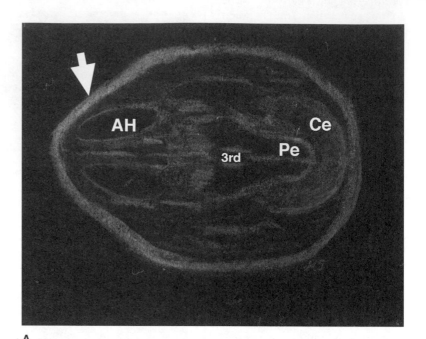

A

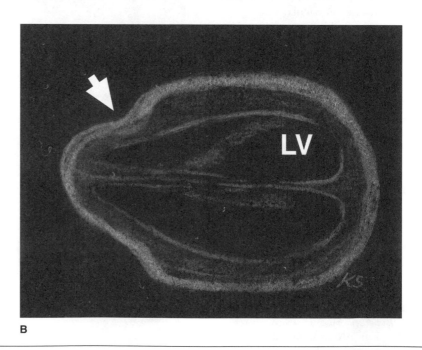

B

FIGURE 18-28. Arnold-Chiari malformation. The anterior portion of the skull has a narrowed shape (arrows), termed a "lemon sign." The cerebellar hemispheres (Ce) form a banana-like shape instead of being two circles. The third and lateral ventricles (LV) are often dilated. Pe = cerebral peduncles.

1. No cortical mantle; a membrane surrounding the fluid where the cortex should be (the dura) can be mistaken for brain tissue.
2. No midline intrahemispheric septum and falx.
3. Visible brainstem and cerebral peduncles and variable amounts of the thalamus and midbrain. No third or fourth ventricular dilation. The brainstem structures protrude into the fluid that replaces the brain in a characteristic fashion (Fig. 18-30).

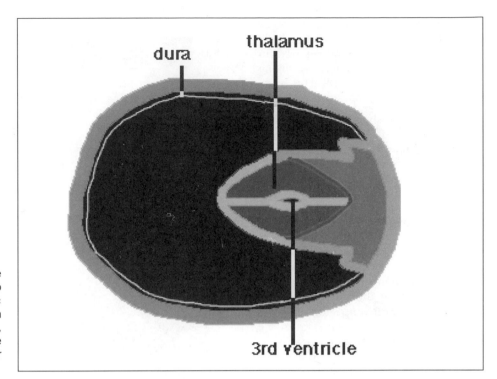

FIGURE 18-29. Hydranencephaly. The brainstem and thalamus protrude into the fluid-filled skull in a characteristic fashion. No cortical mantle is present. In most cases the falx is absent. The dura, a thin membrane that surrounds the brain, is present and may be mistaken for a thin cortical mantle.

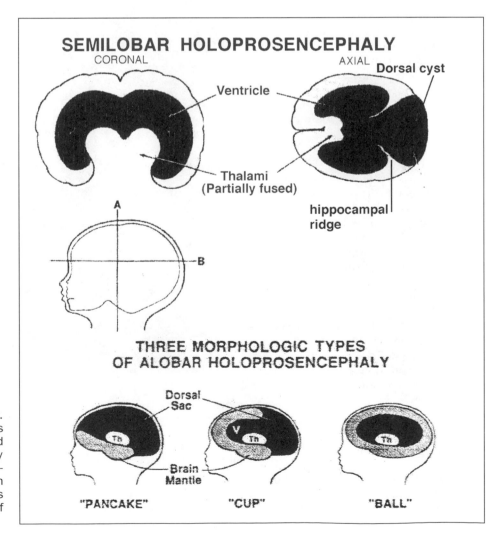

FIGURE 18-30. Alobar holoprosencephaly. (**A**) A single fused horseshoe ventricle is present. Notice the dorsal cyst separated from the main portion of the ventricle by the hippocampal ridge. (**B-D**) Three variants of alobar holoprosencephaly in which the cortex is absent in varying degrees with a single central ventricle (courtesy of David Nyberg).

HOLOPROSENCEPHALY. Holoprosencephaly is a malformation with a dismal prognosis—death if severe, mental retardation if mild (see Fig. 18-30). There is a strong association with trisomy 13. The sonographic features are characteristic:

1. A single horseshoe-shaped ventricle that may be so large that there is virtually no mantle (alobar); a variably sized and asymmetrical horseshoe-shaped ventricle (lobar); or a common ventricle that is fused only posteriorly (semilobar).
2. Fused thalami with no third ventricle visible.
3. A ridge along the lateral border of the ventricle known as the hippocampal ridge.
4. A bulge along the posterior aspect of the common ventricle, known as the dorsal cyst or sac, is seen in the alobar form. Whereas cortical mantle may be seen lining the anterior portion of the skull, none may be seen posteriorly.
5. Absence of corpus callosum and cavum septum pellucidi (see Fig. 18-30).
6. Often unusually close together orbits (hypotelorism) or only a single orbit (cyclops). (See Appendixes 18 and 19.)
7. Often a central cleft palate or cleft lip (see Fig. 18-45C).
8. Often no nose, which is replaced by a proboscis lying above the eyes. If the nose is present a single nostril may be seen.
9. Other anomalies such as clubfoot, omphalocele; also IUGR, since trisomy 13 is a common association.
10. In the milder form, which can be subtle, the only finding is the absence of the septum pellucidum and the cavum septum pellucidum.

DANDY-WALKER CYST. Dandy-Walker cyst is due to a cerebellar abnormality (Fig. 18-31). Mental deficiency is common in survivors. Chromosomal anomalies may be associated. The sonographic features are as follows:

1. Cystic enlargement of the fourth ventricle. The cisterna magna is enlarged above a 10-mm distance. The hypoplastic cerebellum and vermis are separated by a fluid-filled tubular structure which may be small or large and which extends from the fourth ventricle to the cisterna magna.

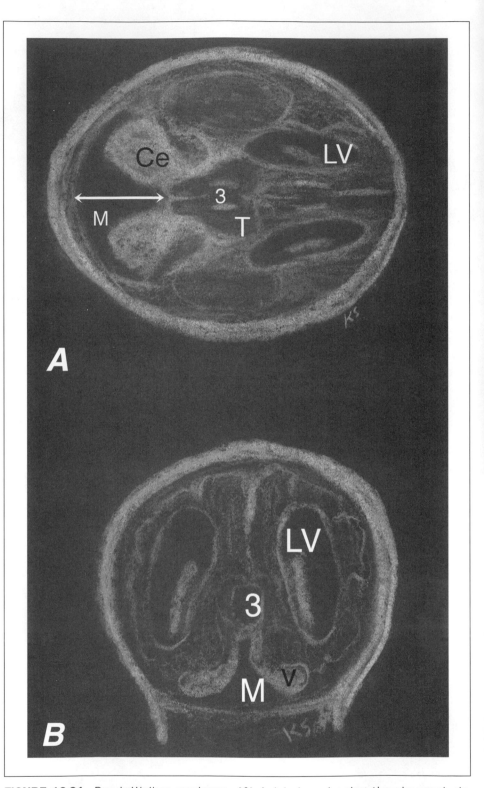

FIGURE 18-31. Dandy-Walker syndrome. (**A**) Axial view showing the abnormal, deformed shape of the cerebellum (Ce), the enlarged fourth ventricle (M), and the dilatation of the third (3) and lateral ventricles (LV). (**B**) Coronal view of Dandy-Walker syndrome showing the abnormal cerebellum and secondary dilation of the third and lateral ventricles.

2. Dilation of the third ventricle and aqueduct may be present.

3. Dilation of the lateral ventricles to a variable degree.

4. The cerebellar lobes, particularly the vermis, are split apart, smaller than usual, and abnormal in shape.
5. Agenesis of the corpus callosum is an important and difficult to diagnose association. If agenesis (see Fig. 18-33) is present, the chance of mental retardation is much increased. Agenesis of the corpus callosum is described later in the chapter.

VEIN OF GALEN ANEURYSM. A large arteriovenous malformation, a vein of Galen aneurysm, causes high-output congestive failure (Fig. 18-32). The lesion is rare and usually fatal at birth, despite surgery. The sonographic features are as follows:

1. Posterior midline pulsatile structure connected to a central tubular fluid-filled space extending posteriorly from above the thalamus to a vein called the straight sinus superior to the cerebellum.
2. Pulsatile flow on Doppler with arterial and venous components within the vein.
3. Numerous collateral arteries supplying the vein will be seen. Attempts to define the number and location of the supplying vessels with color flow should be made.
4. Possible compression of the aqueduct by the cyst causing secondary ventriculomegaly.
5. Enlarged heart and vessels supplying the brain (e.g., the carotid artery).
6. Fetal ascites and pleural effusion are possible.

PORENCEPHALIC CYST AND INTRACRANIAL HEMORRHAGE. Porencephalic cysts are a sequel to an intraparenchymal bleed. A cystic area forms that communicates with the ventricle.

1. The ventricle bulges at the site of a porencephalic cyst.
2. Echogenic clot may be seen in the porencephalic cyst, the brain, or the dilated ventricle.
3. Bleeding into the brain causes an echogenic mass.
4. If any intraventricular bleeding occurs, the ventricles dilate and echogenic clot can be seen within the lateral and third ventricles. Blood can rarely get through the narrow aqueduct of Sylvius and often results in obstruction at this level.

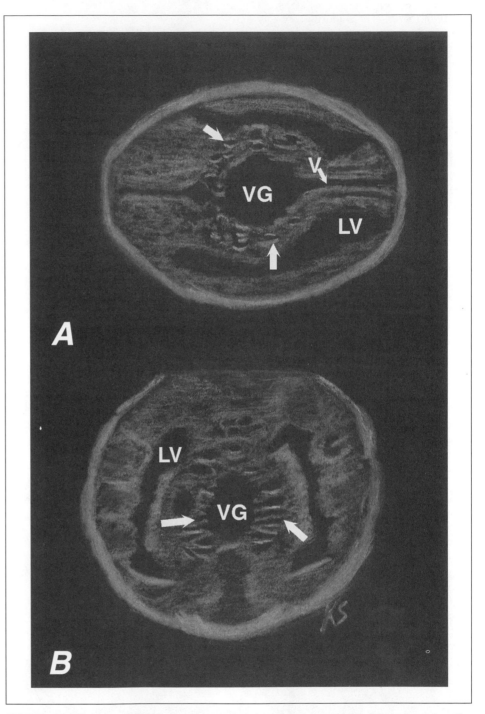

FIGURE 18-32. Vein of Galen aneurysm. Axial and coronal views. Diagram using the standard biparietal diameter approach showing the vein of Galen aneurysm (VG). Note the number of small arteries (white arrow) which are feeding into the large aneurysm. The draining vessel (small arrow) is draining into the sagittal sinus at the posterior aspect of the brain.

ARACHNOID CYST. An arachnoid cyst is a fluid-filled space within the brain substance not communicating with the ventricles. This cystic area can be of any shape. Arachnoid cysts arise from the meninges, so a common location is alongside the tentorum. Secondary hydrocephalus can occur. Infratentorial arachnoid cysts can mimic Dandy Walker if they are in the midline and low, but the vermis and cerebellum will be present.

Agenesis of the Corpus Callosum

Agenesis of the corpus callosum with associated cyst may look awful, but when isolated, does not cause symptoms apart from occasional epilepsy (Fig. 18-33). Agenesis of the corpus callosum is associated with trisomy syndromes, cardiac anomalies, and a number of cranial conditions. If agenesis is present, it usually worsens the prognosis. The sonographic findings are as follows:

1. Increased separation of the lateral ventricles.
2. Enlargement of the occipital horns and atria (colpocephaly). Confusion with hydrocephalus is possible.
3. Upward displacement of the third ventricle.
4. Abnormal gyral pattern. The gyri radiate superiorly from the lateral ventricles rather than lie parallel to the lateral ventricles.
5. Possible superior cystic enlargement of the third ventricle (see Fig. 18-33E).

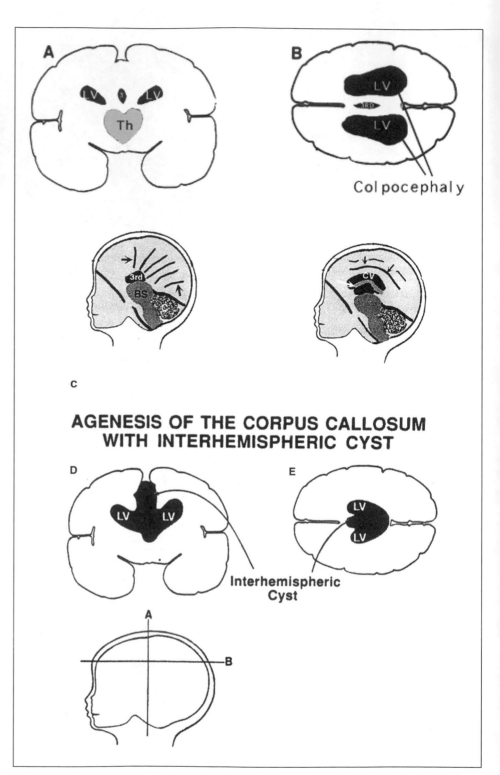

FIGURE 18-33. Agenesis of the corpus callosum. (**A**) Coronal view. Standard form of agenesis of the corpus callosum. Note the high position of the third ventricle (3) located between the lateral ventricles (LV) and lying above the thalamus (Th). (**B**) Axial view. There is posterior dilation of the occipital horns of the lateral ventricles (colpocephaly). (**C**) A sagittal view shows that the gyri (black arrows) are radiating in a vertical fashion rather than horizontally aligned as is usually the case. (**D & E**) Diagrams of the cystic type of agenesis of the corpus callosum. The lateral ventricles are joined by the enlarged third ventricle with a cyst protruding superior to the lateral ventricles.

Intracranial Tumors

Fetal intracranial tumors are rare. Intracranial teratomas are seen as cystic and echogenic areas distributed randomly throughout a greatly enlarged head. Choroid plexus papilloma appears as a bright echogenic mass adjacent to the choroid within the lateral ventricle, with secondary hydrocephalus.

Head and Brain Malformations

Anencephaly

Only the structures at the base of the brain are present in anencephaly. This malformation of the brain is thought to be a consequence of the absence of formation of the skull. The malformation has a different appearance and name depending on when it is detected.

1. At 11 to 13 weeks, acrania is seen (Fig. 18-34B). No skull is formed. Although a normal amount of brain is present, it has an irregular lobular outline since it is unconfined by the skull.
2. At 14 to 16 weeks, exencephaly is present (see Fig. 18-34C). The brain remnant is smaller and it is now obvious that no skull is present.

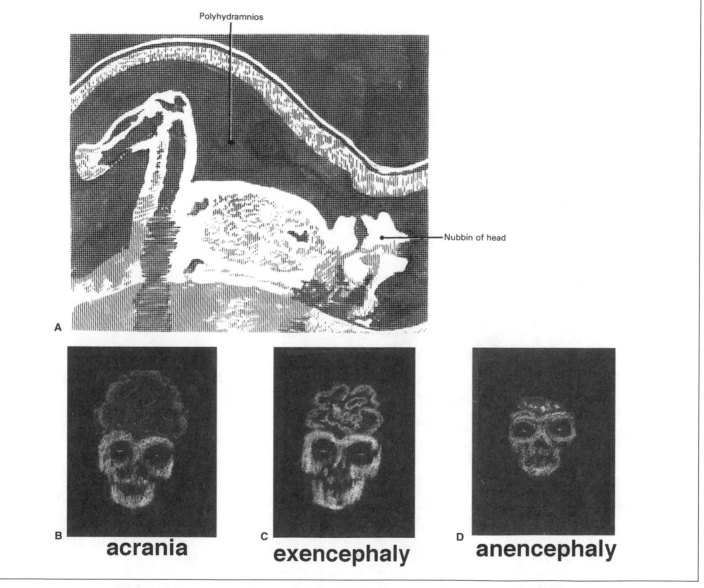

FIGURE 18-34. Anencephalus. (**A**) The fetal head is replaced by a nubbin of tissue, in which the bones of the base of the head can be made out. (**B**) In acrania the skull is absent. All of the brain is present, but tends to protrude to the left or right since nothing confines it. (**C**) In exencephaly some of the brain is absent. Some has been removed, presumably by trauma. (**D**) In anencephaly only a small central bulge occurs above the level of the orbits, which represents the blood vessels in the brain which withstand damage from other structures.

3. From 17 weeks on, anencephaly is present (see Fig. 18-34A and D). A "nubbin" of tissue is visible at the cranial end of the trunk (see Fig. 18-34A). The cerebral hemispheres and cranial vault (skull) are absent. The cranial blood vessels persist and form a vascular mound at the superior aspect of the remaining fetal cranial tissue. When the fetus is supine the facial structures end superiorly with the orbits. When the fetus is prone the fetal head appears to end with the superior aspect of the spine. Polyhydramnios with much fetal movement is present if fetal swallowing is impaired by brain destruction. Anencephaly is associated with spina bifida and iniencephaly.

Iniencephaly

This rare condition is often associated with anencephaly. The fetal head is retroflexed because there are too few cervical vertebra. The cervical vertebra are unfused with a meningocele present (rachischisis).

Microcephaly

The head and brain are too small in microcephaly, resulting in mental retardation. The sonographic findings are not straightforward.

1. The cranium is small. Deciding whether the head is small enough to be of concern is not easy. The head may be quite small (greater than two standard deviations below the mean) as a normal variant. An abnormally low head-to-trunk ratio (three standard deviations or less) strongly suggests that the fetus is microcephalic. Serial sonograms show a progressively small head in comparison to the trunk and limbs. The diagnosis can usually not be made before 24 weeks.

2. Ventriculomegaly with a small head is diagnostic of microcephaly. The ventricles dilate because the brain is becoming atrophic. A normal-sized cranium with enlarged ventricles may well be due to atrophy rather than obstruction.

3. Calcification may be seen alongside the ventricle if the cause of microcephaly is cytomegalic inclusion disease. In microcephaly due to toxoplasmosis there is patchy calcification within the brain.

Mass Arising From the Head or Neck

Encephalocele

1. With encephalocele, a defect is present, usually in the posterior aspect of the skull, through which portions of the brain substance and perhaps the ventricle prolapse (Fig. 18-35A). Usually encephaloceles contain cerebrospinal fluid, but they may contain brain tissue, in which case the prognosis is much worse.

2. The more brain tissue within the encephalocele the worse the prognosis. The head is often small (microcephaly).

3. Secondary hydrocephalus is a common associated finding.

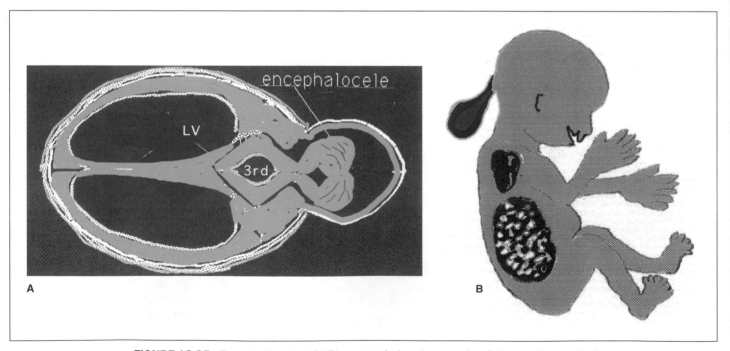

FIGURE 18-35. Encephalocele. (**A**) The encephalocele contains fluid and the cerebellum is in an occipital location in the midline as is usually the case. (**B**) Diagram of a fetus with Meckel-Gruber syndrome showing the encephalocele on a stalk, the enlarged kidney filled with small cysts, the polydactyly, the cleft lip and palate, and the cardiac abnormality. All are features of this syndrome.

4. Look for multiple fingers or toes (polydactyly) and enlarged kidneys containing cysts, the main components of the lethal Meckel-Gruber syndrome (see Fig. 18-35B).

5. A few encephaloceles are on the lateral aspect of the head. Look for an amniotic band if this is the case. Additional features of the amniotic bands such as truncated or swollen limbs, club feet and cleft palate may be seen.

6. A rare form of encephalocele protrudes between the eyes in an anterior location.

Cystic Hygroma

Defective formation of the lymphatic system leads to a build-up of lymph in the neck. Bilateral cysts develop in the neck (Fig. 18-36A and B).

1. In a mild form of cystic hygroma there is a small cystic area in the posterolateral or posterior aspect of the neck. Chromosomal analysis often shows Turner's or Down syndrome when this is an isolated finding. Such cystic hygromas often regress over the course of the pregnancy and disappear.

2. In the more severe form, large cysts on the posterior aspect of both sides of the neck may be in contact with each other (see Fig. 18-36B). The findings of hydrops are present, i.e., pleural effusion, ascites, skin thickening, and pericardial effusion.

3. Severe skin thickening is seen. Multiple septa are seen within the thickened skin, sometimes with small cystic areas where lymph has pooled.

4. When hydrops is present as well as cystic hygroma, the condition is always fatal within a few weeks of diagnosis.

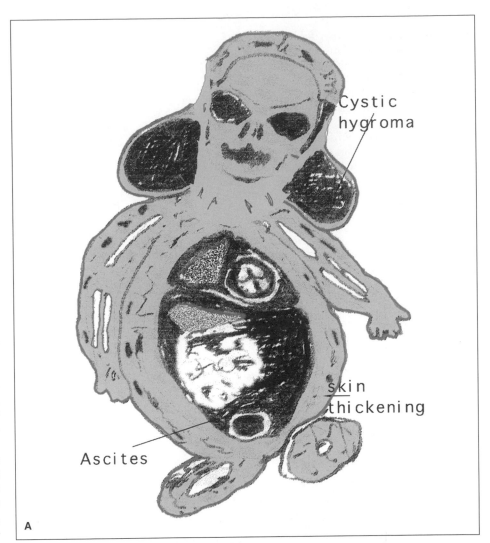

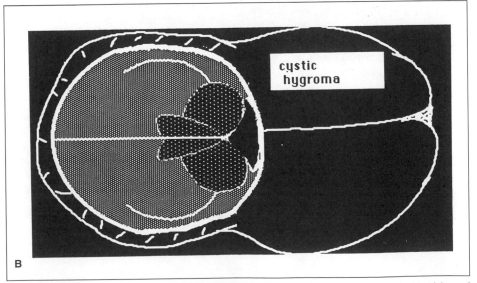

FIGURE 18-36. Lethal cystic hygroma. (**A**) Cystic structures arise from both sides of the neck. There is marked skin thickening with septa present. Ascites and pleural effusions are seen. (**B**) Possible appearance of very severe cystic hygroma. The cystic hygromas balloon out so that they contact each other with only a septum separating them. They may surround the head.

Goiter

1. Enlargement of the thyroid leads to a solid mass on the anterior aspect of the neck, often causing head extension.
2. There is severe polyhydramnios, since swallowing is impeded by the neck mass.
3. A goiter is smooth bordered and evenly textured. The thyroid gland lies on either side of the fetal trachea. Normal standards for thyroid size exist (see Appendix 30).

Teratoma of the Neck

A solid mass of varied echo texture is seen in the anterior neck region when a teratoma of the neck is present. This rare mass usually extends from the jaw to the clavicle.

Limb Shortening

Micromelia is the term used when all limbs and portions of limbs are short. Mesomelia is used when the distal limbs are most short and rhizomelia is used when the proximal long bones are most affected (Fig. 18-37). These different patterns are associated with different types of dwarfism.

When a short limb is found, determine whether all limbs are short or only one or two.

Shortening Confined to a Few Limbs

FAMILIAL RHIZOMELIC LIMB SHORTENING

1. If the humerus and femur are mildly shortened (between the 5th and 10th percentile) look at the parents. It is likely that they will also have short proximal limbs. This is a common normal variant.
2. This finding is associated with Down syndrome. Look for other findings of Down syndrome. If this is the only finding, amniocentesis is not usually recommended.

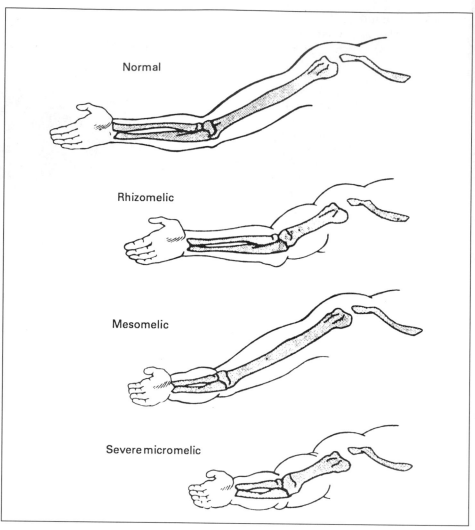

FIGURE 18-37. Diagram showing the different types of limb shortening that can occur. The shortening may be only in the proximal limbs (rhizomelia), only in the distal long bones (mesomelia), or throughout the limbs (micromelia). (Reprinted with permission from R. Romero.)

FOCAL FEMORAL DEFICIENCY

1. One of the femurs is very short and usually angulated at the midportion. The femoral head is sometimes absent.
2. The fibula and sometimes the tibia may also be short or absent. Other long bones such as the arms or opposite femur may occasionally be involved.

MILD OSTEOGENESIS IMPERFECTA
See Figure 18-38.

1. One or more limbs are shortened to a variable extent.
2. The disease tends to affect the lower limbs, notably the femur.
3. The limb is deformed by one or more of the following: bowing; a fracture; a locally thickened midshaft bulge due to callus formation; and overall bony irregularity related to previous fractures.

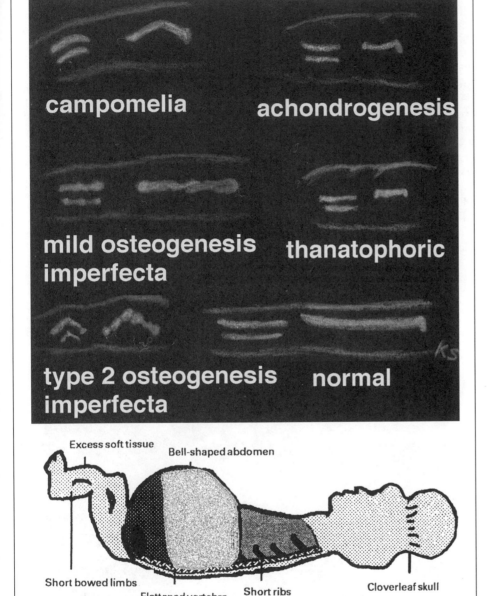

FIGURE 18-38. (A) Long bones in various types of dwarfism. In campomelic dwarfism, the femur is acutely bowed and the tibia is evenly bowed. Both proximal and distal limbs are mildly shortened. In achondrogenesis, all limbs are extremely short with excessive soft tissues. In mild osteogenesis imperfecta, there is some long bone irregularity and thanatophoric dwarfism, limbs are extremely short with a telephone receiver appearance to the femur. In type 2 osteogenesis imperfecta, the limbs are very short. Multiple irregularities and fractures are visible. A normal femur, tibia and fibula are shown for comparison. **(B)** Thanatophoric dwarfism. The limbs are extremely short and bowed. The chest is very small, so the abdomen balloons out. The ribs are very short. In a few examples of thanotophoric dwarfism, there is a bulge off the top of the skull known as a cloverleaf deformity, and the ribs are flattened.

Generalized Limb Shortening

The severity of the limb shortening may be such that the dwarfism is lethal. Lethal dwarfism is present when the limbs are exceedingly short and more importantly when there is severe polyhydramnios and the chest is very small (chest circumference less than .81 of abdominal circumference).

Lethal Dwarfisms

Numerous rare forms of lethal dwarfism exist. Only the most common and easily recognizable forms will be described.

THANATOPHORIC DWARFISM

Thanatophoric dwarfism is the most common lethal dwarfism, with the following features (see Fig. 18-38B):

1. Grossly shortened, bowed limbs. The femur, which is more shortened than the tibia and fibula, usually has a "telephone receiver" shape.
2. Tiny chest with normal-sized abdomen, giving a bell shape to the trunk.
3. Severe polyhydramnios thought to be due to compression of the esophagus by the small chest.
4. Flattened vertebrae. These are difficult to recognize with ultrasound, but can be seen on a fetal x-ray. On ultrasound, the vertebrae appear unduly close together.
5. Redundant soft tissues. It would appear that the normal quantity of soft tissue surrounds a very short limb.
6. A bulge off the top of the head, forming a deformity known as a cloverleaf skull or Kleebattschadel deformity. This is due to the fusion of some of the skull structures. Cloverleaf changes are seen only infrequently, but the head is always large.
7. Short and stubby fingers (triradiate) and feet.

ACHONDROGENESIS

See Figure 18-38A.

1. Findings in achondrogenesis are similar to those in thanatophoric dwarfism.
2. In the most common variety, the spine is very poorly ossified.
3. Thickening of the skin at the back of the neck occurs with even the formation of a cyst. Hydrops may be present.
4. This condition is always lethal.

OSTEOGENESIS IMPERFECTA (LETHAL RECESSIVE FORM)

See Figure 18-38A.

1. The limbs and ribs are very short with multiple fractures, bowing, and irregular contours.
2. The skull is poorly ossified, so the brain is seen too well. Brain structure close to the transducer and the near skull border can be easily seen. Light transducer pressure over the fetal head will deform the skull.
3. The chest is small and there are numerous rib fractures.
4. The spine is poorly ossified.
5. Polyhydramnios may be present if the chest is very small.

Nonlethal Dwarfisms

ACHONDROPLASIA

1. In the usual heterozygous form of achondroplasia the limbs do not become short until after 24 weeks. The proximal limbs are more shortened than the distal limbs (rhizomelic shortening). The head is large and the ventricles may be mildly dilated, as in hydrocephalus.
2. In the homozygous form, where both parents are achondroplastic dwarfs, the limbs are very short and the disease is fatal. It is indistinguishable, except by family history, from thanatophoric dwarfism.

PHOCOMELIA

The long bones are missing in phocomelia, and the hands and feet arise from the shoulder or hips.

Limb/Body Wall Defect Syndrome (Cyllosoma)

The limb/body wall defect syndrome, a lethal multisystem disease, is thought to be due to amnion disruption occurring in the first two months of pregnancy. The components are as follows:

1. A variant of gastroschisis in which the liver as well as the small bowel and possibly the heart are outside the abdominal wall.
2. Myelomeningocele, sometimes with hydrocephalus.
3. Absence of one or more limbs.
4. Gross twisting of the spine (kyphoscoliosis), sometimes with loss of the sacrum (caudal regression).
5. Sometimes amniotic bands are visible.

There is usually oligohydramnios, which, combined with the twisted short spine, makes an examination very difficult.

Blood Tests or Maternal Age Suspicious for Down Syndrome

The triple screen is a combination of the alpha-fetoprotein, estriol, and HCG levels. If the three are elevated above normal maternal blood levels, the risk of Down syndrome is increased. A maternal age of over 35 (some would say 32) also increases the risk of Down syndrome (see Table 18-1).

There are several ultrasonic signs that make the diagnosis of Down syndrome more likely. Absence of these signs diminishes the risk for Down syndrome.

Down Syndrome Signs (Trisomy 21)

1. Short femur and humerus length. If the femur and humerus length are less than .91 of the expected femur or humerus length for the gestational age, the risk of Down syndrome is increased.
2. Thickening of the skin on the back of the neck seen on the cerebellar view. A distance of greater than 6 mm is a strong sign of Down syndrome (see Fig. 14-13). Skin thickening in this area is most pronounced at 11 to 13 weeks, when a long, thin echogenic line along the back of the fetus (called nuchal translucency) is strongly associated with Down syndrome (Fig. 18-39).

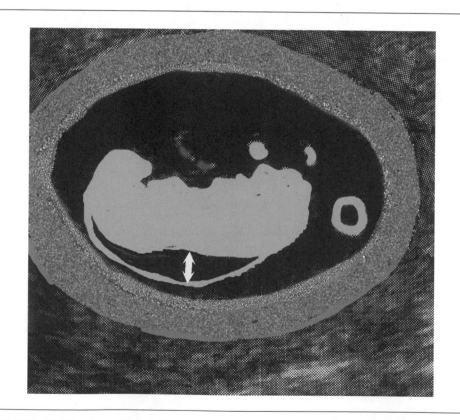

FIGURE 18-39. View of an early gestational sac showing a 9-week pregnancy with nuchal translucency. A thin membrane extends from the back of the head to the rump. If it is separated from the main trunk of the fetus by more than 3 mm (arrow), a strong association with Down syndrome and other chromosomal anomalies exists.

3. Endocardial cushion defect. This form of cardiac anomaly and, to a lesser extent, other congenital heart defects are associated with Down syndrome (see Chapter 20).
4. Duodenal atresia. This type of gastrointestinal obstruction and, to a lesser extent, other types of intestinal obstruction have a strong association with Down syndrome.
5. Echogenic bowel. A localized clump of small bowel, which is as echogenic as neighboring bone, suggests Down syndrome, cytomegalic inclusion disease, ingested blood, or meconium peritonitis, or it may be normal. A weak sign.
6. Sandal toe. The big toe is widely separated from the remaining toes. A weak sign.
7. Small curved middle phalanx of the little finger. A weak sign.
8. Mild renal pelvic dilation to 4 mm or greater. A weak sign.
9. Mild cranial lateral ventricular dilation. A strong sign.
10. Echogenic foci in the chordi tendinae or in the moderator band of the right ventricle. A weak sign.

If the triple screen levels are lowered, then trisomy 18, a lethal chromosomal anomaly, becomes more likely.

Trisomy 18 Signs

The features of trisomy 18 are as follows:

1. Clenched fists with overlapping of the ring finger.
2. Early growth retardation (i.e., in the second trimester).
3. Spina bifida and associated neural crest malformations.
4. Gut containing omphalocele.
5. Choroid plexus cysts. If the only finding is a cyst in the choroid plexus, most consider this insufficient to perform an amniocentesis, whereas others favor amniocentesis. (Our policy is no amniocentesis if the triple screen is normal.)
6. Abnormal fetal heart.

Mass Arising From the Trunk

Omphalocele

See Figure 18-40.

1. Abdominal contents prolapse through the cord insertion site. Liver and/or gut compose the omphalocele. The cord enters the center of the omphalocele.
2. Omphalocele may be a component of the pentalogy of Cantrell. Ectopia cordis, the heart outside the chest, and interrupted diaphragm are other principal components.
3. Other anomalies are present with omphalocele about half the time, particularly cardiac problems.

4. If the omphalocele contents are entirely bowel, there is a strong chance of a chromosomal anomaly.
5. A membrane is seen surrounding the herniated contents.
6. Between 8 and 11 weeks gut normally rotates outside the fetal trunk to give a transitory appearance similar to a gut containing omphalocele.

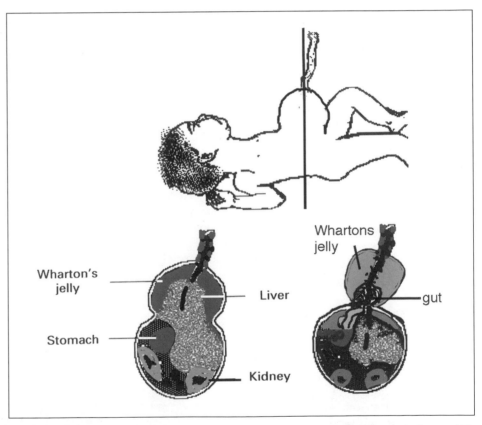

FIGURE 18-40. Omphalocele. The abdominal contents prolapse through the umbilicus into a sac in front of the abdomen. Note the umbilical cord entering the sac. Fluid may surround the liver or gut within the sac. If only gut is present in the sac, there is a strong association with chromosomal anomalies.

Gastroschisis

1. Some or all of the gut escapes through a hole in the right lower abdomen into the amniotic fluid (Fig. 18-41). The liver remains in the abdomen. The cord enters at its normal site. In severe cases, the stomach and/or the bladder can lie outside the abdomen.
2. If the abdominal wall opening is small, the gut within the gastroschisis or in the fetal abdomen may be distended. Gut and stomach dilation are now thought to have little relationship to long-term prognosis.
3. Usually this is an isolated anomaly.
4. No membrane surrounds the gut; it floats freely in the amniotic fluid.

Sacrococcygeal Teratoma

1. Teratomas occur most often in utero adjacent to the sacrum, where they are known as sacrococcygeal teratomas (Fig. 18-42). Arising from the coccyx, they usually extend inferiorly between the legs. They may also infiltrate superiorly, posterior to the bladder.
2. Although they usually contain cysts, many contain solid areas and calcification.
3. Obstruction of the bladder and kidneys may occur if the tumor has an intrapelvic component.
4. Hydrops may develop, thought to be due to vascular shunting through the mass.
5. Some teratomas grow to a huge size so they are as large or larger than the fetus.

Spina Bifida/Myelomeningocele and Related Abnormalities

1. Spina bifida most often occurs in the lumbosacral area, but may be found in the cervical or thoracic area as well (Figs. 18-43 and 18-44). Almost all are posterior to the spine, but they may rarely be anterior.
2. The number and level of involved vertebrae influences prognosis. With higher lumbar vertebra and thoracic vertebra involvement, difficulty walking and inability to sit up are likely.
3. If there is no leg movement and the feet are clubbed, the prognosis is very poor. On some occasions, leg movement is seen in utero, but once surgery has been performed, movement ceases.

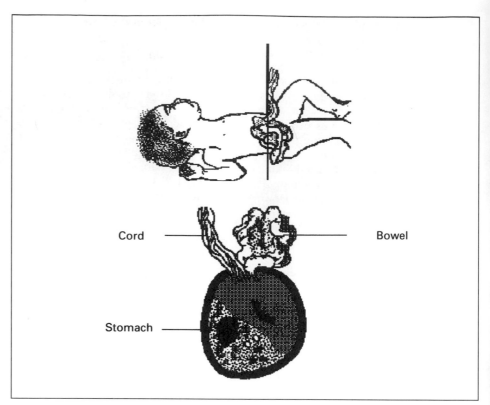

FIGURE 18-41. Gastroschisis. Along the right anterior inferior aspect of the fetal abdomen loops of bowel emerge from the abdomen.

4. After birth, spina bifida causes urological problems, but hydronephrosis and bladder dilation are practically never seen in the fetus.
5. There are various types of spina bifida, some more severe than others:

a. Myeloschisis—low termination of the cord with absent spinal processes and widened interpedicular distance. The skin is open over the defect, but no pouch is present.
b. Meningocele—a pouch containing cerebrospinal fluid, but no nerve tissue. The prognosis is good.

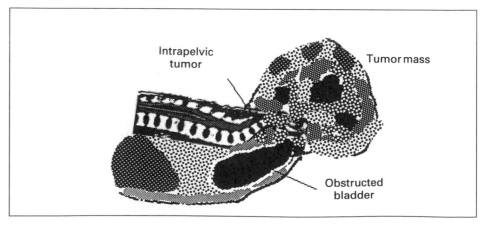

FIGURE 18-42. Sacrococcygeal teratoma. View of the inferior aspect of the fetus showing the large mass protruding from the coccygeal area containing cystic and solid components. There is secondary obstruction at the bladder due to the small intra-abdominal component.

c. Myelomeningocele—a combination of low termination of the cord and a pouch of cerebrospinal fluid containing nerves. The more tissue that is present within the pouch, the worse the prognosis.

6. Ultrasonic findings seen with spina bifida include the following:

a. Spine

In the normal spine three echogenic foci are seen on transverse view—an echo from the posterior vertebral body and the two posterior element ossification centers. These three echoes normally form a triangle on transverse views that widens slightly in the cervical and lumbar areas. In spina bifida the two posterior element echoes are separated and a U shape is formed (see Fig. 18-43).

In a sagittal view of the normal spine two parallel lines of echoes representing the posterior elements and the vertebral body are seen. The posterior elements are absent at the level of the defect. A skin defect or a pouch may be seen posterior to the spine at the defect level (see Fig. 18-44). Try to place the transducer posterior and parallel to the skin to see this bulge or defect. The distal end of the cord can often be seen (see Fig. 18-44). The lumbosacral cord normally ends at L2. In low level myelomeningoceles it ends at approximately L5.

A coronal spinal view will show widening at the level of spina bifida.

Curved echogenic lines representing nerves may be seen within the pouch.

The spine may be flexed and angulated at the level of the defect (a gibbous deformity).

b. Skull. The cerebellum normally forms two round circles. In spina bifida, the cerebellum forms a banana shape. This shape change indicates the Arnold-Chiari malformation, which is almost always present with spina bifida and may occasionally occur as an isolated process (see Fig. 18-28). The cisterna magna will be absent.

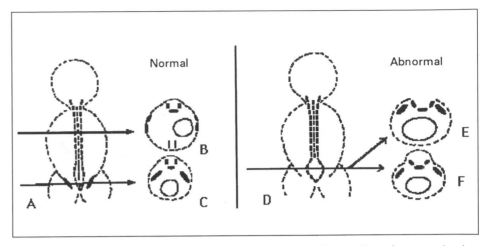

FIGURE 18-43. Spina bifida. (**A**) A longitudinal sonographic section of a normal spine has three components. The vertebral arches from two parallel series of echogenic dots. The width of the space between them widens slightly in the cervical and lumbar areas. In the center is another series of echogenic dots that represents the posterior ossification center of the vertebral bodies. (**B**) On transverse section, a circle of echoes is formed. (**C**) Level of the bladder. (**D**) Longitudinal section. In spina bifida the circle is incomplete, with separation of the posterior element echoes. The space between the arches is widened at the involved level. (**E**) The spina bifida creates a U-shaped gap. (**F**) A fluid-filled sac (a meningomyelocele) may be present.

c. Cerebellum. The skull shape often resembles a lemon, with a flattened anterior portion, also a consequence of the Arnold-Chiari malformation (see Fig. 18-28). This finding may occasionally be seen in the absence of a spinal anomaly.

d. Lateral ventricles. The lateral ventricles and third ventricle may be dilated.

Diastomatomyelia

In a rare variant of spina bifida called diastematomyelia there is widening of the lumbar spine. The cord splits in two around a central bony spur. There is cord tethering. Very disorganized vertebra are seen below the level of the bony spur.

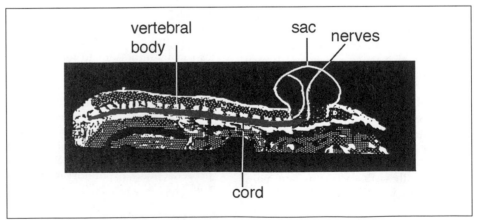

FIGURE 18-44. Sagittal view of the spine with a myelomeningocele. Note the absence of the vertebral ossification centers alongside the myelomeningocele and the tethering of the cord, which ends at the level of the myelomeningocele. Some nerves can be seen entering the myelomeningocele.

Lipoma

If the cord is tethered and no spinal anomaly is seen, look for an echogenic mass in the spinal canal. Such a mass of fatty tissue is termed a lipoma. It is rarely seen in utero.

Vertebral Deformities

Spinal deformities are often found with diabetes mellitus.

1. In hemi-vertebrae the spine is angulated slightly at the level of the deformity and one of the posterior element echoes will be missing.
2. With block vertebra one of the posterior element echoes will be larger than expected and the spine will be slightly angulated.

Caudal Regression

In this condition the spine is too short and some of the vertebra are missing.

1. Find the iliac crests. The upper aspect of the iliac crest corresponds to L5.
2. Sacral vertebra normally extend down from this level. Sometimes in addition to the sacrum some or all of the lumbar vertebra are missing.
3. Club feet with absent leg movement are often found.

Stomach Not Seen

Inability to see the stomach is an important clue that serious pathology exists. Occasionally it is difficult to see the stomach in obese women with normal fetuses. Coincident polyhydramnios makes a normal variant unlikely. When the stomach is absent, look in the chest, face, and neck for cleft palate, tracheoesophageal atresia, and diaphragmatic hernia.

Cleft Lip And Palate

Three forms exist: unilateral, bilateral, and central. Isolated cleft palate without cleft lip is almost impossible to detect with ultrasound in utero. The stomach is usually visible with this anomaly. Often there is a family history of cleft palate.

1. *Unilateral.* An oblique laterally placed gap is seen in the upper lip which may also affect the maxilla (Fig. 18-45A). It extends into the nose. An abnormal hooked nostril is seen on a profile view.

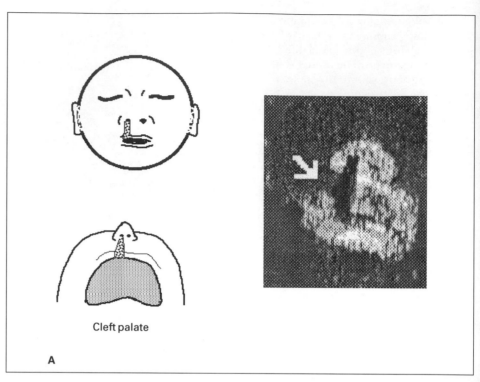

FIGURE 18-45. Cleft palate. (**A**) Diagram showing the location of a unilateral cleft lip and palate and a sonogram showing a unilateral cleft (arrow). (**B**) Bilateral cleft lip and palate. The central component swings anteriorly and forms a mass (upper arrow) that can be mistaken for a tumor or encephalocele on the lower image. L = lip. The two arrows show the bilateral cleft. (**C**) Central cleft palates of the type that occur with holoprosencephaly and trisomy 18. Note the hypoteilorism (close set eyes) and a single nostril.

2. *Bilateral.* A centrally placed mass protrudes immediately below the nose (see Fig. 18-45B). The upper lip and maxilla are interrupted by the mass. Profile views will show the mass protruding beyond the nose. Additional abnormalities should be sought if either of these cleft types are seen. It is especially important to look for amniotic band deformities.
3. *Central.* A gap is seen below the nose in the upper lip and maxilla (see Fig. 18-45C). As a rule, the nose is abnormal and is either absent or there is a single nostril. This type of cleft palate is frequently associated with holoprosencephaly, hypotelorism, and trisomy 13.

Tracheoesophageal Atresia

With tracheoesophageal anomalies the esophagus is partially absent (atresia), but often it connects (by a fistula) to the trachea, which in turn connects with the stomach. This type of anomaly is often not detectable before birth because amniotic fluid can pass into the gut through the fistula.

1. When the connection to the stomach is narrow, a small stomach is seen.
2. If no connection to the stomach exists (10% of cases), the stomach is not seen on ultrasound and there is very severe polyhydramnios.
3. Cardiac, chromosomal, gastrointestinal, genitourinary, and vertebral malformations may also occur.

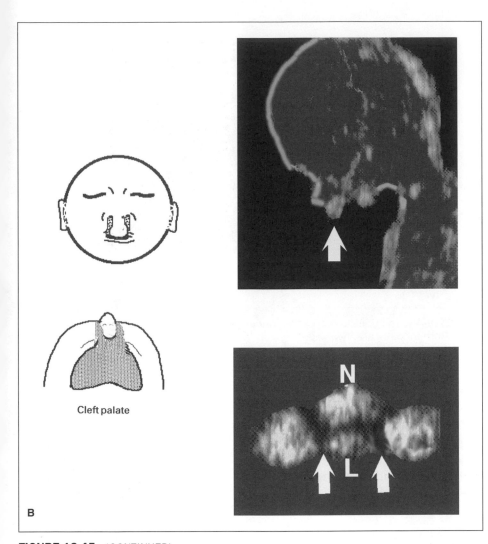

FIGURE 18-45. (CONTINUED)

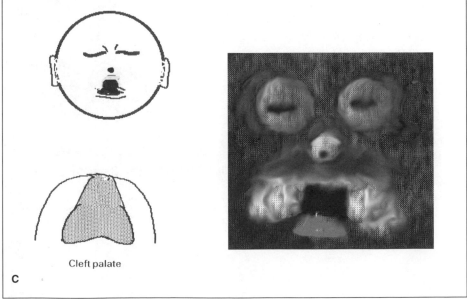

FIGURE 18-45. (CONTINUED)

Diaphragmatic Hernia

Failure to visualize the stomach in its normal location is often due to diaphragmatic hernia. In left-side diaphragmatic hernia the stomach is in the chest. (See also Cyst in the Chest section and Fig. 18-24.)

Hydrops

The features of hydrops fetalis are as follows:

1. Ascites
2. Pleural effusions
3. Pericardial effusion if hydrops is severe
4. Polyhydramnios
5. Thick echogenic placenta
6. Skin thickening

The presence of any two of these features allows the diagnosis of hydrops. Isolated ascites or isolated pleural effusion does not represent ascites. There are two main types: immune hydrops and nonimmune hydrops (see Chapter 17).

Immune Hydrops (Rh Incompatibility)

If the fetus in a first pregnancy has a different blood group from the mother, antibodies develop at delivery when the two circulations mix. In a second pregnancy these antibodies pass through the placenta and destroy fetal blood cells, and the fetus becomes anemic. With the anemia comes heart failure, pleural effusions, ascites, and other problems.

Immune hydrops can be prevented if RhoGAM is given with the first pregnancy, so it is rare today. Treatment of immune hydrops is by fetal blood transfusion. The blood is usually introduced into the umbilical cord by percutaneous umbilical blood sampling (see Chapter 52). Transfusion into the peritoneal cavity is a less desirable alternative.

Nonimmune Hydrops

The sonographic findings with nonimmune hydrops are the same as those with immune hydrops, but are usually much more severe, with gross skin thickening. There are many different causes of nonimmune hydrops:

1. Heart diseases, both congenital anomalies such as endocardial cushion defect and irregular rhythms (arrhythmias or dysrhythmias).
2. Lung problems such as cystadenomatoid malformation or pleural effusion that prevent venous return to the heart.
3. Infections such as toxoplasmosis and cytomegalic inclusion disease.
4. Large placental tumors fed by the blood intended for the fetus.
5. Anemic problems such as twin-twin transfusion syndrome and alpha thalassemia.
6. Gastrointestinal problems such as diaphragmatic hernia and meconium peritonitis.
7. Chromosomal problems such as Down syndrome and triploidy.
8. Masses with arteriovenous shunting such as sacrococcygeal teratoma and vein of Galen malformations.

The basic mechanism of hydrops appears to be anemia or inadequate venous return.

Skin Thickening

Skin thickening is seen with the following conditions:

1. *Macrosomia.* If the fetus is very large (at term over 4000 g, over 90th percentile for weight at other times), the skin usually becomes thickened and echogenic. There is usually polyhydramnios. Such macrosomia occurs in women with diabetes, particularly the form occurring only with pregnancy (gestational diabetes) and in the fetuses of large women (see Chapter 17).
2. *Hydrops.* Skin thickening is one of the features of hydrops. Look for pleural effusions, ascites, pericardial effusion, polyhydramnios, and placentomegaly in addition (see Chapter 17).

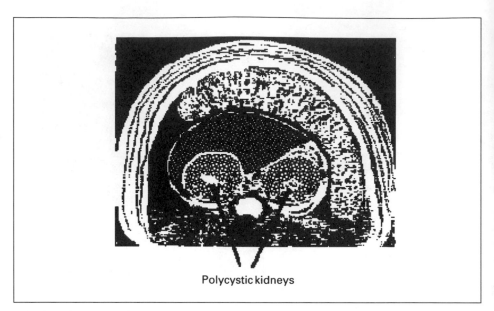

Polycystic kidneys

FIGURE 18-46. In infantile polycystic kidney disease the kidneys are large and echogenic. Both kidneys are involved.

3. *Fetal Death.* A late sign of fetal death is thickening of the skin. Death should have been recognized by absence of fetal heart movement long before this sign is seen (see Chapter 19).

Bilateral Large Echogenic Kidneys

Infantile Polycystic Kidney

See Figures 18-46 and 18-47.

1. The kidneys are much enlarged (see Appendixes 16 and 17) and more echogenic than usual. Usually no cysts are visible.
2. Usually there is severe oligohydramnios or no amniotic fluid if the diagnosis is made after 18 weeks.
3. Infantile polycystic kidney is a recessive genetic condition.
4. A form of polycystic kidney is the essential component of Meckel's syndrome, which also comprises polydactyly (extra digits) and encephalocele (see Fig. 18-35B). In this type of polycystic kidney, small cysts are visible.
5. If an infantile polycystic kidney is seen in utero, it almost always results in stillbirth.

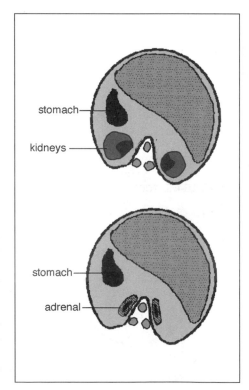

stomach
kidneys

stomach
adrenal

FIGURE 18-47. (A) The normal positions of the adrenal gland and kidney are shown. **(B)** The adrenals are more medial and anterior than the kidneys. The adrenals lie superior to the kidneys.

Adult Polycystic Kidney

Adult polycystic kidney is a dominant condition that can very rarely be detected in utero. Appearances vary from enlarged echogenic kidneys with no obvious cysts to kidneys containing large cysts. Because of the variability in appearance the parents of any fetus with bilateral enlarged kidneys with possible cystic disease should have their kidneys examined.

Bilateral Multicystic Dysplastic Kidney

1. Variable-size visible cysts that are interspersed with echogenic areas are seen in bilateral multicystic dysplastic kidney (see Fig. 18-15). The cysts are larger and more numerous than those occasionally seen with infantile polycystic kidney.
2. Both kidneys may be large.
3. There can be urine in the bladder (persisting from when the kidneys were functioning), but no amniotic fluid will be seen after 18 weeks.
4. The cysts increase in size as the pregnancy progresses and may later start to decrease in size while the fetus is still in utero.

Benign Glomerulosclerosis

The kidneys are mildly enlarged and echogenic but there is a normal amniotic fluid quantity. A normal cortical and medullary pattern can still be seen within the kidney. The prognosis is excellent.

Absent or Small Kidneys

Renal Agenesis

1. When there are no kidneys, there is no amniotic fluid after 15 to 18 weeks and no bladder or kidneys can be seen. Anatomy is difficult to see because of the absence of amniotic fluid.
2. The adrenals assume a flattened discoid shape and tend to be located lower and more lateral than normal (see Fig. 18-47). Since in utero they have an echogenic center, they can easily be mistaken for small kidneys.

3. If no fluid is present it can be hard to decide whether the cause of absent fluid is renal agenesis. Amnioinfusion is a technique that is sometimes performed under these circumstances. A small needle is placed into the amniotic cavity. This may be difficult because there is little or no fluid present. A combination of a dye (indigo carmine) and a sugar-containing fluid is injected into the amniotic space. About 150 cc is usually administered. If the kidneys are present, the fetus will start to swallow and the stomach and bladder will enlarge. The renal areas will become much easier to see because of the surrounding fluid. In the presence of premature rupture of membranes, which is often confused with renal agenesis, fluid leakage through the vagina will occur and sanitary pads will stain blue.

Masses in the Region of the Kidneys

Adrenal Hemorrhage

Hemorrhage in the third trimester may occur spontaneously or as a result of maternal loss of blood pressure. A mass in both adrenals is seen which is evenly echogenic or partly or completely cystic. The mass will be superior to the kidney and posterior to the liver. A rapid change in acoustic texture over a period of days will be seen as the hemorrhage evolves.

Neuroblastoma

This tumor is common at birth, but is usually so small it cannot be seen. It regresses spontaneously. It is usually densely echogenic, but since it is frequently associated with adrenal hemorrhage, it may be evenly echogenic or fluid filled. It is usually seen in the third trimester but has been reported at 20 weeks. Metastases to the liver may be seen.

Renal Tumor

Renal masses are rare and only occur in the third trimester. They are usually mesoblastic nephroma. Typically, these tumors are large and evenly echogenic, but there may be cystic components. They are always associated with severe polyhydramnios.

Fetal Liver Tumors

Several rare liver tumors may occasionally be seen in the third trimester in the fetus. All are extremely vascular. Hemangioendothelioma, the most common, is characterized by large vascular cystic spaces that show up on color flow. Hepatoblastoma are also highly vascular, but appear solid.

Second Collecting System

If there is a duplication of the upper half of the kidney and this is obstructed, an echogenic mass containing cysts will be seen due to the development of multicystic dysplastic changes in the kidney. Alternatively, a cystic lesion may be seen representing all that remains of the duplicated kidney.

Extralobar Sequestration

A portion of the lung forms just above the left adrenal gland. The resulting mass is echogenic with a large supplying artery seen on color flow. Similar appearances to neuroblastoma are seen, but CT scan shows fluid rather than solid tissue.

⭐ PITFALLS

1. *Sacral spina bifida.* Sacral spina bifida is easily missed because the spine ossifies late and curves at this site. Only transverse views may show the abnormality. Apparent spina bifida may be created by angling obliquely and transversely when examining the lower lumbar spine (Fig. 18-48).

2. *Femoral length.* Apparent short limbs can be created if the sonographer is not meticulous about making sure that the longest bone length views are obtained.

3. *Adrenal glands vs. kidney.* The fetal adrenal glands have been mistaken for kidneys in cases of renal agenesis. The adrenals are smaller and more medial and superior than the normal kidney (see Fig. 18-47). There will be no amniotic fluid after 15 to 18 weeks with renal agenesis.

4. *Gut vs. kidney.* Do not mistake gut dilation for a renal cystic anomaly. Renal problems lie in contact with the spine, whereas gut problems lie at a more anterior level.

5. *Gut distention.* Do not mistake normal loops of bowel for pathologically dilated bowel. On some occasions the fetal bowel can reach a width of approximately 8 mm and yet not be pathologically enlarged. An examination on another day will probably show that the fluid-filled loops have disappeared. Peristalsis may be seen in normal gut.

6. *Gut vs. cord.* Gastroschisis may be mistaken for a long redundant umbilical cord. In the normal cord three vessels should be seen, whereas in gastroschisis only a single tube of bowel is seen, and the umbilical cord enters the trunk at another site. Color flow makes recognition of the cord easy.

7. *Pseudohydronephrosis due to distended bladder.* If the bladder is large, secondary dilation of the pelvicalyceal system in the kidneys can occur transiently. This dilation disappears when the fetus voids.

8. *Fetal ear versus mass.* To the inexperienced sonographer the normal ear with its half-circle shape and two ridges can resemble a mass arising from the side of the head.

9. *Physiological gut herniation.* Until 11 weeks, fetal gut herniating into the base of the umbilicus is embryologically normal. If liver is seen as well as gut, suspect omphalocele.

10. *Colon problems in the third trimester.* Colon filled with meconium in the third trimester can be mistaken for cysts. Low-level echoes are seen within the bowel, which can be traced from cecum to rectum. In dehydrated patients the meconium becomes very concentrated and develops an echogenic appearance.

11. *Pseudo-omphalocele.* Undue pressure with the linear array on the fetal trunk may distort the shape of the trunk so that the abdomen protrudes in a fashion that raises the question of omphalocele. When the fetus turns prone or the pressure on the transducer is released, the apparent omphalocele will disappear.

12. *Pseudohydrocephalus.* If the lateral ventricles are examined at an oblique axis, they may appear enlarged. The lateral ventricles and choroid plexus do not change size during the second and third trimester. At any stage the lateral ventricular width at the posterior aspect of the ventricles (atria) should be no more than 10 to 11 mm, and the choroid plexus should be seen.

13. *Pharynx mistaken for a cystic mass in the neck.* The pharynx is sometimes visible as a cystic mass in the neck at the base of the skull (Fig. 18-49).

14. *Retrocerebellar arachnoid cyst vs. Dandy-Walker cyst (DWM).* Both present as a cyst in the posterior fossa. The DWM will compress and splay the cerebellar lobes as it replaces or inserts in the vermis. An extra-axial cyst will compress, but not alter the cerebellum.

15. *Dacryocystocele.* A cyst develops adjacent to the eye. This cystic structure is found medial to the orbit and represents a dilated lacrimal duct. This is a rare finding. The abnormality will disappear once the baby is born.

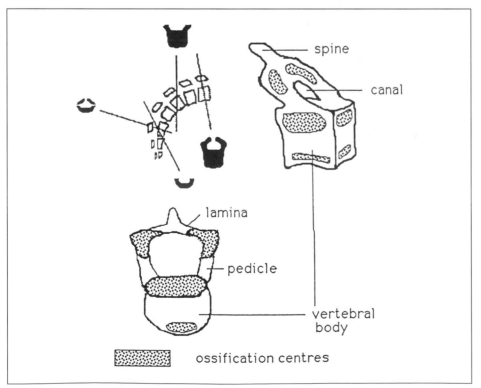

FIGURE 18-48. Diagram showing the fashion in which an oblique view through the lower sacrum and lumbar vertebrae can create an apparent spina bifida.

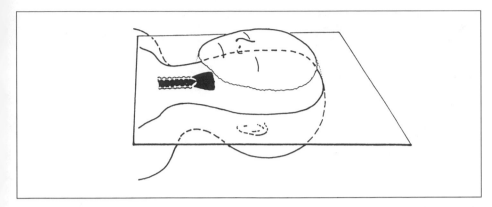

FIGURE 18-49. Diagram showing the fluid in the pharynx that can mimic a cystic mass in the neck.

16. *Pseudoascites.* A small amount of fluid may appear to be present in the fetal abdomen located laterally; this is actually abdominal musculature, and will not be visible around the cord insertion. In true ascites, the liver is seen indenting into the gut.

17. *Pseudopericardial effusion.* A small amount of fluid may appear to be present around the heart. This represents fat. It is difficult to tell a true pericardial effusion from a pseudopericardial effusion, but a finding of an apparent focal thickening of the fluid at any site favors a diagnosis of true pericardial effusion.

18. *Mildly shortened limbs.* In patients with a strong family history of short femur or short humerus, a fetus may have a femur or humerus that is at the fifth percentile. This raises the question of Down syndrome, but more likely it is a familial trait. Look at the parents to see whether they also have a similar configuration.

19. *Mildly small/large head.* It is not uncommon to find a biparietal diameter and head circumference that is below the 10th percentile or above the 90th percentile as a normal variant. A large head with normal intracranial structure is usually familial and a parent will be found to also have a large head. Distinction between a small normal head and microcephaly is difficult and is covered in detail in the segment on microcephaly. Familial small head is usually the case.

20. *Absent stomach.* Sometimes the stomach appears to be absent as a normal variant. At a follow-up study or after a delay the stomach will be seen.

21. *Absent bladder.* On occasion, the bladder will not be seen because it has been completely emptied, although as a rule the fetus does keep some urine within the bladder. Reexamination at the end of the study or at a later date will show the bladder to have some urine within it.

22. *Pseudo clubfeet.* Especially when there is too little fluid, the foot may be very flexed or extended. When the foot is examined at a later time it will assume a normal configuration. In a true clubfoot, the foot should be bent to one side as well as being flexed or extended.

❓ WHERE ELSE TO LOOK

1. *Duodenal atresia.* There is a strong association with Down syndrome, so look at the heart for atrioventricular canal problems (endocardial cushion defect) (see Chapter 20). Chromosomal analysis for trisomy 21 (Down syndrome) is desirable.

2. *Hydrocephalus.* If the obstruction level is below the third ventricle look at the cerebellum for the banana sign of the Arnold-Chiari malformation and look at the spine for a spina bifida.

3. *Gastroschisis with liver outside abdomen.* Look for the features of the limb/body wall complex: caudal regression, spina bifida, kyphoscoliosis, hydrocephalus, and absent limbs.

4. *Infantile polycystic kidney.* Consider the possibility of the Meckel-Gruber syndrome and look for polydactyly and encephalocele.

5. *Unilateral hydronephrosis.* Look for a dilated ureter. Look in the bladder for a ureterocele.

6. *Omphalocele.* Chromosomal analysis is important. Many other anomalies may be present. Look particularly for heart problems and cystic hygroma.

7. *Pleural effusion.* Look for the other features of hydrops: pericardial effusion, ascites, skin thickening, polyhydramnios, and placental thickening.

8. *Ascites.* If ascites is not accompanied by the other features of hydrops, look at the genitourinary tract for an obstructive lesion and at the heart for a cardiac anomaly. Look in the bowel for evidence of meconium peritonitis.

9. *Absent stomach.* Look for diaphragmatic hernia, cleft palate, and a small jaw (micrognathia).

10. *Absent bladder.* Look for the kidneys: there could be renal agenesis.

11. *Facial anomalies.* If hypotelorism and cleft palate are present, look in the skull for holoprosencephaly.

12. *Horseshoe-shaped single ventricle in brain.* Look for facial anomalies.

13. *Severe ureteropelvic junction obstruction.* On a coronal view, displacement of the stomach may be seen if the ureteropelvic junction obstruction is left sided. Impingement on the stomach or bowel may cause polyhydramnios.

14. *Cleft lip.* If cleft lip is found, look for an amniotic band and problems associated with amniotic bands, such as encephalocele and club feet.

15. *Skeletal dysplasia.* If the femur length is below two standard deviations, measure all long bones to rule out a skeletal dysplasia.

16. *Absent kidneys.* If the kidneys are absent in their normal location, look for a horseshoe kidney or pelvic kidney. If the fetus is female, look for cloacal anomalies.

SELECTED READING

Ariyuki, Y., Hata, T., Manabe, A., Hata, K., and Kitao, M. Antenatal diagnosis of persistent right umbilical vein. *J Clin Ultrasound* 23:324–326, 1995.

Benacerraf, B. R. Fetal central nervous system anomalies. *Ultrasound Quart* 8:1–42, 1990.

Bootstaylor, B. S., Filly, R. A., Harrison, M. R., and Adzick, N. S. Prenatal sonographic predictors of liver herniation in congenital diaphragmatic hernia. *J Ultrasound Med* 14:515–520, 1995.

Bowerman, R. A. Ultrasound of the fetal face. *Ultrasound Quart* 11:211, 1993.

Bowerman, R. A. Anomalies of the fetal skeleton: Sonographic findings. *AJR* 164:973–979, 1995.

Bromley, B., and Benacerraf, B. Abnormalities of the hands and feet in the fetus: Sonographic findings. *AJR* 165:1239–1243, 1995.

Bromley, B., Parad, R., Estroff, J. A., and Benacerraf, B. R. Fetal lung masses: Prenatal course and outcome. *J Ultrasound Med* 14:927–936, 1995.

Finberg, H. J., and Clewell, W. H. Ultrasound-guided interventions in pregnancy. *Ultrasound Quart* 8:197, 1990.

Greene, M. F., Benacerraf, B., and Crawford, J. M. Hydranencephaly: US appearance during in utero evolution. *Radiology* 156:779–780, 1985.

Guzman, E. R., Ranzini, A., Day-Salvatore, D., Weinberger, B., Spigland, N., and Vintzileos, A. The prenatal ultrasonographic visualization of imperforate anus in monoamniotic twins. *J Ultrasound Med* 14:547–551, 1995.

McKenna, K. M., Goldstein, R. B., and Stringer, M. D. Small or absent fetal stomach: Prognostic significance. *Radiology* 197:729–733, 1995.

Nyberg, D. A., Mack, L. A., Bronstein, A., Hirsch, J., and Pagon, R. A. Holoprosencephaly: Prenatal sonographic diagnosis. *AJR* 149:1051–1058, 1987.

Nyberg, D. A., Sickler, G. K., Hegge, F. N., Kramer, D. J., and Kropp, R. J. Fetal cleft lip with and without cleft palate: US classification and correlation with outcome. *Radiology* 195:677–684, 1995.

Nyberg, D. Pandya, P. P., Kondylios, A., Hilbert, L., Snijders, R. J. M., and Nicolaides, K. H. Chromosomal defects and outcome in 1015 fetuses with increased nuchal translucency. *Ultrasound Obstet Gynecol* 5:15–19, 1995.

Pilu, G., Sandri, F., Perolo, A., Giangaspero, F., Cocchi, G., Salvioli, G. P., and Bovicelli, L. Prenatal diagnosis of lobar holoprosencephaly. *Ultrasound Obstet Gynecol* 2:88–94, 1992.

Romero, R., et al. *Prenatal Diagnosis of Congenital Anomalies.* Norwalk, CT: Appleton & Lange, 1988.

Rubenstein, S. C., Benacerraf, B. R., Retik, A. B., and Mandell, J. Fetal suprarenal masses: Sonographic appearance and differential diagnosis. *Ultrasound Obstet Gynecol* 5:164–167, 1995.

Rypens, F. F., Avni, E. F., Abehsera, M. M., Donner, C., Vermeylen, D. F., and Struyven, J. L. Areas of increased echogenicity in the fetal abdomen: Diagnosis and significance. *Radiographics* 15:1329–1344, 1995.

Sanders, R. C., et al. (Ed.). *Structural Fetal Abnormalities: The Total Picture.* New York: Mosby-Year Book Publishers, 1996.

Shipp, T. D., Bromley, B., and Benacerraf, B. The ultrasonographic appearance and outcome for fetuses with masses distorting the fetal face. *J Ultrasound Med* 14:673–678, 1995.

Thieme, G. A. Developmental malformations of the fetal ventral body wall. *Ultrasound Quart* 10:225–266, 1992.

19

Fetal Well-Being and Fetal Death

MARY MCGRATH-LING

Sonogram Abbreviations

AF	Amniotic fluid
AFI	Amniotic fluid index
BPP	Biophysical profile
BPS	Biophysical profile score
FHM	Fetal heart motion
FHR	Fetal heart rate
LL	Left lower quadrant
LU	Left upper quadrant
NST	Nonstress test
PI	Placenta
RL	Right lower quadrant
RU	Right upper quadrant
VCR	Videocassette recorder

Key Words

Acoustical Stimulator. Noise-emitting device placed on maternal abdomen to buzz or wake up baby.

Amniotic Fluid Index (AFI). Assessment of the amount of amniotic fluid by measuring and adding the largest vertical pocket in each of the four uterine quadrants.

Biophysical Profile (BPP). An objective test for more accurately diagnosing and subsequently managing fetal oxygen deficiency (hypoxia/asphyxia) consisting of assessment of fluid, breathing, and movements.

Biophysical Profile Score (BPS). All parameters are scored and totalled.

Bradycardia. Slow fetal pulse (less than 110 bpm).

Contraction Stress Test (CST). Fetal heart rate is monitored for accelerations (normal) vs. late decelerations (abnormal) in response to uterine contractions.

Doptone. Detection of fetal heartbeat by Doppler. Usually the fetal heart can be heard by 12 weeks.

Eclampsia. Severe pregnancy-induced hypertension with protein loss in the urine. It may be associated with convulsions.

Fetal Breathing Movement (FBM). When a diaphragm excursion is observed.

Fetal Hypoxia/Asphyxia. Lack of adequate oxygen supply to the fetus.

Fundal Height (FH). Relative height of uterine fundus at various stages of pregnancy.

Intrauterine Growth Restriction (IUGR). Alternative preferable term for intrauterine growth retardation. Term used to describe compromised growth of the fetus.

Kick Count. Maternal assessment of fetal movement by counting kicks felt over a 1-hour period.

Lecithin-Sphingomyelin Ratio (L/S Ratio). A ratio of two of the substances (protein and lipids) that are released into the amniotic fluid by the fetus. Measurement at amniocentesis is used in the assessment of fetal lung maturity.

Maceration. Disintegration of the fetus following death. Debris from a dead fetus can be identified in the amniotic fluid.

Modified Biophysical Profile. Sonographic evaluation of fluid volume only, either by amniotic fluid index (*AFI*) or by largest single pocket done in conjunction with fetal heart rate monitoring (*NST*).

Nonstress Test (NST). Fetal heart rate is monitored in response to fetal movement.

Placental Insufficiency. Poorly performing placenta, usually due to focal infarcts.

Pre-eclampsia. Pregnancy-induced hypertension with urinary loss of protein.

Presyncopal. Prior to fainting.

Respiratory Distress Syndrome (RDS). Infant breathing problem associated with prematurity.

Robert's Sign. Gas in the fetal abdomen following fetal demise.

Spaulding's Sign. Overlapping of the fetal skull bones as the result of fetal death in utero (FDIU).

Tachycardia. Too fast pulse rate (over 180 bpm).

Umbilical Artery Doppler. Doppler evaluation of umbilical arteries to detect abnormal (high-resistance) diastolic flow.

Vanishing Twin. Phenomenon where fetal death of one twin occurs and on subsequent sonograms the dead twin can no longer be seen. This is due to maceration and eventual disintegration and resorption of the dead twin.

THE CLINICAL PROBLEM
Risks to Fetal Well-Being

Many pregnancies are at risk for fetal distress or fetal death. Maternal risks include chronic hypertension, pre-eclampsia, eclampsia, diabetes mellitus (including gestational diabetes), alcohol or narcotics abuse, and systemic diseases such as lupus. Placental problems such as placental insufficiency or abruption may result in fetal distress. Multiple pregnancy, intrauterine growth restriction (IUGR), preterm labor, premature rupture of membranes, and fetal anomalies all result in an increased risk of fetal distress. Pregnancies extending beyond 40 weeks' gestation or a previous history of a stillbirth or fetal distress are also risk factors. High-risk patients are monitored more closely for early detection and appropriate management of fetal distress. In the absence of risk factors, the maternal assessment of decreased fetal movement warrants an ultrasonic look for fetal distress.

Fetal Activity

Fetal activity is easily assessed sonographically. The fetus is most active up to approximately 26 to 28 weeks' gestation. Fetal activity decreases somewhat in the third trimester owing to less available space. It is helpful to ask the mother how much the fetus is moving and whether she has noticed a decrease in activity. Fetal limb and body movements, along with flexion and extension, can be monitored during real-time scanning. The sonographer should always observe fetal movement during any exam and not overlook an inactive fetus. Some unsuspected compromised fetuses may be detected if all third trimester fetal sonograms include assessment of fetal movement. In addition to observing fetal activity, the placenta and amniotic fluid volume should be evaluated and documented.

The Pulse Rate

The normal fetal heart rate is approximately 140 beats per minute (bpm), with the normal range being 110 to 180 bpm after the first trimester (Appendix 28). Brief periods of bradycardia are usually normal if followed by a return to a normal heart rate. However, prolonged (greater than 30 seconds) or continuous bradycardia is reason for concern, and fetal distress should be considered along with other causes of bradycardia such as cord compression due to decreased amniotic fluid, arrhythmias, congenital heart lesions, or complete atrioventricular block (see Chapter 20). Fetal tachycardia (greater than 180 bpm) is caused by a number of fetal and maternal conditions including smoking, certain drugs, anxiety, fetal distress, and arrhythmias (see Chapter 20).

When evidence of fetal ill health is discovered, the obstetrician has the advantage of timing the delivery to optimize the likelihood of a favorable outcome. Ultrasound can greatly impact this management decision with the biophysical profile, which is a useful tool for assessing fetal condition. Good biophysical scores (8–10 out of a possible 10) are associated with a favorable perinatal outcome. A fetus at risk for a poor fetal outcome is monitored at appropriate intervals throughout the remainder of the pregnancy.

Because the biophysical profile results impact the timing of delivery, they are only performed once viability outside the uterus is possible (i.e., 24–26 weeks). The nonstress test is used in conjunction with the ultrasonic biophysical profile. The nonstress test is often nonreactive prior to 28 weeks' gestation and, therefore, is of limited use for that time. Real-time is used to assess amniotic fluid volume, fetal tone, and fetal breathing.

While premature delivery may result in respiratory distress syndrome (RDS) and other complications, the fetus may have a better chance of survival with preterm delivery as opposed to remaining in a hostile intrauterine environment.

Fetal Death

Fetal demise is most common in the first trimester (i.e., spontaneous abortion; see Chapter 12). This chapter will concentrate on the sonographic appearance and diagnosis of fetal death in the second and third trimesters. Fetal death usually occurs in association with the same risk factors that cause fetal distress (discussed earlier). Fetal demise may also result from structural or chromosomal anomalies in the fetus. Cord problems such as cord compression if the cord comes first, cord knots, or the cord twisted around the fetal neck are also responsible for some unexpected fetal deaths.

Fetal death is suspected on the basis of absent maternal perception of fetal movement. Failure to detect fetal heart tones by Doppler or failure of the fundal height to grow may also raise suspicion of fetal death. Frequently, fetal heart pulsations go undetected by Doppler because of maternal obesity, retroverted uterus, excessive fetal movement, or fetal position. Real-time ultrasound is essential for confirming or excluding fetal demise.

TECHNIQUE
Biophysical Profile

The fetus should be observed for up to 30 minutes if necessary to meet the scoring criteria. Most often, a healthy fetus will satisfy all criteria in only a few minutes. Once all the parameters have been observed the exam can be ended.

The mother should be placed in a semi-upright position and made as comfortable as possible. A recumbent left or right lateral position is also acceptable. Having the patient supine may cause compression of the inferior vena cava and resultant presyncopal symptoms. The optimal time for observing an active fetus is after the mother has eaten. If the baby appears to be in a resting state, there are several things the observer can do to enhance fetal activity.

TABLE 19-1. Biophysical Profile Scoring According to Manning and Coworkers

Parameter	Score of 2	Score of 0
Breathing	30 seconds or more of breathing noted in 30-minute period	Less than 30-second period or no breathing in 30 minutes
Movement	3 or more gross body/limb movements in 30-minute period	Less than 3 gross body/limb movements in 30 minutes
Tone	At least 1 episode of flexion or extension with return to normal position in a 30-minute period	Failure to observe any flexion or extension in a 30-minute period
Fluid	One pocket of amniotic fluid measuring 2 cm in both vertical and horizontal planes	Failure to identify fluid pocket measuring 2 cm in any plane
Nonstress test	Negative or reactive test	Less than 2 accelerations of at least 15 bpm

TOTAL POSSIBLE SCORE 10

1. Gentle shaking may awaken or stimulate a resting fetus.
2. Give the mother cold water or a sweetened drink.
3. Have the mother breathe in and out deeply several times.
4. Vary mother's position. Often the mother can tell you which positions the baby does not "like." Those positions will usually result in the most fetal movement.
5. Use an acoustical stimulator to wake up the baby. Sometimes the father's voice will work just as well!

The technique for the biophysical profile described below is based on work by Manning and coworkers (see Selected Reading) and is currently the most widely used by obstetricians.

Scoring Parameters

Each parameter is accorded a score of 0 or 2, as discussed later. There is no score of 1 (Table 19-1).

Nonstress Test

The nonstress test (NST) is an aid in the evaluation of fetal health; the fetal heart rate (FHR) is monitored over a 20-minute period. A normal fetus responds to fetal movement by an increase in fetal heart rate. A reactive (normal) result is when at least two or more accelerations (15 bpm above a baseline) occur in a 20-minute period (Fig. 19-1A). A nonreactive (or positive) nonstress test indicates there have been less than two accelerations of FHR over a 40-minute period (see Fig. 19-1B). If the result for the first 20 minutes is nonreactive, the NST is continued for an additional 20 minutes using artificial (acoustical) stimulation. If fetal movement is followed, after a delay, by a lowered fetal pulse rate, this ominous sign of fetal sickness is called a late deceleration (see Fig. 19-1C). If the results of the NST are negative (reactive), the biophysical score (BPS) is 2. If there are less than two accelerations of at least 15 bpm above the baseline during the NST, the score is 0. The NST is often nonreactive in the normal pregnancy prior to 28 weeks' gestation.

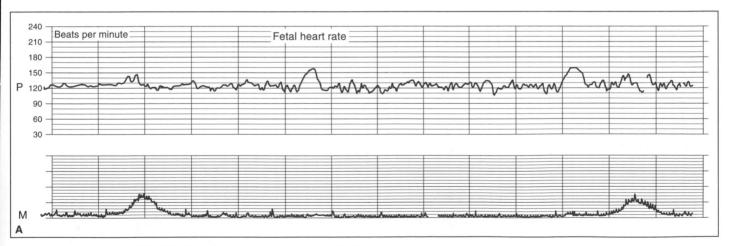

FIGURE 19-1. The nonstress test. (**A**) Normal nonstress test showing fetal movement in the lower tracing and pulse rate in the top. Note that when the uterine movement (M) occurs, on the lower tracing, it is followed by a pulse rate increase (P) on the upper tracing. *(continued)*

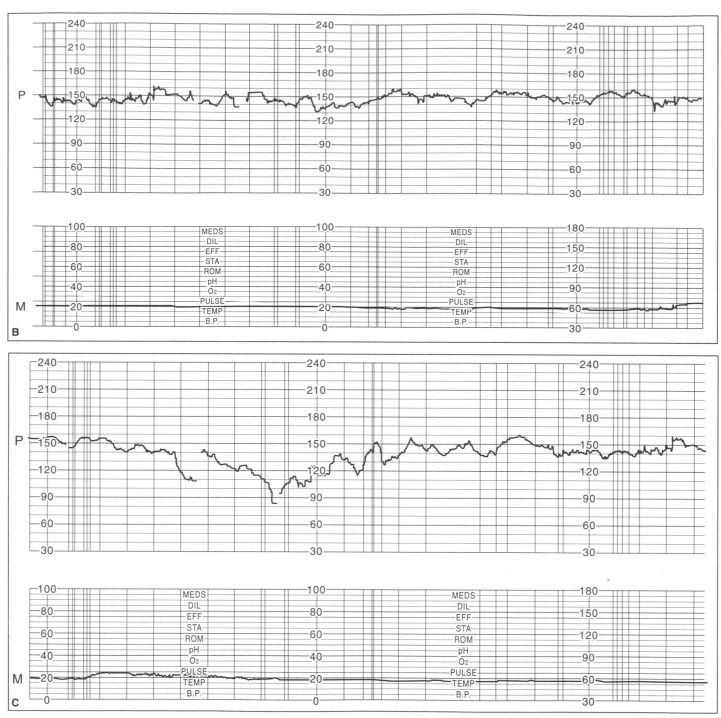

FIGURE 19-1. (CONTINUED) (**B**) Nonstress test showing no movement (M) over a prolonged period, although there is some variation in fetal pulse rate (P). (**C**) Tracing showing little or no movement (M), but some significant decreases in fetal pulse rate (P), known as decels.

Fetal Breathing

Fetal breathing can be identified sonographically by observing the movement of the diaphragm as reflected in stomach and liver movement (Fig. 19-2). Fetal breathing is visible in all normal fetuses from 26 weeks on, but it is intermittent. A prolonged period of fetal breathing, lasting 30 seconds or more, needs to be observed before a biophysical profile score of 2 is given. If fetal breathing is not observed for a 30-second period during the 30-minute observation period, the score for breathing is 0.

Fetal Movement

There should be at least three gross body or limb movements during the 30-minute period for a normal BPS of 2. Less than three body or limb movements scores 0. Only significant body movements are scored. Subtle or very slight movements do not count.

Movement is not always easily assessed in the third trimester because only one segment of the fetus can be observed at a time. A healthy fetus will, nevertheless, demonstrate twisting or kicking movements if it is observed over an adequate period of time. Sometimes a fetus will respond to gentle shaking. If adequate movement is not noted, the fetus can be stimulated by using a noise-producing device. A normal resting fetus will usually respond, whereas a truly sick fetus will not.

Fetal Tone

Flexion and extension movements are monitored. There should be at least one episode of good flexion and extension of fetal limbs or spine followed by return to normal position. Flexion and extension of the arms or legs, arching of the spine, or opening and closing of hands are all good indicators of normal tone for a BPS of 2. Failure to observe any of these movements in the 30-minute period results in a score of 0. This parameter is very closely related to fetal movement; the difference is that specific attention is paid to flexion and extension movements. Caution: if a fetal hand is in an open or limp position for a prolonged period, it is usually a strong indicator of poor fetal tone. Do not overlook this ominous sign.

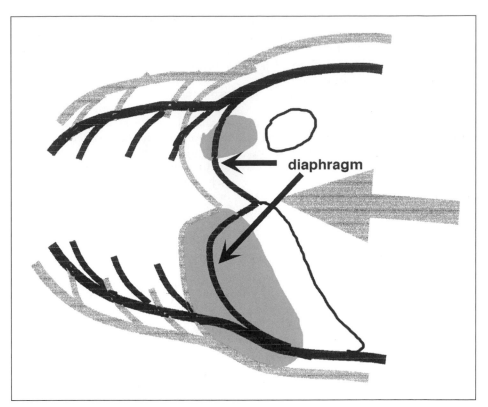

Amniotic Fluid Volume

Assessment of amniotic fluid volume is of crucial importance in establishing fetal well-being or sickness. There should be at least one pocket of amniotic fluid measuring 2 cm in both the horizontal and vertical planes for a BPS of 2. Failure to identify a fluid pocket of at least this size results in a score of 0. Do not include a section of umbilical cord in the fluid pocket when the fluid is minimal as this will give a false negative result.

If there is a fluid pocket of less than 2 cm, oligohydramnios is considered present and severe. Less severe changes in amniotic fluid volume should be noted since the volume rarely decreases enough to meet the zero biophysical profile criteria until fetal demise is imminent. The amniotic fluid can be evaluated by using the amniotic fluid index, the largest vertical pocket, or subjective assessment by an experienced operator.

FIGURE 19-2. Fetal breathing. The normal position is shown in the black lines. As the fetus breathes, the diaphragm, liver, and stomach move up (shown in gray). Changes in the ribs are minimal. Fetal breathing is easiest to see in the coronal position but can also be seen on a sagittal view.

AMNIOTIC FLUID INDEX (AFI). This is currently the preferred method for quantitating amniotic fluid volume.

Fluid is measured vertically in each of the four uterine quadrants and added together to obtain the AFI (Fig. 19-3). The largest pocket in each quadrant is measured. Care must be taken not to include segments of the umbilical cord in the measurement. Sometimes what appears to be fluid is actually coiled cord filling the entire space. Usually adjusting the gain will be adequate to make the distinction between fluid and cord. Sometimes patient habitus makes this distinction extremely difficult, so use color Doppler to define the cord.

A sum of 5 or less indicates significant oligohydramnios, regardless of gestational age. A sum of 20 or more is indicative of polyhydramnios. *If there is a fluid pocket which meets the 2 cm criterion in both the vertical and horizontal planes, a BPS of 2 is assigned even in the presence of oligohydramnios by AFI calculation.*

The amniotic fluid index can be falsely reassuring where there are narrow vertical pockets. Conversely, when wide shallow pockets are present, subjective assessment of fluid volume may prove more useful (Fig. 19-4).

Subjective assessment, although quite accurate when done by an experienced observer, has limitations because it cannot provide quantitative information about trends in fluid volume, particularly if a different monitors the patient in subsequent exams.

LARGEST VERTICAL POCKET. A single pocket of fluid is measured in the vertical plane, not including segments of the umbilical cord. A measurement of less than 2 cm is indicative of oligohydramnios, whereas a pocket of 8 cm or more is representative of polyhydramnios. This technique is most helpful when trying to quantitate fluid volume in the multiple gestation pregnancy or in the assessment of polyhydramnios.

Placental Grading (Vintzelios's Technique Only)

Placental grading is included by Vintzelios and colleagues (Table 19-2) because they have demonstrated an association of grade 3 placentas with abnormal fetal heart rate patterns and abruptio placentae during labor. There are two significant differences between Vintzelios's grading system and that of Manning and coworkers. Minor amounts of breathing or movement can be given a score of 1 by Vintzelios and the placental appearance is scored. If placental grading is included, a placental grade of 0, 1, or 2 equals a BPS of 2 (see Chapter 13). A posterior placenta which is difficult to evaluate is assigned a BPS of 1. A grade 3 placenta is assigned a BPS of 0.

Interpretation of Scores

Assuming normal amniotic fluid volume, a BPS of 8 to 10 is normal; 6 is suspicious for chronic asphyxia; and 0 to 4 is highly suggestive of asphyxia (Table 19-3). The clinical significance of the various components of the biophysical profile varies with both the parameter and gestational age. Vintzelios and colleagues describe the parameters as either acute or chronic markers of fetal asphyxia. The acute markers are fetal heart rate, fetal movement, tone, and breathing, whereas fluid volume and placenta are the chronic markers. Interestingly, the biophysical parameters that appear the earliest in pregnancy are the last to disappear with fetal asphyxia. Fetal tone first appears at 7.5 to 8.5 weeks' gestation. Movement begins at 9 weeks and breathing at 20 to 21 weeks; fetal heart rate control is the last to appear in the late second or early third trimester.

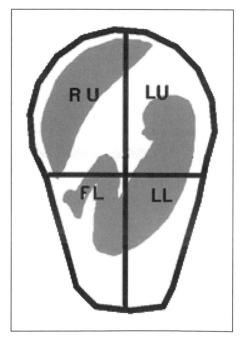

FIGURE 19-3. Amniotic fluid index. The amniotic fluid index is measured by dividing the uterus into quadrants and measuring the longest depth of fluid in each quadrant. The transducer should be positioned longitudinally when the measurement is made.

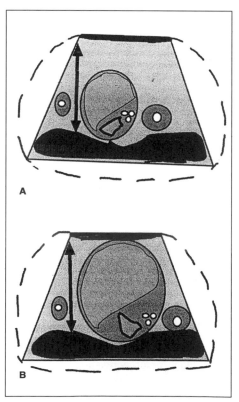

FIGURE 19-4. The amniotic fluid index can be deceptive if the vertical measurement is long but the fluid-filled area is narrow. The same measurement is obtained with a thin, narrow fluid pocket in (**B**) as in the wide pocket seen in (**A**).

TABLE 19-2.   Criteria for Scoring Biophysical Variables According to Vintzelios

Parameter	Score of 2	Score of 1	Score of 0
Nonstress test	5 or more FHR accelerations of at least 15 bpm in amplitude and at least 15 seconds' duration associated with fetal movement in a 20-minute period (NST 2)	2 to 4 accelerations of at least 15 bpm and at least 15 seconds' duration associated with fetal movements in a 20-minute period (NST 1)	1 or 0 accelerations in a 20-minute period (NST 0)
Fetal movements	At least 3 gross (trunk and limbs) episodes of fetal movements within 30 minutes. Simultaneous limb and trunk movements are counted as a single movement (FM 2)	1 or 2 fetal movements within 30 minutes (FM 1)	Absence of fetal movements within 30 minutes (FM 0)
Fetal breathing movements	At least 1 episode of fetal breathing of at least 60 seconds' duration within a 30-minute observation period (FBM 2)	At least 1 episode of fetal breathing lasting 30 to 60 seconds within 30 minutes (FBM 1)	Absence of fetal breathing, or breathing lasting less than 30 seconds within 30 minutes (FBM 0)
Fetal tone	At least 1 episode of extension of extremities with return to position of flexion and also 1 episode of extension of spine with return to position of flexion (FT 2)	At least 1 episode of extension of extremities with return to position of flexion or 1 episode of extension of spine with return to point of flexion (FT 1)	Extremities of extension; fetal movements not followed by return to flexion; open hand (FT 0)
Amniotic fluid volume	Fluid evident throughout the uterine cavity; a pocket that measures 2 cm or more in vertical diameter (AF 2)	A pocket that measures less than 2 cm but more than 1 cm in vertical diameter (AF 1)	Crowding of fetal small parts; largest pocket less than 1 cm in vertical diameter (AF 0)
Placental grading	Placental grade 0, 1, or 2 (PL 2)	Placenta posterior; difficult to evaluate (PL 1)	Placental grade 3 (PL 0)

Note: FHR = fetal heart rate.
Source: Reprinted with permission from Vintzelios, A.M., et al. The fetal biophysical profile and its predictive value. *Obstet Gynecol* 62:271–278, 1983.

TABLE 19-3.   Management Based on Biophysical Profile

Score	Interpretation	Management
10	Normal infant; low risk of chronic asphyxia	Repeat testing at weekly intervals; repeat twice weekly in diabetic patients and patients at ≥42 weeks' gestation
8	Normal infant; low risk of chronic asphyxia	Repeat testing at weekly intervals; repeat testing twice weekly in diabetics and patients at ≥42 weeks gestation; oligohydramnios is an indication for delivery
6	Suspect chronic asphyxia	If ≥36 weeks gestation and conditions are favorable, deliver; if at <36 weeks and L/S <2.0, repeat test in 4–6 hours; deliver if oligohydramnios is present
4	Suspect chronic asphyxia	If ≥32 weeks gestation, deliver; if <32 weeks, repeat score
0–2	Strongly suspect chronic asphyxia	Extend testing time to 120 minutes; if persistent score ≤4, deliver, regardless of gestational age

Reprinted from Manning et al., with permission.

Modified Biophysical Profile

In some instances, the obstetrician may feel that only a modified version of the biophysical profile is necessary (Fig. 19-5). The modified biophysical profile is the sonographic evaluation of fluid volume only, preferably by AFI and FHR monitoring (NST). Instances where this method is indicated include the following:

1. Postterm pregnancies where decreased fluid would warrant induction of labor owing to increased risk of cord compression with resultant fetal compromise or demise.
2. Patients who are receiving indomethacin (which can cause decreased fluid production) for preterm labor; these patients often get baseline and weekly AFIs as a minimum.
3. Some patients with size slightly less than dates who are not strongly suspected of having IUGR but where more prudent observation seems indicated.

Umbilical Artery Doppler

Umbilical artery Doppler can provide useful information about underlying circulatory problems associated with pregnancy. The diastolic portion of the Doppler waveform is related to vascular resistance in the placental bed. The normally low resistance (Fig. 19-6) decreases throughout pregnancy with a resultant increase in the diastolic velocity. In cases of fetal compromise there may be an increase in placental resistance resulting in a decreased, absent (see Fig. 19-6), or reversed flow through the diastolic portion of the Doppler waveform. Various indices have been used for measuring umbilical artery flow but the simplest and most widely used is the A/B ratio:

$$AB = \frac{peak\ systole.}{end\ diastole}$$

The resistive index is also widely used (Appendix 27):

$$RI = \frac{systolic\ flow - diastolic\ flow}{systolic\ flow}$$

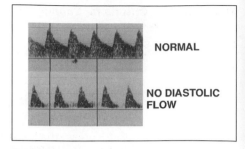

FIGURE 19-6. Normal umbilical artery Doppler and abnormal flow with no diastolic component.

An abnormal umbilical artery waveform is associated with a poor outcome of the pregnancy.

Technique

If color flow is available, the cord is located as close as possible to the fetal abdomen. The gate is placed over one of the arteries and the pulsed Doppler is activated. No attempts are made to obtain a 60-degree angle to the artery since its angle is unknown. If the SD (systole/diastole) ratio is lower than 3 or the resistive index is less than .7, results are considered normal. Levels above these are considered suspicious, but of questionable significance if diastolic flow is seen. If no diastolic flow is seen or there is a reversal of flow in diastole, these are worrying findings of clinical significance. The cranial structures are then analyzed using color flow. The middle cerebral vessels (see Fig. 43-3) are identified and Doppler analysis of the middle cerebral artery is performed. If significant cranial diastolic flow is seen with absent diastolic flow in the umbilical artery, this is an ominous sign that many feel would indicate that early delivery should be performed.

Uterine artery Doppler is also performed in some centers in the 16-to-22-week stage of pregnancy since there is evidence that an abnormal uterine artery Doppler flow at this stage correlates with the development of IUGR later on. This technique is not widely performed in the United States as yet, since there are so many false positive findings.

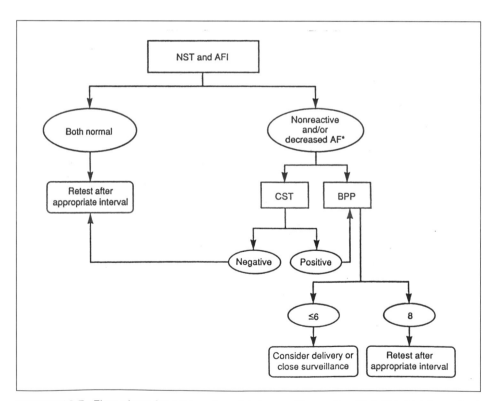

FIGURE 19-5. Flow chart for antepartum fetal surveillance in which the nonstress test (NST) and amniotic fluid index (AFI) are used as the primary methods for fetal evaluation. A nonreactive NST and/or decreased amniotic fluid (AF) are further evaluated using either the contraction stress test (CST) or the biophysical profile (BPP). *If the fetus is mature and amniotic fluid volume is reduced, delivery should be considered before further testing is undertaken. (Adapted from Finberg et al., with permission.)

Fetal Lung Maturity

Fetal lung maturity cannot be predicted by ultrasound appearance. The following parameters increase the likelihood but are *not* indicative of fetal lung maturity:

1. A placental grade of 3
2. Echopenic meconium in the large bowel
3. IUGR (the lungs mature earlier in fetuses with IUGR)
4. Proximal humeral epiphyses seen on ultrasound

The lecithin-sphingomyelin ratio measured in the amniotic fluid is the gold standard for predicting fetal lung maturity.

FETAL DEATH

Real-time examination is the technique of choice for excluding or confirming fetal demise. Fetal heart motion (FHM) can be detected by real-time ultrasound 5 to 7 weeks after the last menstrual period and as early as 4½ weeks by transvaginal sonography (see Chapter 12).

FHM can be difficult to appreciate early in pregnancy since the fetal chest cavity is so small. Monitor flickering can resemble heart motion but will not be limited to the fetal trunk. Document FHM whenever possible by M-mode, videotape, or Doppler. If an M-mode or videocassette recorder (VCR) is not available, or if there is the slightest doubt concerning heart motion, it is best for two observers to witness FHM and agree upon its presence or absence. If there is no fetal heart motion after 2 to 3 minutes of observation, the diagnosis of fetal death in utero can be made.

Sonographic Appearances of Fetal Death

Immediately following death, absent FHM is often the only sonographic sign of fetal demise. Within a couple of days other findings develop (Fig. 19-7).

1. *Subcutaneous edema.* Appears as a double outline with a sonolucent center surrounding the fetus. Skin thickening may also be seen with fetal hydrops or maternal diabetes.
2. *Unnatural fetal position.* Usually the fetus is curled into a tight ball or is in a position of extreme flexion or extension.
3. *Spaulding's sign.* Overlapping of skull bones is seen in labor as a normal phenomenon, but at other times it indicates fetal death. Often the shape of the fetal head becomes grossly distorted following fetal death.

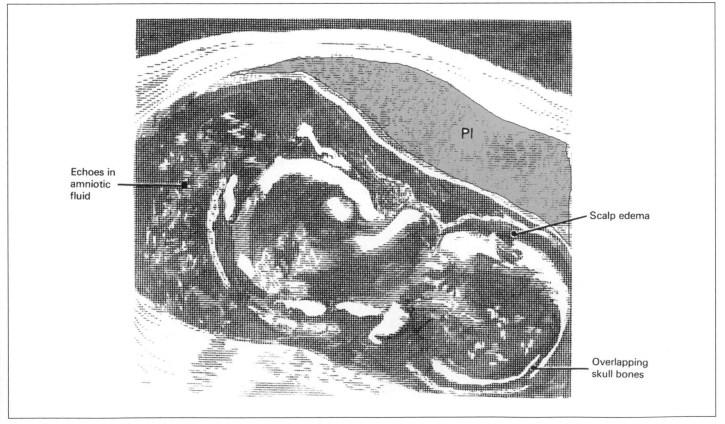

FIGURE 19-7. Signs of fetal death on a B-scan include scalp edema, overlapping of skull bones, unusual fetal position, and extra echoes in the amniotic fluid due to maceration of the tissues.

4. *Loss of definition of structures in the fetal trunk.* Anatomic structures cannot be made out and abnormal echoes start to appear in the fetal brain.
5. *Robert's sign.* Gas develops in the fetal abdomen and may obscure fetal anatomy. Shadowing is seen from a strong echo.
6. *Maceration.* Causes echoes to develop in the amniotic fluid.

PITFALLS

Biophysical Profile

1. *Hiccups.* Prolonged fetal hiccups will make detection of fetal breathing difficult.
2. *Resting fetus.* A false positive BPS result occurs if a normal fetus is observed during a sleep or rest cycle.
3. *Oligohydramnios.* Fetal movement and tone can be difficult to assess owing to cramped space when fluid is decreased. The postterm pregnancy or pregnancies complicated by premature rupture of membranes (PROM) are often more difficult to evaluate.
4. *Subjective calculation.* The assessment of subtle decreases in amniotic fluid may not be appreciated by an inexperienced observer. Calculating the amniotic fluid index makes it less likely that oligohydramnios will be overlooked.
5. *Cord inclusion.* Fluid volume assessment or AFI calculation can be inaccurate when segments of umbilical cord are difficult to see and are thus included in the calculation.

Fetal Death

1. *Transmitted maternal pulse.* Some fetal motion is derived from the maternal aorta. Help clarify that apparent fetal pulsation is maternal by taking the maternal pulse.
2. *Maternal habitus.* Obesity or excessive scarring may make real-time sonography technically suboptimal. Endovaginal sonography may be helpful, especially in first and second trimester pregnancies, but is somewhat limited in the third trimester.
3. *Frame rate.* The use of multiple focal zones decreases pulse repetition frequency, resulting in a significantly lower frame rate. One may fail to demonstrate FHM in a viable fetus if multiple focal zones are used.
4. *Persistence.* Some ultrasound systems have a variable persistence option. Fetal heart motion may be present but undetectable with the persistence on.

SELECTED READING

Gabbe, S. G., Niebyl, J. R., and Simpson, J. L. *Obstetrics: Normal and Problem Pregnancies* (2nd ed.). Churchill Livingstone.

Grant, E. G. Maternal-fetal Doppler sonography: Potential or reality. *Semin Roentgenol* 36:75–86, 1991.

Manning, F. A., Basket, T., Morrison, I., and Lange, I. Fetal biophysical profile scoring: A prospective study in 1184 high-risk patients. *Am J Obstet Gynecol* 140:289, 1981.

Manning, F. A., Harman, C. R., Morrison, I., et al. Fetal assessment based on fetal biophysical profile scoring. *Am J Obstet Gynecol* 162:703, 1990.

Vintzileos, A. M., et al. The fetal biophysical profile and its predictive value. *J Obstet Gynecol* 62:271, 1983.

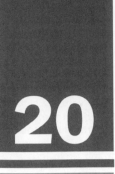

20 ABNORMAL FETAL HEART

MIMI MAGGIO SAYLOR, JOYCE CORDIER

SONOGRAM ABBREVIATIONS

Ao	Aorta
ASD	Atrial septal defect
AV	Atrioventricular
LA	Left atrium
LPA	Left pulmonary artery
LV	Left ventricle
LVOT	Left ventricular outflow tract
MPA	Main pulmonary artery
PA	Pulmonary artery
PDA	Patent ductus arteriosus
RA	Right atrium
RPA	Right pulmonary artery
RV	Right ventricle
RVOT	Right ventricular outflow tract
TAPVR	Total anomalous pulmonary venous return
TOF	Tetralogy of Fallot
VSD	Ventricular septal defect

KEY WORDS

Abdominal Situs. Term used to define whether the heart is on the normal left side or is right sided.

Accutane. An oral drug administered to treat acne. Maternal ingestion may cause complex congenital heart disease in fetuses.

Angiomas. Echogenic masses that can be situated anywhere in the fetal heart. These tumors are thought to resolve spontaneously.

Annulus. A fibrous ring of tissue where the cardiac valves insert.

Aortic Media. The aorta normally has three components to its walls; the adventitia, intima, and media (see Chapter 29). In coarctation, the media is the deformed portion.

Aortic Stenosis. Obstruction of the left ventricular outflow tract; may occur at one or more levels.

Apical. Inferior left portion of the heart at the end of the two ventricles.

Arrhythmia. An irregular heart rate.

Atresia. Congenital absence or pathologic closure of a normal anatomic opening or tube.

Atrial Isomerism. Both atrial chambers have the anatomic characteristics of a right atrium or left atrium.

Atrial Septal Aneurysm. A thin membrane that bows right to left, sometimes seen at the foramen ovale level.

Atrial Septal Defect (ASD). Defect within the septal wall between the right and left atrium.

Atrioventricular Valves. Group name for the two valves that connect between the atrium and ventricle, i.e., the mitral and tricuspid valves.

Bicuspid Aorta. Normally there are three components to the aortic valve. In the bicuspid aorta, there are only two components.

Bradycardia (Fetal). Heart rate of less than 100 beats per minute (bpm).

Cardiomyopathy

Dilated. Abnormal dilatation of the heart causing it to function poorly. Seen with critical aortic valve stenosis and heart failure.

Hypertrophic. An abnormal thickening of the septum and ventricular walls. Can be seen in the fetus of a diabetic mother.

Chordae Tendineae. Small cord that connects the papillary muscles to the atrioventricular valves.

Coarctation of the Aorta. A localized malformation characterized by deformity of the aortic media, causing vessel narrowing. Coarctation usually occurs at or near the junction of the patent ductus arteriosus.

Cone (Conus Arteriosus). Part of the embryonic heart that becomes the outflow tracts of the ventricles for the great arteries.

Contractility. The ability of the cardiac tissue to shorten in response to the appropriate stimulation.

Coronary Sinus. Linear venous structure draining into the right atrium.

Dextro. Right.

Dextrocardia. The heart is located on the right side of the chest. Associated with major cardiac malformations if it is the only structure that is on the wrong side.

Diastole. In diastole, the heart muscles relax and atrial filling occurs. The mitral and tricuspid valves are closed.

Digoxin. Drug administered to the mother to regulate a fetal tachycardia.

Double Outlet Ventricle. Both semilunar valves arise from the same ventricle.

Dysrhythmia. An irregular heart rhythm.

Ebstein's Anomaly. One or more leaflets of the tricuspid valve have been displaced apically into the right ventricle, atrializing a portion of the right ventricle.

Ectopia Cordis

Abdominal Type. A gap in the diaphragm through which the heart protrudes into the abdominal cavity.

Thoracic Type. Displacement of the heart outside the thoracic cavity.

Endocardial Fibroelastosis. Hypertrophy of the wall of the left ventricle and conversion of the endocardium into a thick fibroelastic coat. The cavity of the ventricle is sometimes reduced, but often increased. Often the walls appear echogenic.

Endocardium. The endothelial lining membrane of the heart.

Eustachian Valve. The valve of the inferior vena cava as it enters the right atrium.

Extrasystoles (Premature Beats). Abnormal atrial or ventricular beats.

Foramen Ovale. An opening created by a flap in the fetal atrial septum allowing shunting from the right atrium to the left atrium.

Holt-Oram Syndrome. Absence or partial absence of the radius, thumb, and first metacarpal may be present. An atrial septal defect is the most common cardiac abnormality, but other cardiac defects may be seen.

Hypertrophy. Enlargement, usually used when describing a muscle or a chamber such as the atrium or ventricle.

Hypoplastic. Incomplete development of tissue.

Hypoplastic Left Heart. Incomplete development of the left side of the heart.

Isomerism. Both ventricles or atria have characteristics of a right or left heart structure.

Ivemark's Syndrome. Agenesis of the spleen. Commonly associated with cyanotic heart disease and malposition of the abdominal viscera. The heart is on the right side.

Leaflet. A cusp of a heart valve.

Levo. Left.

Lithium. Women who are treated with lithium for depression have produced offspring with Ebstein's anomaly.

Lupus (Systemic Lupus Erythematous). A disease in which the body's own immune defenses will damage the connective tissue of an organ. It is associated with congenital heart block in the fetus.

Moderator Band. A band of normal tissue in the right ventricle.

Myocardium. The middle and thickest layer of heart wall.

Papillary Muscle. Striated muscle located in the ventricles of the heart.

Patent Ductus Arteriosus. In fetal life, a connection exists between the pulmonary artery and the aorta. This connection is known as the ductus arteriosus. This connection closes shortly after birth in normal infants.

Pentalogy of Cantrell. Ectopia cordis, omphalocele, and a diaphragmatic defect are present. Can be associated with congenital heart disease.

Pericardial Effusion. Accumulation of fluid around the heart within the pericardial sac. This may result from any type of cardiac failure.

Perimembranous. Thin area of the ventricular septum inferior to the aortic root.

Phenylketonuria (PKU) (Maternal). In utero the fetus may be damaged by elevated phenylketonuria levels (amino acids) in the mother. Possible structural defects include growth deficiency and skeletal and cardiac anomalies (tetralogy of Fallot, hypoplastic left heart).

Polysplenia. Two or more spleens are sometimes associated with complex congenital heart disease, with malformation of the abdominal organs and absence of the inferior vena cava.

Premature Closure of the Foramen Ovale. May result in underdevelopment of the left heart depending on time of occurrence in utero.

Pressure Gradient. There is a normal increase in pressure between the atrium and the ventricle and a similar alteration in pressure can occur at other sites such as a narrowed aortic valve, if pathology is present. This change in pressure is known as a pressure gradient.

Pulmonary Stenosis. A narrowing of the pulmonary root or thickening of the pulmonary valve causing obstruction of the right ventricular outflow tract.

Regurgitation. In the normal individual, flow always occurs from the atrium into the ventricle. In patients with diseased hearts, flow may occur from the ventricle back into the atrium during ventricular contraction (systole). This is known as regurgitation.

Rhabdomyoma. Associated with tuberous sclerosis. This is a tumor with homogenous, bright echo texture. It may occupy any part of the ventricular or atrial walls and chambers. Often associated with rhythm disturbances.

Root. Term used in the heart for the origin of the aorta or pulmonary artery.

Semilunar Valve. Valves of the pulmonary and aortic arteries.

Systole. Term used for the segment of the cardiac cycle in which the muscles of the heart contract.

Tachycardia. Heart rate of greater than 180 bpm.

Tetralogy of Fallot (TOF). Four associated findings are perimembranous ventricular septal defect, overriding of the aortic root, pulmonary stenosis (varying from mild valve narrowing to atresia of the valve and artery), and right ventricular hypertrophy (not usually seen in the fetus).

Thrombocytopenia. Too few platelets are present.

Thrombocytopenia With Absent Radius (TAR). An inherited, autosomal disease with bilateral absence of the radii and other limb abnormalities. Atrial septal defects and tetralogy of Fallot are common.

Total Anomalous Pulmonary Venous Return (TAPVR). The pulmonary veins, which normally empty into the left atrium, join to form a confluence that drains into the right atrium or coronary sinus. They may form below the diaphragm and drain into a systemic vein in the abdomen.

Transposition of the Great Arteries

   D-Transposition of the Great Arteries. The main pulmonary artery arises from the left ventricle and the aorta arises from the right ventricle. Ventricular septal defects are common.

   L-Transposition of the Great Arteries (Corrected Transposition). The ventricles are transposed, but are correctly connected to the great arteries. Associated with pulmonary stenosis and congenital heart block.

Truncus Arteriosus. A large ventricular septal defect with one great artery that straddles both ventricles.

Tuberous Sclerosis. A familial disease affecting the brain, skin, kidneys, and other organs. Skin lesions, seizures, and mental retardation are the classical clinical findings. There are varying degrees of severity. Associated with rhabdomyomas.

Turner's Syndrome. A chromosomal abnormality with numerous physical defects, including cystic hygroma, growth retardation, and cardiac defects—most commonly coarctation of the aorta or other left-sided defects.

Ventricular Outflow Tracts. Term used for views of the aorta and the pulmonary artery as they leave the left and right ventricles.

Ventricular Septal Defect (VSD). A gap in the ventricular septum (see Pitfalls). VSD may be the only finding or it may be associated with other cardiac defects.

 THE CLINICAL PROBLEM

Congenital heart disease is found in slightly less than 1% of infants. With an immediate family history or a prior sibling with congenital heart disease, there is an increased risk. Entities associated with congenital heart disease are as follows:

1. Fetal cardiac arrhythmia
2. Chromosomal abnormalities
   a. Turner's syndrome
   b. Down syndrome (trisomy 21)

c. Trisomy 13
d. Trisomy 18
3. Familial disease
   a. Ivemark's syndrome
   b. Holt-Oram syndrome
   c. Thrombocytopenia with absent radius
   d. Family history of congenital heart disease
4. Fetal anomalies
   a. Cystic hygromas
   b. Omphalocele
   c. Nonimmune hydrops
      Pleural or pericardial effusion
      Ascites
      Skin thickening
      Polyhydramnios
      Placentomegaly
   d. Intrauterine growth retardation (see Chapter 16)
   e. Duodenal atresia
5. Maternal disease
   a. Diabetes
   b. Lupus
   c. Alcoholism
   d. Medication
   e. Drug abuse

In the presence of complex congenital heart disease a number of management issues arise. Depending on the severity of the prognosis, the family may elect termination of the pregnancy. Repeat echocardiograms can follow the progression of the disease. Fetuses with complex congenital heart disease are best delivered at a center with a team of pediatric cardiologists, neonatologists, and pediatric cardiac surgeons.

ANATOMY AND PHYSIOLOGY

The heart has four chambers. Blood flows through veins and enters the right atrium from the inferior vena cava and superior vena cava. The right atrium connects to the right ventricle, through the tricuspid valve. The pulmonary valve lies between the right ventricle and the pulmonary artery. The pulmonary artery perfuses the lungs. The pulmonary veins drain from the lungs into the left atrium. The left atrium connects to the left ventricle through the mitral valve. Blood exits from the left ventricle through the aorta past the aortic valve. The right ventricular outflow tract (RVOT) and the left ventricular outflow tract (aorta; LVOT) crisscross each other

Contraction of the heart is initiated at the atrial level. As the atria contract, blood is pushed through the mitral and tricuspid valves into the ventricles. Once the blood is in the ventricles, the ventricles start to contract and the mitral and tricuspid valves close, so blood cannot get back into the atria. When the ventricles contract, blood enters the pulmonary artery and the aorta through the aortic and pulmonary valves, which close as soon as contraction ceases, so blood cannot get back into the ventricles.

The anatomy just described is seen in the infant, child, and adult. In the fetus (Fig. 20-1), since the lungs do not have any function and all blood perfusion comes from the placenta through the umbilical cord, the situation is slightly different. The umbilical arteries join the iliac arteries and send blood into the arterial circulation. The umbilical vein drains blood from the venous circulation through the portal vein and ductus venosus. Two connections exist between the right and left heart circulations. A vessel termed the ductus arteriosus connects the pulmonary artery to the descending aorta. There is a connection between the two sides of the heart at the atrial level through the foramen ovale. The ductus venosus, ductus arteriosus, and foramen ovale close when the cord is clamped and the fetus starts to breathe (see Fig. 20-1).

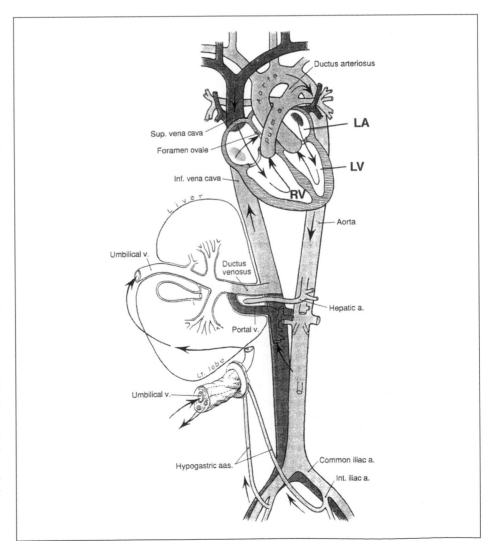

FIGURE 20-1. The fetal circulation.

The right and left cardiac chambers are approximately the same size in the fetus. Disproportion between the right and left chamber sizes may be due to obstruction of blood flow through the ductus arteriosus and foramen ovale or the aorta. Maldevelopment of either the right or left ventricle may not cause any hemodynamic problem in utero because blood flow through other right-to-left communications, such as the ductus arteriosus and foramen ovale, is possible.

◢ TECHNIQUE

First define the fetal position. Correct identification of the right and left side of the fetus is critical (see Chapter 14). The stomach is an ideal landmark once abdominal situs is established. The ideal situation is when the fetal spine is down. The following views assume this position. These views will be oriented differently when the fetus is in different positions, such as spine up.

Four-Chamber View

The fetal heart lies transversely in the chest. Identify the long axis of the spine, then rotate 90 degrees at the level of the thorax; or slide up toward the head from the abdominal circumference. The fetal heart should occupy about one third of the thorax (Fig. 20-2) and is situated to the left in the chest. Angle perpendicular to the ventricular septum (see Pitfalls) to view the thickness and continuity of the septum (Fig. 20-3A and B).

1. The right ventricle (RV) is situated beneath the anterior chest wall. The moderator band is in the RV and the walls are trabeculated. The left ventricular walls are much smoother.
2. The left atrium is nearest to the spine.
3. The ventricular cavities are similar in size. At term, the right side of the heart may be slightly larger than the left side.
4. The atrioventricular valves open during diastole.
5. Tricuspid valve insertion into the ventricular septum is slightly more apical than the mitral valve.

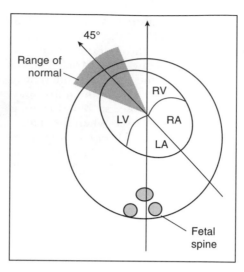

FIGURE 20-2. Diagram showing cardiac axis related to the spine. The normal axis is 45 degrees. A 20 degree variation in either direction is still considered within normal limits.

6. The ventricular septum is continuous. The muscular portion is of equal thickness to the left ventricular wall. The membranous portion is much thinner (see Fig. 20-3B).
7. The foramen ovale bows into the left atrium.
8. The atrial chambers are similar in size.
9. The pulmonary veins can be seen entering the left atrium.
10. The cardiac axis is between 30 and 60 degrees to a line from the spine to the midpart of the chest (see Fig. 20-2).

Long-Axis View of the Left Heart

At the four-chamber, view tilt the scan plane slightly toward the fetal head, pivoting at the apex. The best long-axis view will be obtained when angling from the right side of the heart (see Figs. 20-3B and 20-8). As you angle up toward the aorta, the ventricular septum at this level should be evaluated, as many defects occur in this area (see Ventricular Septal Defects).

1. The aortic valve and root, mitral valve, left ventricle and LVOT should be seen.
2. Part of the right ventricle is present anterior to the aortic root and ventricular septum.
3. The left atrium sits along the posterior wall of the aortic root.
4. The anterior wall of the aortic root is continuous with the ventricular septum.
5. The posterior wall of the aortic root is continuous with the anterior leaflet of the mitral valve.

Pulmonary Artery Arising From the Right Ventricle

Angle slightly more cephalad from the long-axis view of the left heart, pivoting at the apex. The size of the aortic root relative to the size of the pulmonic root can be evaluated as you angle from the long-axis view (see Fig. 20-3C).

1. The pulmonary artery and RVOT can be seen.
2. Branches of the pulmonary artery can be seen.

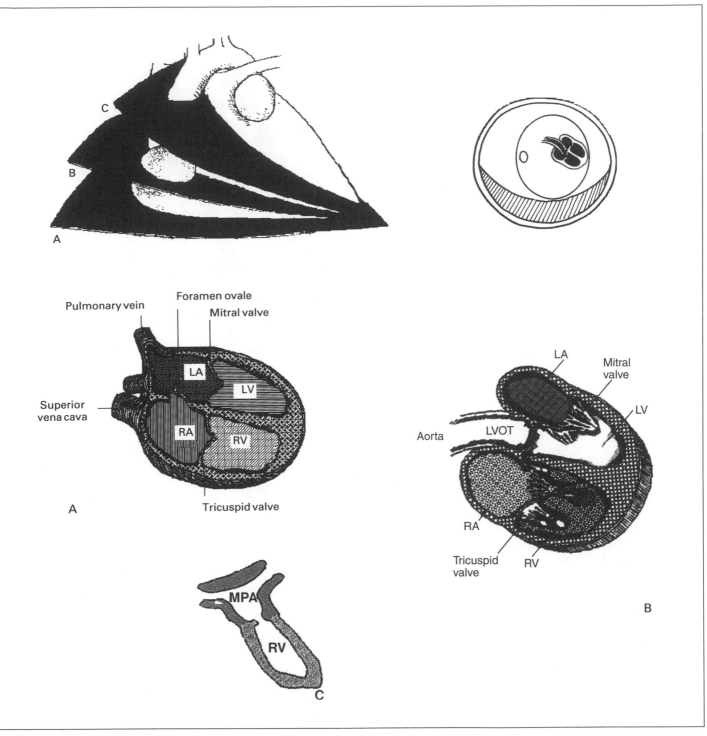

FIGURE 20-3. Diagram at the top left shows the axis at which A, B, and C were obtained. (**A**) Four-chamber view. (**B**) The long axis view of the left heart. (**C**) Pulmonary artery arising from the right ventricle. At the top right is a diagram showing the cardiac position in the fetal chest.

Short-Axis View for Evaluating Chamber Size

Rotate the beam 90 degrees from the four-chamber view. Start at the apex and slide toward the atrioventricular valves (Fig. 20-4B).

1. Obtain a view just below the valves to demonstrate the ventricular chamber size and thickness of the walls compared to the ventricular septum.
2. Angle toward the great vessels. The aortic root should be positioned in the center (Mercedes-Benz sign) (see Fig. 20-4A).
3. The pulmonary artery and root, right atrium, right ventricle, and left atrium wrap around the aortic valve.
4. Branches of the pulmonary artery may be seen.
5. The size of the aortic root compared to the pulmonic root can be evaluated from this view.

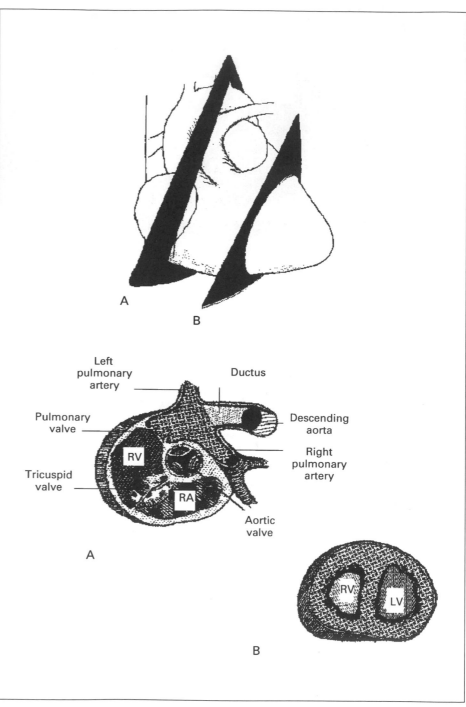

FIGURE 20-4. Diagram of short-axis views. (**A**) Short-axis view for demonstrating the great vessels. (**B**) Short-axis view for evaluating ventricular chamber size.

Aortic Arch Into Descending Aorta

Obtain a long-axis of the fetus and direct the beam through the fetal abdomen to visualize the abdominal aorta (Fig. 20-5). When the spine is up scan laterally on the maternal abdomen and angle under the spine.

1. The aorta exits the left ventricle from the center of the heart.
2. The aortic arch gives rise to the head and neck vessels, which include the innominate, left carotid, and left subclavian arteries.
3. The arch curves toward the spine and continues into the descending aorta.

Patent Ductus Arteriosus

Stay in the long-axis plane. At the aortic arch view slide slightly toward the descending aorta.

1. The pulmonary artery arises from the anterior aspect of the heart (right ventricle) and takes a sharp course straight back toward the descending aorta.
2. The course of the pulmonary artery to the descending aorta (patent ductus arteriosus) resembles the shape of a hockey stick (see Fig. 20-5B).

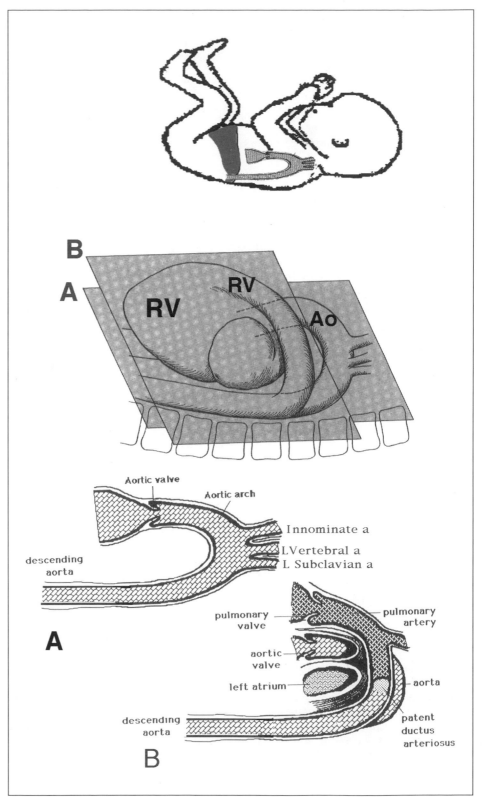

FIGURE 20-5. Diagram of views required to show the aortic arch and pulmonary artery into descending aorta. (**A**) Aortic arch into descending aorta. (**B**) Patent ductus arteriosus and pulmonary artery.

Inferior Vena Cava Entering the Right Atrium

On the long-axis view of the fetus, direct the beam through the ventral wall of the fetus angling toward the right of the spine (Fig. 20-6).

1. The inferior vena cava (IVC) enters the right atrium inferiorly.
2. The superior vena cava (SVC) enters the right atrium superiorly.
3. The ductus venosus and hepatic veins can be seen entering the IVC before the IVC enters the right atrium.

Pulsed Doppler—An Additional Tool

When performing the fetal echocardiogram, pulsed Doppler can add information or reinforce the suspected diagnosis. The same technique limitations that hold true when performing the two-dimensional exam apply when recording the pulsed Doppler exam. For optimal flow patterns, stay parallel to the blood flow.

In utero, the aortic and pulmonic arterial pressures are equal because of the wide connection through the ductus arteriosus. In the presence of ventricular outflow obstruction or in the absence of a ventricular septal defect (VSD), a pressure gradient may cause turbulent flow. Atrioventricular valve regurgitation (e.g., Ebstein's anomaly or atrioventricular canal defect) can be documented with pulsed Doppler.

Color Doppler

Color Doppler is a very useful tool in fetal echocardiography. Some areas in which color Doppler is useful include the following:

1. Confirming normal anatomy in the obese or difficult to scan patient.
2. Confirming a VSD or proving that the suspected area is not a defect.
3. Visualizing pulmonary vein flow with the Doppler scale low for the low-velocity venous flow.
4. Looking for valve regurgitation in a fetus with atrioventricular canal defect or in a fetus with signs of hydrops or heart failure.
5. Visualizing sufficient shunt flow across the patent ductus arteriosus and patent foramen ovale.
6. Confirming flow or absence of flow through valves, vessels, or chambers.

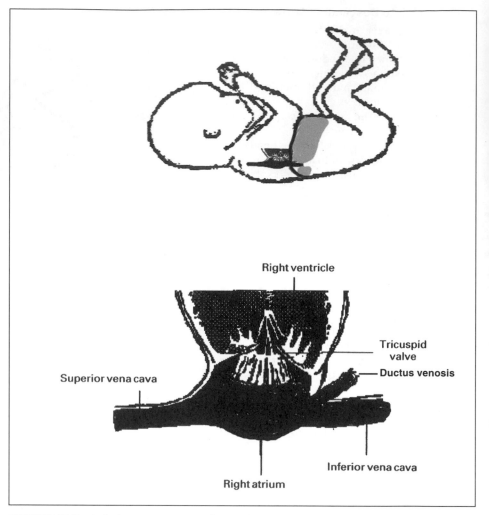

FIGURE 20-6. Inferior vena cava and superior vena cava entering the right atrium.

Measurements

1. Place an m-mode cursor perpendicular to the ventricular septum to measure ventricular chamber size and ventricular wall thickness just below the level of the atrioventricular valves in the four-chamber or short-axis view (Fig. 20-7). Function of the ventricular chambers can be quantitated by m-mode measurements, if there is a concern that function is poor. The right and left ventricular chamber size and wall thickness should be the same until late in the third trimester, when the right ventricular chamber size may be slightly increased compared to the left.

2. Measure the size of the aortic root in the long or short axis. When comparing the size of the two great arteries the short axis is helpful (Fig. 20-8). Once again, symmetry in the size of the pulmonic and aortic root is the expected norm throughout pregnancy, although the pulmonic root may be slightly larger than the aortic root.

Technical Problems

Factors that can affect accurate visualization of a fetal heart are as follows:

3. Decreased or increased amniotic fluid volume can be a problem. Too little fluid prevents ideal visualization of any organ. Too much amniotic fluid can increase the distance between the probe and the fetus, consequently affecting good visualization of the heart.

4. When scanning the fetal heart after 32 weeks, the increased bony deposition of calcium in the ribs and vertebral column can cast a shadow through the heart. The ideal scan is through the anterior chest wall. By staying parallel to the intercostal spaces, good views of the heart can be obtained.

5. In postdate hearts, the right ventricular chamber can be slightly larger than the left ventricle.

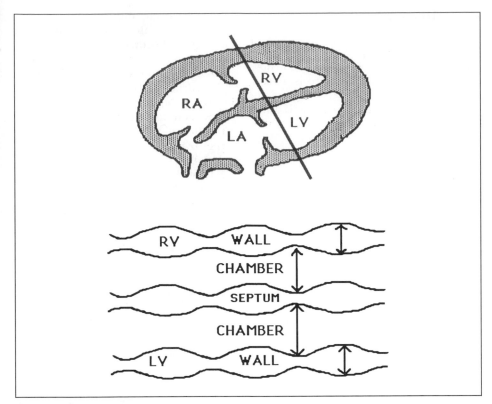

FIGURE 20-7. The placement of a cursor across the ventricular chambers will display the M-mode tracing needed to evaluate ventricular size and wall thickness.

1. Fetal position and increased activity can be quite frustrating when trying to obtain optimum views. Changing the position of the mother by rolling her up on her side can sometimes affect the fetal position. Otherwise, the mother should walk around for awhile. A further attempt at scanning should be made. Emptying or filling the maternal bladder may help.

2. Because of a large body wall, maternal obesity can place anterior reverberations into the chest area. Obesity also increases the distance between the fetus and the probe, making it difficult to optimize visualization of the heart. Don't rule out a lower frequency.

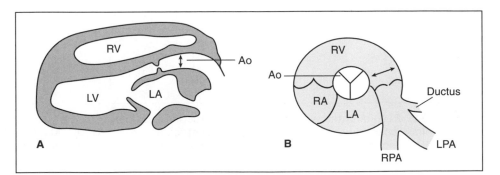

FIGURE 20-8. (A) The aortic root can be measured in the long axis view of the left heart. **(B)** Both great vessels are ideally visualized in the short axis views. Simultaneous measurements can be taken.

Checklist

 PATHOLOGY

Dysrhythmias

Fetal echocardiography is difficult before 16 weeks because the cardiac structures are quite small. If there is a sustained irregular heart rhythm or rate, a more extensive look at the heart is warranted. The normal fetal heart rate varies between 120 and 160 bpm.

1. Record atrial and ventricular contractions simultaneously by directing the m-mode cursor through both the atrial and ventricular walls (Fig. 20-9). Due to the small amplitude of the atrial wall during contraction, this can be difficult to record. Atrial contractions can also be recorded by the arrival (onset) of the A-wave of the tricuspid or mitral valve (Fig. 20-10). The atrial contraction will be followed closely by the ventricular contraction (Fig. 20-11).

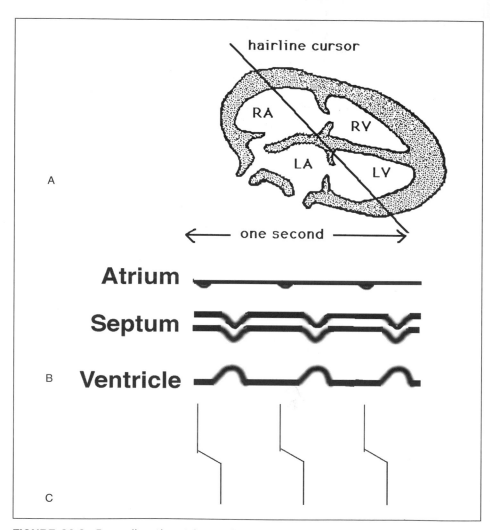

FIGURE 20-9. Recording the atrioventricular contraction sequence. (**A**) A cursor is directed simultaneously through the atrial and ventricular walls. (**B**) The M-mode tracing reveals normal ventricular wall contraction following atrial wall contraction. (**C**) The ladder diagram is helpful in evaluating the contraction sequence.

2. Measure heart rate on the m-mode at the same point on two consecutive beats (see Fig. 20-9). Most pieces of equipment have this capability built in.
3. Check for any signs of hydrops (see Chapter 17). This is associated with fetal cardiac failure and is likely to be present if the dysrhythmia is sustained.
4. Sustained dysrhythmias (especially when hydrops is present) should be followed closely.
5. Dysrhythmias can be associated with structural disease. When both are present, the outcome is often poor.

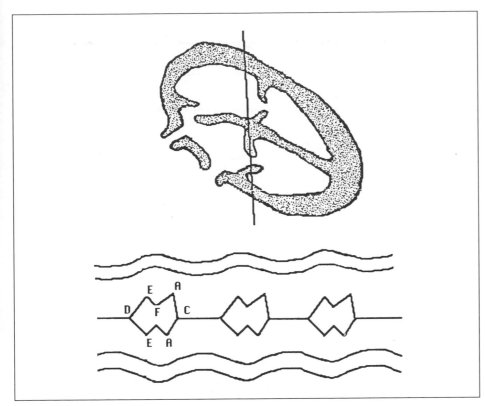

FIGURE 20-10. Onset of the A-wave can also be observed when evaluating atrial contractions. D indicates the end of ventricular systole, E the peak opening of the valve, F diastolic closing, A the peak of atrial systole as the atrium contracts, and C complete valve closure following the onset of ventricular contraction.

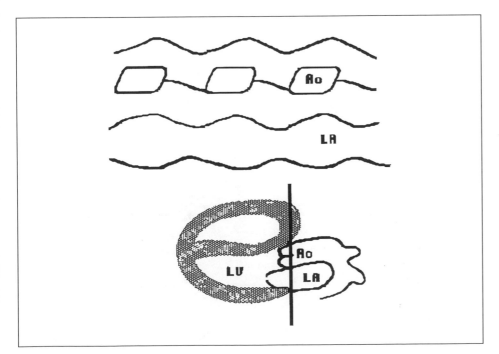

FIGURE 20-11. The atrioventricular contraction sequence can be evaluated angling through a semilunar valve opening and an atrial wall.

Slow Heart Rate

Bradycardia

1. Sinus bradycardia is when the fetal heart rate is less than 100 bpm. The atria and ventricles are beating at a 1:1 ratio (Fig. 20-12).
2. If it is not sustained, it may be normal if seen for brief periods early in pregnancy.
3. Bradycardia can be due to excessive transducer pressure on maternal abdomen.
4. If sustained, it can be due to cord compression or fetal distress.

Complete Heart Block

The ventricles and the atria are not beating at the same rate.

1. Ventricular heart rate is less than 100 bpm, usually 50 to 60 bpm (Fig. 20-13).
2. The ventricle will beat regularly. The atria will beat at a different, generally faster, rate.
3. Fifty percent of fetuses with complete heart block will have structural heart disease.
4. Second-degree heart block is when there is intermittent conduction of atrial beats. The atria will beat twice or three times to a single ventricular beat (2:1 or 3:1).
5. This condition is associated with maternal systemic lupus erythematosus.

Irregular Heart Rate

Premature Atrial Contractions

There will be an early atrial contraction that is either conducted or blocked. When conducted, a ventricular beat will follow. When blocked, a ventricular contraction will not follow (Fig. 20-14).

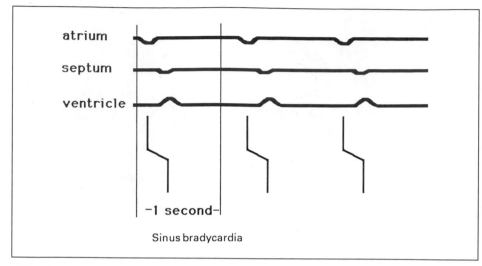

FIGURE 20-12. Sinus bradycardia. A normal one-to-one relationship is seen but the rate is less than 100 beats per minute.

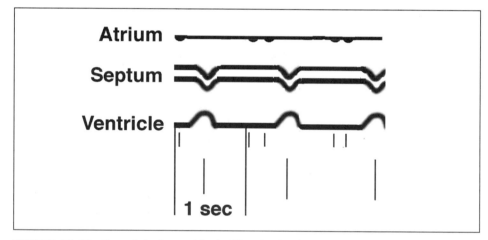

FIGURE 20-13. Complete heart block. The rhythm is totally out of synchronization. The ventricular rate is less than 100 beats per minute.

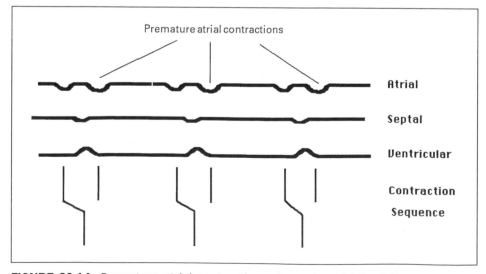

FIGURE 20-14. Premature atrial contractions. An early atrial beat is seen without conduction to the ventricle.

1. Often the foramen ovale is bowed so far into the left atrium that it hits against the atrial wall. This may be the cause of premature contraction of the atrial wall.
2. They can be isolated and occur only occasionally.
3. Bigeminy is when there are two beats then a skipped beat or pause. The beating of atria and ventricles will be in a 1:1 relationship (Fig. 20-15).
4. Trigeminy refers to three beats and a skipped beat or pause.

Premature Ventricular Contractions

A premature ventricular contraction occurs when a ventricular contraction is not preceded by an atrial contraction. Such contractions are usually not of much significance when isolated (Fig. 20-16).

Fast Heart Rate (Tachycardia)

Tachycardia is defined as a heart rate over 180 bpm.

Supraventricular Tachycardia (SVT)

1. The heart rate is over 200 bpm.
2. The ventricles and the atria are beating in a 1:1 ratio (Fig. 20-17).
3. If the SVT is sustained for prolonged periods, it will not be well tolerated and the fetus is likely to develop signs of hydrops. Serial echocardiograms are warranted to follow the heart rate.
4. If sustained maternal drug therapy is used, digoxin is often the first mode of treatment.

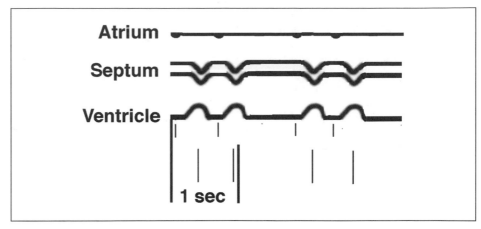

FIGURE 20-15. Atrial bigeminy. Two beats are seen in a one-to-one relationship and then there is a pause.

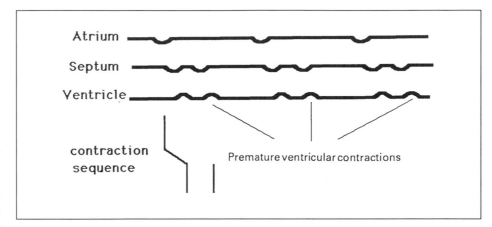

FIGURE 20-16. Premature ventricular contractions. A ventricular contraction precedes an early contraction.

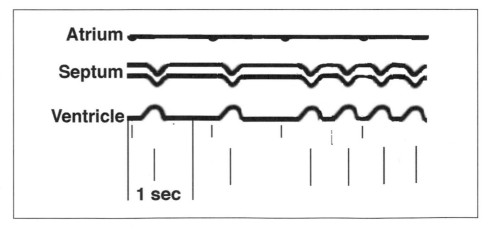

FIGURE 20-17. Supraventricular tachycardia. A normal sinus rhythm increased abruptly from 140 to 200 beats per minute.

Atrial Flutter

1. The atria will beat at a rate of 400 to 600 bpm.
2. The ventricular rate is blocked (not conducted) and will beat two to three times slower than the atria (Fig. 20-18). The ventricular rate is usually 200 to 300 bpm.
3. Long-term atrial flutter is poorly tolerated. The fetus is likely to develop signs of hydrops. Serial echocardiograms are used to follow the heart rate.
4. If the abnormal heart rate persists, maternal drug therapy is used.

Sinus Tachycardia

1. The heart rate is 180 to 190 bpm (Fig. 20-19).
2. The ventricle and the atria are beating in a 1:1 ratio.
3. No treatment is required.

Ventricular Tachycardia

1. The atria beat at a normal rate.
2. The ventricles beat at a rate slightly above the normal heart rate.
3. No treatment is required.

Abnormal Heart Location

Initially exclude any noncardiac cause for the abnormal heart position, such as diaphragmatic hernia, a common cause of apparent dextrocardia.

Apex of the Heart Pointing to the Right (Dextrocardia, Dextroversion)

The fetal heart is situated on the right side of the body with the apex pointing toward the right. If the stomach is also on the right, structural abnormalities are unlikely. If the stomach remains on the left, complex cardiac anomalies are common. The spleen is often absent or has multiple components (Ivemark's syndrome).

Heart Outside the Chest (Ectopia Cordis)

The fetal heart extends outside the rib cage through either the thorax (a sternal defect) or a thoracoabdominal defect (diaphragmatic and abdominal defects) in ectopia cordis.

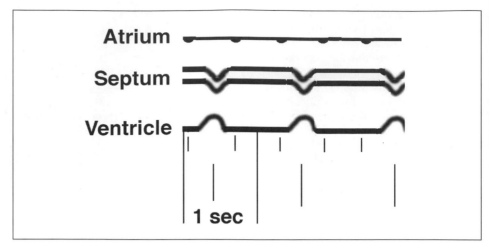

FIGURE 20-18. Atrial flutter—2:1 block. Only every other atrial contraction is conducted to the ventricle.

Associated abnormalities are common and include central nervous system anomalies and skeletal or facial defects, as well as other cardiac defects. When there is malrotation and displacement of the heart, be careful in making the diagnosis of cardiac defects. Apparent cardiac defects may be spurious when there is a diaphragmatic defect, omphalocele, and partial or complete extrathoracic cardiac position (pentalogy of Cantrell). The prognosis associated with the condition is poor; most infants die in the neonatal period. A few have undergone successful surgery.

Enlarged Heart

Heart Failure

The fetal heart chamber size will increase when there is heart failure. Evidence of hydrops with pleural effusion, ascites, and so on may be seen. There are many causes of heart failure, including sustained arrhythmias or critical aortic stenosis.

Pericardial Effusion

Fluid lies outside the cardiac chambers within the pericardium. As the heart beats, variation in the amount of pericardial fluid around the heart can be seen. Look for other components of hydrops when a pericardial effusion is detected. With pericardial effusions, the lungs are displaced posteriorly. Pericardial and pleural effusions are commonly confused. With pleural effusions, the lungs are floating within the fluid.

Thickened Walls, Poorly Contractile Heart

HYPERTROPHIC CARDIOMYOPATHY. The ventricular walls and interventricular septum will be thickened. Depending on the severity, the right, left, or both outflow tracts may be obstructed. This can be associated with maternal diabetes.

DILATED CARDIOMYOPATHY. The heart chambers will be dilated and the walls thin. The heart contracts poorly.

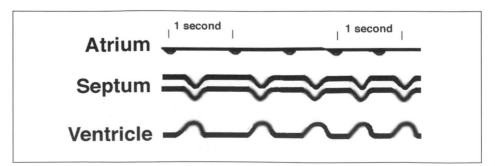

FIGURE 20-19. Sinus tachycardia. A gradual increase in the rate is seen.

ENDOCARDIAL FIBROELASTOSIS. Linear echogenic areas may be found in the heart walls with endocardial fibroelastosis. The heart contracts poorly. Most of the time this is associated with left ventricular outflow obstruction and heart failure. Aortic stenosis is often present.

Echogenic Mass Within the Heart

Myocardial Tumors

Several myocardial tumors have been detected in utero. Cardiac tumors are quite rare; they need to be followed in case obstruction and hydrops develop.

RHABDOMYOMA. This type of tumor appears as an echogenic mass most commonly involving the ventricular walls or ventricular septum and impinging on the ventricular chambers. Rhabdomyoma can also be found in the atrial septum and atrial walls impinging on the atrial chambers. They are more echogenic than the myocardium (Fig. 20-20). Most are small, but they can become as large as 4 or 5 cm in size. Dysrhythmias can occur if rhabdomyomas involve the conducting system.

TERATOMA. These extremely rare tumors have a similar appearance to rhabdomyoma.

ANGIOMYOMAS. Angiomyomas are small, highly echogenic tumors that can be seen anywhere in the heart. They usually resolve on their own.

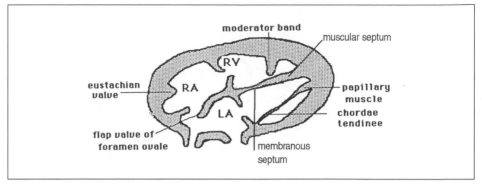

FIGURE 20-21. Normal structures within the fetal heart sometimes present as bright echoes, being mistaken for small tumors.

Normal Structures That Can Appear Echogenic

See Figure 20-21.

1. The *moderator band* is a structure seen at the apex of the right ventricle.
2. *Chordae tendineae* and *papillary muscle* are usually visible in the ventricles toward the apex.
3. The *eustachian valve* can be seen in the right atrium at the entrance of the IVC.

4. The *flap of the foramen ovale* between the two atrial chambers can appear bright. It is rapidly mobile.

Abnormal Four-Chamber Heart

Small Left Heart

HYPOPLASTIC LEFT HEART
See Figure 20-22.

1. The left ventricle, aorta, and LVOT are all small. The tip of the left ventricle will not reach to the apex of the heart.

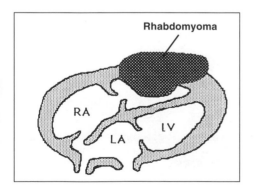

FIGURE 20-20. A rhabdomyoma could be missed if texture changes in the myocardium and symmetry in the chamber size are not evaluated.

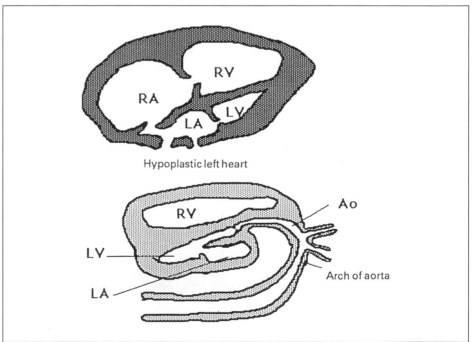

Hypoplastic left heart

FIGURE 20-22. Hypoplastic left heart syndrome. The obvious asymmetry in the four-chamber view can help make the diagnosis (Top). Ascending and transverse aortic arch will be small and difficult to image (Bottom).

2. Most often both the mitral and aortic valves are severely hypoplastic or atretic. Although both valves are usually affected, either one can be normal with the other affected. If the mitral and aortic valves are both affected, their annuli will be small. No valve opening will be seen.

3. The left ventricular walls will be thickened. The atrial septum is usually intact or has a small patent foramen ovale.

4. The right ventricle will form the apex and be enlarged, but structurally normal.

5. When the aortic valve is atretic the ascending and transverse aortic arches are small.

6. On real-time the left heart will be difficult to see in the four-chamber view.

7. The cross-section of the ventricles will show a tiny left ventricle that is not contracting. The aortic arch will be very difficult to image. The ascending aorta will appear to be about the size of a coronary artery. The patent ductus arteriosus will be quite large and easy to confuse for the aortic arch. The origination of the head vessels will be the aortic arch.

8. There will be no flow by color or pulsed Doppler through the left ventricle when the mitral and aortic valves are atretic. Some flow can be detected across the foramen ovale if it is patent. In the transverse aortic arch, color Doppler will demonstrate retrograde flow from the patent ductus arteriosus into the aortic arch.

Small Right Heart

When the right side of the heart is small there is either inlet or outlet obstruction or both.

TRICUSPID ATRESIA (INLET ATRESIA)

1. Either there is a thin membrane in place of the tricuspid valve or there may be a small, hypoplastic valve which does not allow adequate blood flow. Hemodynamically the two function the same. There will be little or no flow through the tricuspid valve by color Doppler.

2. The right ventricle will be small.

PULMONARY ATRESIA (OUTLET ATRESIA)

Outlet atresia will result in pulmonary atresia or severe pulmonary stenosis. A small right ventricle and tricuspid valve annulus usually develop and can be seen on the four-chamber view. Little or no flow through the small tricuspid valve annulus will be seen. Color Doppler will confirm flow or the absence of flow. The pulmonic root will be difficult to visualize. There may be a normal-sized pulmonic root, with a thin membrane between the RVOT and the main pulmonary artery that does not allow flow. Color Doppler is helpful in outlining the pulmonary artery anatomy. Use color Doppler to search for the pulmonary artery if it is not visualized on real-time.

Enlarged Left Heart

Establish whether the entire left heart is enlarged or just the atrium or ventricle.

ENLARGED LEFT VENTRICLE

Aortic Stenosis. Left ventricular outflow obstruction may be present at one or multiple levels. Possible levels include a subvalvular membrane, aortic valve stenosis, and supravalvular stenosis. If the obstruction is mild, a fetal echocardiogram may appear normal. However, if the obstruction is severe, the left ventricle may dilate and function poorly. There may be secondary endocardial thickening (Fig. 20-23).

Color and pulsed Doppler will be helpful in estimating the severity of the stenosis. The color Doppler flow pattern will become turbulent at the point of obstruction.

MITRAL STENOSIS. This is extremely rare as a congenital disease. The valve will appear thickened and echogenic on real-time. Flow velocity by pulsed Doppler will be increased. An enlarged left ventricle will be present.

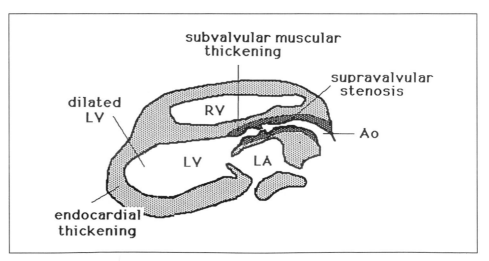

FIGURE 20-23. Aortic stenosis. The long axis view best demonstrates stenosis along the aortic root. One or more of these conditions may be responsible for this entity; endocardial thickening is secondary to the stenosis.

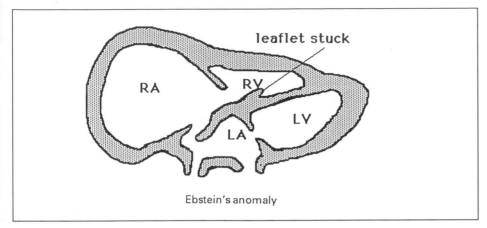

FIGURE 20-24. Ebstein's anomaly. The septal leaflet of the tricuspid valve is positioned lower than normal and is adherent to the ventricular septum. The four-chamber view allows comparison of the mitral position to the tricuspid.

Dysplastic Pulmonary Valve or Pulmonary Atresia. An atretic pulmonary valve will not allow flow to the main pulmonary artery. The rest of the right heart is usually formed normally. There will be a massive amount of tricuspid valve regurgitation causing enlargement of the right atrium. The atrial septum will bow into the left atrium and make the left atrium quite small and difficult to see. The four-chamber view will show the right atrium enlargement. A thin membrane will be seen at the level of the pulmonary valve, and there will be no opening in the membrane. Color Doppler can be used to confirm the lack of flow across the pulmonary valve and will demonstrate the severity of the tricuspid valve regurgitation.

ENLARGED LEFT ATRIUM

Mitral Regurgitation. If severe, mitral regurgitation will cause left atrial enlargement. Mitral regurgitation is common in fetuses with an atrioventricular canal (see Septal Break) (see Fig. 20-32). Another cause of mitral regurgitation is heart failure. Color Doppler will demonstrate a jet of flow into the left atrium when the mitral valve is closed (systole).

Enlarged Right Heart

Establish whether the entire right heart is enlarged or just the atrium or the ventricle.

ENLARGED RIGHT ATRIUM

Ebstein's Anomaly of the Tricuspid Valve. One or more of the tricuspid valve leaflets are displaced into the right ventricle (Fig. 20-24). However, the valve annulus remains at the normal level. The septal leaflet is hypoplastic and adherent to the interventricular septum, whereas the anterior leaflet is larger. There are varying degrees of this anomaly ranging from mild displacement to displacement into the right ventricular apex. The portion of the right ventricle above the valve becomes atrialized (it has to function as an atrium) with consequent enlargement of the right atrium. The amount of tricuspid regurgitation will depend on the severity of the anomaly. Arrhythmias can be associated. On real-time, the four-chamber view will appear abnormal. The tricuspid valve insertion and opening of the valve will be closer to the apex than normal. There will be enlargement of the right atrium. Color Doppler can help identify the opening of the tricuspid valve and demonstrate the severity of tricuspid valve regurgitation.

ENLARGED RIGHT VENTRICLE

Coarctation of the Aorta. Coarctation of the aorta is difficult to detect in utero (Fig. 20-25). A posterior shelf above, below, or at the level of the ductus arteriosus may be imaged. It is infrequently seen in utero. On the four-chamber view the right ventricle may be enlarged. This may be the only finding and it may be subtle. Other findings include VSD, abnormal mitral valve, and bicuspid aortic valve (difficult to detect on fetal echocardiogram). Color Doppler of the aortic arch may help identify a coarctation if there is severe obstruction; although coarctation of the aorta is difficult to identify, hypoplasia of the isthmus (interrupted aortic arch) is more easily identified. The aortic arch will be quite narrow and difficult to identify even with the help of color Doppler. The ductal arch will be large.

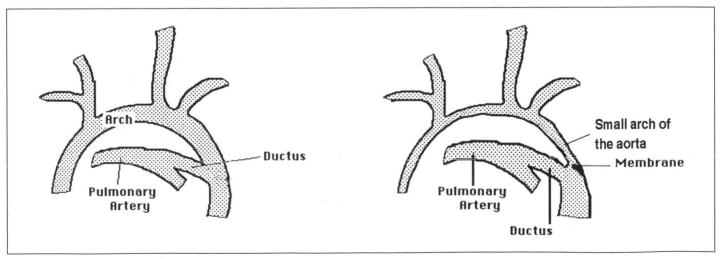

FIGURE 20-25. Coarctation of the aorta. Diagram at the left shows normal aortic arch. Diagram at the right shows coarctation of the aorta with posterior shelf.

Pulmonary Stenosis. Pulmonary valve stenosis is the most common obstructive lesion involving the RVOT (Fig. 20-26). The ventricular septum is intact. If obstruction is mild the valve may appear normal. The right ventricle will function normally. If the right ventricle and the right atrium are dilated, severe obstruction is present. Stenosis can occur at other levels of the right outflow, such as the infundibular portion (before the valve) or the supravalvular portion (after the valve) (see Fig. 20-26). The four-chamber view may appear normal if there is mild obstruction. If the obstruction is severe, the right heart may be enlarged. Measure the diameter in the cross-section of the aortic and pulmonic roots (see Fig. 20-4). Color flow Doppler will identify the point of the obstruction and any evidence of tricuspid valve regurgitation. The severity of the obstruction can be estimated with continuous wave Doppler.

Tetralogy of Fallot. Four findings are always present with tetralogy of Fallot (TOF) (Fig. 20-27):

1. A large perimembranous VSD that is anterior and to the right of the tricuspid valve.
2. An enlarged aortic root overriding the VSD. The aorta is more rightward than normal.
3. Some type of pulmonary stenosis. There is a wide spectrum of pulmonary disease that ranges from mild pulmonary valve stenosis to pulmonary atresia. The valve may be thickened and stenotic or the entire RVOT may be quite small without a discrete point of obstruction.
4. Right ventricular hypertrophy. This is not always present in fetal life. The presence or absence of right ventricular hypertrophy depends on the severity of the pulmonary disease. The four-chamber view may appear normal. The right ventricle may be enlarged. Measure the pulmonary and aortic valve annuli. Color Doppler will identify the pulmonary anatomy, especially if it is small and difficult to see on real-time.

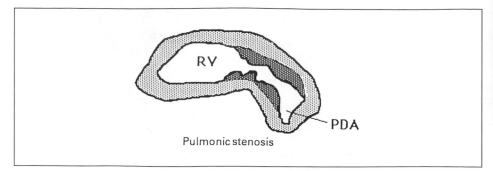

FIGURE 20-26. Pulmonary stenosis. Thickening and/or narrowing of the right ventricular outflow tract, thickening of the pulmonary valve, and narrowing of the pulmonary artery may be present.

Single Ventricle (Univentricular Heart).

A single ventricle heart defect is due to maldevelopment of the interventricular septum. The atrioventricular junction is connected to one chamber in the ventricular area of the heart. There may be one or two atrioventricular valves, which can be seen on a four-chamber view. No interventricular septum will be seen. Both the aorta and pulmonary arteries will originate from the ventricle, although there may be a small, nonfunctioning ventricle giving rise to one of the great arteries. In this situation a VSD will be present.

Inability to Visualize Continuity of the Great Arteries From the Ventricular Outflow Tracts
Small Aortic Root

For discussion of hypoplastic left heart, see the pertinent information presented earlier under Small Left Heart. For discussion of aortic stenosis, see the pertinent information presented earlier under Enlarged Left Heart.

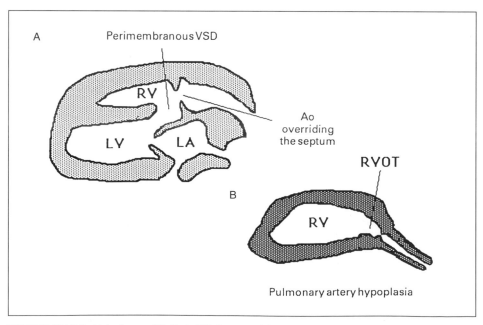

FIGURE 20-27. Tetralogy of Fallot. (**A**) An overriding aorta will be associated with a ventricular (perimembranous) septal defect in tetralogy of Fallot. It is important to obtain the best long-axis view possible because this distortion can be technical (see Pitfalls). (**B**) As one angles more superiorly from the long-axis view, pivoting at the apex, the root of the pulmonic artery will appear hypoplastic in extreme cases of tetralogy of Fallot.

Small Pulmonic Root

For discussion of pulmonic stenosis and tetralogy of Fallot, see the pertinent information presented earlier under Enlarged Right Heart.

Double Outlet Right or Left Ventricle

With double outlet of the right or left ventricle, both the great arteries arise from one ventricle with bilateral coni. A large VSD will be present (Fig. 20-28). The four-chamber view may appear normal or one of the ventricles will appear enlarged. When angling toward the great arteries from the four-chamber view, both great vessels will arise from one of the ventricles. Color Doppler will help identify the blood flow pattern from the ventricles to the great arteries.

Truncus Arteriosus

Truncus arteriosus (Fig. 20-29) consists of the following findings:

1. Outlet VSD
2. Single semilunar valve
3. Common arterial root that overrides the ventricular septum

The arterial root usually originates from the two ventricles equally. It can originate more from one ventricle than the other. The truncal valve (semilunar valve) may have one to six leaflets. It can have normal flow, regurgitation, or stenosis. There are three types of truncus arteriosus. In all three types the pulmonary artery comes off the aorta. It can be the main pulmonary artery or one or both of the branches of the pulmonary artery. The position of their origin determines the type.

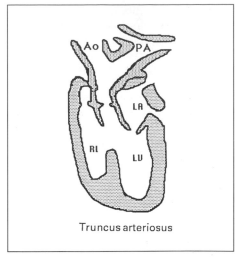

FIGURE 20-29. Truncus arteriosus. A large ventricular septal defect with a single great artery is well shown.

A four-chamber view at the level of the atrioventricular valves can appear normal. When angling toward the great arteries from the four-chamber, a large VSD will be present. One great artery will override the VSD. The artery will be larger than normal. A pulmonary artery must be imaged originating from the aorta to make this diagnosis. This is the only way to differentiate truncus arteriosus from tetralogy of Fallot with pulmonary atresia. Color Doppler will show flow from both ventricles into one great artery. It will also show flow from the aorta into the pulmonary artery and help identify this anatomy.

Total Anomalous Pulmonary Venous Return (TAPVR)

The pulmonary veins join to form a "pulmonary venous confluence" and drain into the right atrium rather than the left atrium. The confluence can (1) vary in position and be posterior and separate from the left atrium; (2) be superior to the left atrium and drain into the right atrium, coronary sinus, or superior vena cava via a vertical vein; or (3) be inferior to the left atrium or inferior to the diaphragm and drain into the inferior vena cava.

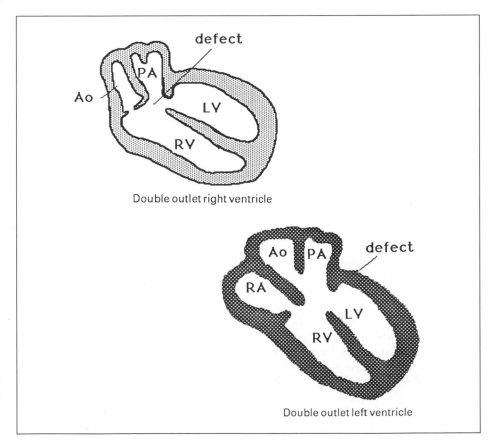

Double outlet right ventricle

Double outlet left ventricle

FIGURE 20-28. Double outlet ventricle. Simultaneous visualization of both semilunar valves is seen in the same long-axis plane.

On a four-chamber view the left heart will appear smaller than the right. There will be a cystic, vascular structure where the pulmonary vein confluence is located. Pulmonary veins can be difficult to visualize. Color Doppler will help confirm the diagnosis. The color Doppler scale should be set to a low velocity to detect the low venous velocity. There can be partial anomalous pulmonary venous return. This is associated with a sinus venosus ASD. One or two of the right pulmonary veins drain into the right atrium. Again, this is a difficult diagnosis to make in utero.

D-Transposition (Dextro-Transposition) of the Great Arteries

The anterior right ventricle gives rise to the aorta and the posterior left ventricle gives rise to the main pulmonary artery (Fig. 29-30). VSD and pulmonary stenosis can be associated. The four-chamber view at the level of the atrioventricular valves will appear normal. In the long-axis view of the heart, the two great arteries will be parallel when leaving the heart. To make the diagnosis, the anterior aorta must give rise to the head vessels and the posterior pulmonary artery must bifurcate. Color Doppler will help track the great vessels.

L-Transposition (Levo-Transposition; L-Loop; Corrected Transposition) of the Great Arteries

The ventricles are transposed, but are correctly connected to the great arteries. The right atrium is connected to the morphologic left ventricle and the pulmonary artery. The left atrium is connected to the morphologic right ventricle and the aorta. The aorta is to the left of the pulmonary artery most of the time. The aorta and pulmonary artery will be parallel exiting the heart. Circulation is hemodynamically correct. This can be associated with other defects, most commonly pulmonary stenosis, congenital heart block, abnormalities of the tricuspid valve, and VSD. To make the diagnosis, identify the morphology of the atria, ventricles, and great arteries. The ventricle on the left of the fetus has the characteristics of a right ventricle (tricuspid valve closer to the apex and a moderator band).

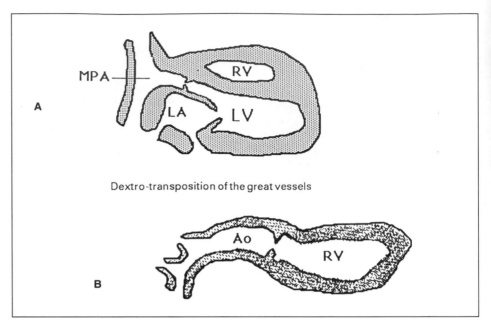

FIGURE 20-30. Dextro-transposition of the great vessels. (**A**) The early bifurcation of the pulmonary artery arising from the left ventricle is seen in dextro-transposition of the great vessels. (**B**) The aortic root will be continuous with the right ventricle.

Septal Break

Atrioventricular Septal Defect; Atrioventricular Canal; Endocardial Cushion Defect)

There is a wide spectrum of atrioventricular septal defects (AVSD). A common atrioventricular valve will have superior and inferior bridging leaflets with one or two valve orifices. In a partial form, the common valve leaflet will be displaced downward and connect to the crest of the muscular septum, allowing shunting only across a primum ASD (see Fig. 20-31B). When the valve is free-floating in a complete form (not attached to the atrial or ventricular septum), shunting occurs above and below the valve level (see Fig. 20-31A). On four-chamber view the mitral and tricuspid valves will appear to be one leaflet crossing or attaching to the ventricular septum at the same level. The ventricles may be of equal size or one may be larger than the other. The short axis at the level of the atrioventricular valves will demonstrate the anatomy of the valves.

Color Doppler will demonstrate the flow across the atrial or ventricular septum. With a large defect there will not be much flow across the septum because the pressure in the two sides of the heart will be equal. Regurgitation of the mitral and tricuspid valves is common. Color Doppler will help quantitate the amount.

ATRIAL ISOMERISM. An atrioventricular canal defect can be a feature of either left or right atrial isomerism. Both atrial chambers assume the same anatomic characteristics, for example, both atria are structured as a right atrium or a left atrium. The IVC is often not seen with left atrial isomerism.

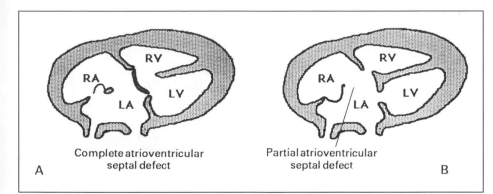

FIGURE 20-31. Atrioventricular septal defect. (**A**) Complete atrioventricular septal defect. There is an inlet ventricular septal defect, ostium primum atrial septal defect, and common atrioventricular valve leaflet. (**B**) Partial atrioventricular septal defect. Ostium primum atrial septal defect with common atrioventricular valve leaflet.

Ventricular Septal Defect

Morphologically the ventricular septum is divided into two segments: the membranous portion is the small thin portion inferior to the aortic root (Fig. 20-32B) and the muscular septum is divided into three portions: (1) the inlet portion which is at the level of the atrioventricular valves (see Fig. 20-32A); (2) the outlet or infundibular portion which is the anterior portion at the level of the semilunar valves; and (3) the muscular septum which extends from the membranous portion to the apex (see Fig. 20-32D). VSDs are common. There can be more than one VSD in the same or different portions of the septum. They are often associated with other types of congenital heart disease.

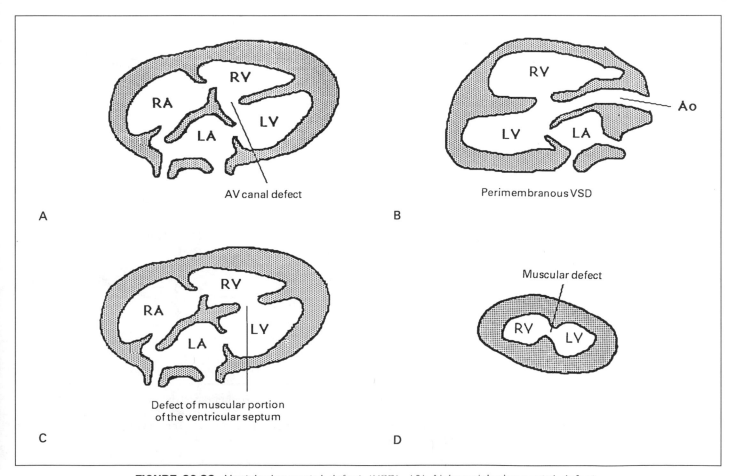

FIGURE 20-32. Ventricular septal defect (VSD). (**A**) Atrioventricular septal defect. Defect of the inlet ventricular septum. (**B**) Perimembranous VSD. Best demonstrated in the long axis view. Thin portion of ventricular septum missing. Edge of the muscular septum may appear bright. (**C**) Muscular VSD. Can occur anywhere in the muscular portion of the ventricular septum. Best imaged when perpendicular to the septum. (**D**) Muscular VSD can be imaged from the short axis of the ventricles. Small defects may be difficult to image without color Doppler.

On a real-time view there will be persistent drop-out in the septum and there should be echogenic borders to the VSD. To best identify number, size, and location of the VSD, multiple views are necessary. The four-chamber view is valuable if you are careful to sweep from anterior to posterior in the heart. It is helpful to be perpendicular to the septum for best visualization of the VSD, to avoid false positives (see Fig. 20-34B).

Color and pulsed Doppler are helpful in confirming the presence or absence of a VSD. Being perpendicular to the septum will also enhance the Doppler signal. Color Doppler is especially helpful in demonstrating multiple small defects (Swiss cheese defects) of the muscular septum.

Atrial Septal Defect

The atrial septum is divided into three portions:

1. The most superior portion is the sinus venosus portion of the septum. Defects in this portion are associated with partial anomalous pulmonary venous return.
2. The midportion (area of the fossa ovalis) of the septum is the secundum portion (Fig. 20-33A). This is the most common area for defects to occur. Because the foramen ovale is patent in fetal life, it is difficult to diagnose a defect in this portion prenatally. An aneurysm of this area can occur (see Fig. 20-33B).
3. The most inferior portion is the ostium primum portion (see Fig. 20-33C). A defect in this portion is associated with AVSDs. A four-chamber view that is perpendicular to the atrial septum will demonstrate drop-out of the atrial septum. Color Doppler will demonstrate flow across defect. If an ASD at this site is demonstrated, other associated defects must be ruled out.

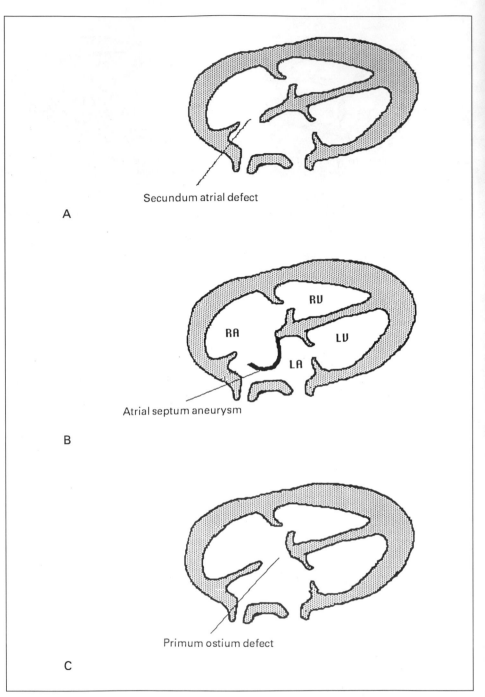

FIGURE 20-33. Atrial septal defects. (**A**) Secundum atrial defect. The central part of the atrial septum is missing. (**B**) Atrial septal aneurysm. A bowing of the membrane can be visualized. (**C**) Ostium primum atrial defect. The lower portion of the atrial septum is not seen.

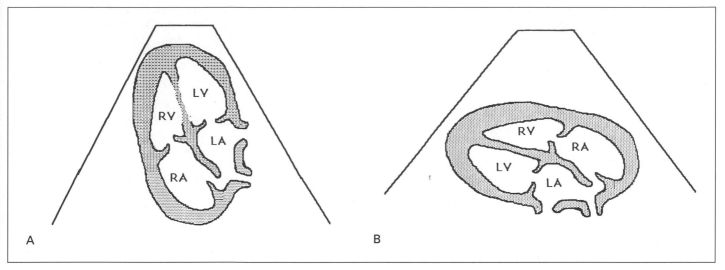

FIGURE 20-34. (**A**) Angling through the apex of the heart in the four-chamber view will create dropout at the antrioventricular. (**B**) To avoid this artifact, try to obtain the four-chamber view by angling through the lateral aspect.

PITFALLS

1. *Cardiac situs.* One of the first steps should be to determine the right and left sides of the fetus. First, see whether the cardiac axis is in the same direction as the stomach; then make sure both are not on the wrong side.

2. *Cardiac location and anomalies.* If the cardiac apex is shifted, determine the reason for the shift (e.g., pleural/pericardial effusion, omphalocele, ectopia cordis, diaphragmatic hernia). Careful attention to the cardiac anatomy is also important.

3. *Pericardial vs. pleural effusion.* A pericardial effusion will push the lungs posteriorly, whereas with a pleural effusion the lungs float within the fluid.

4. *Pseudo pericardial effusion.* False-positive pericardial effusion can sometimes be diagnosed. A thin sonolucent rim around the heart is a normal finding. Serial echocardiograms will show it unchanged. A pericardial effusion must be seen in more than one view.

5. *Echogenic spot in the heart.* There may be a bright echogenic spot in the left or right ventricle (see Fig. 20-21). It is a normal variant when part of the chordae tendineae or papillary muscle. Use multiple views to confirm this is the position of the bright spot. These echogenic foci are associated with an increased risk for Down syndrome.

6. *Eustachian valve.* The eustachian valve or the flap of the foramen ovale may appear as an echogenic line within the atrium.

7. *Possible cardiac tumor.* If there is a question of a cardiac tumor in one of the cardiac walls or chambers, change to a different position. To make a positive diagnosis demonstrate the tumor in more than one view.

8. *Ventricular wall thickness.* Differentiating between normal heart wall thickness and heart wall pathology may be difficult. Different views of the heart walls and m-mode measurements may be helpful.

9. *Excessive transducer pressure.* Excessive pressure on the maternal abdomen may cause episodes of bradycardia. Release the pressure and the heart rate should return to normal.

10. *Patent ductus arteriosus vs. aortic arch.* The ductus arteriosus and the aortic arch can be mistaken for each other on the long-axis view of the fetus. The aortic arch has the appearance of a candy cane with a tight, rounded curve and the three head vessels originate superiorly. The ductus arteriosus resembles a hockey stick with a wider, flatter curve (see Fig. 20-5B).

11. *Pseudo VSD due to transducer angle.* In the four-chamber view, angle through the lateral aspect of the heart instead of the apex to avoid drop-out and fabrication of an appearance resembling a VSD (Fig. 20-34). Also use color Doppler to confirm the diagnosis.

12. *Right heart mildly enlarged.* Close to term this is normal; however it is important to image the aortic arch for a possible coarctation and image the pulmonary vein flow into the left atrium.

13. *Taking time.* Most important to a good fetal echocardiogram is to take your time. False-positives can occur when the fetus is in a difficult-to-image position. Have Mom walk around and empty or fill her bladder, and then try again.

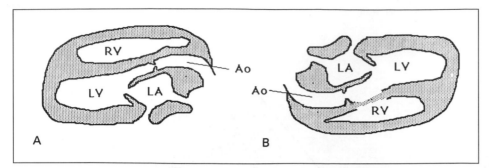

FIGURE 20-35. Left ventricular outflow tract (LVOT). (**A**) Scan through the right side of the heart if possible to obtain the LVOT. (**B**) When scanning through the left side of the heart to obtain the LVOT, the appearance of override of the aorta can be created.

14. *Pseudo overriding aorta.* If possible obtain the long axis of the LVOT by scanning through the right heart. Remember, the ventricular septum thins out at the aortic root (Fig. 20-35).

We are grateful to Kathy Reed, M.D., for allowing us to adapt Figures 20-3, 20-4, 20-5, 20-5, 20-6, and 20-28 from her book and for her comments on the chapter. Jean Kan, M. D., provided extremely valuable editorial help.

SELECTED READING

Allan, L., Sharland, G., and Cook, A. *Color Atlas of Fetal Cardiology.* Barcelona: Mosby-Wolfe, 1994.

Divon, M. Y., Yeh, S. Y., Zimmer, E. Z., Platt, L. D., Paldi, E., and Paul, R. H. Respiratory sinus arrhythmia in the human fetus. *Am J Obstet Gynecol* 151:425—428, 1985.

Fyfe, D. A., Meyer, K. B., and Case, C. L. Sonographic assessment of fetal cardiac arrhythmias. *Semin Ultrasound, CT MRI* 14:286—297, 1993.

Reed, K. L., Anderson, C. F., and Shenker, L. *Fetal Echocardiography: An Atlas.* New York: Alan R. Liss, 1988.

Smith, R. S., Comstock, C. H., Kirk, J. S., and Lee, W. Ultrasonographic left cardiac axis deviation: A marker for fetal anomalies. *Obstet Gynecol* 85:187—191, 1995.

21 SONOGRAPHIC ABDOMINAL ANATOMY

IRMA WHEELOCK TOPPER

SONOGRAM ABBREVIATIONS

Ao	Aorta
Azv	Azygos vein (ascending lumbar vein)
Ca	Celiac artery
CBD	Common bile duct
CHa	Common hepatic artery
CHD	Common hepatic duct
CIa	Common iliac artery
Cr	Crus
Du	Duodenum
GBl	Gallbladder
Gda	Gastroduodenal artery
Hea	Hepatic artery
Hev	Hepatic vein
IMa	Inferior mesenteric artery
IMv	Inferior mesenteric vein
IVC	Inferior vena cava
K	Kidney
L	Liver
LGa	Left gastric artery
LGv	Left gastric vein
LHev	Left hepatic vein
LPv	Left portal vein
LRa	Left renal artery
LRv	Left renal vein
MHev	Middle hepatic vein
P	Pancreas
PHa	Proper hepatic artery
Ps	Psoas muscles
Pv	Portal vein
QL	Quadratus lumborum
RA	Rectus abdominis
RGv	Right gastric vein
RHev	Right hepatic vein
RPv	Right portal vein
RRa	Right renal artery
RRv	Right renal vein
S	Spine
SGv	Splenogastric vein
SMa	Superior mesenteric artery
SMv	Superior mesenteric vein
Spa	Splenic artery
Spv	Splenic vein
St	Stomach

Since the bony landmarks visible with other imaging modalities are not available and gas may limit the ultrasound field of view, recognizing normal anatomic landmarks is crucial for proper orientation. Vascular landmarks are the most important in defining location, but normal muscular structure and organ position must also be known.

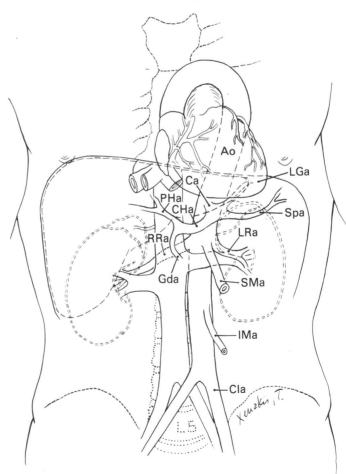

FIGURE 21-1. Commonly visualized vessels arising from the aorta are the celiac artery, splenic artery, left gastric artery, common hepatic artery, proper hepatic artery, gastroduodenal artery, right and left renal arteries, superior mesenteric artery, inferior mesenteric artery, and below the bifurcation at the level of the fourth lumbar vertebra, the right and left iliac arteries. Only the portion of the aorta below the diaphragm is visualized on an abdominal study.

KEY WORDS

ARTERIES

Aorta (Abdominal). Main trunk of the arterial system (Fig. 21-1; see also Fig. 21-5). It is anterior to the spine and bifurcates into the right and left common iliac arteries at the level of the umbilicus.

Celiac Artery (Axis, Trunk). Arises just below the liver from the anterior aorta and is only 2 to 3 cm in length (Fig. 21-2; see also Figs. 21-1 and 21-5). It almost immediately divides into the splenic, left gastric, and common hepatic arteries.

Femoral Arteries. These vessels, seen in the inguinal regions, can be traced into the upper leg (see Fig. 46-1). A branch—the profunda femoris—originates just below the inguinal ligament.

Gastroduodenal Artery. Originates from the common hepatic trunk and supplies the stomach and duodenum (Fig. 21-3; see also Figs. 21-1 and 21-2). It is a landmark delineating the antero-lateral aspect of the head of the pancreas.

Hepatic Artery (Common). Originates from the celiac trunk (see Figs. 21-1 and 21-2). Supplies the stomach, pancreas, duodenum, liver, gallbladder, and greater omentum. Divides into the proper hepatic and gastroduodenal arteries.

Hepatic Artery (Proper). Originates from the common hepatic artery and supplies the liver and gallbladder (see Figs. 21-1 and 21-2); runs medial to the common bile duct and anterior to the portal vein into the liver within the porta hepatis.

Iliac Arteries. Originate from the aorta at the level of the bifurcation and extend toward the groin (see Fig. 21-1). Both are normally 1.5 cm in diameter at origin.

Inferior Mesenteric Artery. Originates from the abdominal aorta close to the umbilicus (see Fig. 21-1). Supplies the left portion of the transverse colon, the descending and sigmoid colon, and part of the rectum. It is not usually seen on the sonogram except at its origin.

Left Gastric Artery. Arises from the superior margin of the celiac axis and can be seen for only 1 or 2 cm (see Figs. 21-1 and 21-2); supplies the stomach.

Popliteal Artery and Vein. Can be seen posterior to the femoral and tibial condyles running alongside each other (see Fig. 46-1). The popliteal arteries are approximately 1 cm in diameter.

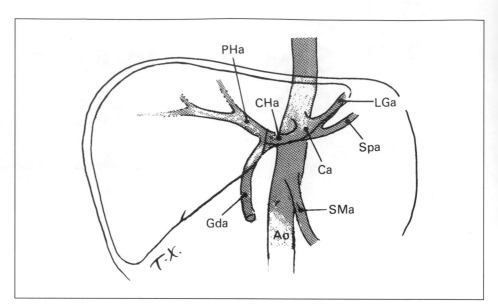

FIGURE 21-2. The vessel leaving the aorta closest to the diaphragm is the celiac artery. This vessel is a 1- to 2-cm trunk that bifurcates into the splenic and hepatic arteries. The hepatic artery again bifurcates into the proper hepatic artery and gastroduodenal artery. The superior mesenteric artery arises from the anterior surface of the aorta at a level just inferior to the celiac artery. The less frequently visualized left gastric artery originates from the celiac artery.

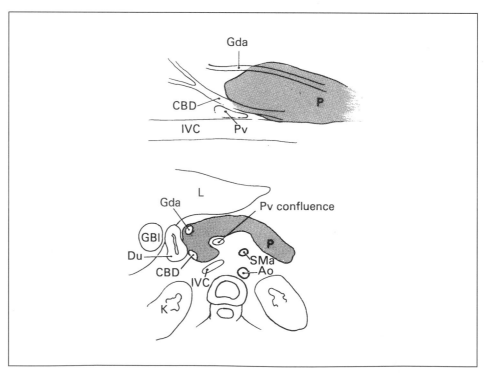

FIGURE 21-3. The gastroduodenal artery outlines the antero-lateral margin of the head of the pancreas, whereas the common bile duct marks the postero-lateral margin. (**A**) Longitudinal scan. (**B**) Transverse scan.

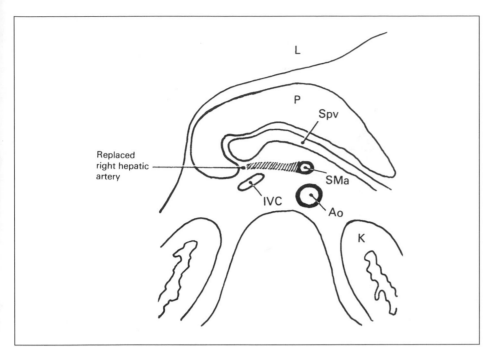

FIGURE 21-4. At the level of the splenic vein and pancreas, a normal variant can sometimes be visualized. The replaced right hepatic artery originates from the superior mesenteric artery to supply the liver.

Renal Arteries (Right and Left). Originate from the abdominal aorta at about the level of the superior mesenteric artery (see Fig. 21-1); the right renal artery runs posterior to the inferior vena cava. They supply the kidney, adrenals, and ureters and are often best seen when the patient is in the appropriate decubitus position.

Replaced Right Hepatic Artery. A variant hepatic arterial supply originating from the superior mesenteric artery (Fig. 21-4).

Splenic Artery. Originates from the celiac trunk (see Figs. 21-1, 21-2, and 21-5). Supplies the pancreas, spleen, stomach, and greater omentum and runs superior to the body and tail of the pancreas throughout most of its course. It is a quite tortuous vessel and may be difficult to visualize completely on one section.

Superior Mesenteric Artery. Originates from the anterior abdominal aorta just below the celiac axis and runs parallel to the aorta (Fig. 21-5; see also Figs. 21-1 to 21-4). Supplies the small bowel, cecum, ascending colon, and part of the transverse colon, and is a major landmark for localization of the pancreas.

FIGURE 21-5. Oblique view, showing the relationship of the portal vein, inferior vena cava, and aorta to the kidneys and gallbladder. The major branches of the portal vein, hepatic artery, and common hepatic duct in relationship to the porta hepatis are shown.

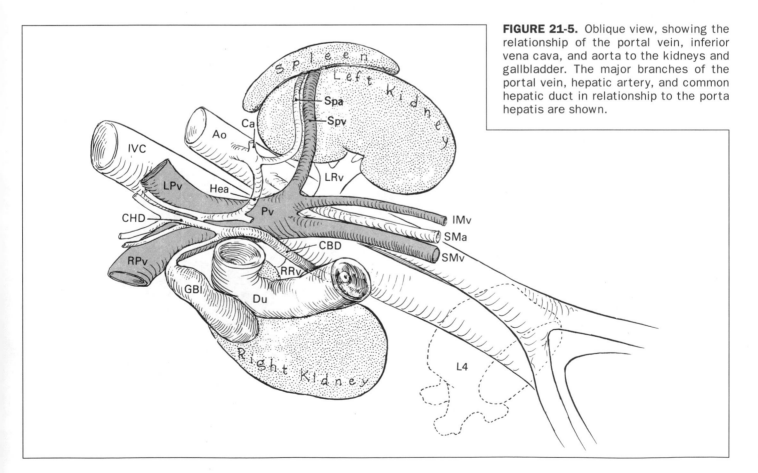

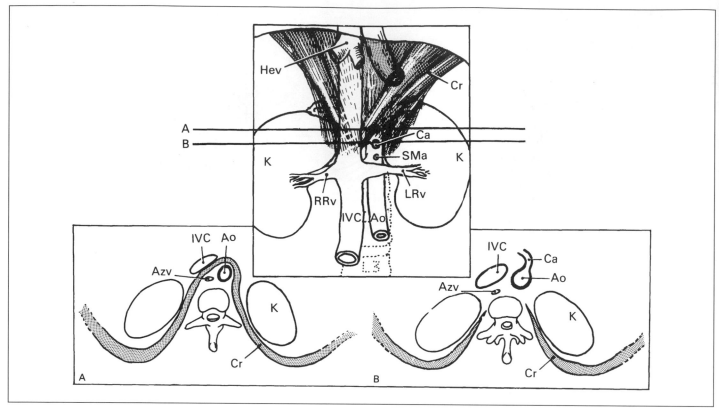

FIGURE 21-6. The crus of the diaphragm can be visualized anterior to the aorta above the level of the celiac artery. Below that level it extends along the lateral aspects of the vertebral columns only. (**A**) A transverse section at a higher level shows the crus posterior to the inferior vena cava and anterior to the aorta. The infrequently visualized azygos vein is seen posterior to the crus. (**B**) At a lower level, transversely, the crus is seen only at the lateral vertebral margins extending posteriorly.

VEINS

Azygos Vein. Lies posterior to the inferior vena cava and is not usually seen unless the patient has congestive heart failure or portal hypertension (Fig. 21-7).

Collaterals. Vessels that develop when portal vein pressure is increased (e.g., by thrombosis) (see Fig. 21-6). Collaterals are seen in the region of the pancreas, around the esophagogastric junction (anterior to the upper portion of the aorta), and in the porta hepatis (Fig. 21-7).

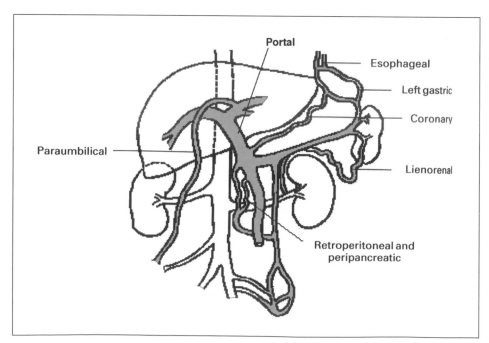

FIGURE 21-7. Diagram showing some of the collateral routes established when portal hypertension exists. The paraesophageal, left gastric, coronary, paraumbilical, lienorenal, retroperitoneal, and peripancreatic collaterals are demonstrated.

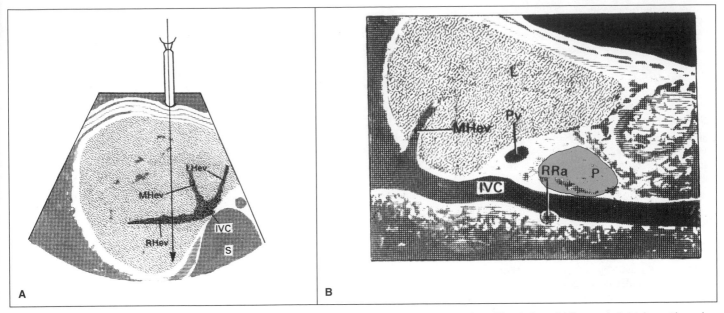

FIGURE 21-8. Hepatic veins. (**A**) Transverse view, using a slightly cephalad angulation. The left, middle, and right hepatic veins can be imaged as they empty into the inferior vena cava just beneath the right diaphragm. (**B**) Longitudinal view. The middle hepatic vein is shown as it empties into the inferior vena cava at the level of the right diaphragm. The main branch of the portal vein is seen in its extrahepatic location just superior to the head of the pancreas. The right renal artery is visualized posterior to the inferior vena cava.

Confluence. The junction of the superior mesenteric vein, splenic vein, and portal vein (see Figs. 21-5 and 21-9).

Coronary Vein. Connects the splenic vein to the region of the esophagus (see Fig. 21-7). Can be seen in only 10 percent to 20 percent of normal people, and measures less than 4 mm. Dilates in portal hypertension.

Femoral Veins. Lie medial to the femoral arteries in the groin and are larger than the arteries. Normally compress easily and do not pulsate. Can be traced along the medial aspect of the thigh toward the popliteal fossa (Figs. 45-2 and 45-3).

Hepatic Veins. Drain the liver and empty into the inferior vena cava just below the diaphragm (Figs. 21-8 and 21-9; see also Fig. 21-14). They have poorly defined borders and branch away from the diaphragm. There are three main veins, of which two, the left and the middle, have a common trunk into the inferior vena cava.

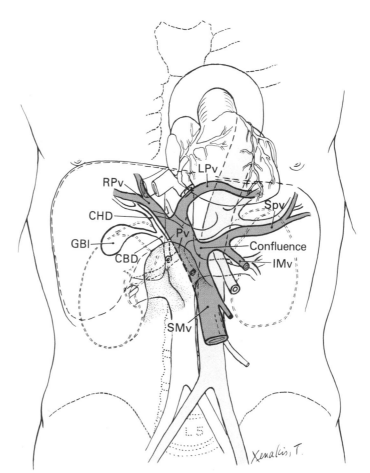

FIGURE 21-9. The splenic vein and superior mesenteric vein join (at the confluence) to form the main portal vein. The portal vein then branches into the liver, forming the left portal vein and the right portal vein.

Inferior Mesenteric Vein. Vein of highly variable size (see Fig. 21-9). It is usually small and runs to the left of the superior mesenteric vein to join the splenic vein.

Inferior Vena Cava. Returns blood from the lower half of the body and enters the right atrium of the heart (see Figs. 21-5, 21-6, and 21-8B). There is a marked change in caliber with respiration (Fig. 21-10).

Paraumbilical Vein. Not normally visible but can be seen in portal hypertension as a sonolucent center in the ligamentum teres (Fig. 21-7).

Portal System. Composed of the superior and inferior mesenteric veins, splenic vein, and portal vein.

Portal Vein. Collects blood from the digestive tract and empties into the liver (see Fig. 21-9). Formed by the junction of the splenic vein and the superior mesenteric vein. A large left branch supplies the left lobe of the liver (see Fig. 21-9). The right portal vein has a major branch coming off just superior to the gallbladder (Fig. 21-11). Portal veins have echogenic borders and branch away from the porta hepatis.

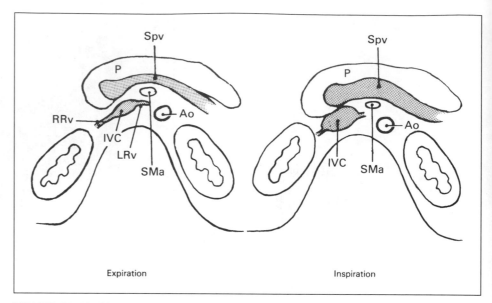

FIGURE 21-10. Venous structures should dilate at the end of deep inspiration or Valsalva's maneuver. This can help confirm the venous nature of the vessels or perhaps to enlarge the vein to make it easier to image.

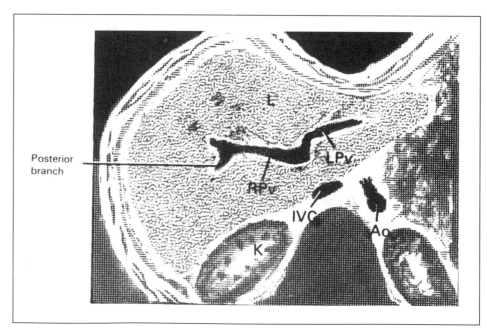

FIGURE 21-11. Transverse view within the liver. The portal vein branches into the left and right portal veins. The right vein again bifurcates the posterior branch supplying the posterior right lobe of the liver.

Renal Veins. Drain the kidneys and empty into the inferior vena cava (Fig. 21-12; see also Figs. 21-5 and 21-6). The left is much longer than the right and may be dilated before it passes between the superior mesenteric artery and the aorta, a condition that should not be confused with adenopathy.

Splenic Vein. Collects blood from the spleen and part of the stomach (see Figs. 21-4, 21-5, and 21-9). It runs posterior to the middle of the pancreas to join the superior mesenteric vein, forming the portal vein, and is a pancreatic landmark.

Superior Mesenteric Vein. Drains the cecum, transverse and sigmoid colons, and small bowel (see Figs. 21-5, 21-9, and 21-12). Ascends in the mesenteric sheath just anterior to the aorta to join the splenic vein at the "confluence" behind the head of the pancreas. It too is a pancreatic landmark.

OTHER LINEAR STRUCTURES

Crus of the Diaphragm. A tubular muscular structure seen anterior to the aorta and posterior to the inferior vena cava above the level of the celiac axis and superior mesenteric artery (see Fig. 21-6).

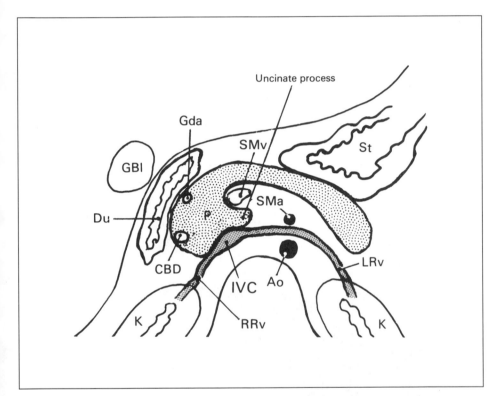

FIGURE 21-12. Many vascular structures can be visualized on a transverse section in the midabdomen. The inferior vena cava gives rise to the right and left renal veins; the latter passes between the aorta and the superior mesenteric artery. Anterior to the inferior vena cava lies the superior mesenteric vein. The pancreas can be imaged anterior to these vessels. The gastroduodenal artery and the common bile duct assist in outlining the lateral margin of the head of the pancreas. When empty, the walls of the antrum of the stomach and the duodenum are seen as echo-free linear structures. The gallbladder is lateral to the duodenum.

Fissure Between the Right and Left Lobes of the Liver (Main Lobar Fissure). Seen only between the gallbladder and the right portal vein (Fig. 21-14).

Hilum of the Spleen. Echogenic structure in the center of the medial border of the spleen; it represents the site of vessel entrance.

Ligamentum Teres. Echogenic structure in the left lobe of the liver (a remnant of the ductus venosum) in which the umbilical vein runs (see Figs. 21-13 and 21-14).

Ligamentum Venosum. Echogenic line anterior to the caudate lobe of the liver (see Figs. 21-13 and 21-14).

Porta Hepatis. Echogenic region surrounding the portal veins, hepatic artery, and common bile duct where all these structures enter the liver.

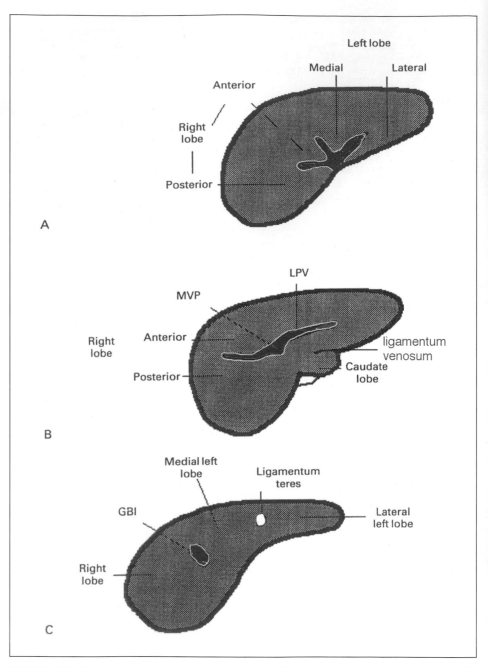

FIGURE 21-13. Series of transverse views of the liver to show vascular supply at different levels. Level **A** is taken close to the diaphragm and shows the hepatic veins. Level **B** is taken in midliver and shows the left and right portal veins. Level **C** is taken at the level of the gallbladder. Venous structures should dilate at the end of deep inspiration.

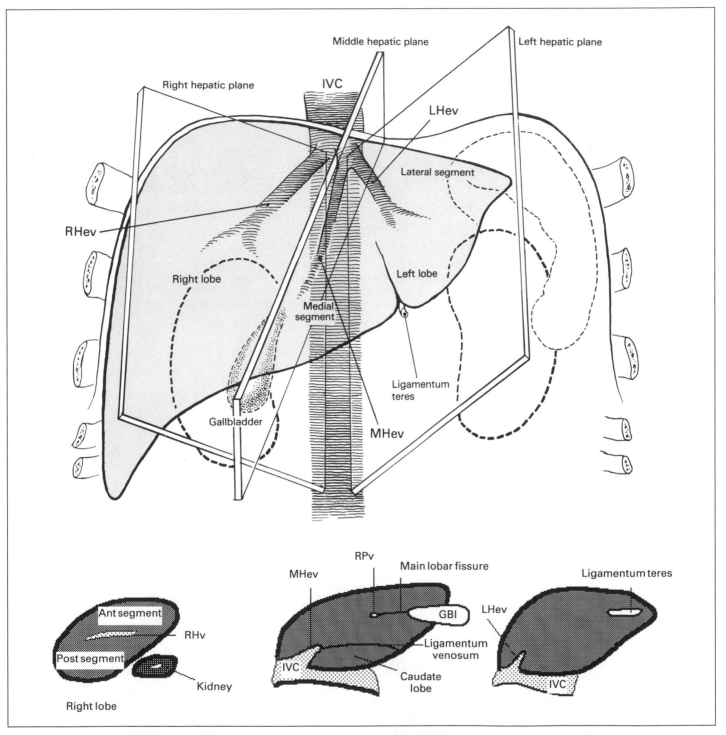

FIGURE 21-14. Overall view of the upper abdomen showing the liver, spleen, gall-bladder, and kidneys. The hepatic veins represent the divisions between the lobes and segments of the liver. The middle hepatic vein divides the right and left lobes of the liver. The left hepatic vein separates the medial and lateral segments of the left lobe; the right hepatic vein separates the anterior and posterior segments of the right lobe of the liver. The gallbladder represents the inferior end of the separation between right and left lobes of the liver; the ligamentum teres represents the inferior end of the separation between the medial and lateral segments of the left lobe.

ANATOMY

Gut

The gut has three principal manifestations (Fig. 21-15).

Empty Gut

When the gut is empty an echogenic center is surrounded by a thin sonolucent ring (e.g., the antrum of the stomach usually has this appearance), which should not exceed 4 mm in thickness.

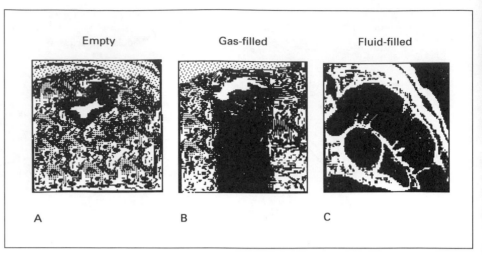

FIGURE 21-15. Gut can have a number of different manifestations. (**A**) When empty, there is an echo-free wall around an echogenic center. (**B**) When gas-filled, there is acoustic shadowing. (**C**) When fluid-filled, one may be able to make out the haustral markings of the colon or valvulae conniventes of the small bowel in the wall of the fluid-filled bowel.

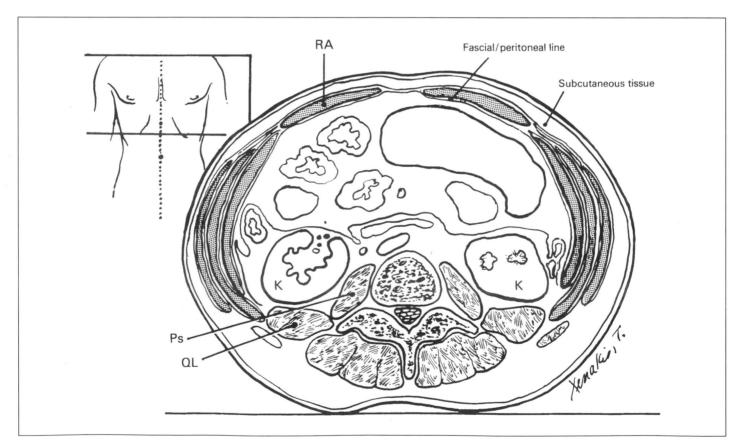

FIGURE 21-16. The rectus abdominis muscles lie on either side of the midline, anteriorly deep to the subcutaneous tissues. The psoas and quadratus lumborum muscles are shown in transverse section.

Gas-Filled Gut

When the gut is gas filled, acoustic shadowing is present. The shadow has an irregular border, a poorly defined source, and some internal echoes, or, alternatively, it forms a banding pattern (see Chapter 53).

Fluid-Filled Gut

When the gut is filled with fluid, sausage-shaped, fluid-filled structures are seen. Sometimes one can make out the valvulae conniventes of the small bowel or the haustral markings of the large bowel if there is a large amount of fluid in distended loops of bowel.

Muscles

Some large muscles form a sort of framework on which the intra-abdominal structures lie.

Psoas Muscles

The psoas muscles lie alongside the spine and join the iliacus muscles in the pelvis (Fig. 21-16; see also Fig. 21-17).

Quadratus Lumborum

The quadratus lumborum muscles form the posterior wall of the abdomen behind the kidneys (Fig 21-17; see also Fig. 12-16).

Internal and External Oblique Muscles

The internal and external oblique muscles form the anterior and lateral walls of the abdomen.

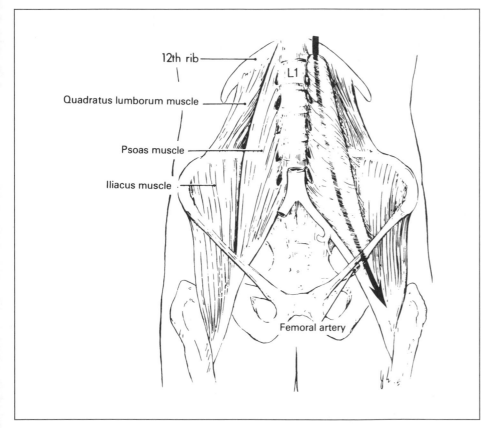

FIGURE 21-17. Diagram showing the normal location of the psoas, iliacus, and quadratus lumborum muscles.

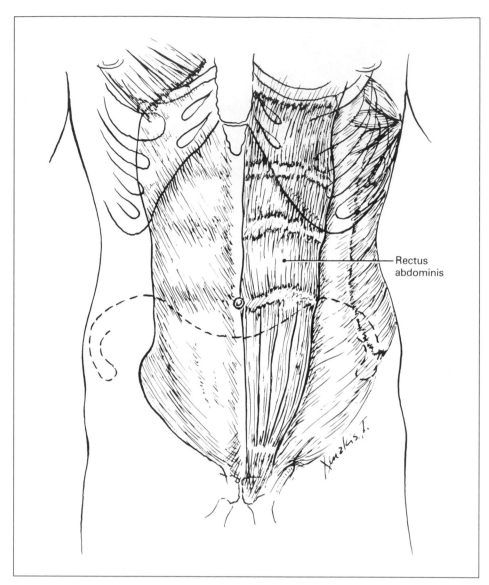

FIGURE 21-18. Diagram showing the location of the rectus abdominal muscles.

SELECTED READING

Carlsen, E. N., and Filly, R. A. Newer ultrasonic anatomy in the upper abdomen. *Journal of Clinical Ultrasound* 4:85, 1976.

Chafetz, N., and Filly, R. A. Portal and hepatic veins: Accuracy of margin echoes for distinguishing intrahepatic vessels. *Radiology* 130: 725–728, 1979.

Curry, R. A., and Tompkins, B. B. *Ultrasonography: An Introduction to Normal Structural and Functional Anatomy.* Philadelphia: WB Saunders, 1995.

Filly, R. A., and Laing, F. C. Anatomic variation of portal venous anatomy in the porta hepatis: Ultrasonographic evaluation. *Journal of Clinical Ultrasound* 6:73–142, 1978.

Heap, S. W. The cross-sectional anatomy of the vessels and ducts of the upper abdomen. *Australas Radiol* 24:32, 1980.

Netter, F. H. *Digestive System: Upper Digestive Tract. Part I, Vol. 3. CIBA (The Collection of Medical Illustrations).* New York: CIBA Pharmaceuticals, 1987.

Ralls, P. W., Quinn, M. F., and Rogers, W. Sonographic anatomy of the hepatic artery. *AJR* 136:1059–1063, 1981.

Sample, W. F. Techniques for improved delineation of normal anatomy of the upper abdomen and high retroperitoneum with grayscale ultrasound. *Radiology* 124:197–202, 1977.

Rectus Sheath

The rectus sheath muscles lie along the anterior aspect of the abdomen and are an important site of hematoma and abscess development (Fig. 21-18; see also Fig. 21-16).

Pelvic Musculature

See Chapter 7.

✳PITFALLS

1. Excessive pressure with the transducer can collapse the walls of vessels so that they become invisible.
2. Expiration views may not allow visualization of vessels such as the inferior vena cava that can be seen on end inspiration.
3. Catheters may be confused with pathology. They are seen as linear parallel echoes or echogenic areas with shadowing.

EPIGASTRIC PAIN (UPPER ABDOMINAL PAIN)

22

Pancreatitis?

ROGER C. SANDERS, MARY MCGRATH LING

SONOGRAM ABBREVIATIONS

Ao	Aorta
Ca	Celiac artery, axis
CBD	Common bile duct
CD	Common duct
CHD	Common hepatic duct
Du	Duodenum
GBl	Gallbladder
Gda	Gastroduodenal artery
Hea	Hepatic artery
IVC	Inferior vena cava
K	Kidney
L	Liver
LRv	Left renal vein
P	Pancreas
PD	Pancreatic duct
Pv	Portal vein
RRv	Right renal vein
SMa	Superior mesenteric artery
SMv	Superior mesenteric vein
Sp	Spleen
Spa	Splenic artery
Spv	Splenic vein
St	Stomach

KEY WORDS

Amylase. See *Serum Amylase.*

Epigastrium. Upper abdominal region overlying the area of the stomach; adj., *epigastric.*

Hemorrhagic pancreatitis. Form of inflammation of the pancreas associated with much bleeding into the pancreas.

Hyperlipidemia. Congenital condition in which there are elevated fat levels that cause pancreatitis.

Ileus. Dilated loops of bowel that do not show any evidence of peristalsis. Ileus is associated with many abdominal problems (e.g., pancreatitis, sickle cell crisis, prolonged bowel obstruction).

Pancreatic Ascites. If a pancreatic pseudocyst bursts, the fluid pools in the same sites as ascites but contains dangerous enzymes. This is a very rare event.

Pancreatic Pseudocyst. Accumulation of pancreatic juice within or outside the pancreas.

Pancreatitis. Inflammation of the pancreas.

    Acute. Edematous swelling of the pancreas with severe upper abdominal pain.

    Chronic. Chronic changes due to repeated attacks with resultant fibrosis, stone formation, and permanent damage.

    Hemorrhagic. Greatly swollen pancreas with inflammation and bleeding.

    Phlegmonous. Very severe form of pancreatitis in which the whole pancreas becomes swollen and full of fluid; there is spread of the inflammatory process into the neighboring structures.

Peptic Ulcer Disease (PUD). An ulcer of the stomach or duodenum.

Serum Amylase. An enzyme that is elevated at some point during the clinical course of acute pancreatitis. It may also be elevated in other conditions such as penetrating peptic ulcer.

Uncinate Process. Portion of the head of the pancreas that lies posterior to the superior mesenteric vein.

Urinary Amylase. Enzyme that remains elevated longer than serum amylase in patients with acute pancreatitis.

◆≫ THE CLINICAL PROBLEM

Epigastric pain, whether acute or chronic, is frequently caused by peptic ulcer or pancreatitis. Acute cholecystitis and hepatic disorders such as abscesses may also be characterized by epigastric pain (see Chapter 24). A rarer cause of epigastric pain is an aortic aneurysm (see Chapter 29). Uncomplicated peptic ulcer has no useful sonographic features, but fortunately all the other diseases do.

Acute Pancreatitis

Alcoholics and patients with blunt mid-abdominal trauma, gallbladder stones, and congenital conditions such as hyperlipidemia are predisposed to the development of acute pancreatitis. Pain can be so intense that exploratory surgery is often considered, although the best treatment is nonsurgical. A sonographic diagnosis of pancreatitis may prevent unnecessary surgery.

The serum amylase level is commonly elevated in acute pancreatitis, although this finding is not specific for this condition. Because pancreatitis may be associated with ileus, gas may be present in large quantities. Acute pancreatitis may lead to the following complications: (1) pancreatic pseudocyst; (2) pancreatic abscess; (3) pancreatic ascites; or (4) common bile duct obstruction.

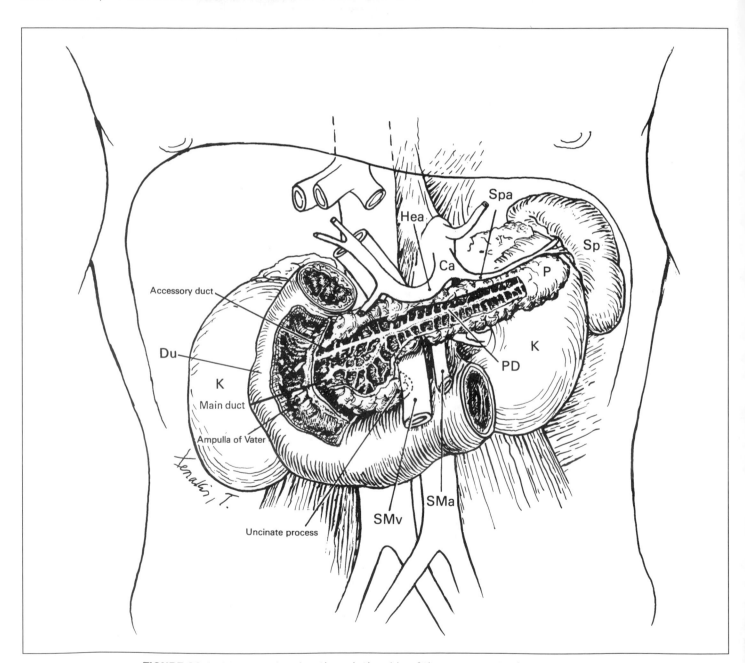

FIGURE 22-1. Diagram showing the relationship of the pancreas to the celiac artery, duodenum, kidneys, and spleen. Note that the pancreatic duct runs through the center of the pancreas to the papilla (ampilla) of Vater. The splenic artery lies superior to the pancreas.

Although the sonographic findings in acute pancreatitis may be disappointingly normal, a baseline sonogram is still worthwhile so complications such as a pseudocyst may be recognized.

Computed tomography has proved to be superior to ultrasound in the average patient when the pancreas is the focus of investigation, but ultrasound is preferred in children and in lean patients who have little abdominal and retroperitoneal fat.

Chronic Pancreatitis

Patients with chronic pancreatitis present with pain similar to that which occurs in acute pancreatitis, but the pain is more persistent and not as severe. The condition occurs most frequently in alcoholics after multiple episodes of acute pancreatitis. In addition, the liver may be a poor acoustic window owing to fatty changes.

Pseudocysts

Fluid collections (commonly termed *pseudocysts*) occur frequently with pancreatitis. These collections are the result of the pancreatic edema that develops in pancreatitis. Such collections may breech their thin covering owing to autodigestion of the pancreas and neighboring organs by enzymes. Collections are commonly found within the following structures:

1. Lesser sac
2. Anterior pararenal space
3. Liver
4. Spleen
5. Mediastinum
6. Mesentery

Ultrasound can be useful for detection of pseudocysts, serial follow-up of the evolution of a collection, and diagnostic aspiration or therapeutic percutaneous drainage of a collection.

Pancreatic Carcinoma

A history of weight loss, chronic severe abdominal pain, and possible epigastric mass suggests carcinoma of the pancreas. Except for lesions involving the ampulla and common duct (see Chapter 25), symptoms are of such late onset that curative surgical treatment is almost always impossible owing to local invasion or metastatic spread.

Because this grim disease is notorious for lymphatic and hematogenous spread, which has usually occurred by the time of diagnosis, the sonographer should not only evaluate the biliary tree but also search for enlarged lymph nodes and metastases to the liver. Ultrasound can be used to accomplish the following:

1. Detect the presence of a mass, particularly if the distal pancreatic duct is dilated
2. Delineate the size of the tumor
3. Establish the degree of local and metastatic spread
4. Guide percutaneous biopsy of a mass

Pancreas Divisum

Pancreas divisum is characterized by failure of the ventral and dorsal portions of the pancreas to fuse so they are both drained by separate ducts that do not communicate.

One duct can be selectively obstructed and cause pain. This unusual condition is seen in young women. There are pharmacologic tests with secretin, a hormone that stimulates pancreatic secretions, that can be used in association with ultrasound to help make this diagnosis.

ANATOMY

The pancreas is a long, thin gland that lies posterior to the stomach and the left lobe of the liver. It is divided into the head, neck, and body and a tail that usually abuts on the spleen.

An understanding of pancreatic anatomy is based upon the relationship of the pancreas to the vessels that surround the pancreas (Figs. 22-1 and 22-2) (see Chapter 21).

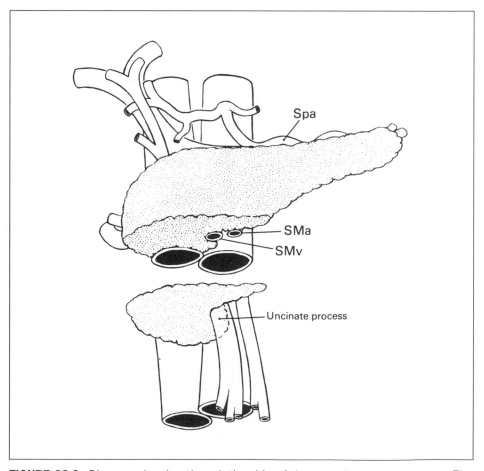

FIGURE 22-2. Diagram showing the relationship of the vessels to the pancreas. The exploded view through the uncinate process shows the relationship of the superior mesenteric artery and the vein to the uncinate process.

Vessels and Ducts

Superior Mesenteric Vein

The superior mesenteric vein is located posterior to the neck of the pancreas and anterior to the uncinate process (Fig. 22-3; see also Figs. 22-1 and 22-2). This is a valuable landmark because its anatomic relationship to the pancreas is a constant one.

Inferior Vena Cava

The inferior vena cava lies posterior to the head of the pancreas in most people (see Figs. 22-2 and 22-3).

Splenic and Hepatic Arteries

The splenic artery traverses the superior margin of most of the pancreas (the body and tail) to enter the splenic hilum (see Figs. 22-1, 22-2, and 22-3C). This vessel is usually quite tortuous. The hepatic artery courses to the right from the celiac axis and enters the liver.

Splenic Vein

Located posterior to the center of the body and the tail of the pancreas, the splenic vein joins the superior mesenteric vein to form the portal vein (see Figs. 22-2 and 22-3B and C).

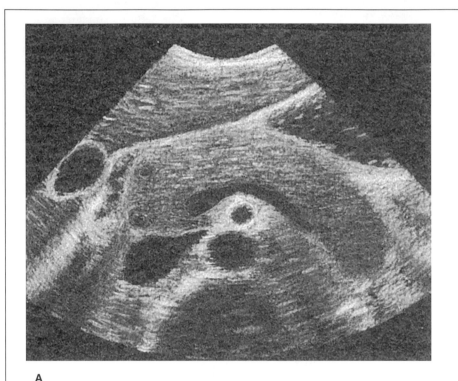

A

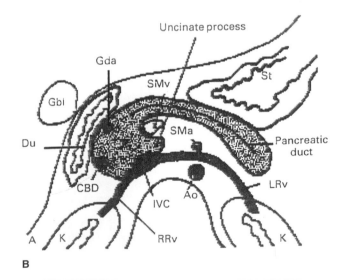

B

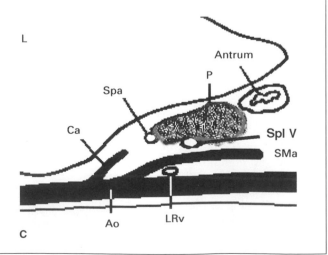

C

FIGURE 22-3. (**A**) Diagrammatic view of the transverse section of the pancreas showing the common bile duct and gastroduodenal artery. (**B**) Transverse section. The uncinate process lies between the superior mesenteric vein and the inferior vena cava. The gallbladder, duodenum, and pancreas form a constant threesome. The superior mesenteric vein lies medial to the head of the pancreas. The gastroduodenal artery and common bile duct lie in the lateral aspect of the head of the pancreas. (**C**) Diagram showing the relationship of the pancreas to the splenic vein, splenic artery, and superior mesenteric artery.

Superior Mesenteric Artery

The superior mesenteric artery is visible on transverse views as a sonolucent dot surrounded by an echogenic area posterior to the body of the pancreas (see Figs. 22-2 and 22-3). It runs anterior to the aorta and is not in contact with the uncinate lobe of the pancreas. The superior mesenteric artery originates approximately at the level of the pancreas.

Left Renal Vein

The left renal vein runs approximately 1 cm posterior to the body of the pancreas between the superior mesenteric artery and the aorta (see Fig. 22-3).

Common Bile Duct

The common bile duct runs in the posterior lateral portion of the pancreatic head (Figs. 22-4 and 22-5; see also Fig. 22-3).

Gastroduodenal Artery

The gastroduodenal artery, a branch of the hepatic artery, lies in the anterior lateral portion of the head of the pancreas (see Figs. 22-3 and 22-4) and can sometimes be seen coursing caudally on a longitudinal scan.

Pancreatic Duct

The pancreatic duct (Wirsung duct), which has a maximum normal diameter of 2 mm, extends through the pancreas. An accessory duct may also be seen (see Figs. 22-1 and 22-3). The duct may change in size over the course of the exam and can be as large as 3 to 4 mm shortly after a meal.

Ampulla/Papilla of Vater

The entrance of the pancreatic duct and the common bile duct into the duodenum is called the ampulla of Vater (see Fig. 22-1). As it enters the duodenum, a small bump called the papilla of Vater is formed.

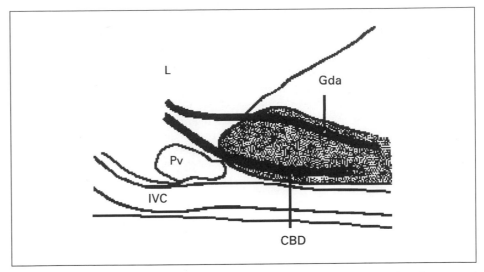

FIGURE 22-4. Longitudinal section through head of the pancreas showing the normal location of the gastroduodenal artery and common bile duct.

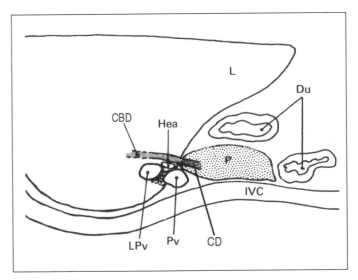

FIGURE 22-5. Diagram of the structures in the porta hepatis showing the common duct (CD) passing anterior to the hepatic artery and the main and left portal veins passing into the head of the pancreas. The distal position of the common bile duct is termed "common duct" because the junction of the cystic duct and the common hepatic duct cannot usually be seen and this anatomically defines the site of origin of the common bile duct.

Relationship to Other Organs

The relationship of the gallbladder, duodenum, and head of the pancreas to other organs remains constant. The gallbladder lies to the right of the third part of the duodenum, which in turn lies to the right of the head of the pancreas. The pancreatic head may lie to the left of the inferior vena cava. The tail of the pancreas is of variable length and may not reach the splenic hilum. The antrum of the stomach lies anterior and somewhat inferior to the pancreas.

Although the pancreas usually has an oblique axis with the head inferior to the tail, the axis is variable and the gland is often horizontal. As a rule, the left lobe of the liver acts as an ultrasonic window for the pancreas (Figs. 22-6 and 22-7).

Texture

The pancreas in most adults is a little more echogenic than the liver. In older people the pancreas may be especially echogenic owing to fatty changes. In fact, the normal pancreas in older people is so echogenic that it is difficult to distinguish from the surrounding retroperitoneal fat. In children, on the other hand, the normal pancreas may be less echogenic than the liver.

◣ TECHNIQUE

Demonstration of the pancreas can present a challenge even to the best sonographer.

Routine Technique

Mapping the pancreas in the longitudinal plane will reveal the oblique direction of the pancreas. Be sure to demonstrate all borders of the pancreas sagittally in at least three views. Find the pancreas anterior to the aorta and to the inferior vena cava to get an idea of its axis, and then direct the transducer obliquely along this axis to show the vascular landmarks (see Figs. 22-2 and 22-6). Angling in a caudal fashion through the liver is desirable. It will show the vascular landmarks in a consistent fashion and will allow comparison with the liver for texture assessment (see Fig. 22-7C). High-frequency transducers (5.0 or 7.5 MHz) may be necessary to scan a superficially situated pancreas.

Gas Problems

If there is gas overlying the pancreas, water in the stomach can provide an acoustic window for the pancreas. Instruct the patient to drink at least 12 ounces of water, preferably in the right-side-up decubitus position. Allow sufficient time to eliminate air bubbles (2–5 minutes). Begin imaging the pancreatic tail through the fundus of the stomach in the right-side-up position. Next, roll the patient supine, allowing water to fill the stomach, visualizing the pancreatic body. Finally, turn the patient left side up for adequate visualization of the pancreatic head using the distended gastric antrum and c-loop of the duodenum as an acoustic window (see Fig. 22-7). Fat may be administered as for a gallbladder examination (e.g., Neocholex) to prevent peristalsis and stomach emptying. Water is given immediately after fat administration. Glucagon can be used instead of fat.

Performing the scan with the patient in an erect position may increase the chances of demonstrating the pancreas because the liver descends from beneath the ribs and can be used as an acoustic window. Placing the patient in the right posterior oblique or left posterior oblique position may also shift bowel gas away from the pancreas. Angulation of the transducer in a transverse plane either cephalad or caudad may circumvent pockets of gas (see Fig. 22-7C).

Substances such as methylcellulose are being commercially tested as ultrasonic contrast media. When they are ingested, they remain in the bowel and act as an acoustic window to see the pancreas and gut wall.

Pancreas Versus Duodenum

Watching for peristalsis is useful in distinguishing the bowel from a mass, particularly in the region of the head of the pancreas where the duodenum and the pancreas can look very similar.

Do not administer fat, but turn the patient onto the right-side-up position so the bulb fills with water.

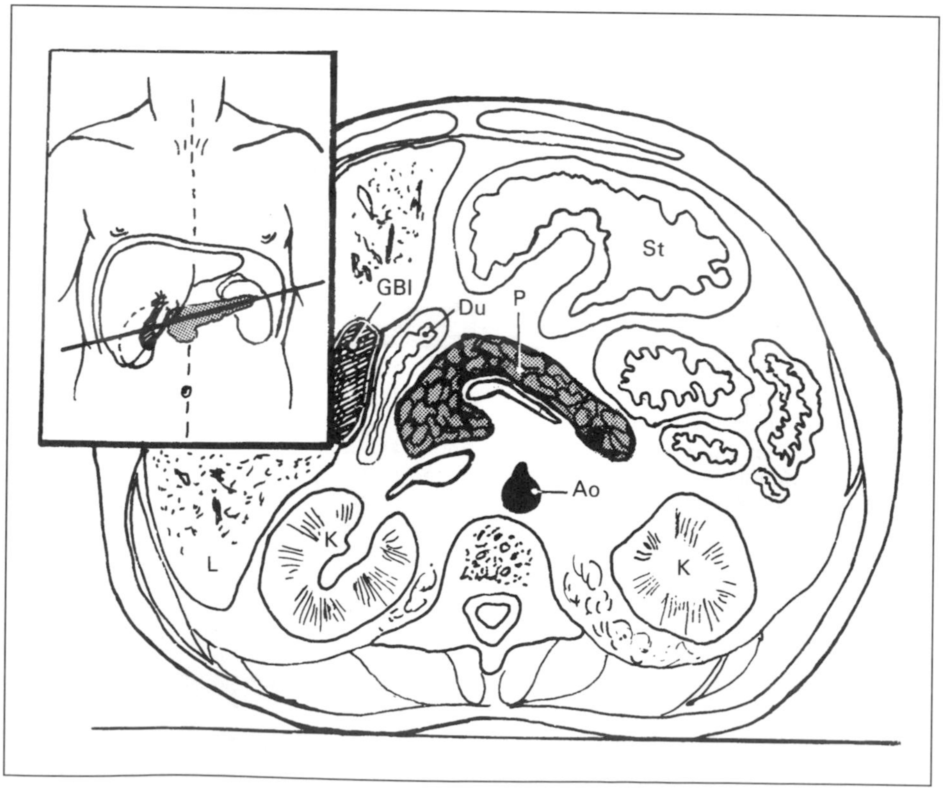

FIGURE 22-6. Transverse section showing the usual axis of the pancreas in relation to the duodenum, gallbladder, kidneys, and stomach.

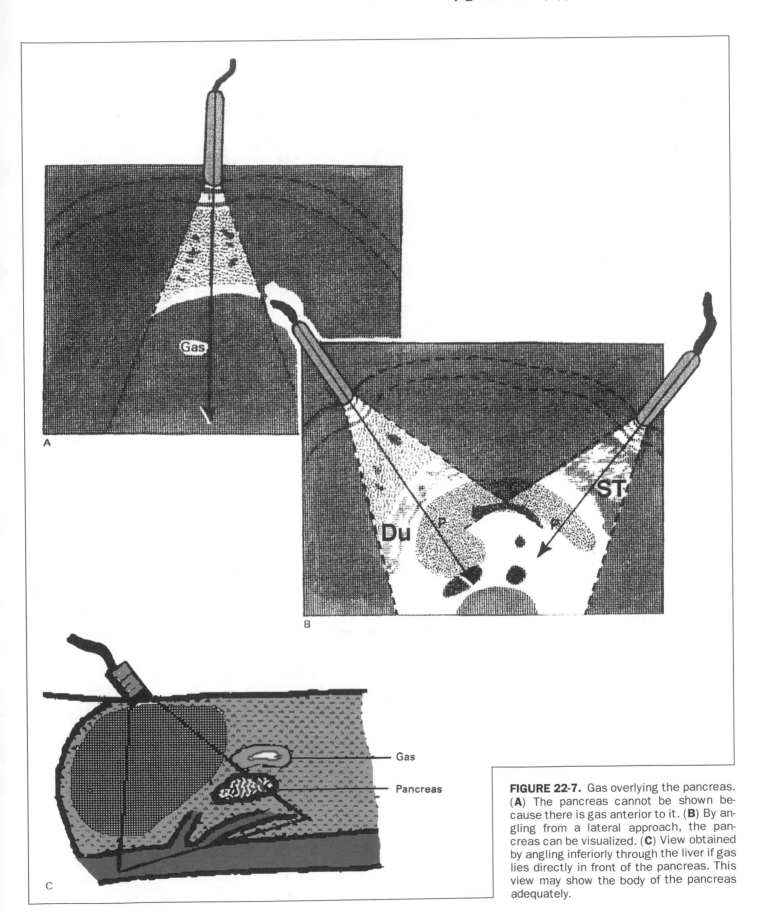

FIGURE 22-7. Gas overlying the pancreas. (**A**) The pancreas cannot be shown because there is gas anterior to it. (**B**) By angling from a lateral approach, the pancreas can be visualized. (**C**) View obtained by angling inferiorly through the liver if gas lies directly in front of the pancreas. This view may show the body of the pancreas adequately.

Possible Pseudocyst Versus Stomach

Filling the stomach with tap water will allow the sonographer to distinguish the stomach from a cystic mass such as a pseudocyst in the left upper quadrant. Tap water will be echogenic at first owing to microbubbles but will later become echo-free. When pancreatitis is suspected, the patient often has a nasogastric tube in position and cannot be given fluids. However, water may be injected through the nasogastric tube and later withdrawn after optimal views of the pancreas have been obtained.

Displaying the Pancreatic Tail

The left-side-up position looking through the kidney should be routine when the sonographer is searching for a pancreatic pseudocyst, because pseudocysts will slip into the available space, which is often obscured by the stomach. The tail of the pancreas may also be demonstrated in the prone position using the spleen and left kidney as a window.

 PATHOLOGY

Acute Pancreatitis

During an initial attack of acute pancreatitis, the findings include the following:

1. *Focal tenderness.* The pancreas may have a normal appearance.
2. *Textural changes.* The pancreas is less echogenic than normal.
3. *Enlargement* (Fig. 22-8). May be focal or diffuse. A width of more than 3 cm for the head and tail is considered indicative of enlargement owing to edema or inflammation. Smaller increases in size can indicate pancreatitis if the pancreas was originally diminutive. The shape appears swollen with rounding off of the borders. However, no changes may be seen in an atrophic pancreas. The pancreas may be massively enlarged if phlegmonous or hemorrhagic pancreatitis is present.
4. *Focal enlargement.* Focal enlargement is possible with local widening and sonolucency in focal acute pancreatitis.

When acute pancreatitis is superimposed on chronic pancreatitis, ultrasonic changes may not be seen.

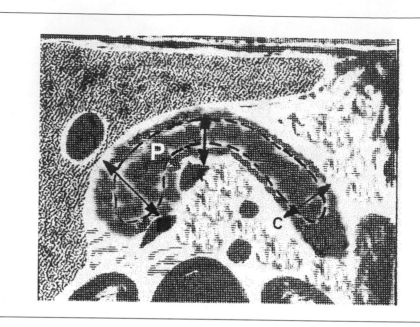

FIGURE 22-8. In pancreatitis the pancreas swells and becomes more sonolucent than usual. The dotted lines show the normal size of the pancreas; the arrows (**A**, **B**, **C**) show the increase that occurs with pancreatitis. The pancreas is normally considered to have an upper size limit of 1.5 cm at the level of the body and of 3 cm at the head and tail.

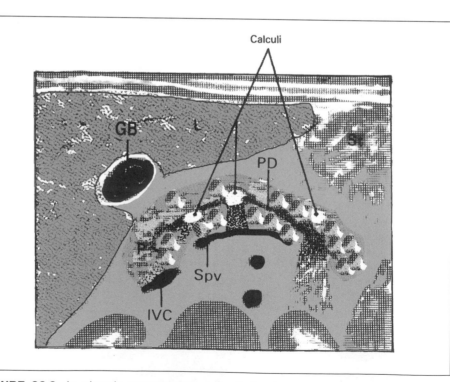

FIGURE 22-9. In chronic pancreatitis, calculi develop within the pancreas (some with acoustic shadowing), and the pancreatic duct enlarges. The outline of the pancreas is more irregular, and its overall echogenicity is increased.

Acute pancreatitis can be present with normal measurements if the pancreas was originally small.

Chronic Pancreatitis

See Figure 22-9. There are four ultrasonic features of chronic pancreatitis:

1. *Irregular pancreatic outline*
2. *Dilatation of the pancreatic duct* (over 2 mm)
3. *Calculi*, identified as small groups of dense echoes, often with acoustic shadowing
4. *Focal enlargement* with patchy groups of echoes; appearance can be similar to an uncinate mass

In the more advanced stages, there is a generalized decrease in the size of the pancreas with increased echogenicity because of fibrosis. Acute-on-chronic pancreatitis may show features of both conditions.

Pseudocyst

A pseudocyst usually appears as a circular, echo-free mass with good through transmission. The most common location is in the lesser sac anterior to the tail of the pancreas (Fig. 22-10). The head of the pancreas is the next most common site. Less frequently, pseudocysts may have internal echoes, fluid-fluid levels, or irregular borders, particularly when hemorrhage or infection is present.

Pseudocysts may be multiple and may dissect into neighboring structures, notably the liver, spleen, or mediastinum. Septation within a pseudocyst may be seen. Infection can occur but may not alter the sonographic pattern.

An effort should be made to see wall thickness—surgeons prefer a well-defined wall, but it is usually not visible. An immediate preprocedure scan is desirable because a pseudocyst may spontaneously rupture prior to drainage.

Pancreatic Cancer

Typically, there is a hypoechoic mass that is less echogenic than the surrounding pancreas in pancreatic cancer. The mass may be too small to cause changes in the pancreatic outline, but can be recognized by the irregular borders and a difference in acoustic texture (Fig. 22-11).

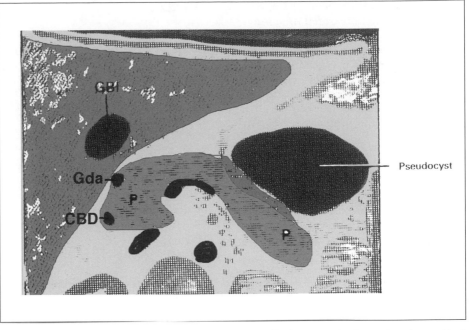

FIGURE 22-10. Pancreatic pseudocysts are usually large, echo-free structures that lie in the region of the lesser sac. They show good through transmission. They can lie in many other locations.

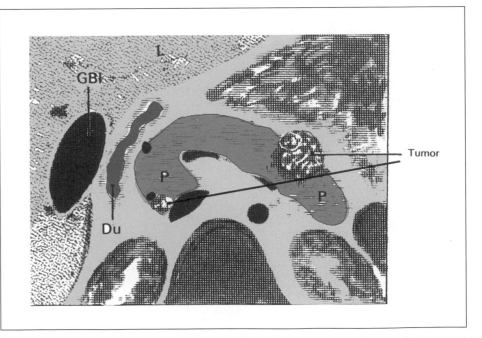

FIGURE 22-11. Pancreatic carcinomas are generally less echogenic than the normal pancreas, with irregular borders. They can develop anywhere in the pancreas, but when located in the pancreatic head, their presence soon becomes evident by causing biliary duct obstruction.

Often a mass in the head of the pancreas is better demonstrated on a longitudinal view since the caudal extent may be several centimeters below the splenic vein. Subtle cancers may involve the uncinate process, and therefore tend to be overlooked. Common bile duct obstruction or pancreatic duct obstruction is common with carcinoma of the pancreas.

Cystadenomas

Cystadenomas are rare neoplasms that may be benign or malignant and may be recognizable because they contain cysts. They may be confused with pancreatic pseudocysts. The microcystic form may present as a hypoechoic mass.

Islet Cell Tumors

Islet cell tumors are unusual and produce a hormone that causes hypoglycemic episodes. They can grow to a large size before clinical presentation if they do not produce hormones, and are generally echo-free.

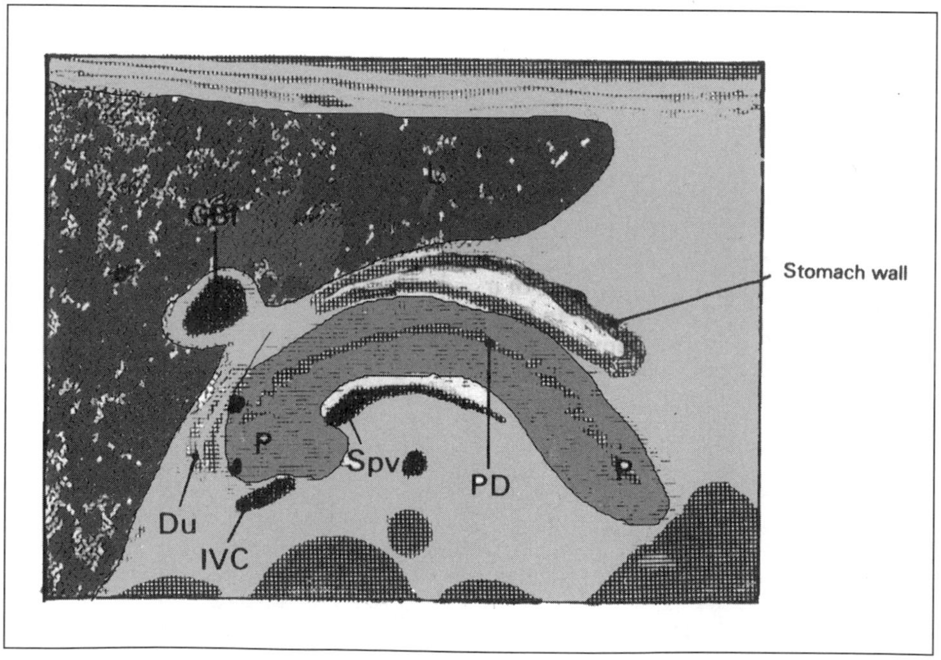

✴ PITFALLS

1. *Posterior wall of the stomach vs. pancreatic duct.* The posterior wall of the stomach can be mistaken for the pancreatic duct. However, the stomach wall can be traced around the entire outline of the stomach (Fig. 22-12).
2. *Fatty changes vs. chronic pancreatitis.* The pancreas becomes more echogenic with age owing to fatty changes. Do not confuse normal aging changes, where the outline remains smooth, with chronic pancreatitis, which causes an uneven pancreatic echogenicity. Echogenicity of the pancreas is hard to assess when the patient has an abnormal liver (e.g., fatty liver), since echogenicity assessment is based on comparison with the liver.
3. *Bowel vs. pseudocyst.* Cystic structures near the pancreas are not always pseudocysts. Make sure that the cystic structure is not a fluid-filled stomach or colon.

4. *Splenic artery vs. pancreatic duct.* The splenic artery may be confused with the pancreatic duct and occasionally runs through the center of the pancreas. Examine it with real-time and color Doppler to see if the apparent duct connects with the celiac axis and pulsates.
5. *Gallbladder vs. pseudocyst.* Confusion between a gallbladder and a pseudocyst may occur; a gallbladder will contract with fat administration, but a pseudocyst will not. Pseudocysts may develop where the gallbladder used to lie after cholecystectomy. Make sure the patient has had a cholecystectomy if you see a cyst in this area; remember scars from a laparoscopic cholecystectomy may not be evident.
6. *Duodenum vs. head of pancreas.* The duodenum may be mistaken for a mass in the head of the pancreas when the gut contents have similar texture to the pancreas. Using real-time, identify the location of the common duct and the gastroduodenal artery. Give the patient fluid by mouth to identify the duodenum.
7. *Pancreatic calcification vs. gut.* Calcifications in the pancreatic head and body may resemble air in the gut if one is not careful to follow landmarks and recognize borders between the pancreatic head and duodenum.
8. *Caudate lobe vs. pancreatic mass.* The caudate lobe may extend medially in a fashion that raises the question of a pancreatic neoplasm. Careful sonographic analysis will show that the caudate lobe connects to the liver and is separate from the pancreas.
9. *Uncinate process vs. pancreatic mass.* The uncinate process posterior to the superior mesenteric vein may be relatively large as a normal variant. A portion of duodenum may extend into this area, making one concerned about a pancreatic mass. Use water to highlight the duodenum.
10. *Fluid in colon vs. acute pancreatitis.* The transverse colon runs anterior to the pancreas, so fluid within the transverse colon can be mistaken for the pancreas.

FIGURE 22-12. The posterior wall of the stomach can be mistaken for a dilated pancreatic duct if the site of the pancreas is not carefully identified. The posterior wall of the stomach does not reach as far to the right as the pancreatic duct.

11. *Fluid in lesser sac vs. pancreatic duct.* When fluid accumulates primarily in the lesser sac, it can be mistaken for a massively dilated pancreatic duct. However, pancreatic tissue will not be seen on both sides of the supposed duct.

12. *Horseshoe kidney vs. pancreas.* The isthmus of a horseshoe kidney can resemble the body of the pancreas. It will be located at the lower level and will be directly adjacent to the aorta and inferior vena cava. The normal pancreas is separated from the aorta by a fat-filled space containing the mesenteric vessels.

 WHERE ELSE TO LOOK

1. If a *mass* in the head of the pancreas is noted, make sure that the common bile duct, intrahepatic ducts, gallbladder, and pancreatic duct are not obstructed and dilated.

2. A *mass* in the pancreas may be a carcinoma. Look for liver metastases and para-aortic or porta hepatis nodes.

3. If *pancreatitis* is found, look for the other stigmata of alcoholism or cholecystitis, such as the following:

    a. Altered liver texture due to cirrhosis, hepatitis, or fatty liver

    b. Splenomegaly

    c. Portal hypertension, shown by dilated splenic, portal, superior mesenteric, and coronary veins, as well as evidence of collaterals (extra vessels around the pancreas). Use Doppler or color flow to determine direction of flow in the portal vein.

    d. Ascites that may be caused by liver disease or pancreatic ascites (e.g., a ruptured pseudocyst)

    e. Gallstones or tenderness directly over the gallbladder with or without a dilated common duct

4. If the *pancreatic duct* is dilated, make sure that there is not an obstructing mass in the pancreas.

SELECTED READING

Bowie, J. D., and MacMahon, H. Improved techniques in pancreatic sonography. *Seminars in Ultrasound* 1:170–178, 1980.

Gimenez, A., Martinez-Noguera, A., Donoso, L., Catala, E., and Serra, R. Percutaneous neurolysis of the celiac plexus via the anterior approach with sonographic guidance. *AJR* 161: 1061–1063, 1993.

Goldstein, H. M., and Katragadda, C. S. Prone view ultrasonography for pancreatic tail neoplasms. *AJR* 131:231–234, 1978.

Jeffrey, B., and Ralls, P. Sonography of the Abdomen. New York: Raven, 1995.

John, T. G., Greig, J. D., Carter, D. C., and Garden, O. J. Carcinoma of the pancreatic head and periampullary region: Tumor staging with laparoscopy and laparoscopic ultrasonography. *Ann Surg* 221:156–164, 1995.

Junewick, J. J., Grant, T. H., Weiss, C. A., and Piano, G. Celiac artery aneurysm: Color Doppler evaluation. *J Ultrasound Med* 12:355–357, 1993.

Kosuge, T., Makuuchi, M., Takayama, T., Yamamoto, J., Kinoshita, T., and Ozaki, H. Thickening at the root of the superior mesenteric artery on sonography: Evidence of vascular involvement in patients with cancer of the pancreas. *AJR* 156:69–72, 1991.

Lumkin, B., Anderson, M. W., Ablin, D. S., and McGahan, J. P. CT, MRI and color Doppler ultrasound correlation of pancreatoblastoma: A case report. *Pediatr Radiol* 23:61–62, 1993.

Maringhini, A., Ciambra, M., Raimondo, M., Baccelliere, P., Grasso, R., Dardanoni, G., Lanzarone, F., Cottone, M., Sciarrino, E., and Pagliaro, L. *Pancreas* 8:146–150, 1993.

Marks, W. M., Filly, R. A., and Callen, P. W. Ultrasonic evaluation of normal pancreatic echogenicity and its relationship to fat deposition. *Radiology* 137:475–479, 1980.

Shawker, T. H., Garra, B. S., Hill, M. C., Doppman, J. L., and Sindelar, W. F. The spectrum of sonographic findings in pancreatic carcinoma. *J Ultrasound Med* 5:169–177, 1986.

23

RIGHT UPPER QUADRANT MASS

Possible Metastases to Liver

NANCY SMITH MINER, ROGER C. SANDERS

SONOGRAM ABBREVIATIONS

Ao	Aorta
Bl	Bladder
Ca	Celiac artery
CD	Common duct
D	Diaphragm
GBl	Gallbladder
Hea	Hepatic artery
Hev	Hepatic vein
Ip	Iliopsoas muscle
IMv	Inferior mesenteric vein
IVC	Inferior vena cava
K	Kidney
L	Liver
LHev	Left hepatic vein
MHev	Middle hepatic vein
Pv	Portal vein
RHev	Right hepatic vein
RPv	Right portal vein
RUQ	Right upper quadrant
S	Spine
Sp	Spleen
Spa	Splenic artery
St	Stomach

KEY WORDS

Adenopathy. Multiple enlarged lymph nodes.

Alpha-Fetoprotein. Biochemical marker that, when elevated, may indicate liver metastases.

Ameboma. Abscess caused by amebic infection. Common in Mexico and southern United States.

Budd-Chiari Syndrome. Thrombosis of the hepatic veins. Associated with ascites and liver failure.

Carcinoembryonic Antigen (CEA). Biochemical tumor marker that, when elevated, may indicate liver metastases.

Caudate Lobe. Lobe of the liver that lies posterior to the left lobe and anterior to the inferior vena cava.

Cold Defect. Area of decreased radionuclide uptake on nuclear liver-spleen scan.

Courvoisier's Sign. A right upper quadrant mass with painless jaundice implies that there is a carcinomatous mass in the head of the pancreas that is causing biliary duct obstruction. The palpable mass is due to an enlarged gallbladder.

Echinococcal Cyst. Infected cyst caused by hydatid disease. Frequently calcified. Seen in individuals who are in contact with sheep and dogs.

Hemangioma. Benign tumor of the liver that is highly vascular, making biopsy dangerous.

Hepatoblastoma. Liver tumor that is common in childhood.

Hepatoma (Hepatocellular Carcinoma). Tumor of the liver that is associated with end-stage cirrhosis. Common in the Far East and Africa, where toxins from certain fungi can precipitate the disease.

Hydatid. See *Echinococcal Cyst*.

Ligamentum Teres. Echogenic focus in the left lobe of the liver; remnant of the fetal umbilical vein (see Fig. 23-1).

Quadrate Lobe. Obsolete term for the medial segment of the left lobe of the liver.

Riedel's Lobe. Change in shape that occurs when the right lobe of the liver is longer than usual but the left is smaller—a normal variant.

◆》 THE CLINICAL PROBLEM

Patients can present with a right upper quadrant mass for a great variety of reasons. Palpable causes include everything from enlarged organs to primary or metastatic tumors. Hepatomegaly can result from infection, leukemia, anemia, congestive heart failure, or portal hypertension. These are often accompanied by splenomegaly. An important underlying cause of hepatomegaly is a malignancy.

Liver tumors or metastases may be suspected because biochemical tumor markers (carcinoembryonic antigen and alphafetoprotein) or liver function test results are elevated. Alternatively, a patient may be referred because a previous computed tomography (CT) scan or other imaging technique raised a question.

CT is usually the first modality used in the United States when metastases are suspected because it produces a more comprehensive survey of the liver and is not as operator-dependent as ultrasound. The kind of problems referred to ultrasound from CT are generally lesions which are difficult to characterize as cystic or solid. A CT scan performed without contrast can yield ambiguous results that ultrasound can resolve. Some tumors can be seen with ultrasound but not with CT.

Primary liver tumors may also be suspected in cirrhotic patients experiencing a rapid downhill course if liver function tests become rapidly worse. Delineation of the precise site of a primary liver tumor is important because it influences surgical resectability. If both right and left lobes are involved, a tumor cannot be resected. The margins between the individual segments of each lobe can be defined with ultrasound, both preoperatively and intraoperatively.

ANATOMY

Liver Position

The major structure in the right upper quadrant (RUQ) is the liver. This more-or-less triangular organ hugs the right diaphragm. The gallbladder hangs from its inferior aspect, and the right kidney lies to the right posteriorly (see Fig. 23-1). The porta hepatis (a fibrous structure containing the hepatic artery, the portal vein, lymph nodes, and the common bile duct) enters the liver from its inferior aspect close to the midline. Adjacent to the porta hepatis are the duodenum, gallbladder, and head of the pancreas. The inferior vena cava (IVC) runs through the posterior aspect of the liver to the right of the midline. The aorta lies just to the left of the midline behind the left lobe of the liver.

Lobes of the Liver

The liver is divided into three lobes: right, left, and caudate (Fig. 23-1). A fissure known as the ligamentum teres, in which lies a remnant of the fetal umbilical vein, appears to be a logical separation between the right and left lobes, but in reality it separates the left lobe into two segments. The medial segment of the left lobe (the one closest to the right lobe) was formerly known as the quadrate lobe. This is now an obsolete term.

The division between the right and left lobes is visible sonographically only where certain anatomic landmarks appear (see Fig. 23-1):

1. *Main lobar fissure.* This shows up on ultrasound as an echogenic line superior to the gallbladder, which seems to connect the right portal vein to the gallbladder fossa.
2. *Middle hepatic vein.* More superiorly, the middle hepatic vein runs between the right and left lobes.

The left lobe is divided into medial and lateral segments superiorly by the left hepatic vein and more inferiorly by the ligamentum teres. Between those two points, the segment of the left portal vein that turns sharply anterior marks the division between the medial and lateral segments of the left lobe. The right lobe is divided into anterior/posterior segments by the right hepatic vein. The caudate lobe, which has its own blood supply, is posterior to and separated from the left lobe by the ligamentum venosum, which is an echogenic interface posterior to the left lobe.

The porta hepatis is the site where the portal vein, common bile duct, and hepatic artery (the portal triad) enter the liver. It is located just anterior and lateral to the IVC (see Fig. 23-1). It extends into the liver until the point at which the left portal vein takes off from the main portal vein.

Liver Shape

The normal shape of the liver varies considerably with the shape of the patient. Barrel-chested people—those with a large antero-posterior (AP) diameter—often have small left lobes that taper off before they reach the midline, and deep right lobes that are not very long. Slim people (small AP diameter) have left lobes that may extend well into the left upper quadrant and right lobes that can extend below the costal margin. Although this length could constitute hepatomegaly in someone else, it may be normal in a long, lean patient.

Normal liver contour should be smooth with no focal bulges, apart from a subtle rounding of the caudate lobe.

The hepatic arteries and portal venous structures are described in Chapter 21, Sonographic Abdominal Anatomy, and in Chapter 25, Abnormal Liver Function Tests, Jaundice; see Chapter 25 for a description of the biliary tree.

■ TECHNIQUE

Because the liver is such a large organ, the responsibility of viewing it in its entirety lies with the sonographer. A systematic approach to demonstrating various landmarks aids in ensuring that the transducer has indeed covered the territory. Bear in mind that a surgical approach to treatment relies heavily on an accurate description of which lobes are involved with the pathology. It is therefore crucial to include the necessary anatomic landmarks on a liver sonogram.

A sector scanner or curvilinear scanner with a small footprint is the optimal tool because it allows good visualization through the ribs, where access is limited. A suggested scanning pattern is outlined below.

Basic Scanning of the Right Upper Quadrant

Longitudinal Views

Longitudinal views should include sections through the midline, lateral left lobe, aorta, and IVC. To scan the midline in a longitudinal view start in the subxiphoid area. *On every longitudinal cut, angle superiorly and inferiorly to see both margins of the liver (and pancreas, when possible), even if this means additional pictures.*

Obtain views of the following:

1. The *lateral left lobe* by sweeping left until there is no more left lobe. Document the *left hepatic vein,* however tiny it appears on this view, and demonstrate the long axis of the *aorta* and the *superior mesenteric artery.*
2. The *IVC,* making sure you have documented the *head of the pancreas,* the *portal vein,* and the *middle hepatic vein.* You may be able to do this on one image, probably two.
3. A *texture comparison* between the pancreas and liver. Often this is easiest to document on a longitudinal view through the left lobe.
4. The *ligamentum venosum.* Document the *caudate lobe* (see Fig. 23-1) on this scan.
5. The *ligamentum teres* (see Fig. 23-1).
6. The *portal triad.* Include the *right portal vein,* the *hepatic artery,* and a segment of the *common duct* (see Figs. 21-5 and 25-1).
7. The *main lobar fissure.* Show a section demonstrating the right portal vein, the main lobar fissure, and the gallbladder fossa (see Fig. 23-1).
8. The *gallbladder* (see Chapter 24).
9. The *right lobe.* Multiple scans to demonstrate *texture.*
10. The *diaphragm.* Include images that show the diaphragm so that there is evidence that the dome of the liver has been scanned. Check above and below the diaphragm for fluid.
11. The *right kidney.* Demonstrate renal size. Obtain an image that also shows the right lobe of the liver for *texture comparison* purposes and enough images to rule out a renal mass or hydronephrosis.

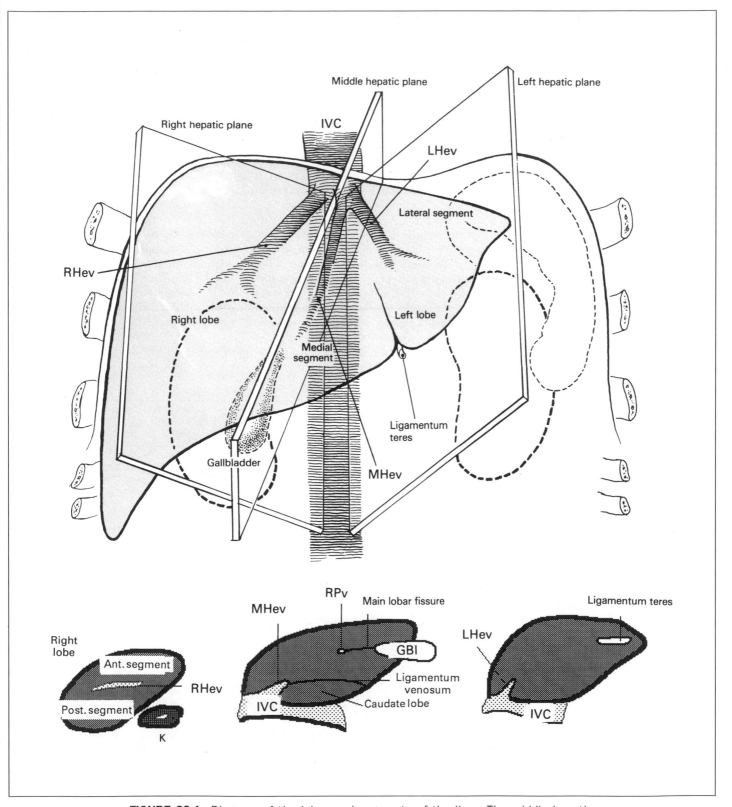

FIGURE 23-1. Diagram of the lobes and segments of the liver. The middle hepatic veins separate the left and right lobes of the liver. The main lobar fissure is part of this division. The left hepatic vein and ligamentum teres separate the lateral and medial segments of the left lobe. The right hepatic vein separates the anterior and posterior segments of the right lobe superiorly while the main lobar fissure separates them inferiorly. The caudate lobe can be seen posterior to the ligamentum venosum.

Transverse Views

Begin in the subxiphoid area. Obtain views of the following:

1. The *left lobe of the liver*, including the *left portal vein*, by angling superiorly.
2. The *hepatic veins* in transverse section. All three should be demonstrated, not necessarily on the same image. Trace them to the *IVC*.
3. The *spleen*, by sweeping inferiorly and scanning through the left flank, to give a general idea of its size.
4. The *pancreas*. Use the left lobe of the liver as an acoustic window and for texture comparison purposes. Include the inferior margin.
5. The *ligamentum teres* and the *midportion of the liver*.
6. The *ligamentum venosum* and *caudate lobe* on a transverse section.
7. The *right lobe*. Document the following structures and survey all of the liver texture in between:
   a. The *portal vein* including the *bifurcation*.
   b. The *gallbladder* (see Chapter 24).
   c. The *kidney* (on a transverse view of the liver) for *texture comparison* purposes.
8. The *gallbladder, duodenum,* and *common bile duct* in a single *head of the pancreas* view.
9. The *right kidney*, on additional transverse views.
10. The *subhepatic space* and *paracolic gutter*.

The structures described above can be demonstrated in a variety of views in addition to the longitudinal and transverse. Follow these general guidelines: (1) adjust the transducer to obtain the long axis of vessels or the kidney; and (2) scan the patient in oblique supine, decubitus, or even upright position if it facilitates visualization.

You *must* scan between the ribs if you are to demonstrate the lateral margin of the liver properly. Using various intercostal points, in both longitudinal and transverse planes, also gives the beam a better vantage point to use the liver for a window. Often this is the best way to find the long axis of the common duct. You can angle the beam around the duodenum to get a transverse view of the head of the pancreas.

Trying to demonstrate hepatomegaly with ultrasound can be tricky, because in an adult the liver will not fit on one image. It is not acceptable to extrapolate the measurements if the liver is enlarged, because the clinician may be using serial scans to mark the progress of the treatment. Find a landmark in the midclavicular line, perhaps the gallbladder or right portal vein, and always measure at that same level on subsequent scans (Fig. 23-2). If your equipment allows you to "match up" two halves of an image for a larger field size, do so. Split the image at the renal sinus to help determine where to start the second image. Use a linear array to help line up the anatomy if possible; do not worry about the picket-fence appearance of the ribs—this picture is for accuracy, not beauty. Otherwise, measure from the diaphragm to a designated structure (e.g., the neck of the gallbladder) on the first scan, then from the structure to the liver edge on the second scan.

See Chapter 25, Abnormal Liver Function Tests, Jaundice, for a discussion of how to obtain Doppler tracings of the portal and hepatic venous systems. Both duplex and color flow can be useful in defining the anatomy and pathology of the right upper quadrant.

Respiration

Scanning on inspiration is often helpful when examining the right upper quadrant, but not always. The relationship of the anatomy to the ribs is so variable from patient to patient that scanning should be tried at different stages of respiration. In those patients whose abdomen falls sharply away from the ribs, it can be quite helpful to ask the patient to take in a breath while pushing out his or her abdomen. This can bring structures such as the left lobe and pancreas down into view.

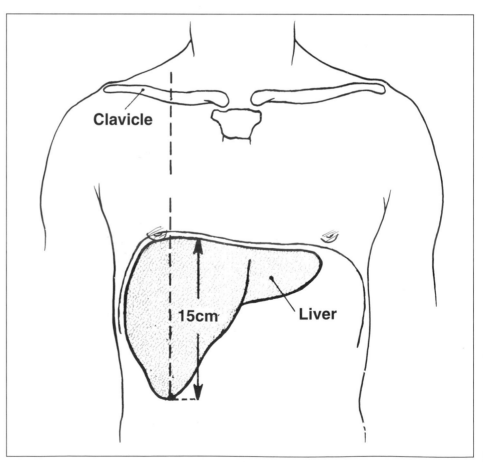

FIGURE 23-2. Diagram showing the site for measurement of liver size. The length is measured in the midclavicular line.

Scanning Masses

When scanning to rule out a right upper quadrant mass, begin, as always, by looking in the chart and talking to the patient. Check the CT report or other relevant studies, especially previous ultrasounds, then try to palpate the mass. The patient can usually tell you how it is most easily felt.

Effect of Masses on Anatomy

Once a tumor is located, determine its effect on the surrounding anatomy. Is it displacing vessels? Is it obstructing ducts or ureters? Has it invaded the bile ducts, hepatic arteries, or portal vein? Trace the vessels to their origins to make sure they are not involved. Use pulsed Doppler or color flow when necessary.

Characterization of Masses

Make sure that you have determined the correct origin of the mass. For instance, if a mass is in the region of the adrenal gland, follow the perinephric fat around the kidney and see whether it encloses the mass, thereby affirming that it is retroperitoneal. If the mass is of hepatic origin, the perinephric fat will come between it and the kidney (Fig. 23-3).

Usually it is impossible to be specific about the nature of a mass; one must be content with documenting as many characteristics of it as possible. Most pieces of equipment allow for different levels of enhancement; experiment with different preprocessing and postprocessing modes, including color filters, to help delineate subtle textural changes. Doppler and color flow may be of help in determining whether a mass is vascular; they are not always.

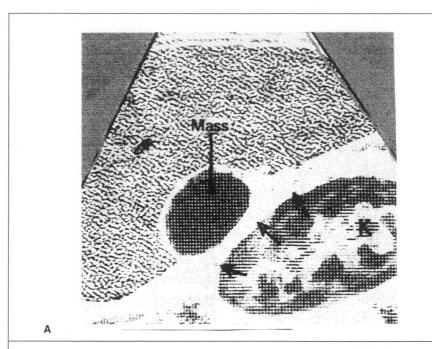

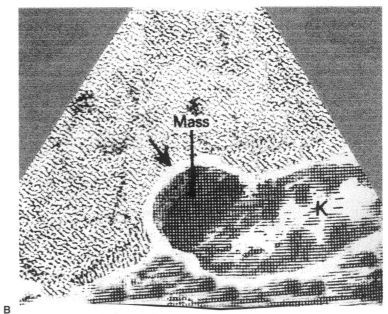

FIGURE 23-3. The retroperitoneal fat line anterior to the kidney and posterior to the liver (arrows) shows whether a mass is intraperitoneal or retroperitoneal. The line is displaced posteriorly, (**A**) by intraperitoneal lesions, and anteriorly, (**B**) by retroperitoneal masses.

◆ PATHOLOGY

Hepatomegaly

The liver is considered enlarged if it measures more than 15 cm in length at a point midway between the spine and the right side of the body (see Fig. 23-2). The left lobe does not extend very far across the midline and is usually smaller in patients with a large AP diameter.

If the organs are in a normal relationship, a simple assessment of liver enlargement can be made by noting whether the inferior aspect of the liver extends well below the right kidney. However, this rule will not work if the kidney is situated close to the diaphragm, as it is in patients with a large AP diameter (see Pitfalls).

Hepatomegaly may be due to single or multiple masses. Hepatomegaly can also be caused by diffuse liver disease, notably fatty liver and acute hepatitis or lymphoma. The liver is also large in patients with chronic passive congestion. In such cases there will be a generalized alteration in sonographic appearance (described in Chapter 25).

Liver Cysts

Liver cysts are rather common and may be multiple. They usually have no internal echoes. Smooth borders are usual, but an irregular outline and septum may be seen.

Multiple cysts are also seen in about half of patients with autosomal dominant polycystic renal disease. Like ordinary cysts, they are generally asymptomatic, not usually affecting liver function tests. The liver will be enlarged and the cysts are multiple, varying in size and shape throughout the liver. Any liver cyst can cause fever or pain if it becomes infected or hemorrhagic; internal echoes or septa may then develop.

Metastases

Metastases are almost always multiple. Common patterns include the following:

1. *Bull's eye.* An echogenic center with a surrounding echopenic area (Fig. 23-4).
2. *Echopenic.* Less echogenic than the neighboring liver (see Fig. 23-4).
3. *Echogenic.* More echogenic than the surrounding liver. (The echogenicity may be due to calcification within the mass; see Fig. 23-4; see also Pitfalls). This type of metastasis is often associated with malignancy of gastrointestinal origin.

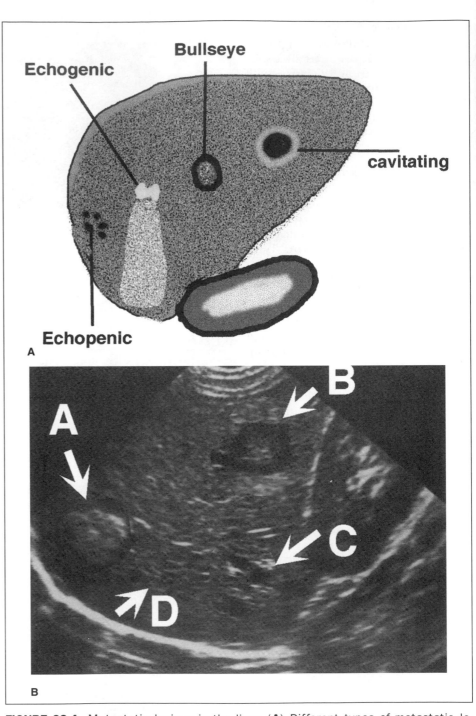

FIGURE 23-4. Metastatic lesions in the liver. (**A**) Different types of metastatic lesions that may occur in the liver include bull's eye, echogenic, echopenic, and cavitating. Cystic lesions may also be seen. (**B**) Liver with several different metastatic lesions within. Type A is echogenic with shadowing as commonly derived from the colon. Type B is bull's eye metastasis. Type C is a group of echopenic metastases. D shows several echopenic areas as is seen with lymphoma.

4. *Cystic.* Rare and impossible to distinguish sonographically from a benign cyst.
5. *Diffuse.* Numerous echopenic lesions throughout the liver. This appearance raises the question of lymphomatous infiltration or neoplasm related to acquired immunodeficiency syndrome (AIDS).
6. *Necrotic.* Fluid-filled center with thick, irregular walls.

If there is a mass found in the right upper quadrant, it is useful to use color and then pulsed Doppler to determine whether there is flow present. Malignancies usually exhibit flow. Several flow patterns may be helpful in defining metastases, such as flow surrounding the tumor (basket pattern), flow centrally in the tumor (spot pattern), the "vessels-within-the-tumor" pattern, and flow between tumors (detour pattern). However, attempts to correlate these patterns with specific tumors are of limited value, because the internal vascularity patterns of some metastases, some hemangiomas, and focal nodular hyperplasia tend to overlap. In general, lower-velocity shifts are indicative of hemangiomas, whereas high-velocity shifts are more compatible with malignant lesions.

One feature useful in detecting a malignancy, although not pathognomonic, is a hypoechoic halo around isoechoic or hyperechoic lesions in the liver. Various types of malignant lesions exhibit these rims, which have proven histopathologically to be due to an extratumoral rim of compressed liver tissue. In extremely uniform tumors this sign may not be present.

In patients being evaluated for surgical liver resection, either for a liver transplant or curative resection for some sort of cancer, the exact number and location of hepatic lesions are of paramount importance. Use of duplex or color flow Doppler may be helpful for detection. Careful attention to vascular landmarks and a precise description of their relationship to lesions will make the sonogram report valuable to the clinician.

For a discussion of intraoperative liver scanning see Chapter 52, Guidance Techniques.

Primary Malignant Liver Tumors

1. *Malignant hepatoma* (hepatocellular carcinoma). The most common malignant liver tumor. Single, multifocal, or even diffuse, it usually presents in Western cultures as the sequela to alcoholic cirrhosis. Very common in Asian and African cultures, in patients with chronic hepatitis B, and in those exposed to toxic fungi in certain foods. The smaller lesions tend to be echopenic, but become increasingly echogenic and complex as they increase in size.

   Invasion of the portal (more common) or hepatic (less common) venous system may occur. Color flow imaging can be helpful in demonstrating heightened vascular flow surrounding and branching within these vascular tumors. In a patient with severe cirrhosis, this may help to distinguish the malignancy from the nodular changes of cirrhosis.
2. *Fibrolamellar hepatoma.* A vascular tumor that is generally echogenic and often contains a central scar seen as an echogenic line or region.
3. *Cystic mesenchymoma.* See Chapter 28, Pediatrics.
4. *Hepatoblastoma.* See Chapter 28, Pediatrics.
5. *Hemangioendothelioma.* See Chapter 28, Pediatrics.

Benign Tumors

1. *Hemangiomas.* These appear as a brightly echogenic focus with smooth borders, often with a subtle echopenic center. Usually small, they may be multiple. *Cavernous hemangiomas,* usually larger, are variable in echo pattern and size. Although highly vascular, hemangiomas do not exhibit a pathognomonic pattern on duplex or color flow Doppler, because the flow is venous. The flow is usually so slow that it is hard to see at all, even with power Doppler.

2. *Adenoma.* Generally echogenic, they can have variable echo patterns and do not always remain benign adenomas, so patients may be surgical candidates. Usually seen in women and associated with oral contraceptive use.
3. *Focal nodular hyperplasia.* Generally echopenic (may be echogenic, or of mixed echogenicity). This mass sometimes contains a central bright linear echo, the "scar sign." Correlation with nuclear medicine studies is helpful in narrowing down this diagnosis.

Budd-Chiari Syndrome

The Budd-Chiari syndrome, which is caused by clot in the hepatic veins or IVC, is a rare cause of an enlarged and tender liver. Because the hepatic veins are usually visualized so well on ultrasound, color flow Doppler is a good way to evaluate for thrombosis. The normal veins show up blue in the traditional orientation (denoting flow away from the transducer, into the IVC). Demonstration of collaterals, absence of flow, and disruptions in the normal triphasic flow pattern of the hepatic veins may indicate thrombosis (see Pitfalls). Normal flow patterns for liver vessels are shown in Figure 25-8.

Hematomas

Usually occurring after trauma or surgery, hematomas undergo the following changes:

1. *When fresh,* they are echo-free.
2. *Within a few hours,* there are low-level echoes.
3. *Within a few days,* they develop sonolucent areas.
4. *Eventually,* they become echo-free.

Subcapsular hematomas appear as a rim around the lateral aspect of the liver and look confusing at two points in their evolution: when they are fresh and echogenic they can be confused with the liver, and when they are longstanding and echopenic they can resemble ascites (Fig. 23-5).

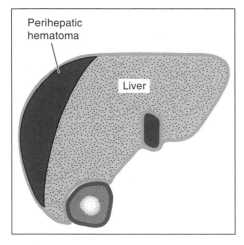

Perihepatic hematoma

Liver

FIGURE 23-5. A relatively recent hematoma seen just below the diaphragm would have a similar acoustic appearance to the liver; this older one has become sonolucent.

Porta Hepatis Nodes

Nodes can cause a right upper quadrant mass, particularly when they are clustered in the porta hepatis. If large enough, they can displace the portal vein and obstruct the common duct. Typically, they are not limited to the porta hepatis but surround and straighten the celiac axis and the superior mesenteric artery; the abdominal search must then be extended to cover all areas that could show lymphadenopathy. If nodes are caused by lymphoma, they are generally echo-free. A lymph node, just anterior to the portal confluence, may be seen as a normal variant (see Pitfalls).

Gallbladder

If the cystic duct or common duct is obstructed, the gallbladder may become so enlarged that it is palpable. A right upper quadrant mass coupled with jaundice and absence of pain is known as Courvoisier's sign; it indicates obstruction of the common duct, usually caused by carcinoma of the pancreas.

Gastrointestinal Tumors

Mesenteric masses such as carcinoma of the colon or stomach may lie immediately adjacent to the liver but feel as if they are of hepatic origin. The typical appearance of a gastrointestinal mass with an echogenic center and an echo-free rim is described in Chapter 30.

Pancreatic Pseudocyst

Pancreatic pseudocysts can originate in most areas of the abdomen and may migrate to the right upper quadrant (see Chapter 22).

Renal Masses

Very large renal tumors or severe hydronephrosis may appear as right upper quadrant masses (see Chapter 32). This may shift the focus of the study to the genitourinary system, but if a renal tumor is present, one must look for accompanying ascites, adenopathy, and metastases. Wilms' tumor and neuroblastoma are two retroperitoneal tumors that occur chiefly in children and infants; these also present as right upper quadrant masses (see Chapter 28).

Adrenal Gland

A mass located above the right kidney may arise from the liver, adrenal gland, or retroperitoneal tissue. A fat line separates the retroperitoneum from the peritoneum (see Fig. 23-3). This line is displaced posteriorly by intraperitoneal masses such as hepatic lesions and anteriorly by masses originating in the retroperitoneum.

Any right upper quadrant mass of questionable origin necessitates a search for a normal separate adrenal gland to prove that the adrenal is not involved (see Chapter 39).

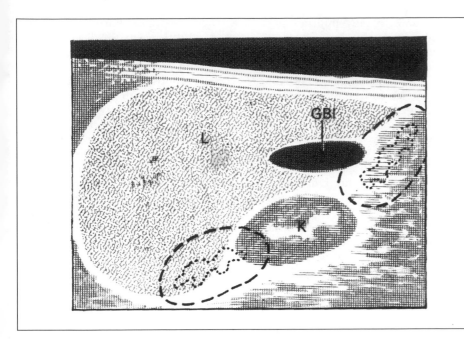

FIGURE 23-6. A kidney with a lower pole tilted anteriorly may be palpable and may be clinically mistaken for a pathologic mass.

Abdominal Wall

Make sure that the mass is not in the abdominal wall. Occasionally lipomas and other superficial masses can be mistaken for intra-abdominal structures. Look for the peritoneal fascial planes to help make this distinction (see Chapter 29).

★ PITFALLS

1. *Kidney axis.* The axis of the right kidney is variable, and occasionally the lower pole may be tilted anteriorly, making it palpable even though there is no mass present (Fig. 23-6).

2. *Riedel's lobe.* Riedel's lobe is a normal variant of liver shape in which an unusually large right lobe of the liver causes a false impression of hepatomegaly (Fig. 23-7); however, the left lobe is very small.

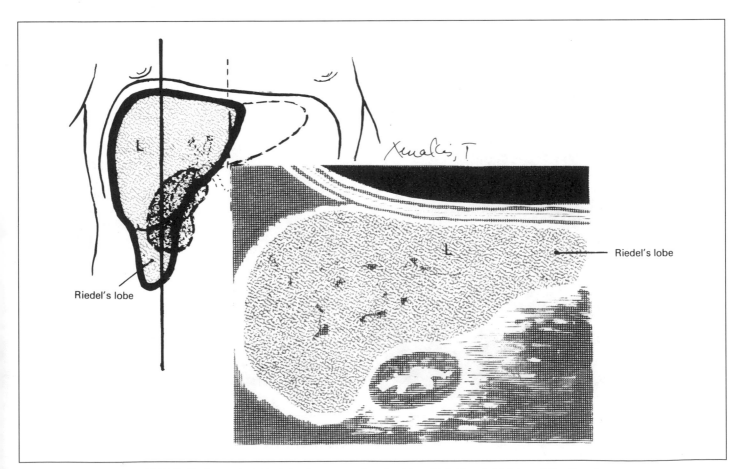

FIGURE 23-7. A Riedel's lobe is a normal variant in which the right lobe of the liver is larger and the left lobe is smaller than usual. The overall size is within normal limits.

3. *Ligamentum teres.* This remnant of the fetal umbilical vein is a fibrous structure surrounded by fat. It appears as an echogenic lesion in the left lobe of the liver in the transverse plane, and can be mistaken for a focal hemangioma or echogenic metastatic lesion (Fig. 23-8). In the sagittal plane, the ligamentum teres appears as a long, echogenic linear structure coursing inferiorly from the ascending left portal vein.

4. *Dilated hepatic vein vs. cysts.* On longitudinal scans, cystic structures with poorly defined walls in the right lobe of the liver may represent hepatic veins. A transverse view will show that the apparent cyst is a tubular structure draining into the IVC (Fig. 23-9). Enlarged hepatic veins are often associated with congestive heart failure. These may be worth labeling on short-axis views if they appear to be cysts.

5. *Fat-free area.* In fatty infiltration of the liver, the overall liver parenchyma is more echogenic than it should be by comparison with the kidney (see Chapter 25). There may be patchy areas free of fat that are *less* echogenic and can be mistaken for metastases. However, fat-free areas usually have smooth borders, and vessels run through them undistorted; a typical location is just anterior to the right portal vein.

6. *Diaphragmatic leaflet.* The diaphragm may appear to be double in certain segments owing to its insertion into the ribs. The right triangular ligament can be visualized between the liver and diaphragm in patients with ascites.

7. *Hypoechoic caudate and posterior left lobes.* Owing to absorption and attenuation by fissures or the left portal vein, the caudate lobe and the posterior aspect of the left lobe of the liver may be less echogenic than the rest of the liver; the caudate lobe also has a different blood supply which may be unaffected by pathology that alters echogenicity in the other lobes. This appearance is a normal variant.

8. *Gut vs. metastasis.* Portions of the gut may lie between the liver and the diaphragm (Chilaiditi syndrome), causing acoustic shadowing. These bowel loops may be confusing. Try to confirm with peristalsis. Scan through the patient's side with the patient lying supine to bring the beam anterior to the air in the gut.

9. *Ascites vs. subcapsular hematoma.* Echo-free subcapsular hematomas surrounding the liver can be mistaken for ascites (see Fig. 23-5). Ascites may move if the patient changes position. Free fluid is also often seen in other places, such as the cul-de-sac.

10. *No color flow in hepatic veins.* This is not always indicative of thrombus. Patency may be obscured by a scarred and shrunken cirrhotic liver, or a swollen one.

11. *Hemangioma vs. metastasis.* Hemangiomas are usually isolated and asymptomatic. Often echogenic, they can vary in appearance much like metastases. Consider the clinical history; hemangiomas also tend to have lower velocity shifts then metastases, but at this writing the findings with duplex and color Doppler overlap enough between the two entities that Doppler is too limited to use for a specific diagnosis.

12. *Node in porta hepatis.* At the entrance to the porta hepatis, just superior to the portal confluence, one can see a node that can be as large as 2 cm in normal patients. This is probably a normal variant if no adenopathy is seen elsewhere.

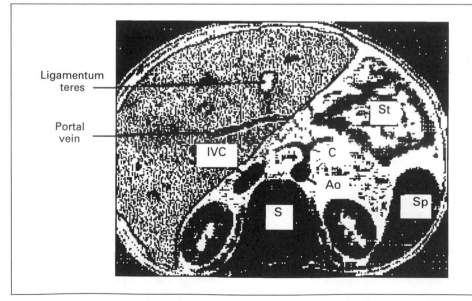

FIGURE 23-8. An echogenic focus in the left lobe of the liver, sometimes associated with acoustic shadowing, represents the ligamentum teres—a normal variant and remnant of the fetal umbilical vein.

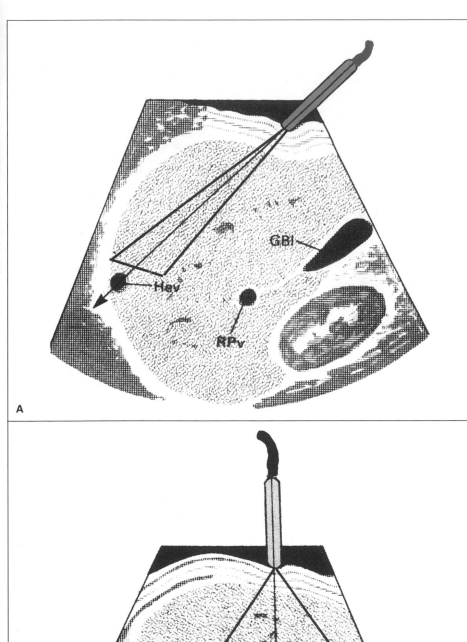

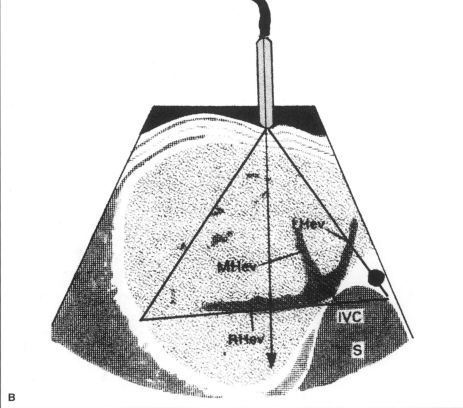

1. If a malignancy or a metastatic lesion is found, the rest of the patient's abdomen and pelvis should be surveyed for evidence of adenopathy, primary lesions, or ascites.
2. If echogenic metastatic lesions are seen, look throughout the bowel for a target lesion that suggests carcinoma of the colon or stomach (see Chapter 30).
3. If polycystic liver disease is seen, examine the kidneys, which are certain to show signs of the disease. Note any compression of the IVC. Also examine the pancreas and spleen, which on rare occasions have cysts with polycystic liver disease.
4. If subcapsular hematoma is suspected around the liver, check for similar appearance around the spleen and check the abdomen for other collections of blood.
5. If the liver is enlarged, look for associated splenomegaly.

FIGURE 23-9. Dilated hepatic veins. A sonolucent structure in (**A**), close to the diaphragm within the liver, may not represent a cyst. A transverse view, (**B**), shows that this structure actually represents a dilated right hepatic vein.

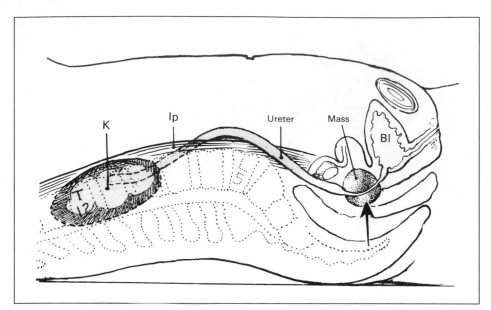

FIGURE 23-10. If the kidney is obstructed, look along the course of the ureter to detect the cause of obstruction, for example, a pelvic mass.

6. If the mass turns out to be a dilated hydronephrotic kidney, try to identify the cause of the obstruction in the pelvis or along the course of the ureter (Fig. 23-10).

7. If the mass is a greatly dilated gallbladder, look for the site and nature of the obstruction of the biliary tree. Be sure to evaluate the pancreatic head and common duct.

8. If porta hepatis nodes are found, look for splenomegaly and evidence of malignancy in other areas of the abdomen.

SELECTED READING

Kane, R., and Eustace, S. Diagnosis of Budd-Chiari syndrome: Comparison between sonography and MR angiography. *Radiology* 195:117–121, 1995.

Knol, J. A., Marn, C. S., Francis, I. R., Rubin, J. M., Bromberg, J., and Chang, A. Comparisons of dynamic infusion and delayed computed tomography, intraoperative ultrasound, and palpation in the diagnosis of liver metastases. *Am J Surg* 165:81–88, 1993.

Marks, W. M., Filly, R. A., and Callen, P. W. Ultrasonic anatomy of the liver: A review with new applications. *J Clin Ultrasound* 7:131–146, 1979.

Mukai, J. K., Stack, C. M., Turner, D. A., Gould, R. J., Petasnick, J. P., Matalon, T. A. S., Doolas, A. M., and Murakami, M. Imaging of surgically relevant hepatic vascular and segmental anatomy. Part 1. Normal anatomy. *AJR* 149:287–292, 1987.

Mukai, J. K., Stack, C. M., Turner, D. A., Gould, R. J., Petasnick, J. P., Matalon, T. A. S., Doolas, A. M., and Murakami, M. Imaging of surgically relevant hepatic vascular and segmental anatomy. Part 2. Extent and resectability of hepatic neoplasms. *AJR* 149:293–297, 1987.

Needleman, L. M. Diffuse benign liver disease. In *Gastrointestinal Sonography* (Clinics in Diagnostic Ultrasound Series, Vol 23). New York: Churchill Livingstone, 1988.

Nino-Murcia, M., Ralls, P. W., Jeffrey, R. B., et al. Color flow Doppler characterization of focal hepatic lesions. *AJR* 160:515–521, 1993.

Nisenbaum, H. L., and Rowling, S. E. Ultrasound of focal hepatic lesions. *Semin Roentgenol* 30:324–346, 1995.

Numata, K., Tamaka, K., Mitsui, K., et al. Flow characteristics of hepatic tumors at color Doppler sonography: Correlation with angiographic findings. *AJR* 160:515–521, 1993.

Solomon, M. J., Stephen, M. S., Gallinger, S., and White, G. H. Does intraoperative hepatic sonography change surgical decision making during liver resection? *Am J Surg* 168:307–310, 1994.

Stone, M. D., Kane, R., Bothe, A., Hessup, J. M., Cady, B., and Steele, G. D. Intraoperative ultrasound imaging of the liver at the time of colorectal cancer resection. *Arch Surg* 129:431–436, 1994.

Wernecke, K., Henke, L., Vassallo, P., von Bassewitz, D. B., Diederich, S., Peters, P. E., and Edel, G. Pathologic explanation for hypoechoic halo seen on sonogram of malignant liver tumors: An in vitro correlative study. *AJR* 159:1011–1016, 1992.

24 RIGHT UPPER QUADRANT PAIN

NANCY SMITH MINER

SONOGRAM ABBREVIATIONS

Ao Aorta

CBD Common bile duct

GB,GBl Gallbladder

IVC Inferior vena cava

K Kidney

L Liver

Pv Portal vein

S Spine

KEY WORDS

Acute Abdomen. Sudden onset of abdominal pain. Causes include appendicitis, perforated peptic ulcer, strangulated hernia, acute cholecystitis, pancreatitis, and renal colic.

Adenomyomatosis. A chronic gallbladder condition causing right upper quadrant pain with several sonographic manifestations, the most common being multiple, small polypoid masses arising from the gallbladder wall.

AIDS. Acquired immunodeficiency syndrome (see Chapter 26).

Amebiasis. Infection with amebic parasite, common in Mexico, the southern United States, and warm climates.

Ameboma of the Liver. Abscess caused by amebiasis.

Cholangitis. Inflammation of a bile duct.

Cholecystitis. Inflammation of the gallbladder.

> **Acute.** Usually caused by gallbladder outlet obstruction.

> **Chronic.** Inflammation persisting over a longer period.

Choledochojejunostomy. Surgical procedure in which the bile duct is anastomosed to jejunum; food and air may reflux into the bile ducts.

Choledocholithiasis. Gallstone in a bile duct.

Cholelithiasis. Gallstones in the gallbladder.

Cholesterosis (Cholesterolosis). Variant of adenomyomatosis in which cholesterol polyps arise from the gallbladder wall.

Hartmann's Pouch. Portion of the gallbladder that lies nearest the cystic duct where stones often collect.

Junctional Fold. Septum usually arising from the posterior mid-aspect of the gallbladder; a normal variant.

Murphy's Sign. Tenderness when an inflamed gallbladder is palpated clinically, usually on deep inspiration.

Phrygian Cap. Variant gallbladder shape in which the fundus of the gallbladder is separated from the body of the gallbladder by a junctional fold.

Pyogenic. Producing pus.

Rokitansky-Aschoff Sinuses. Multiple pouches in the wall of the gallbladder.

Sphincterotomy. Procedure in which the sphincter of Oddi is widened surgically. Gas will reflux into the bile ducts.

WES (Wall Echo Sign). Sonographic pattern seen when the gallbladder is filled with stones.

◆» THE CLINICAL PROBLEM

Right upper quadrant (RUQ) pain, either chronic or acute, may be caused by disease in the gallbladder, liver, porta hepatis, pancreas, right kidney, adrenal gland, lung, or diaphragmatic pleura. Differential diagnosis is sometimes difficult and often requires the use of many modalities, including the history and physical examination, laboratory tests, computed tomography (CT) scans, nuclear medicine, and ultrasound. Important physical signs and symptoms include the presence or absence of jaundice, acute pain, fever, and vomiting.

Ruling out gallstones is perhaps the most common indication for a right upper quadrant scan. Although stones in the gallbladder and ducts certainly can cause pain, often they are asymptomatic. Because choledocholithiasis may be indicated by increases in liver function tests before any pain is experienced, this condition will be discussed in Chapter 25. The clinician is asking for concrete evidence from the sonographer before referring the patient to a surgeon: Does the gallbladder have stones? A thickened wall? Fluid around it? Is it locally tender? Is it enlarged? Is there biliary tree dilatation?

When right upper quadrant pain is acute, rapid and accurate diagnosis on an emergency basis may be crucial. Many of the internal disasters that precipitate an acute abdomen, such as renal colic with secondary hydronephrosis and pancreatitis, are readily detectable with ultrasound. Others, however, such as perforated ulcer, are not.

Because of the proximity of the gallbladder and pancreas to the right hemidiaphragm, patients with cholecystitis and pancreatitis sometimes experience referred pain in the right shoulder area. Pain may also be referred into the right upper quadrant from inflammation of the diaphragmatic pleura. Thus, the finding of an unsuspected pleural effusion by sonography may shift the focus of the work-up to the chest. Pyelonephritis and renal stones (see Chapter 33), as well as liver tumor or abscess, may present as right upper quadrant pain.

Sometimes, right upper quadrant pain is the result of chronic disease, as when oncology patients get viscous bile from prolonged stasis and develop acute acalculous cholecystitis or gallstones; or when AIDS patients develop cholangitis. Right upper quadrant abnormalities may be incidental findings in these patients because the pain may not be marked, or because the signs and symptoms get buried in a very complex clinical picture. These patients require a careful search for any problem that can be treated to alleviate pain.

ANATOMY
Gallbladder

The gallbladder is situated on the inferior aspect of the liver, medial and anterior to the kidney, and lateral and anterior to the inferior vena cava. The main lobar fissure is a sonographic landmark leading to the gallbladder fossa, seen as an echogenic line (Fig. 24-1) that runs from the right portal vein to the gallbladder. The gallbladder is pear shaped and varies in size. It may contain a kink (the junctional fold) close to the neck (Fig. 24-2). It is divided into the fundus (the distal tip area), the body, and the neck (Hartmann's pouch is that portion of the gallbladder between the junctional fold and the neck). The gallbladder has an echogenic wall that should not be more than 3-mm thick. See Chapter 25, Abnormal Liver Function Tests, Jaundice, for anatomy of the biliary tree.

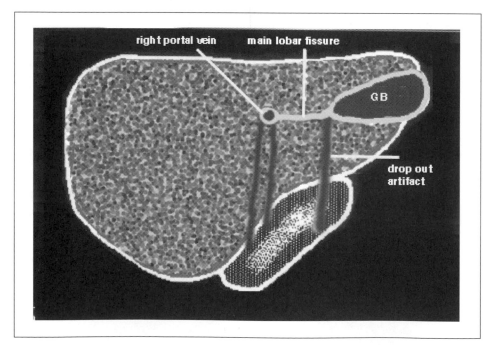

FIGURE 24-1. Diagram showing the main lobar fissure between the right portal vein and the gallbladder. Note the refractive acoustic shadowing from the gallbladder wall and the portal vein wall. There is no echo source for these areas as there would be if a gallstone were present.

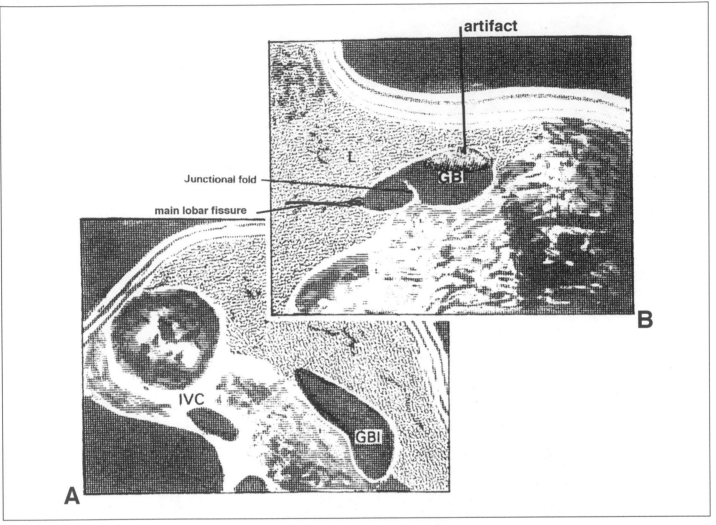

FIGURE 24-2. Reverberation artifacts. (**A**) Reverberations are a common problem in the anterior aspect of the gallbladder (artifact). The gallbladder is easily located by following the main lobar fissure from the right portal vein to the gallbladder fossa. The fold at the neck of the gallbladder could cause confusion if caught in a plane that demonstrated only a portion of it. (**B**) Increasing the gallbladder's distance from the transducer by turning the patient in a decubitus position moves the gallbladder wall into the focal zone of the transducer and decreases reverberations. The decubitus position allows the fundus to fall and the kink to straighten out.

◼ TECHNIQUE

Patient Preparation

Gallbladder studies should be performed when the patient is fasting. Water (and oral contrast for CT, which has only a weak contracting effect on the gallbladder) is permitted, but be sure the patient is not scheduled for other exams for which he or she should be without fluids such as an upper gastrointestinal series.

Even if the gallbladder is not present, abdominal sonograms benefit from the patient's fasting; there is less air in the stomach and it makes a better window if there is a need to fill it with water.

Transducer

The two most important things to remember in scanning gallbladders are to use a transducer with a high frequency and to set the electronic focus at the back wall where stones collect. The frequency must be adequate to penetrate the entire organ, but you may need to change the transducer from the one used to demonstrate the right lobe of the liver or you can obliterate subtle shadowing.

Patient Position

Supine Position

The gallbladder is first examined with the patient in a supine position using a sector or curvilinear scanner. Try to obtain long-axis views by varying the obliquity of the transducer until the maximum length of the gallbladder is seen. Scan through the short axis of the gallbladder, beginning at the neck and sweeping through the fundus. It is often necessary to angle caudally through the body to demonstrate the entire fundus well; it can be tucked up under the bowel.

Decubitus Position

It is *mandatory* to obtain additional gallbladder views in the decubitus (right side up), prone, or erect position because stones may be missed if only supine views are obtained (see Fig. 24-2). They might be small and therefore undetectable along the back wall. Changing position can pile stones together and create enough volume to produce shadowing. The decubitus position allows the liver to act as an acoustic window for visualization of the gallbladder. Stones and gravel will fall into the most dependent portion—usually the fundus—whereas polyps or adherent stones will stay put. Sludge will only gradually level off in the bottom.

Prone Position

If the most dependent part of the gallbladder becomes obscured by bowel on a decub, or if there are no stones seen on supine and decubitus views, persist and try a prone view. Position the transducer on the patient's side and scan coronally through the liver when the patient is in a decubitus position, then watch while the patient rolls flat (or flatter) onto the stomach. It's important not to let the patient get settled in the prone position before visualizing the gallbladder, because the advantage of this position is in seeing the "snowflakes" falling as the patient turns. Sometimes this picks up stones that layered and were undetectable on other views.

Upright Position

This is awkward for both patient and sonographer, but in patients with a small, high liver and large AP diameter, it may be the best alternate view. Don't just sit the patient up on the stretcher; the bowel may push up in front of the gallbladder (Fig. 24-3). Have the patient stand and brace against the stretcher. Don't waste all this effort—be sure to scan the pancreas while the patient is upright. In patients with this build, it's often the best way to get an acoustic window, and so worth the trouble.

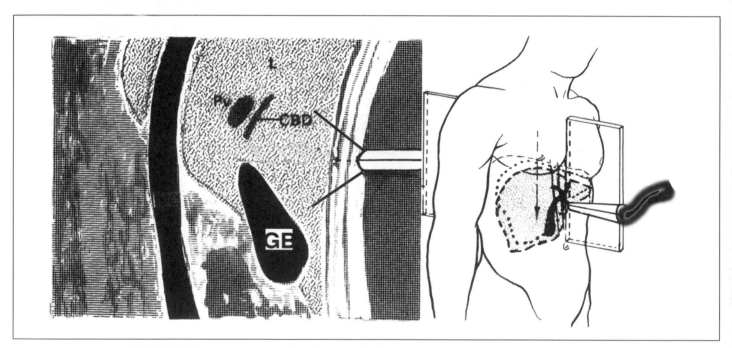

FIGURE 24-3. Gravity and redistribution of abdominal organs allows better access to the liver, gallbladder, and pancreas when the patient is upright.

Local Tenderness

Getting a positive ultrasonic Murphy's sign is an excellent indicator that right upper quadrant pain is indeed localized to the gallbladder. Press the transducer subcostally over the gallbladder and ask the patient if that hurts. (The answer is irrelevant if you are scanning between ribs.) Because this is a somewhat subjective assessment: double check a positive result by pressing in the epigastric region and right lower quadrant. If these areas also hurt, this is not a valid Murphy's sign, although the gallbladder may still be the source of the pain.

If uncertain, turn the patient into a decubitus position and let the gallbladder move into the midline. Press on the gallbladder in the new location and see whether it still hurts. If it doesn't hurt here, where the transducer may have even better access, think again and check the right kidney for stones, or the liver for abscess.

PATHOLOGY

Gallstones

Gallstones are seen with acute and chronic cholecystitis but may be found in symptom-free patients as well. They may have several different sonographic appearances.

Gallstone With Shadowing

A stone surrounded by bile appears as a dense echogenic structure within fluid. The density of the stone will absorb and reflect sound, so that a column of acoustic shadowing is seen posterior to the gallstone (Fig. 24-4).

Shadowing from a stone is "clean" with sharp borders and few internal echoes, whereas shadowing from air is less well defined with more echoes, that is, soft or "dirty" (Fig. 24-5).

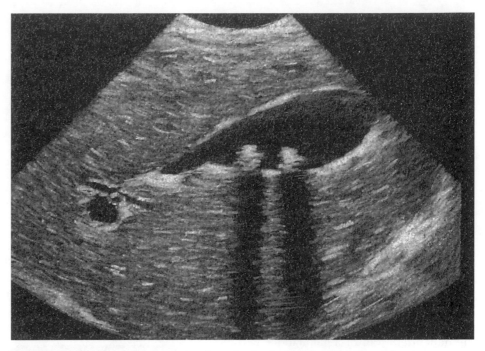

FIGURE 24-4. Two gallstones showing shadowing. Note that the echo sources are within the gallbladder.

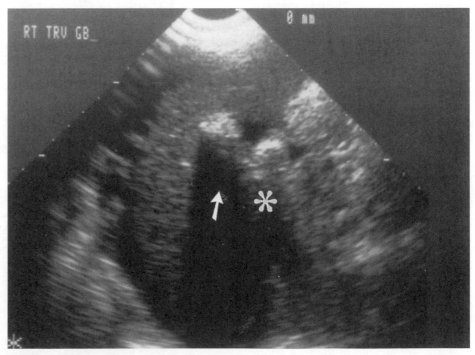

FIGURE 24-5. Gallstone in the gallbladder casts a "clean" shadow (arrow). Nearby is bowel forming a "dirty" shadow (*).

Gallstones Without Shadowing

See Figure 24-6. Very small stones may not be associated with acoustic shadowing using standard transducers. If an echogenic focus (a possible stone) can be shown to move when the patient is repositioned—for example, in the left lateral decubitus or prone position—the lesion is a stone; if the focus does not move, the echoes probably represent a polyp or a septum, although stones can be adherent and immobile.

Gravel

If many small stones are present, they will layer out in the most dependent portion of the gallbladder. It is impossible to discern each separate stone; an irregular pattern of echoes is displayed along the posterior wall of the gallbladder. Shadowing may or may not be seen. Gravel will layer out immediately along the dependent wall of a gallbladder in the decubitus position.

Gallbladder Filled With Stones

Sometimes when the gallbladder contains many stones, no echo-free bile can be seen around them. The stones appear as a group of dense echoes with acoustic shadowing located near the liver edge but within the liver on all views. Because this condition looks suspiciously like a gas-filled duodenum, it can represent a diagnostic problem (Fig. 24-7), and special techniques are required:

1. Make sure another candidate for gallbladder is not visible somewhere else in the right upper quadrant.
2. Trace the main lobar fissure to the gallbladder fossa to prove that this is the gallbladder, as opposed to the duodenum.
3. Change the patient's position. This may cause stones to settle in the dependent portion of the gallbladder and a thin layer of bile to appear across the top (see Fig. 24-7).
4. Have the patient drink water; peristalsis will be seen in the true duodenum.
5. Evaluate the acoustic shadow. Air causes shadowing that has a less well-defined pattern than dense stones (see Fig. 24-5). The borders of a shadowed area caused by stones are generally sharper and more clearly outlined than those caused by gas.

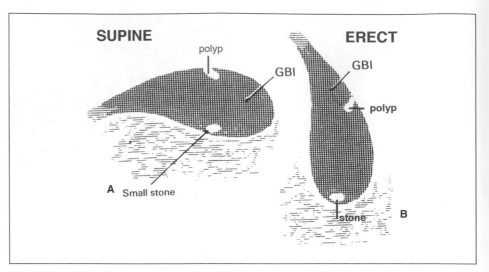

FIGURE 24-6. (**A**) Because this stone is small, shadowing is not seen. The stone should not be mistaken for a polyp. (**B**) The stone falls into the dependent fundus on the erect view.

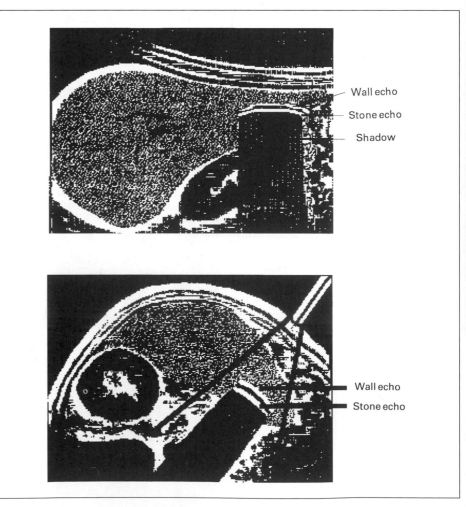

FIGURE 24-7. Acoustic shadowing. Top: Clear, well-defined shadowing is evidence that this is a gallbladder full of stones and not gas shadowing from adjacent structures (the wall echo sign). (There is an echo from the gallbladder wall and from the layer of stones.) The shadowing arises within the liver contour. Bottom: If a gallbladder full of stones is examined on a decubitus view, a thin layer of bile may appear, supporting the diagnosis of gallstones.

6. Look for the wall echo sign (WES; see Fig. 24-7). Echoes are seen both from the wall of the gallbladder and from the layer of stones. By contrast, air in the duodenum will be right against the mucosa.

Stones as a Fluid Level

Occasionally stones float and will be seen as a fluid level within the gallbladder, particularly when the gallbladder contains radiographic contrast material. The stones appear singly or as an irregular echogenic line floating in the bile; when the patient's position is changed, the floating line re-forms.

Adherent Stones

Small adherent stones may appear as echoes in the gallbladder with or without shadowing. If the echoes do not change position with alternate views, the possibilities include adherent stones, gallbladder polyps, or a tumor. Color Doppler, at a high sensitivity setting, may show flow in small intraluminal tumors.

Viscid Bile (Sludge)

Viscid bile usually causes low-level echoes in the dependent portion of the gallbladder akin to those seen with numerous small stones but unaccompanied by shadowing. The fluid level associated with viscid bile is usually not entirely horizontal. If the patient is placed in the erect or decubitus position, the fluid level takes several minutes to reaccumulate (Fig. 24-8), whereas many small stones almost immediately fall into a dependent site. Viscid bile is seen mainly in patients with obstructive jaundice, liver disease, hyperalimentation, or sepsis. A focal area of viscid bile can simulate a polyp or nonshadowing stone. Gallstones with definite shadowing may be mixed in with the sludge.

Acute Cholecystitis

When a patient has acute right upper quadrant pain, acute cholecystitis must be considered. If the patient's most tender area turns out to be exactly where the gallbladder is located, this information should be documented for the clinician because it indicates acute cholecystitis (sonographic Murphy's sign). Pain may be the only finding suggestive of cholecystitis because this condition is not always accompanied by gallstones (acute acalculous cholecystitis).

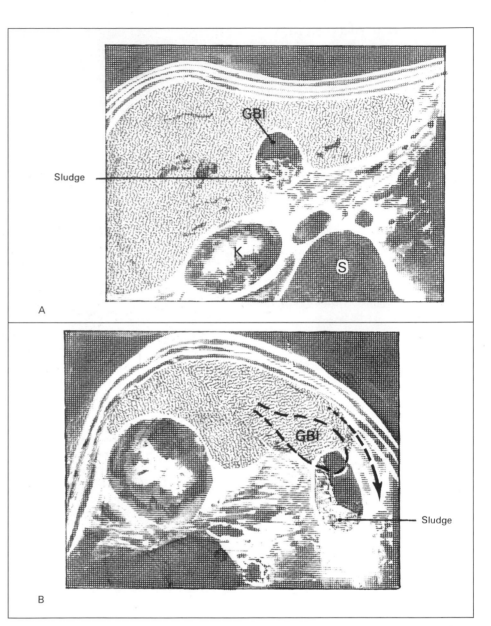

FIGURE 24-8. Presence of sludge. (**A**) Irregular echoes in the posterior aspect of the gallbladder, forming a poorly defined fluid level, suggest the presence of sludge. (**B**) If the patient is placed in a decubitus position, the sludge does not re-form a fluid-fluid level for many minutes.

Checking to see whether a patient has local tenderness over the gallbladder should be part of a routine gallbladder or right upper quadrant examination. If the gallbladder is palpable, it is usually obstructed. A nuclear medicine hepatobiliary scan may be used to establish whether or not the cystic duct is obstructed. However, because the radioisotope cannot enter a flaccid, bile-filled gallbladder, it produces false-positive results in patients on treatment protocols that include parenteral nutrition, large doses of narcotics, antibiotics, or long-term fasting.

Sonographic signs of inflammation include the following:

1. Cholelithiasis
2. Focal tenderness over gallbladder (Murphy's sign)
3. Wall thickening (over 3 mm) and irregularity
4. Fluid in pericholecystic space
5. Gas in the gallbladder

Wall Thickening

Wall thickening is not specific for acute cholecystitis. Diffuse wall thickening can be seen in patients with AIDS, sepsis, hepatitis, congestive heart failure, or ascites. The wall thickening seen in ascites is uniformly echogenic, whereas in acute cholecystitis there is usually an echopenic rim. Striated wall thickening has been associated with acute gangrenous cholecystitis and AIDS (Fig. 24-9). The "wall" should not be more than 3-mm thick; if the outermost echogenic interface is included (solid arrow in Fig. 24-9), the normal thickness should not exceed 5 mm.

Perigallbladder Fluid Collection

A discrete fluid collection, which represents a small abscess, may be seen around the gallbladder, often near the fundus. This is the most definitive evidence of acute cholecystitis (see Fig. 24-9).

Gas in the Gallbladder

With emphysematous cholecystitis the gallbladder or gallbladder wall is filled with gas, which reflects sound back and forth in a reverberation pattern. The appearance is therefore different from that of a gallbladder filled with stones, which blocks the sound completely. The gallbladder will be acutely tender.

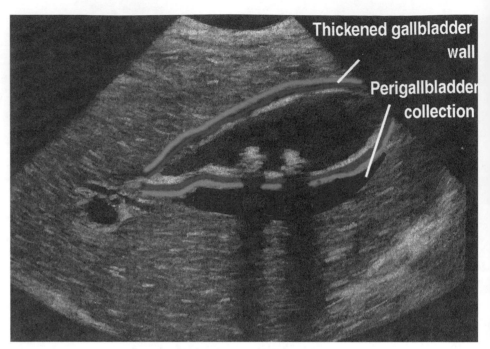

FIGURE 24-9. Acute cholecystitis. The gallbladder wall is thickened and there is a perigallbladder collection. A gallstone is present. The gallbladder was very tender.

Adenomyomatosis

Adenomyomatosis is considered a noninflammatory disease of the gallbladder wall, with hyperplasia and intramural diverticula (Rokitansky-Aschoff sinuses). It causes mild recurrent right upper quadrant pain. There are three sonographic appearances:

1. Multiple septa within the gallbladder
2. Multiple polyps in the gallbladder
3. Multiple "comet effects"—ring-down artifacts resulting from small stones or cholesterol crystals forming in the intramural diverticula (Fig. 24-10)

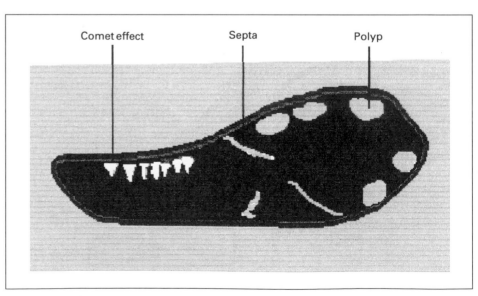

FIGURE 24-10. Adenomyomatosis. Small stones in the gallbladder wall cause the comet effect diagnostic of adenomyomatosis. Septa may be seen. Small polyps are common.

Carcinoma of the Gallbladder

On rare occasions, carcinoma of the gallbladder causes pain; more often it is an unexpected finding on a study performed for other reasons. Possible appearances include the following:

1. Gallbladder partially or completely filled with solid material
2. Focal thickening of the gallbladder wall
3. Stones usually present

Nongallbladder Causes of Right Upper Quadrant Pain

Abscesses

Abscesses in the liver usually have an echopenic center with good through transmission and a thickened wall; sometimes the collapsed wall shows up as an echogenic focus in the liver after drainage of the abscess. Some pyogenic abscesses exhibit low-level echoes on high-gain settings. Necrotic liver tumors also have fluid-filled centers and may be confused with abscesses, but they generally have thicker walls. Color flow may help depict flow in vessels in the wall of an abscess. The subhepatic and subphrenic spaces are also common sites for abscesses, particularly in the postoperative patient. Multiple small abscesses with echogenic centers are seen in immunosuppressed patients owing to fungal infection (Fig. 24-11).

Echinococcal (Hydatid) Cysts

Echinococcal cysts, round or oval in shape, are caused by the parasite *Echinococcus granulosus* and can have any one or a combination of the following appearances (Fig. 24-12):

1. Simple cyst with a parallel line (a laminar membrane) inside the wall. Loose, mobile debris may be seen ("falling snowflakes")
2. Cyst containing smaller daughter cysts; these can deflate and the walls cave in to form the "drooping lily sign" (see Fig. 24-12)
3. Homogeneous material filling cyst or surrounding internal contents
4. Calcifications within; calcified walls
5. Collapsed cyst within the "parent" cyst
6. Echogenic, with or without the other signs; poor acoustic enhancement

A second type, alveolar echinococcus, is seen principally in the Far East. Masses have irregular borders and are echopenic, resembling a neoplasm.

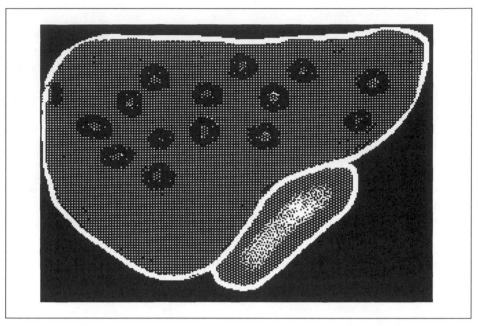

FIGURE 24-11. View showing multiple fungal abscesses within the liver. They are echopenic but have an echogenic center.

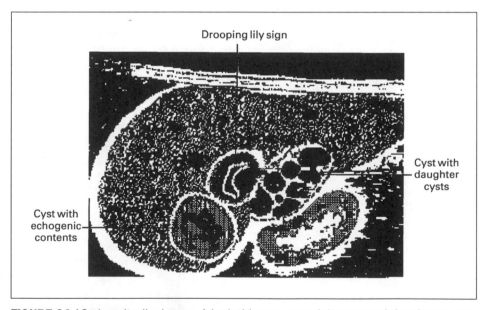

FIGURE 24-12. Longitudinal scan. A hydatid cyst, containing several daughter cysts, lies at the inferior aspect of the liver and displaces the kidney and its surrounding fat line posteriorly. Other types of hydatid appearances—the drooping lily sign and a cyst with echogenic contents—are seen.

Perihepatic Fluid Collections

A collection of fluid on either side of the diaphragm is an important finding and should be easily shown on longitudinal scans through the liver.

A pleural effusion appears as an echo-free, wedge-shaped area superior to the diaphragm on a longitudinal view (see Fig. 47-2). Transversely there is an echo-free rim above the diaphragm. A subdiaphragmatic collection, which may be less well defined, is an area of decreased echogenicity inferior to the diaphragm.

Subphrenic fluid can be differentiated from a pleural effusion (Fig. 24-13) on transverse views. In the latter, the diaphragm will be adjacent to the liver, not separated by fluid. The bare area prevents fluid from lying between the diaphragm and the liver in the midline, whereas a pleural effusion may extend posterior to the heart alongside the spine.

Pyelonephritis

The tenderness may be localized to the kidney. The kidney itself can look normal even when acute inflammation (pyelonephritis) is present. There may be a focal swollen, relatively echopenic area of the kidney that represents an area of acute pyelonephritis. Renal calculi may be seen with or without hydronephrosis and can be the cause of right upper quadrant pain (see Chapter 33).

Pancreatitis

Although the patient complains of right-sided pain, the tenderness may be caused by pancreatitis. The pancreas will be swollen and more sonolucent than normal if pancreatitis is acute (see Chapter 22).

PITFALLS

1. *Artifact vs. stone.* Scattered echoes adjacent to the anterior wall of the gallbladder may be due to reverberation, and near the posterior wall of the gallbladder they may be due to the partial volume effect (see Chapter 53). To diminish these artifacts:
   a. Be sure the electronic focus on the sector scan is set at the correct level; this is operator-dependent on most real-time equipment.

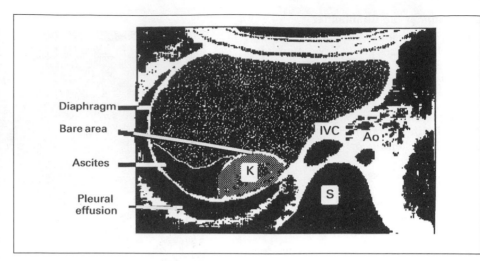

FIGURE 24-13. A transverse scan above the xiphoid shows a collection of pleural fluid above the diaphragm. Some ascites is seen below the diaphragm outlining the "bare area."

   b. Use a transducer with the correct focal zone and frequency. A short focus, high frequency is usually correct.
   c. Change the position of the patient to obtain a decubitus or erect view, thereby increasing the distance between the gallbladder and the transducer. This will eliminate near-field reverberation artifacts (see Fig. 24-2).
   d. Lower the overall gain to decrease echogenicity, producing an artifact-free gallbladder. Remember that a good setting for viewing the gallbladder may not be appropriate for imaging other soft-tissue organs.

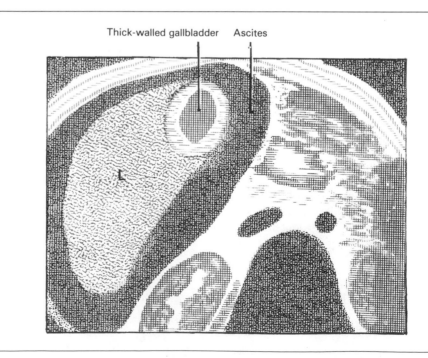

FIGURE 24-14. Ascites, even in very small quantities, can cause a thick gallbladder wall.

2. *Apparently absent gallbladder.* When the gallbladder is small, it can be missed entirely. The main lobar fissure is seen at the right portal vein bifurcation, running directly to the gallbladder fossa, serving as a guide.

3. *Polyp vs. nonshadowing stone.* Acoustic shadowing can be enhanced by using a high-frequency transducer, which places the stone in the correct focal zone. Overgaining can obscure shadowing. Changing patient position helps determine whether a polyp or a stone is present by demonstrating a change in the stone's location.

4. *Gallbladder wall thickening.* Although wall thickening is suggestive of acute cholecystitis, other possible causes include the following:

   a. A recent meal, which causes subsequent gallbladder contraction
   b. Ascites (Fig. 24-14)
   c. Hypoalbuminemia
   d. Hepatitis and other hepatic dysfunction
   e. Some chemotherapeutic drugs
   f. AIDS
   g. Chronic heart failure

5. *Food in the gallbladder.* Following a choledochojejunostomy or sphincterotomy, where a communication between the gallbladder and the gut is created surgically, it is possible for food or gas to reflux into the gallbladder; there may even be acoustic shadowing owing to gas in the gallbladder or biliary tree.

6. *Kink or septum in the gallbladder.* Gallbladders often fold over on themselves or contain a septum, usually in the region where the neck and body meet (the junctional fold). If only a portion of the septum is seen on a single cut, it can resemble a gallstone or polyp in the dependent portion of the gallbladder (Fig. 24-15A). A decubitus or erect view can straighten out a folded gallbladder and reveal that a suspected stone is only a kink.

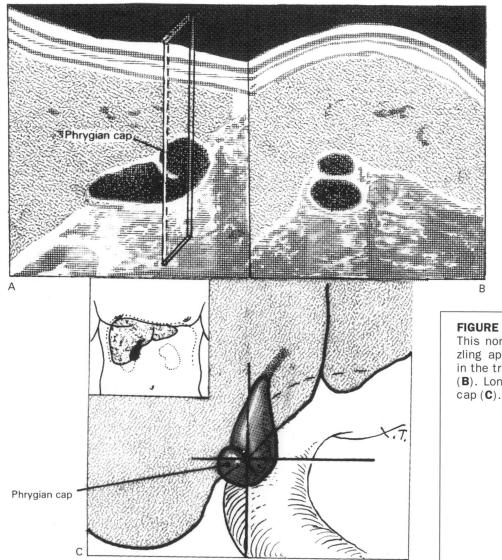

FIGURE 24-15. Phrygian cap variant. This normal variant can produce a puzzling appearance, especially if scanned in the transverse plane shown in (**A**) and (**B**). Long-axis views should include the cap (**C**).

7. *Phrygian cap.* Sometimes a septum develops in the fundus of the gallbladder, forming a "Phrygian cap." This is a normal variant (Fig. 24-15).

8. *Portal vein collaterals mimicking a perigallbladder collection.* A sonolucent space medial to the gallbladder in the region of the porta hepatis can be caused by multiple collaterals from portal vein hypertension. Flow will be seen on Doppler if a Valsalva maneuver is performed, or they should light up on color flow.

9. *Refractive shadowing mimicking stones.* An apparent shadow at the neck of the gallbladder with no echogenic focus at its source is due to refraction of the beam from the wall (see Fig. 24-1).

10. *Surgical clips mimicking gallbladder with calculi.* Clips at the site of cholecystectomy can shadow and resemble stones. Look at the patient's incisions and check the chart. Remember that the gallbladder can be removed from appendectomy incisions or laparoscopically.

? WHERE ELSE TO LOOK

If gallstones are found, look for dilatation of the biliary tree (see Chapter 25).

SELECTED READING

Babb, R. R. Acute acalculous cholecystitis: A review. *J Clin Gastroenterol* 15:238–241, 1992.

Khuroo, M. S., Zargar, S. A., and Mahajan, R. Echinococcus granulosus cysts in the liver: Management with percutaneous drainage. *Radiology* 180:141–145, 1991.

Leopold, G. Gallbladder and bile duct abnormalities in AIDS: Sonographic findings in eight pts. *AJR* 150:123–127, 1988.

Romano, A., van Sonnenberg, E., Casola, G., Gosink, B., Withers, C., McCutcheon, J. A., Starinsky, R., and Alon, Z. Gallbladder size: Is it affected by oral intake of water or dilute contrast medium? *J Ultrasound Med* 13:435–438, 1994.

ABNORMAL LIVER FUNCTION TESTS

Jaundice

NANCY SMITH MINER, ROGER C. SANDERS

25

SONOGRAM ABBREVIATIONS

A	Ascites
Ao	Aorta
Ca	Celiac artery
CBD	Common bile duct
CD	Common duct
Du	Duodenum
GB,GBl	Gallbladder
H	Heart
Ha, Hea	Hepatic artery
IMv	Inferior mesenteric vein
IVC	Inferior vena cava
K	Kidney
L	Liver
LPov	Left portal vein
P	Pancreas
PE	Pleural effusion
Pv	Portal vein
RPov	Right portal vein
S	Spine
SMa	Superior mesenteric artery
SMv	Superior mesenteric vein
Spa	Splenic artery
Spv	Splenic vein

KEY WORDS

ALT (SGPT). Alanine aminotransferase. Enzyme greatly increased in alcoholic hepatitis and moderately increased in jaundice and cirrhosis.

Ampulla (or Papilla) of Vater. Duodenal entrance of the common bile and pancreatic ducts.

AST (SGOT). Aspartate aminotransferase. Enzyme elevated in acute hepatitis and cirrhosis.

Biliary Atresia. Condition in which the bile ducts become narrowed; affects infants a few months old.

Bilirubin. Yellowish pigment in bile formed by red cell breakdown. Causes jaundice if present in increased amounts, and is elevated in all types of jaundice. Can be measured in the urine and serum. Elevation of direct bilirubin level is usually caused by obstructive jaundice.

Cavernous Transformation of the Portal Vein. The portal vein becomes thrombosed and is replaced by numerous collaterals.

Cholangiocarcinoma. A malignant tumor arising from the bile ducts.

Choledochal Cyst. A fusiform dilatation of the common duct that causes obstruction. This congenital condition is usually found in children but may be diagnosed in adults also.

Choledocholithiasis. Stones in the biliary tree.

Cirrhosis. Diffuse disease of the liver with fibrosis. Causes portal hypertension. May be caused by too much alcohol, chronic cardiac failure, or autoimmune disease.

Collaterals. Sometimes known as varices. Dilated veins that appear when portal hypertension is present. Seen principally in the region of the porta hepatis and pancreas.

Common Duct. Term used to describe the common hepatic and common bile ducts. Because the cystic duct junction is not seen ultrasonically, this less-specific term covers both structures.

Coronary Vein. A vein that comes off the splenic vein in the midline and courses superior and to the left; only seen on ultrasound in patients with portal vein hypertension.

Courvoisier's Sign. A right upper quadrant mass with painless jaundice implies that there is a carcinomatous mass in the head of the pancreas that is causing biliary duct obstruction. The palpable mass is due to an enlarged gallbladder.

Fatty Infiltration. Diffuse involvement of the liver with fat; occurs with alcoholism, obesity, diabetes mellitus, steroid administration, jejunoileal bypass, and malnutrition.

GGT. Gamma globulin. Blood product increased in hepatocellular disease.

Glisson's Capsule. Layer of fibrous tissue that surrounds the bile ducts, hepatic arteries, and portal veins within the liver as they travel together; also surrounds the liver.

Glycogen Storage Disease. Several related congenital diseases in which fat-related substances are abnormally deposited within the liver.

Hemolytic Anemia. Anemia resulting from a destruction of the red blood cells. It is either congenital or can be acquired from a variety of causes including infections such as strep and staph.

Hepatitis. Inflammation of the liver due to viral infection. Disease may be acute or may become chronic after an acute episode.

Hepatocellular Disease. Diffuse disease affecting the liver parenchyma such as cirrhosis, fatty infiltration, or hepatitis.

Hepatofugal. Portal vein flow away from the liver. This pattern can be seen in patients with severe portal hypertension.

Hepatopedal. Normal portal vein flow, toward the liver.

Jaundice (Icterus). Yellow pigmentation of the skin due to excessive bilirubin accumulation. The severity of disease can be judged by the appearance of the sclera (white of the eye).

Klatskin Tumor. A ductal cancer at the bifurcation of the right and left hepatic ducts that can cause asymmetrical obstruction of the biliary tree.

Porta Hepatis. Portion of the liver in which the common bile duct, hepatic artery, and portal vein run alongside each other as they leave or enter the liver. Adenopathy can develop here.

Portal Hypertension. Increased portal venous pressure usually due to liver disease (e.g., cirrhosis); leads to dilatation of the portal vein with splenic and superior mesenteric vein enlargement, splenomegaly, and formation of collaterals. The condition can be caused by portal vein thrombosis.

Presbyductia. The common bile duct gradually increases in size with age, and in the elderly can be large (over 7 mm) but not obstructed.

Primary Biliary Cirrhosis. Autoimmune disease of women, not related to alcohol, with unimpressive sonographic appearances. In more severe cases, looks like other forms of cirrhosis.

Pruritus. Itching. It may be due to excess bilirubin and is found in patients with obstructive jaundice.

Regenerating Nodule. Area of tissue (as in a diseased liver) which is repairing itself, thus exhibiting normal texture.

Schistosomiasis. Parasitic disease, involving the portal venous system, common in Middle Eastern countries.

Serum Enzymes. AST (aspartate aminotransferase), GGT (gamma glutamyltransferase), ALT (alanine aminotransferase), LDH (lactic acid dehydrogenase), Alk. Phos. (alkaline phosphatase). These are liver enzymes released from damaged hepatic cells. They are elevated with both obstructed bile ducts and intrinsic liver disease. However, the alkaline phosphatase level is higher in obstruction, whereas the others are higher in intrinsic liver disease.

Sphincter of Oddi. The muscle contracting around the papilla of Vater.

Sphincterotomy. Surgical procedure in which the common duct entrance into the duodenum is widened at the sphincter of Oddi.

Valsalva Maneuver. The patient takes a deep inspiration and holds it while bearing down.

Varices. See *Collaterals.*

THE CLINICAL PROBLEM

There are three basic mechanisms by which jaundice occurs: red blood cells are destroyed, the liver becomes diseased, or intrahepatic or extrahepatic ducts become obstructed.

Red Blood Cell Destruction

Destruction of red blood cells in hemolytic anemias results in jaundice; red cells are destroyed so rapidly that an elevated bilirubin results. The spleen and the liver, the principal sites of red blood cell removal, may be enlarged.

Hepatocellular Disease

Hepatocellular disease causes impaired hepatic cell function and cell death, which leads to a build-up of bilirubin and elevates the serum enzymes AST, ALT, and GGT. Alcoholic liver disease is the most common form; it progresses from alcoholic hepatitis to fatty liver to cirrhosis. There are many other causes of hepatocellular disease such as congestive heart failure and infection.

Intrahepatic cholestasis is an arrest of bile excretion at a level above the bile ducts within the cells. Not sonographically visible, it is treated by medical means, not surgically.

Obstruction of Intrahepatic or Extrahepatic Ducts

The ducts dilate proximal to the site of obstruction. Unlike hemolytic anemia or hepatocellular disease, obstruction of the biliary system is treated surgically.

The major bile components whose serum levels are elevated when bile excretion is blocked are urine and serum bilirubin, serum cholesterol, and serum alkaline phosphatase. However, biochemical tests for obstruction may be misleading because severe nonobstructive liver disease can also elevate these enzymes.

Common causes of obstructed bile ducts include gallstones and choledocholithiasis, tumors in the pancreas, or tumors in the bile ducts, such as Klatskin tumors. In the infant and small child two other important obstructive processes occur. Biliary atresia, a condition in which the bile ducts narrow, is thought to result from infection. The narrowing occasionally occurs outside the liver, in which case operative anastomosis of the gut to the bile duct helps. A choledochal cyst is a fusiform dilatation of the bile duct, and the bile ducts above the "cyst" are dilated. This condition may also be discovered later in life and is treated surgically.

Ultrasound helps the clinician to decide whether jaundice is a surgical or a medical problem. Hemolytic anemia and diffuse liver disease are medical problems, whereas obstruction requires a drainage procedure.

ANATOMY

Diagnosis of biliary obstruction requires an intimate knowledge of the normal vascular structures within the liver (Fig. 25-1).

Biliary Tree

Normally, one may see only a small segment of the biliary tree within the liver—the common duct, a term used by ultrasonographers to describe the common hepatic duct and the common bile duct. As the duct crosses the portal vein, it is still probably common hepatic. However, it is difficult to see on ultrasound where the cystic duct from the gallbladder joins it to form the common bile duct; the compromise term is common duct. Distally, in the head of the pancreas, it is reasonable to assume that you are seeing the common bile duct.

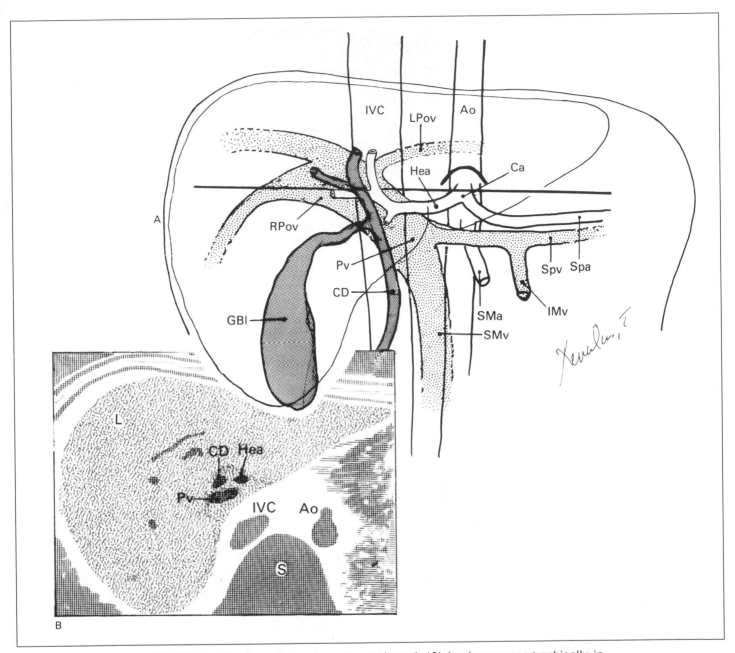

FIGURE 25-1. The transverse plane drawn through (**A**) is shown sonographically in (**B**). The portal triad—the portal vein, common bile duct, and hepatic artery—are intrahepatic at this level. (**A**) demonstrates the relationship between the portal vein, formed by the union of the superior mesenteric vein and splenic vein, with the hepatic artery and bile ducts, which are anterior to the portal vein. The left branch of the portal vein usually leaves the main branch anterior to the inferior vena cava or medial to it.

Sonographically, the common duct lies just to the right of the hepatic artery, and both run anterior to the portal vein throughout their course in the porta hepatis (Fig. 25-2; see also Fig. 25-1).

Branches of the peripheral biliary tree can occasionally be seen normally outside the porta hepatis area as very thin tubular structures lying anterior to portal veins. The walls of the bile ducts are echogenic, and they branch in a tortuous fashion.

The normal width of the common bile duct increases about 1 mm per decade (e.g., a 4-mm duct would be appropriate for a 40-year-old patient and an 8-mm duct for an 80-year-old patient).

Following cholecystectomy, the common duct usually reverts to its normal size. Occasionally it remains dilated when it is not obstructed. If it is dilated and the patient is symptomatic, administer fat and see whether it enlarges, thus demonstrating obstruction. This test works well despite the absence of the gallbladder.

Portal Veins

The portal vein (Figs. 25-3 and 25-4) has to be distinguished from the common duct. It has echogenic walls and branches toward the diaphragm. The right branch bifurcates superior to the gallbladder. The left branch may appear as a double line of echoes in the left lobe of the liver because the lumen is so small. Smaller branches are rarely seen. On Doppler, a normal portal vein shows a monophasic flow pattern, as it flows continuously into the liver. This direction of flow is termed *hepatopedal* (see Fig. 25-8A). With a traditional color flow orientation, this would be encoded in red.

Hepatic Veins

Hepatic veins (Figs. 25-5 to 25-7; and see Fig. 25-3) are easily differentiated from bile ducts and portal veins. They are not surrounded by an echogenic wall, although the posterior wall of the right hepatic vein, which is perpendicular to the beam, often appears bright. Hepatic veins branch in the direction of the feet. They originate close to the diaphragm, and can be traced into the inferior vena cava.

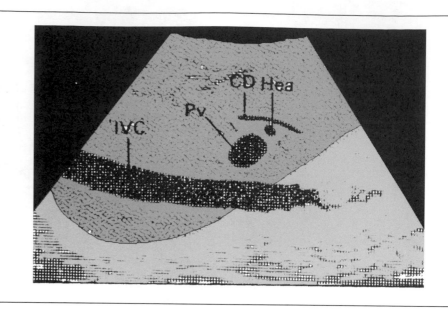

FIGURE 25-2. Supine longitudinal view. The common bile duct in the region of the porta hepatis lies anterior to the portal vein and the right hepatic vein.

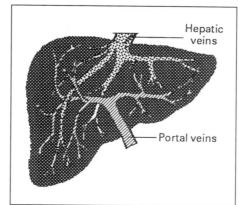

FIGURE 25-3. Diagram showing the relationship of the portal and hepatic veins.

FIGURE 25-4. Right costal margin views showing segments of the portal veins within the liver (arrow). Note the echogenic outlines of the portal veins and the ascending portion of the left portal vein.

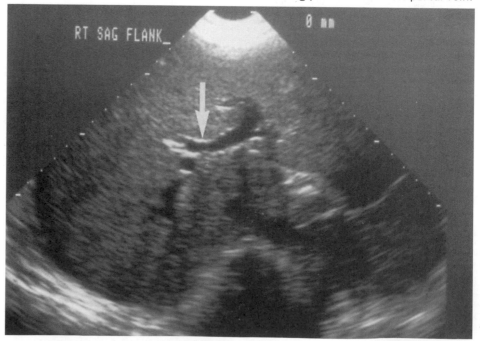

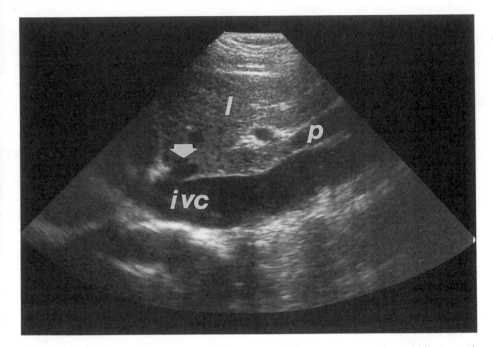

FIGURE 25-5. Longitudinal view showing the inferior vena cava, the middle hepatic vein (upper arrow), and the porta hepatis (p).

Because the direction of flow is away from the transducer, it is traditionally blue on color flow. On duplex Doppler, the flow below the baseline peaks twice, corresponding with the movements of the tricuspid valve. Then there is a transient flow reversal, shown as a peak above the baseline, which corresponds to atrial contraction (see Fig. 25-6B).

Hepatic Arteries

The common hepatic artery takes off from the celiac axis and courses over the anterior, superior edge of the pancreas, then (after giving off the gastroduodenal artery) runs cephalad as the proper hepatic artery into the porta hepatis. It runs anterior to the portal vein and to the left of the common duct. Then the right hepatic artery crosses between the common duct and the portal

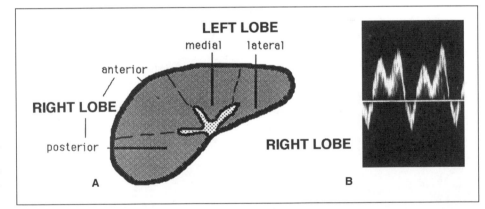

FIGURE 25-6. (**A**) Transverse view showing the right, middle, and left hepatic veins and their relationship to the liver anatomy. Inset (**B**) is the typical Doppler pattern in the hepatic veins.

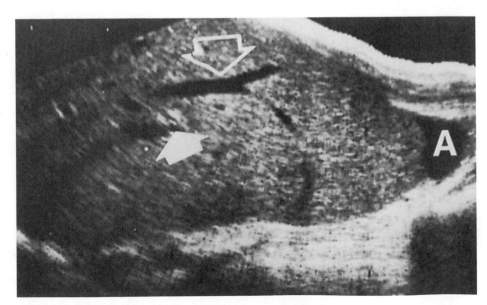

FIGURE 25-7. Longitudinal view showing the middle hepatic veins (open white arrow), which bifurcate toward the feet. Note small collection of ascites (**A**) and the portal vein (solid arrow).

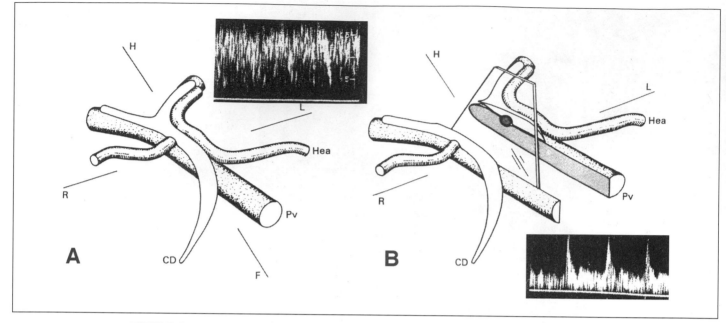

FIGURE 25-8. The relationship of the portal vein, the hepatic artery, and the common duct are demonstrated. Notice that the hepatic artery runs between the common duct and the portal vein and is seen on a standard section through the porta hepatis. Inset is the typical Doppler pattern within the portal vein (left) and on the right, the typical hepatic artery Doppler pattern. H = head, R = right, L = left, F = foot. (Reprinted with permission from Berland, L., and Foley, D. Porta hepatis sonography discontinuation of bile ducts from artery with pulsed Doppler anatomic center. *AJR* 138 : 833, 1982.)

vein (Fig. 25-8). It may double back on itself (Fig. 25-9). Hepatic arteries can be a source of confusion in the region of the porta hepatis because they might be mistaken for a dilated common duct, since they can reach 8 mm in diameter.

Color flow or duplex Doppler will easily make the distinction by showing flow if the vessel is hepatic artery. Because the flow is toward the liver, it will show up red on the traditional color orientation; however, it should be a lighter red than

the portal vein because of its higher velocity of flow. Duplex Doppler shows a typical low-resistance arterial pattern (see Fig. 25-8B).

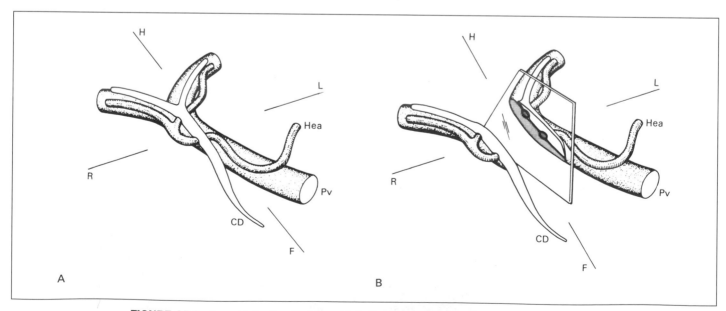

FIGURE 25-9. A variant situation in which the hepatic artery bends to the right and then turns back to the left again. (Reprinted with permission from Berland, L., and Foley, D. Porta hepatis sonography: discontinuation of bile ducts from artery with pulsed Doppler anatomic center. *AJR* 138 : 833, 1982.)

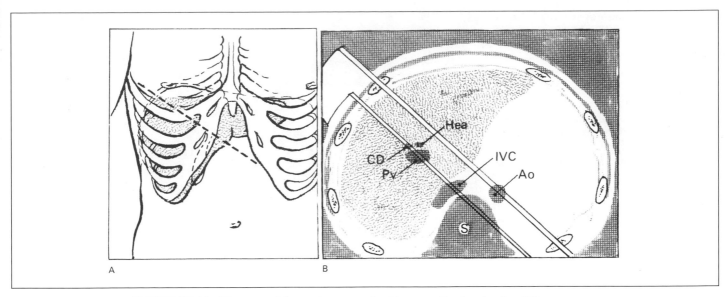

FIGURE 25-10. The two oblique views required to scan the long axis of the common duct are illustrated here. Not only is the path made oblique from a straight longitudinal plane, but the transducer is angled in from the patient's side, throwing the ducts and portal vein into the same plane as the inferior vena cava (see also Fig. 25-11 and 25-2).

▨ TECHNIQUE

Intrahepatic Common Duct

Because the common duct courses in a plane that is somewhat perpendicular to the right costal margin, a parasagittal plane is required to visualize more than a small piece of it. Turning the patient up toward his or her left side (into a left posterior oblique position) is helpful in using the liver to provide a better acoustic window (Figs. 25-10 and 25-11). The standardized place to measure the lumen is where the common duct crosses anteriorly over the right portal veins and right hepatic artery (see Fig. 25-2). Sometimes the duct is most accessible on the decubitus view, when the gallbladder is being checked for layering stones.

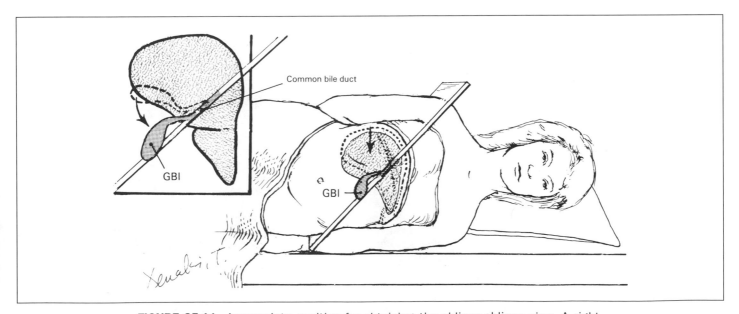

FIGURE 25-11. Appropriate position for obtaining the oblique-oblique view. A right-side-up decubitus position allows the liver to fall medially, often providing easier access to the common duct. The gallbladder can be viewed at the same time for layering of stones.

The distal duct cannot usually be seen in the same plane (Fig. 25-12).

Distal CBD

The axis of the common bile duct changes from oblique to sagittal at the superior margin of the pancreas (see Fig. 25-12). Scan in the sagittal plane, angling under the duodenum if necessary, to see the proximal intrapancreatic portion. At this point, the duct curves laterally and disappears into the sphincter of Oddi.

A transverse plane is needed to investigate this most distal part of the duct. Because this view is often so important in helping determine the level of obstruction, it pays to make a real effort to show the distal duct and surrounding pancreatic head as well.

Gas in the antrum and duodenum is the primary problem to overcome. An erect right posterior oblique position (RPO) helps displace the air. If there is still a problem, have the patient drink 16 oz of water and rest in a right lateral decubitus for 2 to 3 minutes, then rescan in the erect RPO position, transversely (see Fig. 25-12).

Questionable Obstruction

Occasionally it is unclear whether a duct is "borderline" enlarged or if the large size is just a consequence of old age (presbyductia). Postcholecystectomy patients sometimes continue to have ducts which seem dilated but not obstructed. In these cases it is helpful to assess the biliary dynamics rather than rely on size alone. One method is to measure the duct during quiet respiration, then again at maximal Valsalva maneuver. A nonobstructed duct will decrease at least 1 mm in diameter at the level of the portal vein during full inspiration; during the Valsalva maneuver an obstructed duct should not change size.

Another method is to administer a fatty meal. A normal duct will stay the same size or decrease in caliber, while an abnormal duct either remains unchanged or increases in caliber.

Peripheral Ducts

Peripheral ducts will only be seen if they are dilated (Fig. 25-13). There is a characteristic tortuous appearance of biliary structures, with noticeable acoustic enhancement. It is important to examine the entire liver parenchyma, because isolated segmental biliary obstruction can occur.

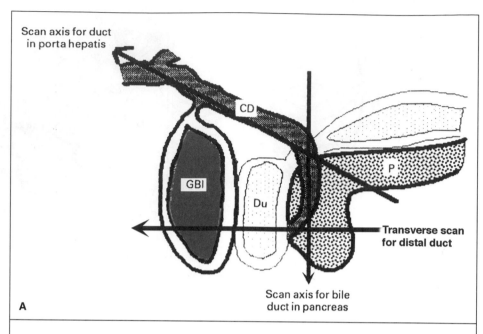

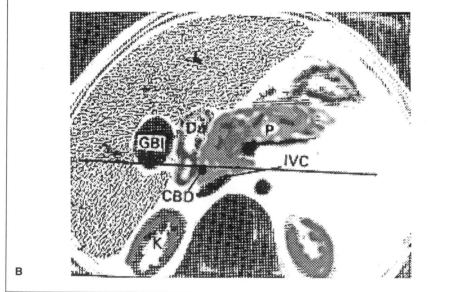

FIGURE 25-12. (**A**) Scanning the common duct. The scan plane used for the common duct in the head of the pancreas is along the same plane as the inferior vena cava, angling slightly laterally. The common duct angles inferiorly shortly before it enters the pancreas. The arrow pointing left shows the scan plane for the porta hepatis. The vertical arrow shows the scan plane in the head of the pancreas region. (**B**) The transverse plane is appropriate for showing the common duct in the head of the pancreas. The common bile duct can be dilated owing to obstruction at this level even if the intrahepatic ducts are normal. Masses occur in the inferior portion of the head of the pancreas, which can be hard to see on long-axis views of the pancreas but are often visible on this view, which is more inferior.

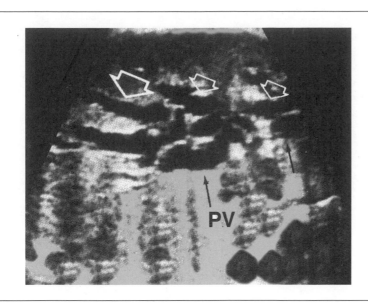

FIGURE 25-13. Peripheral dilated bile ducts are seen (white arrows) anterior to the portal vein and branches (black arrows). Note the acoustic enhancement posterior to the ducts.

Doppler Imaging of Hepatic Vessels

Vessels in the liver are often perpendicular to the beam, making it difficult to maintain a Doppler angle of less than 60 degrees. Creative positioning is called for here, depending on the patient's body habitus. For example, turning the patient left side down and scanning from the right side may be a helpful approach. The portal vein can be scanned sagittally, as though one were scanning for the common duct; presence and direction of flow can be established. However, if ruling out thrombus is the object, try to scan subcostally in order to see the entire vessel.

Beware: A poor angle can create the impression of hepatofugal flow, suggesting a false diagnosis of portal hypertension.

The common hepatic artery can usually be seen from an oblique intercostal approach; hepatic veins are accessible subxyphoid. The veins are usually being assessed for patency; however, cirrhosis and hepatomegaly often compress them so they can't be seen on real-time. Duplex Doppler is then impossible, but sometimes these hepatic veins will still show up with color Doppler.

Lower-frequency transducers are often necessary to get adequate penetration for Doppler examination of the adult abdomen. A 2.25-MHz transducer will increase the Doppler sensitivity greatly, with little degrading effect on the resolution.

◆ PATHOLOGY
Diffuse Liver Disease

Diffuse parenchymal liver disease has a number of sonographic features, although one can rarely make a specific diagnosis. There are generally no mass effects, such as displaced vessels, with diffuse disease. The sonographic appearance of some conditions, such as fatty liver or alcoholic liver disease, can improve rapidly when the primary cause is removed. The following are the most typical patterns.

Fatty Infiltration

The liver becomes enlarged with fatty infiltration. It shows a fine stippled echogenicity. Visualization of portal vein walls and the right hemidiaphragm (even with a low-frequency transducer) is difficult owing to increased acoustic attenuation. Comparing liver echogenicity to that of the right renal parenchyma helps to assess the degree of fatty infiltration (Fig 25-14). The liver parenchyma is normally only slightly more echogenic than the kidney. With severe fatty infiltration, the acoustic impedance can be so great that it is difficult to penetrate more than a few centimeters of liver, completely obscuring any posterior structures.

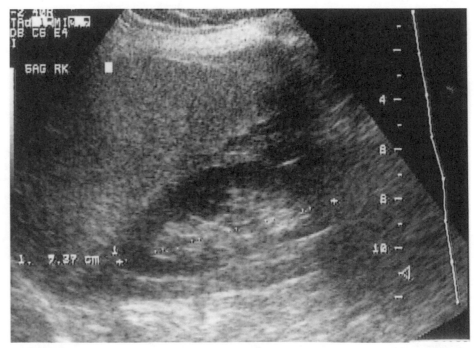

FIGURE 25-14. Fatty liver. The liver is enlarged and has a much coarser echogenic texture than normal and poor acoustic transmission. Note the very echogenic kidney in contrast to the densely echogenic liver.

Early Alcoholic Liver Disease

Subtle changes in shape indicate the presence of alcoholic liver disease. The edge of the right lobe becomes rounded (see Fig. 25-7). A large left lobe or a prominent caudate lobe may herald the development of textural abnormalities, which often progress to acute hepatitis.

Acute Hepatitis

In acute hepatitis the portal vein borders are more prominent than usual. This is said to be a consequence of an overall decreased liver echogenicity. The liver and spleen are enlarged, and the gallbladder wall is often markedly thickened.

Chronic Hepatitis

Changes similar to those typical of fatty infiltration are seen in chronic hepatitis, but the degree of sound attenuation is not as great and the liver is not as large. However, the left and caudate lobes may be large relative to the right lobe.

Cirrhosis

In cirrhosis, the liver is more echogenic, decreases in size, and starts to develop a nodular border. In longstanding, end-stage cirrhosis, the liver is small and very echogenic (Fig. 25-15). It may be outlined by ascitic fluid. One portion of the liver may have a different echogenicity from the remainder and form a bulge, probably representing a regenerating nodule. These patients also have portal hypertension and splenomegaly.

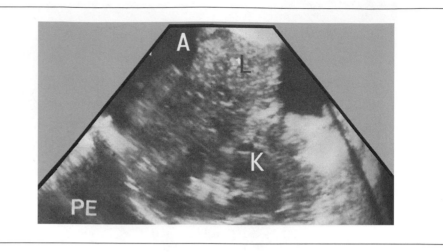

FIGURE 25-15. Cirrhotic liver. The liver is small, has a knobby margin (arrow), and many increased internal echoes. Note pleural effusion and ascites surrounding the liver.

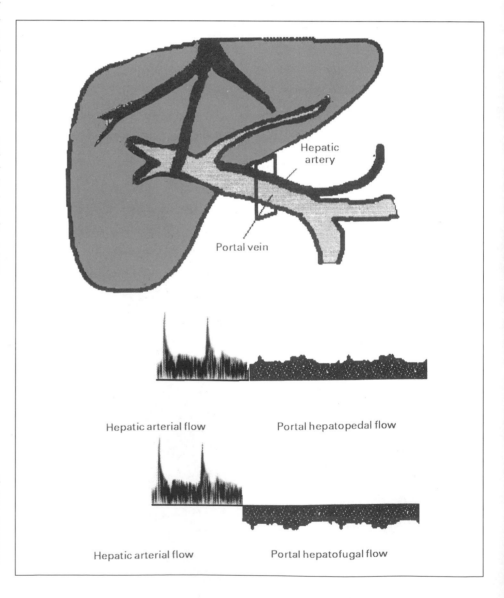

FIGURE 25-16. The Doppler patterns were obtained at the boxed site in the hepatic artery. In normal hepatopedal flow, the hepatic artery and portal vein both flow in the same direction, toward the liver. In hepatofugal flow, the artery still flows toward the liver but the vein flows away from the liver.

Portal Hypertension

Increased pressure in the portal vein is a consequence of liver fibrosis or of portal vein obstruction by clot or tumor. The most common cause of intrahepatic portal hypertension is cirrhosis. Features of portal hypertension include the following:

1. Splenomegaly
2. Portal vein dilated to greater than 1.3-cm diameter (Note: Portal vein size may return to normal if collateral circulation develops.)
3. Recanalization of the paraumbilical veins within the ligamentum teres. The ligamentum teres is the remnant of the umbilical vein in the fetus and still contains small vessels that dilate when the intrahepatic pressure increases.
4. Collaterals. These are seen as small tortuous vessels in the porta hepatis, around the gastric fundus, in the pancreatic bed, and in the splenic hilum. Doppler and color flow help in determining that these are vessels. The portal vein may become thrombosed and replaced by numerous small collaterals. This is known as cavernous transformation of the portal vein.
5. Dilation of the splenic vein, the superior mesenteric vein, and sometimes the coronary vein
6. Ascites
7. In a small number of cases, reversal of flow in the portal vein on duplex or color Doppler flow

The blood in the portal vein and hepatic artery normally flows in the same direction, into the liver (hepatopedal). In severe portal hypertension, flow in the portal vein is reversed, toward the feet (hepatofugal) (Fig. 25-16). Color flow makes this change in direction obvious; a Doppler cursor through both vessels simultaneously demonstrates that the direction of flow is no longer the same in both vessels.

The ligamentum teres runs from the ascending left portal vein to the anterior surface of the liver. Trace it from the left portal vein on longitudinal scans (see Fig. 23-1) and magnify to demonstrate recanalization. Use color to demonstrate the presence and direction of the flow.

Portal and Splenic Vein Thrombosis

Portal vein thrombosis may precipitate a sudden deterioration in the condition of a patient with portal hypertension. Some causes of thrombosis development within the portal or splenic vein are as follows:

1. Portal hypertension
2. Tumor compression or involvement
3. Pancreatitis causing compression
4. Trauma
5. Sepsis

Sonographic features can include the following:

1. Nonvisualization of the vessel
2. Clot within the lumen
3. Echo-free clot appearing normal but showing no flow on duplex Doppler or color flow
4. Collaterals, which will develop in the porta hepatis (cavernous transformation of the portal vein)
5. Marked splenomegaly

Color Doppler can confidently establish that a portal vein is patent, but a small percentage of "no flow" cases may be false-positives due to sluggish flow or technical considerations (see Pitfalls for technical considerations).

Hemolytic Anemia

In most types of hemolytic anemia the only sonographic changes are enlargement of the liver and spleen. Gallstones may be present. If hemolytic anemia is caused by lymphoma, there may be nodal enlargement.

Infiltrative Disorders

Most infiltrative disorders such as glycogen storage disease cause a diffuse increase in echogenicity throughout the liver and overall liver and spleen enlargement. In the pediatric age group, focal echopenic masses can be seen in some of these disorders.

Biliary Obstruction

Bile Duct Measurements

If the liver function tests suggest obstruction, the most sensitive area to check for biliary obstruction is at the level of the common bile duct.

The width of the common duct is usually measured at the point at which it crosses the portal vein anterior to the hepatic artery (Fig. 25-17).

Only the lumen is measured. In the adult, a crude rule is that there is a 1-mm increase per decade. A 2-mm duct is normal in a 20-year-old and a 9-mm duct is normal in a 90-year-old. In a child under 1 year, the duct should always be less than 1.6-mm; and the diameter should not exceed 2.5 to 3 mm during childhood and early adolescence. Children's ducts have been shown to be distensible and change size during daily fluctuations in bile flow, but in general the duct is about the same caliber as the hepatic artery while the child grows.

FIGURE 25-17. Oblique-oblique view. The width of the normal lumen of a common duct at this level should be measured intraluminally.

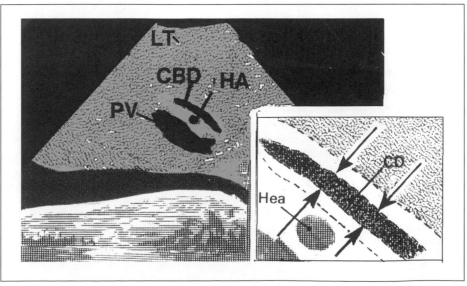

If an adult's common duct is top normal or slightly enlarged, additional techniques using a fatty meal or a Valsalva maneuver are described in the technique section.

Criteria for Dilated Ducts

Recognizing biliary obstruction by ultrasound is a matter of distinguishing the biliary ducts from the portal and hepatic veins and the hepatic arteries, and knowing what constitutes a normal duct size.

The following criteria can aid in correct identification of biliary ducts.

1. Biliary ducts run *anterior* to the *portal veins.*
2. When biliary ducts are dilated, a distinctive pattern is created that has been dubbed the "double barrel shotgun" or "parallel channel" sign (see Fig. 25-13). Two tubular structures, the portal vein and the bile duct, are seen running in parallel.
3. Unlike portal veins, bile ducts branch repeatedly, are tortuous, and show acoustic enhancement (see Fig. 25-13). Suspicious tubular structures should be traced to their origins to ensure that they are part of the biliary system and not hepatic arteries. Color flow will help determine whether you are looking at a vessel or a duct.
4. Dilated peripheral ducts often splay out from a central point, giving them a star-like appearance (see Fig. 25-13).
5. Unlike blood in the vessels which attenuates sound, bile transmits it, so there is acoustic enhancement posterior to dilated biliary ducts.
6. Unlike hepatic veins, obstructed bile ducts will not dilate with a Valsalva maneuver; they stay the same. Normal ducts usually decrease in size.

Causes of Biliary Dilatation

Stones in Bile Ducts

Most stones can be seen if views of the distal common duct are obtained. An area of acoustic shadowing with an echogenic source represents a stone. The obstructing stone may not be seen, but other stones in the proximal dilated duct may be visible. Most stones lie in the distal-most portion of the common duct, best shown by the technique shown in Figure 25-12.

Mirizzi Syndrome

In this condition the obstructing stone lies in the cystic duct or Hartmann's pouch, adjacent to and compressing the common bile duct. There is secondary dilatation of the peripheral bile ducts and the gallbladder. It can be difficult to decide whether the stone is in the cystic or common duct. However, it would be unlikely for a stone in the common duct in such a proximal location to cause a dilated gallbladder.

Think of this syndrome if you see an enlarged gallbladder and dilated peripheral ducts. The diagnosis is made if you show that the stone is indeed in the cystic duct and not in the common bile duct. The common bile duct, which is entirely distal to where the cystic duct joins, should be normal in caliber, whereas the intrahepatic common hepatic duct is enlarged. The surgical management of Mirizzi syndrome can be technically difficult because there is a chance that the common duct will be inadvertently sliced.

Bile Duct Tumors

Rarely, a tumor may be seen within a bile duct (a cholangiocarcinoma), almost always where the common hepatic duct bifurcates into the right and left ducts (Klatskin tumor; Fig. 25-18). The bile ducts are dilated proximal to the tumor. Such peripheral dilation can easily be missed if casual technique is used. The segment of duct that is usually documented anterior to the portal vein would remain normal in size.

Oriental Pyocholangitis (Recurrent Pyogenic Cholangiohepatitis)

Oriental pyocholangitis is seen in the Far East and in people of Asian descent in America. The common bile duct is massively dilated and contains much echogenic sludge and calculi; the intrahepatic ducts can contain multiple soft stones, which may not shadow. These patients have recurrent infections of the biliary tree.

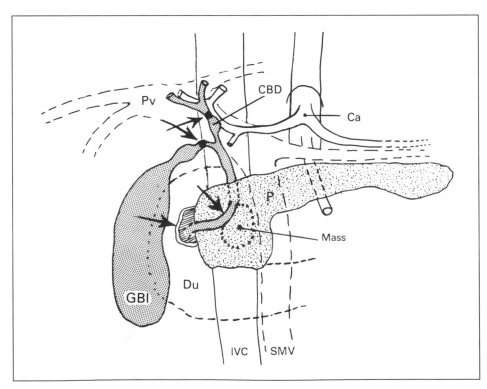

FIGURE 25-18. Arrows indicate some potential sites of obstruction in the biliary tree. Stones may lodge in these sites causing shadows that can be seen if scanned with the correct focal zone and frequency. Another source of biliary obstruction is a mass in the head of the pancreas. The most superior arrow points to the usual site of Klatskin tumors (tumors of the biliary tree).

AIDS Cholangitis

In some patients with AIDS, the bile duct dilates even though it is not obstructed. The walls of the bile ducts become thickened, and the distal common bile duct sometimes tapers.

Caroli's Disease

Segments of the biliary tree are dilated, although not obstructed, and look like tubular cysts in Caroli's disease. Because it is associated with infantile polycystic kidney disease, a casual observer may mistake them for unusually shaped liver cysts; look for communications between the ducts. Intrahepatic biliary stones may or may not be present.

Choledochal Cysts

Choledochal cysts are usually diagnosed in children, and are easy to see sonographically. With real-time one can see a cystic structure in the right upper quadrant inferior to the liver. The common duct is seen entering this structure, and there may or may not be biliary duct dilatation elsewhere. The gallbladder is seen separately from the cyst (Fig. 25-19).

Hepatic Duct Calculi

Stones may develop in the gallbladder and then reflux into the biliary tree to cause focal dilatation of a segment of the biliary tree. These patients present with pain rather than jaundice; the liver function tests are atypical since the bulk of the biliary tree is unaffected.

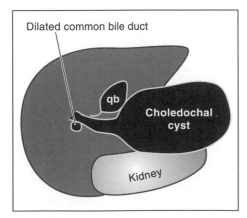

FIGURE 25-19. Choledochal cyst. A dilated bile duct is seen entering a choledochal cyst on a longitudinal scan of the right upper quadrant. The gallbladder is seen separately; the main lobar fissure may be useful in locating it.

Biliary Atresia

In biliary atresia, which occurs in children 3 to 6 months old, the bile ducts, even when dilated, are still very small and can only just be seen. Even obstructed ducts can be only 1 to 2 mm in diameter. The biliary tree is affected by biliary atresia to a variable degree. Whether or not the gallbladder is seen depends on the site of obstruction. An absent gallbladder favors this disease.

Metastatic Tumor

Focal metastatic deposits can block peripheral bile ducts, causing secondary bile duct dilatation. Multiple metastases or lymphomatous deposits can be a cause of jaundice, although no dilated ducts may be visible.

Ascaris

These are worms primarily seen in tropical climates which are ingested and gravitate to the biliary tree or gallbladder. They appear as long, tubular, *moving* structures on real-time.

PITFALLS

1. *Pseudo bile duct obstruction*
   a. *Portal vein bifurcation.* Superior to the gallbladder, the right portal vein bifurcates into two large branches. For a short distance they run parallel to each other and mimic the appearance of a dilated bile duct and portal vein.
   b. *Hepatic artery.* The hepatic artery runs anterior to the portal vein in close proximity to the common bile duct. The artery occasionally reaches a size of over 6 mm and can be mistaken for a dilated duct. However, it is pulsatile and can be traced to the celiac axis. Color flow or duplex Doppler can help make the distinction. Sometimes, the hepatic artery runs anterior to the common duct, as a normal variant which can cause confusion. Patients with cirrhosis and portal hypertension can have abnormally large intrahepatic arteries, which look like dilated intrahepatic ducts; these will readily show flow with color or duplex Doppler.
   c. *Neck of gallbladder (Hartmann's pouch).* The neck of the gallbladder sometimes lies anterior to the common bile duct, and on some views it may appear to be separate from the body. It can thus be mistaken for a dilated duct if not traced into the body of the gallbladder.
   d. *Postcholecystectomy residual duct dilatation.* After surgery, the common duct may remain large even after obstruction has been relieved. Ask for the patient's surgical history. This may be important particularly after laparoscopic cholecystectomy, when the scars may be unnoticeable. A fatty meal will contract these ducts.

2. *Gas in the biliary tree versus stones.* If communication is free between the biliary tree and the gastrointestinal tract (e.g., following a sphincterotomy), gas can reflux into the biliary tree and cause pockets of acoustic shadowing that resemble stones. However, the following should be noted:
   a. The shadowing is "dirty" and contains echoes.
   b. It is located at the anterior (nondependent) aspect of the gallbladder and in the peripheral ducts; air tends to prefer the left branch of ducts because the left is anatomically superior and anterior; air rises.
   c. There will be a change in location when the patient changes position.

3. *Pseudo diffuse liver disease.* By causing coarse echoes in the parenchyma, a high-frequency transducer used with high gain can make the liver look as if it is abnormal due to diffuse liver disease. If you have to scan with maximum gain settings and the TGC at its peak, consider that you may be using a transducer with too high a frequency. Comparison between the liver and kidney will show whether the increased echogenicity is genuine. The normal kidney parenchyma is only slightly less echogenic than the liver. Also, the diaphragm may be poorly seen if too high a frequency is used, making it appear as though there is fatty infiltration.

4. *Splenomegaly causing large splenic, superior mesenteric, and portal veins.* Splenomegaly due to causes other than portal hypertension can result in a dilated portal venous system, but no collaterals will be seen.

5. *No flow in portal vein* (false-positive portal vein thrombus). If no flow is detected in the portal vein (particularly in the absence of other relevant clinical features of portal vein thrombosis) make *certain* that it is not due to technique. Patients with low flow velocity can have all the signals in the portal vein wiped out by high wall filter settings. Increase sensitivity by making sure your angle isn't too perpendicular to the vessel. If the patient is holding his or her breath, the Valsalva effect may eliminate slow flow altogether. Also, consider postprandial scanning in a patient who has been fasting, as eating may increase portal vein flow.

❓ WHERE ELSE TO LOOK

1. *Obstructed bile ducts.* It is essential to trace a dilated duct to the point of obstruction (see Fig. 25-18). Often the obstruction is in the region of the pancreas. Mass lesions such as carcinoma of the pancreas, a pseudocyst, or focal pancreatitis are often responsible. One may see a stone within an obstructed duct; look then for stones in the gallbladder. Rarely, obstructed ducts are due to extrinsic pressure from nodes in the region of the porta hepatis, which can be demonstrated.

2. *Hepatocellular disease.* Diffuse textural changes within the liver are usually caused by alcoholic liver disease. When these changes are found, look for other sequelae of alcoholism: (1) a pancreatic pseudocyst or pancreatitis; and (2) portal hypertension with splenomegaly, enlarged superior mesenteric and splenic veins, visible collaterals, and ascites.

3. *Hemolytic jaundice.* If the jaundice appears to result from hemolytic anemia with an enlarged liver and spleen, look for enlarged nodes, because there may be underlying leukemia or lymphoma.

SELECTED READING

Bressler, E. L., Rubin, J. M., and McCracken, S. Sonographic parallel channel sign: A reappraisal. *Radiology* 164:343–346, 1987.

Feldstein, V. A., and LaBerge, J. M. Hepatic vein flow reversal at duplex sonography: A sign of transjugular intrahepatic portosystemic shunt dysfunction. *AJR* 162:839–841, 1994.

Grant, E., Schiller, V., Millener, P., Tessler, F., Perrella, R., Ragavendra, N., and Busuttil, R. Color Doppler imaging of the hepatic vasculature. *AJR* 159:943–950, 1992.

Green, C. L., Angtuaco, T. L., Shah, H. R., and Parmley, T. H. Gestational trophoblastic disease: A spectrum of radiologic diagnosis. *Radiographics* 16:1371–1384, 1996.

Hernanz-Schulman, M., et al. Common bile duct in children: Sonographic dimensions. *Radiology* 195:193–195, 1995.

Joseph, A. E. A., and Saverymuttu, S. H. Editorial: Ultrasound in the assessment of diffuse parenchymal liver disease. *Clin Radiol* 44:219–221, 1991.

Kane, R., and Eustace, S. Diagnosis of Budd-Chiari syndrome: Comparison between sonography and MR angiography. *Radiology* 195:117–121, 1995.

Ladenheim, J. A., Luba, D. G., Yao, F., Gregory, P. B., Jeffrey, R. B., and Garcia, G. Limitations of liver surface US in the diagnosis of cirrhosis. *Radiology* 185:21–24, 1992.

Laing, F. C., et al. Biliary dilatation: Defining the level and cause by real-time US. *Radiology* 160:39–42, 1986.

Lin, D. Y., Sheen, I. S., Chiu, C. T., Lin, S. M., Kuo, Y. C., and Liaw, Y. F. Ultrasonographic changes of early liver cirrhosis in chronic hepatitis B: A longitudinal study. *J Clin Ultrasound* 21:303–308, 1993.

Matsui, O., Kadoya, M., Takahashi, S., Yoshikawa, J., Gabata, T., Takashima, T., and Kitagawa, K. Focal sparing of segment IV in fatty livers shown by sonography and CT: Correlation with aberrant gastric venous drainage. *AJR* 164:1137–1140, 1995.

Quinn, R. J., et al. The effect of the Valsalva maneuver on the diameter of the common hepatic duct in extrahepatic biliary obstruction. *J Ultrasound Med* 11:143–145, 1992.

Ralls, P. W. Color Doppler sonography of the hepatic artery and portal venous system. *AJR* 155:517–525, 1990.

Ralls, P. W., et al. The use of color Doppler sonography to distinguish dilated intrahepatic ducts from vascular structures. *AJR* 152:291–292, 1989.

Richter, J., Zwingenberger, K., Ali, Q. M., Lima, W. D. M., Dacal, A. R. C., DeSiqueira, G. V., Doehring-Schwerdtfeger, E., and Feldmeier, H. Hepatosplenic schistosomiasis. Comparison of sonographic findings in Brazilian and Sudanese patients. Correlation of sonographic findings with clinical symptoms. *Radiology* 184:711–716, 1992.

Wachsberg, R. H., Needleman, L., and Wilson, D. J. Portal vein pulsatility in normal and cirrhotic adults without cardiac disease. *J Clin Ultrasound* 23:3–15, 1995.

Zwiebel, W. J., Mountford, R. A., Halliwell, M. J., and Wells, P. N. T. Splanchnic blood flow in patients with cirrhosis and portal hypertension: Investigation with duplex Doppler US. *Radiology* 194:807–812, 1995.

FEVER OF UNKNOWN ORIGIN (FUO)

Rule Out Abscesses

26

NANCY SMITH MINER, LISA SIMMONS

SONOGRAM ABBREVIATIONS

Ao	Aorta
Bl	Bladder
GB	Gallbladder
H	Hematoma
Ip	Iliopsoas muscle
IVC	Inferior vena cava
K	Kidney
L	Liver
LHev	Left hepatic vein
MHev	Middle hepatic vein
P	Pancreas
RAt	Right atrium
RHev	Right hepatic vein
RK	Right kidney
S	Spine
Sp	Spleen
St	Stomach
Ut	Uterus

KEY WORDS

Abscess. Localized collection of pus.

AIDS. Acquired immunodeficiency syndrome. A disorder caused by the human immunodeficiency virus (HIV) which increases susceptibility to opportunistic infections, such as candidiasis.

Anemia. Too few red blood cells. Causes include decreased blood cell formation, blood cell destruction, and bleeding.

Candidiasis. A fungal infection with the organism *Candida albicans*. Occurs in patients who are immune-compromised or have been on multiple antibiotics.

Cholangitis. Infection of the biliary tree.

Cystitis. Infection of the bladder.

Cytomegalovirus (CMV). A common airborne virus which can become pathogenic in patients with AIDS.

Fever. A rise above the normal body temperature. Normal in most people is 98.4°F, 37°C.

Gossyphiboma. A sterile collection surrounding a sterile sponge inadvertently left behind during surgery.

Gutters (Paracolic). Areas in the flanks lateral to the colon where ascites and abscesses can form.

Hematocrit. The volume of erythrocytes packed by a centrifuge in a given volume of blood.

Hemolysis. Breakdown of red blood cells with release of hemoglobin into the plasma.

Hemorrhage, Hematoma. Collection of blood.

Immunosuppressed. Term describing a patient being treated with drugs or suffering from an illness that decreases the body's response to infection, for example, steroids or anticancer drugs.

Leukocyte. White blood cell; its primary function is to defend the body against infection.

Leukocytosis. An increase in the number of leukocytes.

Lymphadenopathy. Enlarged lymph nodes.

Morison's Pouch. Space between the right kidney and the liver where ascites may lie or an abscess may develop.

Murphy's Sign. Localized tenderness over the gallbladder, greatest on full inspiration.

Pneumocystis Carinii Pneumonia (PCP). An unusual bacterial pneumonia common in AIDS patients.

Prostatitis. Infection of the prostate.

Pyogenic. Producing pus.

Pyrexia. Fever.

Sepsis. The presence of pathogenic microorganisms or their toxic products in the blood. The patients is usually febrile but may be hypothermic and in shock.

Septicemia. Infection in the blood.

Staging. Demonstration of the areas that are involved in a malignancy. The more areas that are involved, the more severe the staging grade.

Subphrenic. Under the diaphragm.

Subpulmonic. Under the lung but above the diaphragm.

THE CLINICAL PROBLEM

Fever is a common manifestation of a great many illnesses and often arises from an easily identifiable source such as a postoperative wound infection. However, when the cause is not so well defined, sonography can be useful in detecting many of the other causes of fever. Before beginning a study in a patient with fever of unknown origin (FUO), the history and laboratory data in the patient's chart should be checked for evidence suggesting any of the possibilities mentioned below (see also Key Words). Understanding the patient's history will help the sonographer concentrate on the most appropriate areas.

Abscesses

Wound infection in the postoperative patient is a common problem. The accompanying symptoms may be masked by the administration of antibiotics and analgesics. Infections usually start approximately on the fifth postoperative day and develop into an abscess approximately on the tenth postoperative day.

Patients at risk for abscess are diabetics, those with hematoma, those with connective tissue disorders, the immunosuppressed, and those with cancer.

Organ Inflammation

Infection may progress to actual abscess formation or may be limited to organ inflammation. The following conditions may induce fever, yet there may be no localizing clinical signs. Sonographic findings may be present.

1. Hepatitis
2. Pyelonephritis
3. Cholecystitis
4. Cholangitis
5. Pancreatitis
6. Cystitis
7. Prostatitis

Tumors

Some tumors (especially hypernephroma, lymphoma, and hepatoma) cause fever and leukocytosis, characteristics that are similar to those of infections.

Postoperative Collections

Patients who have recently undergone surgery may develop a fluid pocket at the incision site. Cesarean section, hysterectomy, and renal transplant are often followed by collection development that may be a hematoma, urinoma, abscess, lymphocele, or seroma. Hematomas also follow anticoagulant therapy. They may be suspected when a drop in the patient's hematocrit is present.

Gossyphiboma

This sterile collection due to a retained surgical sponge has a distinctive appearance on ultrasound (Fig. 26-1).

AIDS

The acquired immunodeficiency syndrome (AIDS) is a disease transmitted through bodily fluids such as blood and semen. It has many sonographic manifestations and is due to an infection with a virus known as human immunodeficiency virus (HIV). A patient with AIDS does not pose a risk of infection to a sonographer unless blood from the infected individual contacts a bleeding surface or mucous membrane on the sonographer. Infections are alleged to have taken place through the conjunctiva of the eye and the mucous membrane of the mouth from blood that splashed from the patient at the time of surgery or biopsy. It is therefore essential to wear a mask and eyeguard if a puncture procedure is being performed on an AIDS patient. Otherwise, contact with AIDS patients is not dangerous and routine universal precautions are adequate.

AIDS almost exclusively affects members of four groups: (1) homosexuals; (2) intravenous drug abusers; (3) hemophiliacs and those who have had multiple blood transfusions; and (4) individuals who have intercourse with an AIDS-infected person. AIDS is also widespread in Haiti and East Africa.

To diagnose AIDS, an HIV test must be performed. This test can be administered only if the patient agrees, since there is a social stigma to a diagnosis of AIDS and relatively limited treatment that can be offered. It is, therefore, not uncommon for a hospital patient to have undiagnosed AIDS, which is why universal precautions have become the standard in hospital practice (see Chapter 56).

Typical presenting symptoms in patients with AIDS are as follows:

1. Fever
2. Lymphadenopathy
3. Weight loss
4. Diarrhea
5. Right upper quadrant pain
6. Clinical evidence of abdominal masses
7. Gastrointestinal hemorrhage
8. Gastrointestinal obstructions

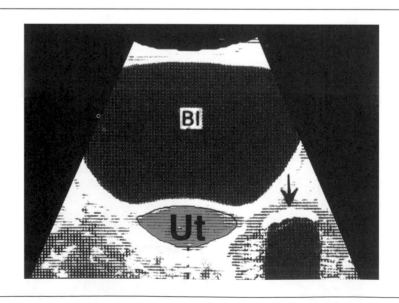

FIGURE 26-1. A transverse view of the female pelvis with a left-sided tubo-ovarian abscess. The abscess contains air, which rises to the top and casts a strong acoustic shadow. Retained sponge (gossyphiboma) would be another cause of the same sonographic appearance.

Many infections are more common in patients with AIDS than in patients with normal immune systems. These include the following:

1. Pneumocystis carinii
2. Candidiasis
3. Cytomegalovirus
4. Herpes simplex virus
5. Mycobacterium avium complex (MAC)

Rare neoplasms are more frequent with AIDS, such as Kaposi's sarcoma and unusual lymphomas (e.g., Burkitt's lymphoma).

ANATOMY

See the relevant chapters for each organ.

◣ TECHNIQUE

Routine Views

1. Start by examining the patient in a supine position. Scan along the inferior vena cava and aorta to make sure that enlarged nodes are not present.

2. On longitudinal sections, examine the liver, right diaphragm, right kidney, subhepatic space, and gallbladder area (Fig. 26-2). Make sure that the diaphragm moves well and that no pleural effusions are present. If a psoas problem is being considered (i.e., pain in the psoas area when the leg is moved), get longitudinal sections of the psoas by scanning medially to the kidney.

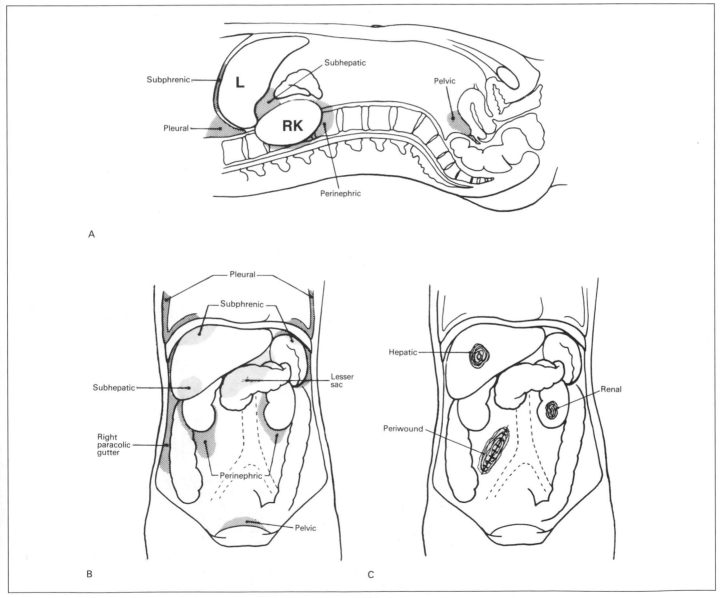

FIGURE 26-2. (A,B) A number of spaces exist in the abdomen where fluid may collect. Common sites for fluid collection are the pelvic, subphrenic, subhepatic, paracolic gutter, and lesser sac areas. Fluid may collect around the kidneys or in the pleural space. **(C)** Sites where abscesses may form are the spaces already mentioned, as well as within the liver or kidney and around incisions.

3. Using a transverse approach, start at the xiphoid and sweep down to the umbilicus, watching for nodes around the inferior vena cava and the aorta. Look in the lesser sac area around the pancreas and in the paracolic gutters (see Fig. 26-2) for collections. This is also the time to examine the perinephric spaces and to look in the renal pelves for adenopathy.

4. With the bladder moderately full, look in the pelvis for ascites, nodes, or a pelvic abscess. Be sure to include the iliopsoas muscles; these may contain an abscess or hematoma or may be surrounded by nodes. If the patient is male, check the prostate and seminal vesicles for enlargement (see Chapter 35. If the patient is female, check the uterus and ovaries (see Chapter 7). An overdistended bladder may compress and displace pathology into inaccessible sites.

5. Turn the patient left side up and look in the region of the left hemidiaphragm. Vary the inspiration until the diaphragm appears in the costal space—often deep inspiration is helpful—and rule out collections above and below. Look at the spleen, the left kidney, and the perinephric area, including the psoas muscles. All are possible sites for abscesses. This left coronal view is also the best way to evaluate the space between the left kidney and the aorta for nodes (Fig. 26-3).

6. In a postoperative patient, examine the incision area. If the incision is recent, use a sterile approach, as described in Chapter 56. Use sterile gel on the skin. To avoid causing pain, scan only adjacent to the wound and angle under it with the beam. A water-path technique may help if the area is extremely sensitive. Depending on how open the wound is, it may be possible to put a stand-off pad or water-filled glove over it, allowing the transducer more direct access to the site. There are also sterile membranes, gel-film skin barriers that can be used to cover the wound for scanning (see Chapter 56).

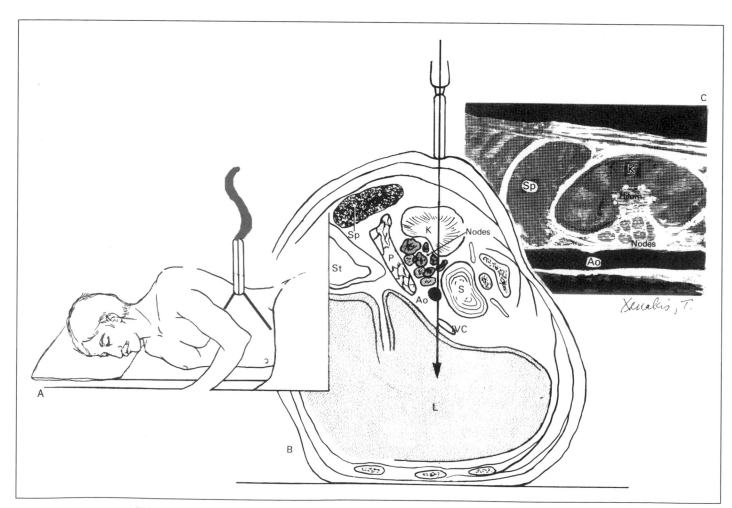

FIGURE 26-3. Left-side-up decubitus view shows a cluster of nodes in the left renal hilum. (**A**) This patient was scanned in a right anterior oblique position. (**B**) A section through the hilar region shows the relationship in a transverse plane. (**C**) Left-side-up sagittal section.

7. Examining the contents of a collection may require a higher-frequency transducer to distinguish between artifact and true septa or debris. Also, changing the patient position can help in two ways: debris will often float and resettle in the dependent portion, and air inside a collection will rise to the top, allowing access through what is perhaps a better acoustic window.

8. A gas-filled abscess may be difficult to distinguish from gut. Give fluid by mouth or rectum. If this does not help, try scanning from a lateral approach with the patient supine so that you get behind the gas (Fig. 26-4).

9. Sometimes a subfascial hematoma can follow cesarean sections (Fig. 26-5). Good near-field visualization is imperative, so use a short focus, high-frequency transducer—linear, curvilinear sector, or sector with a stand-off pad if necessary. Set the electronic focus just below the fascial plane. Look for the rectus muscles to determine whether the collection is posterior to them; if this is difficult at the region of the hematoma, start more laterally and trace the posterior surface of the rectus muscles medially. A lower-frequency transducer will be necessary to evaluate the areas posterior to the bladder.

10. The following special techniques may be valuable in difficult circumstances.

   a. Diaphragm obscured. Often, the left diaphragm is difficult to see owing to lung interference. If this is the case and the patient is lying in a decubitus position, roll the patient back to the supine position and reach around to scan through the ribs. Use whatever degree of inspiration is needed to bring the diaphragm into view. This can keep the lungs out of the field.

   b. Small liver. If the liver is small and high and the edge is obscured by gas, perform intercostal scans from a level superior to the liver edge. This places the beam more perpendicular to this interface. Turning the patient left side down, or upright, is also helpful in making more liver visible.

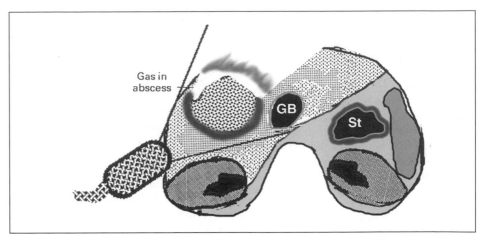

FIGURE 26-4. Abscess in the liver with gas rising to the anterior margin. Scan from a postero-lateral approach with the patient in a supine position so the beam passes behind the gas.

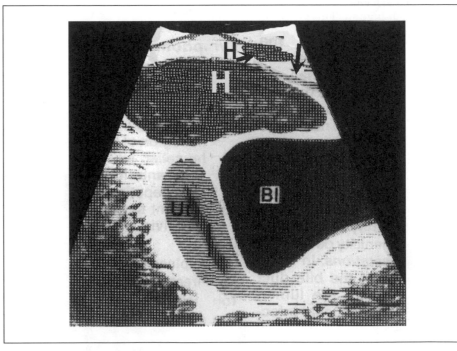

FIGURE 26-5. A postoperative pelvis. A hematoma in the abdominal wall is present (black H). A subfascial hematoma (white H), which is much larger, is also shown. Although the hematoma is echolucent, it does not transmit sound quite as well as a known fluid-filled structure, such as the bladder. The fascia can be seen (arrow).

c. Possible pelvic abscess. When trying to find an abscess that could be located between loops of bowel, watch any suspicious area patiently for a few minutes with real-time, or return to it occasionally to see if it has changed shape or size. If peristalsis is seen, the question is answered; however, because the sigmoid colon is often inactive, a water enema may be required. Use only enough water to cause flow through or around the questionable mass. Unfortunately for the patient, the bladder must remain distended enough to allow for an adequate acoustic window. When using a water enema technique, it is often just as informative to watch the water being drained back into the bag as it was to watch it go in. This gives you a second chance to watch for activity in the questionable area without requiring the patient to go through any extra discomfort.

◆ PATHOLOGY
AIDS: Sonographic Manifestations

1. *Masses.* Nodal masses in the usual node sites (i.e., para-aortic and porta hepatis regions) are common. Lymphadenopathy may develop in other sites that are not routine (e.g., within the liver and kidney).

2. *Kaposi's sarcoma.* Kaposi's sarcoma is normally located in the limbs, but in the presence of AIDS, primary tumors and metastatic lesions may involve the abdomen, the testes, and the liver. Bulky para-aortic nodes are common.

3. *Renal manifestations.* Patients with AIDS develop an AIDS-related nephritis. The kidneys become much enlarged and densely echogenic. Renal enlargement may occur before the increased echogenicity develops.

4. *RUQ.* In AIDS patients who present to ultrasound for right upper quadrant imaging because of fever, abdominal pain, and elevated alkaline phosphatase, the biliary tree should be scanned carefully for signs of AIDS cholangitis. The initial feature of AIDS cholangitis may be thickening of the bile duct mucosa, followed by stricture formation and resultant intrahepatic ductal dilatation. Gallbladder wall thickening in patients with AIDS is a common sonographic finding. Acalculous cholecystitis may be diagnosed sonographically by the presence of gallbladder wall edema and a positive sonographic Murphy's sign.

5. *Fungal and parasitic infections.* Unusual infections, such as cryptococcosis, are common. Abscesses may develop in any part of the abdomen. These abscesses may contain pus that is densely echogenic and can be confused with a tumor. Multiple abscesses may be present in the liver or spleen that, if fungal, may have an echopenic periphery to an echogenic center (see Chapter 23).

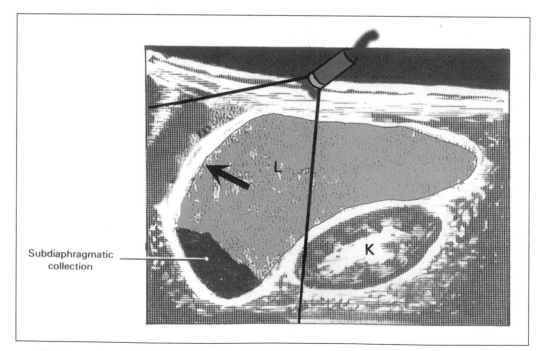

FIGURE 26-6. Right longitudinal section. A subphrenic abscess is shown. Subhepatic, perinephric, and subphrenic collections can all elevate and/or immobilize the diaphragm (arrow).

Subdiaphragmatic collection

6. *Hepatosplenomegaly.* The liver and spleen are often massively enlarged, especially in HIV-infected children. Patients with AIDS may well have complications of alcoholism or intravenous drug abuse (e.g., an abnormal pancreas and evidence of portal hypertension).

7. *Abdominal malignancies.* Cancers such as non-Hodgkin's lymphoma are more common in patients with AIDS than in the general population. Ultrasound is helpful in identifying hepatic lesions in patients with AIDS-related lymphomas, which may appear as large confluent masses or scattered hypoechoic nodular densities throughout the liver. Abdominal lymphadenopathy is also common in the AIDS patient.

Abscesses

Location

There are a number of potential spaces in the abdomen where fluid can collect and where abscesses commonly form. Abscesses tend to collect in spaces around organs and may displace structures or render them immobile (Fig. 26-6; see Fig. 26-2).

1. *Right subphrenic space.* Between the diaphragm and the dome of the liver.
2. *Subhepatic space (Morison's pouch).* Between the inferior posterior aspect of the liver and the right kidney.
3. *Left subphrenic space.* Between the spleen and the left hemidiaphragm.
4. *Lesser sac.* A large potential space mainly anterior to the pancreas and posterior to the stomach.
5. *Pelvis cul-de-sac.* Posterior to the uterus and anterior to the rectum.
6. *Paracolic gutters.* Along the flanks, lateral to the colon.
7. *Perinephric space.* There are various spaces around the kidneys. These are described in detail in Chapter 31, Renal Failure.
8. *Intrahepatic* (Fig. 26-7)
9. *Intranephric*
10. *Psoas area* on either side of the spine medial to the kidney
11. *Region of an incision*

Remember that infection can originate in a site remote from the region where the abscess eventually settles.

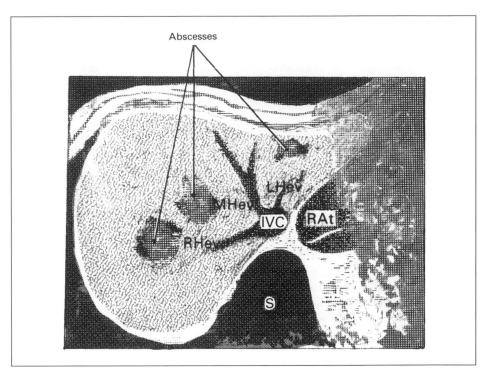

FIGURE 26-7. Multiple hepatic abscesses are seen in a right costal margin view of the liver.

Sonographic Appearance

Abscesses can appear predominantly fluid filled with thick, irregular walls. The amount of through transmission depends on the quantity and composition of the fluid. The contents of an abscess may resemble a dense mass; there are no typical features that consistently set abscesses apart from other entities.

Multiple abscesses may also be found within organs such as the liver (see Fig. 26-7) or the kidney. Less frequently, they are found in the spleen and in the prostate. In alcoholics, a pancreatic pseudocyst may become infected, forming a pancreatic abscess. Abscesses in the mesentery may resemble bowel; local tenderness can help identify them. Those surrounded by gut often resemble fluid-filled loops of bowel with irregular shapes (see Technique). See Chapter 30 for a discussion of appendicitis.

Watch for the following:

1. *Local tenderness.* This may not be present if the patient is immunosuppressed.

2. *Gas.* When there is gas inside an abscess, shadowing varies with the amount and location of the gas (see Figs. 26-1 and 26-4). Gas is a suspicious finding when it occurs in an unlikely location, such as in the liver or kidney parenchyma, or the abdominal wall. Correlation with a computed tomography (CT) scan or an abdominal radiograph is helpful. A radiograph is often the precursor of the sonogram, suggesting, for example, an elevated diaphragm. Scan from a posterior angle in the supine position if there is gas in the abscess so the gas does not obscure the beam as it would if scanning from an anterior approach (see Fig. 26-4).

3. *Debris.* Some collections contain debris, which can appear to be solid and homogeneous but may float or settle in a dependent portion to create a fluid-fluid level. To distinguish from a solid mass, turn the patient and observe the movement of the debris.

Draining an Abscess

Aspiration of an abscess under ultrasonic control is of considerable help in clinical management because it allows identification of the responsible microorganism and may permit curative drainage (Chapter 52).

Inflammatory Changes

Most organs respond to infection in a similar fashion, and without abscess formation. In the involved area, the organ becomes swollen and more sonolucent. Local tenderness is present and should be noted by the sonographer.

Diaphragmatic Mobility

Real-time will allow the demonstration of the mobility of a hemidiaphragm, which is decreased when inflammation is present or when flanked with fluid. If assessing for paradoxical motion, watch both sides simultaneously. This is especially easy in an infant; if the patient is on a respirator, take care to observe the motion briefly with the patient breathing on his or her own if possible. Diaphragmatic paralysis may be overlooked if the patient is on the respirator. Since ultrasound is portable, it may be used for this purpose in the intensive care unit.

Gossyphiboma

A retained sponge has a very distinctive appearance: a dense linear echo in the midgut area with well-defined shadowing seen at the site of tenderness (see Fig. 26-1).

Hepatomas and Hypernephromas

Hepatomas and hypernephromas are acknowledged causes of fever (see Chapters 23 and 32).

Hematomas

Hematomas, whether occurring postoperatively or due to trauma, can cause fever.

Appearance

Hematoma appearances change rapidly. When fresh, hematomas are usually echofree. Within a few hours, they generally become echogenic. After a few days, they become partially echopenic, and when older, they may become so echopenic again that a subcapsular hematoma may be mistaken for ascites.

Location

Depending on the type and location of surgical procedure or trauma, hematomas can form in many different locations. Some common sites for hematoma formation following gynecologic surgery are in the cul-de-sac, in the broad ligament, adjacent to the surgical site, in the anterior abdominal wall, and in the myometrium (see Fig. 26-5).

Hematomas occurring after cesarean delivery can be divided into three types (see Fig. 26-5): superficial wound hematomas, subfascial hematomas, and bladder-flap hematomas. Patients are usually febrile and have a drop in hemoglobin.

1. The superficial variety is anterior to the rectus muscles (see Chapter 29) and involves the incision.
2. The subfascial type is posterior to the rectus muscles and much more serious, requiring surgical intervention. This space is anterior to the bladder but extends into the retropubic area, and 2500 mL of fluid can collect before a mass may be palpable (see Fig. 26-5).
3. A bladder-flap hematoma begins at the incision in the lower uterine segment behind the bladder, but it is covered by a fold of peritoneum that was disrupted during the surgery. Although bleeding is usually confined by the "flap," it can spread along the broad ligaments into the retroperitoneum.

Following a renal transplant, hematomas may form in a subcapsular location, in the perinephric area, or in the retroperitoneum.

Hematomas generally resolve, but they may also develop into abscesses. Hematomas tend to spread along fascial planes rather than break through tissue planes as abscesses do (see Fig. 29-13). If the hematoma is due to trauma, ask the patient's advice on where to start your search.

1. *Bowel vs. abscess.* Examine the area for several minutes with real-time, perform a water enema, or give fluid by mouth. Go back repeatedly to a worrisome area; if it is gut, it often changes. Be careful to duplicate the exact scan plane each time.
2. *Gossyphiboma vs. persistent bowel gas.* Depending on location, try a water enema to decide whether you are dealing with a stubborn gas pocket in bowel or a sponge. It may be necessary to rescan on another day to see whether there is no change; CT is also an option since retained sponges have a specific CT appearance.
3. *Fat deposits.* In obese patients, there may be a deposit of deep subcutaneous fat in the midepigastric region that can resemble an abscess. This fat is symmetrical on both sides of the midline and has well-defined borders.
4. *Ascites vs. abscess/hematoma.* A localized area of ascites may be mistaken for an abscess or echo-free hematoma. Place the patient in the erect, Trendelenburg, or decubitus position: ascites will shift, but an abscess or hematoma will not.
5. *Reverberation problems (pseudo bladder).* "Mirror" reverberations may create apparent fluid collection deep in the pelvis behind the bladder. The following maneuvers may show the "collection" to be an artifact (see Fig. 53-16).
   a. Scanning through a different part of the bladder or through the psoas muscles may cause the suspicious area to change size or disappear, since this will change the distance between the transducer and the bladder border.
   b. Measuring the distance from the skin to the center of the collection may show that the supposed collection lies well behind the patient's back.

❔ WHERE ELSE TO LOOK

1. If nodes are present, look for neoplasm or splenic enlargement due to lymphoma.
2. If one abscess is seen, look for more.
3. If a neoplasm is seen, look for metastases.

Selected Reading

Bechtold, R. E., Dyer, R. B., Zagoria, R. J., and Chen, M. Y. M. The perirenal space: Relationship of pathologic processes to normal retroperitoneal anatomy. *Radiographics* 16:841–854, 1996.

Juimo, A. G., Gervez, F., and Angwafo, F. F. Extraintestinal amebiasis. *Radiology* 182:181–183, 1992.

Keane, M. A. R., Finlayson, C., and Joseph, A. E. A. A histological basis for the sonographic snowstorm in opportunistic infection of the liver and spleen. *Clin Radiol* 50:220–222, 1995.

Molmenti, E. P., Balfe, D. M., Kanterman, R. Y., and Bennett, H. F. Anatomy of the retroperitoneum: Observations of the distribution of pathologic fluid collections. *Radiology* 200:95–103, 1996.

Pantongrag-Brown, L., Nelson, A. M., Brown, A. E., Buetow, P. C., and Buck, J. L. Gastrointestinal manifestations of acquired immunodeficiency syndrome: Radiologic-pathologic correlation. *Radiographics* 15:1155–1178, 1995.

Pastakia, B., Shawker, T. H., Thaler, M., O'Leary, T., and Pizzo, P. A. Hepatosplenic candidiasis: Wheels within wheels. *Radiology* 166:417–421, 1988.

Weiner, M. D., et al. Sonography of subfascial hematoma after cesarean delivery. *AJR* 148:907–910, 1987.

27

PALPABLE LEFT UPPER QUADRANT MASS

ROGER C. SANDERS

SONOGRAM ABBREVIATIONS

Ad	Adrenal gland
Ao	Aorta
D	Diaphragm
GBl	Gallbladder
IVC	Inferior vena cava
K	Kidney
L	Liver
P, Pa	Pancreas
PPs	Pancreatic pseudocysts
R	Ribs
Sp	Spleen
St	Stomach

KEY WORDS

Gaucher's Disease. One of the group of "storage" diseases in which fat and proteins are abnormally deposited in the body, typically in the liver, spleen, and bone marrow.

Myeloproliferative Disorder. Term referring to chronic myeloid leukemia, myelofibrosis, and polycythemia vera—a spectrum of hematologic conditions associated with a large spleen. Sometimes one entity will change into another.

Pancreatic Pseudocyst. Fluid collection produced by the pancreas during acute pancreatitis.

Pheochromocytoma. A hormone-producing adrenal tumor.

Portal Hypertension. A rise in the pressure of the venous blood flowing into the liver through the portal venous system, causing an increase in the size of the portal, splenic, and superior mesenteric veins and of the spleen. If portal hypertension is severe, additional vessels known as collaterals develop around the pancreas (see Fig. 21-7).

Splenomegaly. Enlargement of the spleen.

Subphrenic Abscess. An abscess lying under the left or right diaphragm. Such abscesses commonly follow a surgical procedure in the area, for example, an operation on the stomach.

THE CLINICAL PROBLEM

Splenomegaly

The most frequent left upper quadrant mass is an enlarged spleen. Splenomegaly occurs in a wide variety of disease states.

1. *Infectious diseases* such as tuberculosis, malaria, infectious mononucleosis ("mono"), and subacute bacterial endocarditis (SBE) are often accompanied by an enlarged spleen. (The spleen is occasionally the site of an abscess, particularly with SBE or any other bacteremic state.)
2. *Myeloproliferative disorders* such as myelofibrosis may be characterized by splenomegaly.
3. Splenomegaly occurs when the veins draining the spleen are obstructed, as in *portal hypertension* or *splenic vein thrombosis.* Both pancreatic cancer and pancreatitis can cause splenic vein thrombosis.
4. *Metastases* may occur in the spleen; however, the spleen is not often the site of neoplastic involvement.
5. *Lymphoma* and *leukemia* may involve the spleen directly or cause splenomegaly as a secondary phenomenon because blood production is disorganized.
6. *Storage disorders* such as Gaucher's disease may cause splenomegaly.

Fluid-Filled Masses

A left upper quadrant fluid-filled mass is quite common and may be (1) a renal mass such as hydronephrosis or a large renal cyst; (2) a splenic cyst; (3) an adrenal cyst; or (4) a pancreatic pseudocyst.

Neoplasms

Neoplastic masses in the left upper quadrant include (1) retroperitoneal sarcomas; (2) adrenal tumors, which are usually small (e.g., metastases, pheochromocytoma) but occasionally become large; and (3) pancreas and kidney cancers, which can spread into the left upper quadrant and cause a palpable abdominal mass.

The surgical approach is dictated by the origin and nature of the mass. Cysts may be treated conservatively or by cyst puncture rather than by surgery.

Abscesses

The left subdiaphragmatic region is a common site for abscess collections, particularly in postoperative patients following removal of the spleen or stomach operations.

ANATOMY

Spleen

The spleen is the predominant organ in the left upper quadrant. It lies immediately under the left hemidiaphragm and may be difficult to see because of gas in the neighboring lung and ribs. It lies superior to the left kidney and lateral to the adrenal gland and the tail of the pancreas. The left lobe of the liver is often in contact with the spleen.

The splenic texture is more echogenic than the liver or kidney. A group of high-level echoes in the center of the spleen at its medial aspect represents the splenic hilum at the entrance of the splenic artery and vein.

Adrenal Glands

See Chapter 39.

 ## TECHNIQUE

Left Side View (Coronal)

The left-side-up position (right lateral decubitus) is the preferred position for investigating the left upper quadrant (Fig. 27-1). Angle the transducer somewhat obliquely so that it passes between the ribs. Place a pillow or a wedge under the patient to improve access to the left kidney (see Chapter 31). To identify your location, find the left kidney; the spleen will be superior to it. There should normally be nothing between the spleen and the left hemidiaphragm. Make sure the scan plane allows visualization above the diaphragm as well.

Transverse Views

Transverse views are also obtained in the left-side-up position. The best access route is often far posterior. Administering fluids by mouth or through a nasogastric tube helps to define the stomach and its margin. Placing the patient in the supine position and scanning from the lateral aspect helps if lung interference is a problem.

 ## PATHOLOGY

Splenomegaly

As one gains experience with sonography, it becomes obvious when the spleen is enlarged on real-time, but criteria for documenting enlargement are still unsatisfactory. A good rule of thumb is as follows: if the transducer has a 90-degree angle and the superior/inferior border of the spleen cannot fit on an image, the spleen is enlarged. Beware of this method if the patient has a small AP diameter, because their liver and spleens are often flatter and long as a normal configuration.

Splenic echogenicity may be altered when the spleen is enlarged. If it is less echogenic than usual, one should think of lymphoma; if more echogenic, consider myelofibrosis or infection.

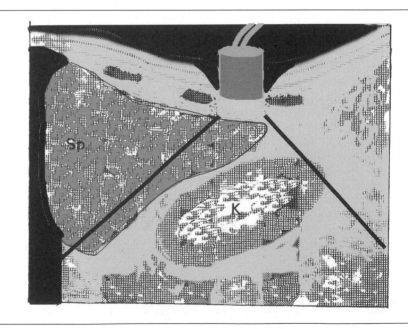

FIGURE 27-1. Left-side-up view of the spleen and left kidney. Ribs partially obscure the spleen and kidney.

Focal Splenic Masses

Though unusual, focal lesions may occur in the spleen. Abscesses usually have irregular borders and some internal echoes; they may show shadowing associated with gas. In immunocompromised patients, multiple echopenic abscesses with echogenic centers may be seen in both the liver and the spleen (see Fig. 23-15). Metastatic lesions, which are rare, resemble those seen in the liver.

Cysts

If the left upper quadrant mass is a cyst, make sure you know the organ of origin.

1. *Splenic cysts* should have a rim of splenic parenchyma around them (Fig. 27-2). An upright position may help to show the complete cyst. Splenic cysts may contain many internal echoes and septa. Administer water to the patient to distinguish the stomach from a medially located cyst.
2. *Renal cysts* arise from the kidney, and there is usually a clawlike portion of renal parenchyma surrounding the cyst (Fig. 27-3). The kidney may become very large with hydronephrosis. Differentiation of hydronephrosis from a cyst is simple in most instances (see Chapter 31).
3. *Pancreatic pseudocysts* usually show some connection with the pancreas; they generally displace the spleen superiorly and the kidney inferiorly (see Fig. 27-2).
4. *Adrenal cysts* and masses displace the spleen anteriorly, the kidney inferiorly, and the pancreas anteriorly (Fig. 27-4B). Adrenal cysts may have a calcified border; if so, the rim of the mass lesion will be densely echogenic, and through transmission will not be seen (see Chapter 39).

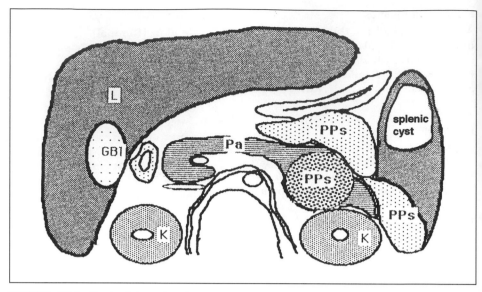

FIGURE 27-2. Typical location for pancreatic pseudocysts. Pancreatic pseudocysts are shown in the pancreas, in the lesser sac, and lateral to the left kidney. Pancreatic cysts are usually echo-free, but can contain internal echoes. A cyst in the spleen is also shown.

Subphrenic Abscess

A fluid collection located in the splenic site following splenectomy or between the diaphragm and the spleen may represent a left subphrenic abscess. These abscesses may be difficult to see because this area is so inaccessible unless, as is common, there is a coincident pleural effusion.

An infected hematoma often develops where the spleen used to lie. Bowel may fall into the splenectomy site. Have the patient drink some water to distinguish the two. Look for pleural effusions above the diaphragm.

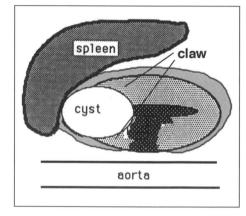

FIGURE 27-3. A renal cyst at the upper pole of the left kidney showing the "claw" effect with renal parenchyma around the cyst.

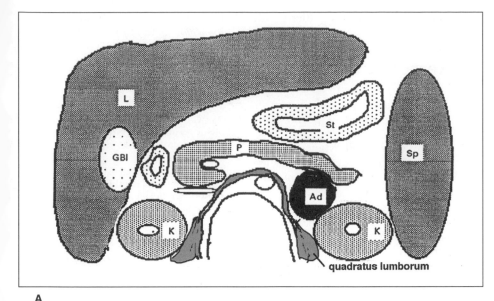

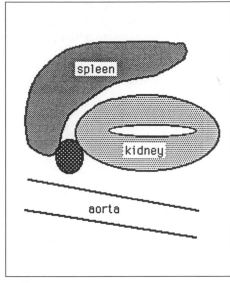

A

B

FIGURE 27-4. Adrenal mass. (**A**) An adrenal mass (Ad) displaces the spleen laterally, the kidney posteriorly, and the pancreas anteriorly. (**B**) On a coronal view an adrenal mass will displace the kidney inferiorly, the spleen superiorly, and the aorta medially.

Solid Mass

If the mass is solid, displacement of the adjacent organs will indicate its origin.

1. *Retroperitoneal sarcomas* will displace the kidney, spleen, and pancreas anteriorly.
2. *Pancreatic neoplasms* will lie superior to the kidney but will displace the spleen anteriorly.
3. *Renal neoplasms* will lie inferior to the spleen and pancreas.
4. *Accessory spleen* appears as a small round solid mass adjacent to the spleen.

⭐ PITFALLS

1. *Left lobe of the liver vs. perisplenic collection.* The left lobe of the liver may extend superior to the spleen, especially if a partial hepatectomy has been performed. Trace the suspect mass into the normal liver. Follow the left portal vein into the suspect mass. The liver is a little less echogenic than the spleen. There is virtually no interface between the two.
2. *Stomach vs. left upper quadrant collection.* The stomach may look like a left upper quadrant fluid collection. Give fluid by mouth, and peristalsis will be seen.

3. *Spleen vs. effusion.* The spleen may resemble a pleural effusion if the sonographer is not careful to establish where the kidney lies, because in an obese patient, a more or less horizontal diaphragm may not be imaged adequately. If there is any difficulty in determining what represents the diaphragm, have the patient sniff. The diaphragm will move if it is not paralyzed.
4. *Splenic hilum.* An echogenic area at the site where the splenic vein and splenic artery enter the spleen, the hilum can be mistaken for a neoplasm. Real-time and color Doppler will show vessels in this area.
5. *Subphrenic vs. subpulmonic collection.* It may be difficult to distinguish a subphrenic from a subpulmonic collection if the diaphragm is not easily seen. Distinguishing between the spleen and a pleural effusion is the key to recognizing the collection site. The kidney lies just below the spleen and is a useful landmark.

6. *Inverted diaphragm.* If the left diaphragm is inverted by a left pleural effusion, an apparent left upper quadrant cystic mass may develop. A longitudinal section will show the true site of the diaphragm and reveal that the cystic area—the pleural effusion—is intrathoracic (Fig. 27-5).
7. *Accessory spleens.* Additional round or ovoid echopenic circular masses may be seen around the spleen, representing accessory spleens. The acoustic texture will be the same as the spleen.
8. *Calcified granulomas* form echogenic foci, often with acoustic shadowing within the spleen, and are relatively common. In the United States, they

usually indicate that the patient had histoplasmosis in the past.

 WHERE ELSE TO LOOK

1. If *splenomegaly* is present:
   a. Examine the liver for evidence of diffuse liver disease, portal and splenic vein enlargement, and collaterals with portal hypertension.
   b. Note whether nodes are present in association with splenomegaly and lymphoma.
2. If the mass appears to be a *pancreatic pseudocyst*, look for the stigma of alcoholism elsewhere and evidence of pancreatitis in the remainder of the pancreas.

3. If the left upper quadrant mass is *hydronephrosis*, look for the cause of obstruction in the pelvis along the course of the ureter.

SELECTED READING

Goerg, C., Schwerk, W. B., and Goerg, K. Splenic lesions: Sonographic patterns, follow-up, differential diagnosis. *Eur J Radiol* 13:59–66, 1991.

Siniluoto, T. M. J., Tikkakoski, T. A., Lahde, S. T., Paivansalo, M. J., and Koivisto, M. J. Ultrasound or CT in splenic diseases? *Acta Radiol* 35:597–605, 1994.

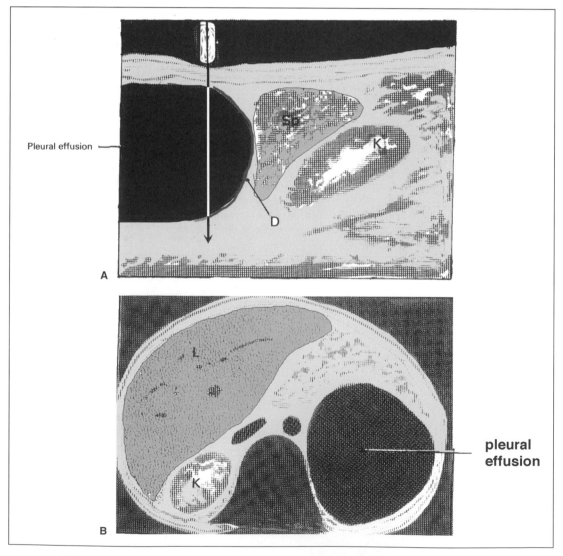

FIGURE 27-5. Pleural effusion. (**A**) A very large pleural effusion may appear as a left upper quadrant mass. The diaphragm may be inverted, and the spleen and kidney may be displaced inferiorly. (**B**) On a transverse view a large pleural effusion inverting the diaphragm can look like a large cyst.

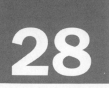

28 PEDIATRIC MASS

ROGER C. SANDERS

SONOGRAM ABBREVIATIONS

K Kidney

L Liver

KEY WORDS

Adrenal Hemorrhage. Hemorrhage into the adrenal gland, usually occurring in the first few days of life and causing a large hematoma that is often mistaken for a kidney mass. It resolves spontaneously, often with development of calcification.

Aniridia. Congenital absence of a portion of the eye (the iris). Associated with Wilms' tumor.

Beckwith-Wiedemann Syndrome. Congenital anomaly in which many organs of the body, such as the tongue, are enlarged. Associated with Wilms' tumor and liver tumors.

Biliary Atresia. Neonatal condition in which the biliary ducts are very small. It can involve the intrahepatic or extrahepatic biliary tree. It may be a consequence of infection. Jaundice is present.

Choledochal Cyst. Congenital focal dilatation of a segment of the biliary tree.

Enteric Duplication. Congenital duplication of the gut. The involved segment does not usually connect with the remainder of the bowel. Thus, this segment becomes filled with fluid and presents as a mass.

Hemihypertrophy. Congenital condition in which half of the body is larger than the other side. Associated with Wilms' tumor.

Hepatoblastoma. Liver tumor that is particularly common in small children.

Hydrops. The gallbladder is markedly enlarged and the cystic duct is functionally obstructed, although often nothing can be found upon surgical exploration. This self-limiting condition occurs in association with some childhood illnesses, for example, Kawasaki's syndrome, and following surgical procedures.

Hyperlipidemia. Congenital disease with increased lipids in the blood.

Intussusception. Obstructed bowel coiled on itself. Seen particularly in children. The walls are thickened.

Kawasaki's Syndrome. Mucocutaneous lymph node syndrome. This viral illness is associated with hydrops of the gallbladder and occurs in epidemics.

Meningocele. Cystic dilatation of the spinal canal at the site of a bony defect. May appear as an abdominal mass in the neonate when it protrudes anterior to the sacrum.

Mesenteric Cyst (Omental Cyst). Cyst filled with lymph found in the mesentery that presents as an asymptomatic abdominal mass.

Mesoblastic Nephroma. Rare, benign tumor of the kidney occurring in neonates; it rarely metastasizes, but needs immediate surgical resection.

Multicystic (Dysplastic) Kidney. Unilateral renal cystic disease that develops in utero. The commonest neonatal mass. May be found later in life as an incidental finding.

Neonate. Infant in the first 4 weeks of life.

Neuroblastoma. A malignant tumor usually arising in the adrenals between birth and the age of 5 years; the child may have gait and eyesight problems ("dancing eyes and dancing feet") or metastatic bone lesions rather than an abdominal mass.

Precocious Puberty. Disease affecting young girls in which they start to menstruate and develop breasts prematurely. Often due to an ovarian tumor.

Pyloric Stenosis. A predominantly male disorder. The pylorus (the exit of the stomach) is narrowed and the wall is thickened. May cause projectile vomiting in infants.

Rhabdomyosarcoma. Sarcomatous muscle tumor that occurs in childhood and has a particular affinity for the bladder and heart.

Stillbirth. Child born dead on delivery.

Teratoma. Usually benign mass composed of elements of most tissues in the body, notably skin, hair, bone, and especially teeth. May occur anywhere in the abdomen, but in the infant it is found predominantly in the sacrococcygeal area. Usually discovered at birth.

Ureterocele. Dilatation of the distal ureter as it inserts abnormally into the bladder. A "cobra head" deformity develops owing to a stenosis.

Ureteropelvic Junction Obstruction (UPJ). Type of renal obstruction in which there is a block at the upper end of the ureter just below the renal pelvis. Thought to be congenital in origin, it is often detected first in neonates.

Vacuum Immobilization Device. An infant immobilization device in which a plastic membrane, distended with air, surrounds and fixes the child, preventing movement.

Wilms' Tumor. Malignant kidney tumor that generally occurs between the ages of 1 and 6 years. Usually presents as an abdominal mass. Associated with hemihypertrophy, aniridia, and the Beckwith-Wiedemann syndrome.

◆》》 THE CLINICAL PROBLEM

The spectrum of masses in the neonate or small child is different from that in the adult. Most, but not all, masses require surgical intervention; the timing and extent of the operation are influenced by the sonographic finding.

Neonatal Masses

Renal Masses

The most common mass is a multicystic (dysplastic) kidney. This mass is not hereditary and probably is a consequence of in utero obstruction. Congenital hydronephrosis due to ureteropelvic junction obstruction is the next most common mass. These two lesions, both fluid-filled, must be distinguished from a rare kidney tumor (mesoblastic nephroma). If the mass is fluid filled, the child can undergo an operation when older and healthier, but if it is a solid tumor, surgical resection should be performed immediately.

Adrenal Hemorrhage

Adrenal hemorrhage, usually detected not at birth but a few days later, may be confused with a renal tumor. However, the sonographer should be able to tell that the mass is adrenal in location. Adrenal hematomas usually occur in children who have undergone a difficult delivery. They may be associated with unusual laboratory findings and hematocrit drop rather than with an abdominal mass. Adrenal hematomas resolve spontaneously.

Other Masses

Other, rarer causes of neonatal abdominal masses are enteric duplication, ovarian cysts (which are surprisingly often found near the liver in neonates), mesenteric cysts, choledochal cysts (see Chapter 25), and teratomas. Teratomas most often arise from the buttocks in a sacrococcygeal location. They extend into the pelvis. Anterior sacral meningocele, a fluid-filled outpouching of the spinal canal, can be confused with a sacrococcygeal teratoma.

Pyloric stenosis, a cause of "projectile vomiting" predominantly in male children a few months old, is caused by muscle thickening around the exit of the stomach.

Older Children

In the 1-to-5-year-old child the most common masses are again related to the kidney, with Wilms' tumor and neuroblastoma being most frequent. Rhabdomyosarcomas occur most commonly in the region of the bladder, but may be found at any site in the abdomen. Hepatoma, hepatoblastoma, and other liver tumors are rare but do occur in this age group.

ANATOMY

Kidney

Because the cortex is more echogenic in infants than in adults, the renal pyramids in infants are prominent and may be mistaken for cysts (Fig. 28-1A). The perirenal and intrarenal fat is almost absent, so the sinus and capsular echoes are barely seen. Tables showing normal kidney sizes of children are available (see Appendix 32).

Adrenal Gland

In neonates and small children, the adrenal gland is about one third the size of the kidney and has an echogenic linear center.

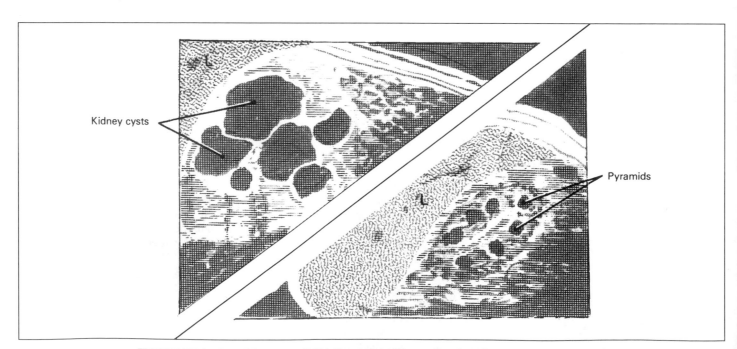

FIGURE 28-1. Renal "masses." (**A**) Neonatal kidney, showing the relative absence of capsular and sinus echoes due to a normal paucity of fat. Note the prominence of the pyramids, which have been mistaken for cysts in this age group. (**B**) Multicystic kidney. The kidney is replaced by cysts of varying sizes that do not communicate. The largest cysts are often more lateral in location.

Biliary Tree

The bile ducts in small children are normally smaller than those in adults. Bile ducts, except for the common duct, are abnormal if they are visible in the first year of life.

Pancreas

The pancreas is much less echogenic in children than it is in adults; it has about the same echogenicity as the liver in young children. It slowly increases in echogenicity as the child becomes older. It is also relatively larger than in adults.

Liver and Spleen

The liver and spleen are normally larger in relation to other abdominal organs in small children than in adults.

Uterus

The prepubertal uterus is about 3- to 4-cm long in the neonate. Fluid may be seen in the endometrial cavity in the neonate owing to the effects of the mother's hormones.

Ovary

The ovaries in the neonate may contain follicles. In the 2 to 3 years before puberty, cysts may be seen in the ovary. The normal ovary at other prepubertal ages is about 1 cm in diameter and does not contain cysts.

◪ TECHNIQUE

Sonographer's Approach to Children

1. Maintain steady eye contact.
2. Speak with a soft voice.
3. Do not talk about sonographic findings in front of the child, although some children respond well to having their anatomy discussed. "This long tube is a vessel. It has *blood* in it."
4. Allow the child to become familiar with the room and the system.
5. Feed small infants with a nipple—bottle or breast—during the study. Scheduling an examination after sleep and food deprivation may help make this effective.
6. Have the parents hold the child. Lying the mother on the stretcher with the child on top may help.
7. Use warm gel.

8. Toddlers are often impressed into cooperation with the dramatic announcement that they are going to be *on T.V.*
9. Show small children something dynamic (e.g., angle under the xiphoid and watch the heart beat) to interest them in the procedure.

Immobilization

The neonate can usually be examined by having an adult restrain the shoulders and legs so that the baby falls asleep or at least lies quietly. With a 2-to-4-year-old, cooperation must be obtained before you touch them with the transducer.

Drape the parents over the child's limb if you must, but first try distracting the child with casual conversation about day care or Sesame Street.

Older children should be shown the system before you perform the examination so that they won't feel threatened by the equipment. Encouraging the child to switch on instrumentation to see himself or herself on TV is helpful. If there is a separate hand control, the child can participate. Asking the child to erase the image from the screen also induces cooperation. If all else fails, perform the study while the child is screaming but is still relatively immobile before taking another breath. Cine loop can be very helpful here.

If it is uncertain whether a mass arises in the kidney, adrenal, or liver, the sling position (Fig. 28-2) may be helpful. Don't hesitate to perform the study with the child draped over a parent. Small children may be reassured if the parent lies on the examining table with the child lying supine on top of the parent during the examination.

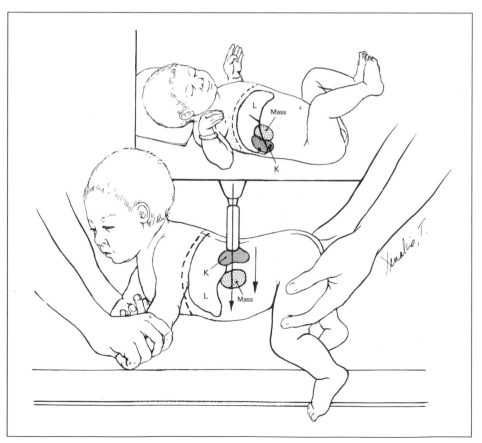

FIGURE 28-2. Diagram showing the sling position that can be used with infants and small children for assessment of a mass. The infant is held in the air by two assistants while scanning is performed. This position will cause a mass to drop away from the adjacent organ.

Sedation

Sedation may very rarely be necessary in a child who has had long-term hospitalization and distrusts anyone in a white uniform. Chloral hydrate, fentanyl (Sublimaze), and ketamine are useful sedative drugs.

Keeping the Neonate Warm

Remember that the neonate must be kept warm. A heating pad or heat lamp is desirable. Small infants should not be uncovered for more than 15 minutes. Always check the bladder first and take a picture before it empties.

Transducer Contact

Obviously, the transducer of choice will always be the one with the highest frequency and the smallest footprint adequate to the task. In a neonate, this may mean using a small parts transducer: don't discount these just because they may happen to be linear arrays. Remember that the near field will be excellent, and much of the right upper quadrant may be visible by angling up under the costal margin. Take advantage of that huge breath that may preclude a scream, and do a sweep. Then go back with the cine loop and record at a more leisurely pace. Also, if there is a large lesion such as a Wilms's tumor, it will be possible to place adjacent images side-by-side to get a more accurate measurement.

Often with very tiny people it is necessary to use a stand-off pad to see a structure that is very superficial, such as the left kidney. If a commercially produced one is not available, put warm water (slowly, to keep air bubbles to a minimum) into a glove and tie it off. This should provide enough distance to keep the kidney out of the very near field and into a reasonable focal zone. With a sector's pie-shaped image, it also places the kidney into a wider section of the image, showing more of the organ. Be sure to use lots of warm gel on both sides of the pad—the skin and the transducer sides—to ensure good contact.

Adrenals

Although adrenal sonograms are rarely requested in adults, it is not uncommon to follow adrenal hemorrhage in neonates with ultrasound. The right adrenal is easily seen through the liver at a level just superior to the upper pole of the kidney—think of the abdominal circumference in the neonate. It lies so medially that it seems to hug the spine under the inferior vena cava, and the limb visible on this view appears almond-shaped. Once localized, you can turn the transducer 90 degrees to show another plane, capping the upper pole. The left adrenal is most easily seen in the sagittal plane, tucked into the space created by the meeting of the left kidney, spleen, and aorta. Scan through the left side with the baby either supine or left side up. Again, change planes after imaging it in one plane; however, on transverse views the stomach tends to shadow the region, so use a very posterior approach.

◆ PATHOLOGY

Multicystic (Dysplastic) Kidney

Multicystic kidney is a unilateral process unless the child is stillborn. Multiple cystic structures of varying size and shape with no evidence of renal pelvis or parenchyma are noted (see Fig. 28-1B). Some cysts may be so small that they are visualized as echoes rather than as fluid-filled structures. These may erroneously be thought to be dense parenchyma.

Hydronephrosis

The appearance of hydronephrosis is the same in children as in adults, although the pelvis is usually more prominent and there may appear to be only a single cystic structure. The amount of parenchyma varies with the severity and duration of the condition. If the obstruction is at a low level, the ureter can be seen posterior to the bladder or in the region of the kidney, but usually hydronephrosis in this age group is caused by ureteropelvic junction obstruction (UPJ). With a UPJ, the pelvis is dilated and the ureter is obstructed where it joins the pelvis. This condition is thought to be congenital.

If the ureter can be seen, examine the bladder for a ureterocele (see Chapter 31). A ureterocele is a cystic structure within the posterior aspect of the bladder. If a ureterocele is present, it is commonly associated with a double collecting system with a hydronephrotic upper segment. The lower segment may look normal or may also be dilated owing to reflux.

Adrenal Hemorrhage

Adrenal hemorrhages are in most instances echogenic at first. Cystic areas rapidly develop, and within 2 to 3 weeks the mass is echo-free (Fig. 28-3). Eventually calcification will be apparent on plain radiographs. A steady shrinkage in size occurs as this progression takes place. Usually the condition is bilateral.

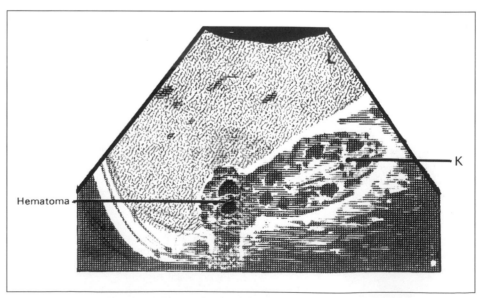

FIGURE 28-3. Adrenal hematoma. There is a mass superior to the kidney, which contains several echo-free areas. It is posterior to the retroperitoneal fat line.

Intussusception

In intussusception (see Chapter 30) one portion of the bowel, usually the terminal ileum, is surrounded by bowel that normally lies more distally. A mass causing obstruction is created by the bowel coiled within itself. Peristalsis pushes the more-proximal bowel into the mass so that the mass has a sleeve-like shape. On the transverse view, the walls of both layers of bowel can be seen (Fig. 28-4).

Color flow shows arteries in each layer of bowel on a transverse view of the intussusception. Intussusception can be cured if fluid is infused rectally so the blocking bowel is pushed toward the stomach. Such a procedure is often done under fluoroscopic control, but ultrasound can be used as the monitoring technique.

Pyloric Stenosis

An epigastric mass is present with pyloric stenosis with an echogenic center and sonolucent walls, resembling the target sign of bowel wall thickening (see Chapter 30). The pyloric mass can be visualized connected to the stomach. Measurements are made of the wall thickness (Fig. 28-5). A wall thickness of greater than 4 mm and pyloric length of greater than 1.5 cm indicates pyloric stenosis. The mass is located to the right of midline just below the gallbladder. Placing water in the stomach through a nasogastric tube makes identification of the stomach more obvious. Usually, the much enlarged, fluid-filled stomach lies to the left of the pylorus.

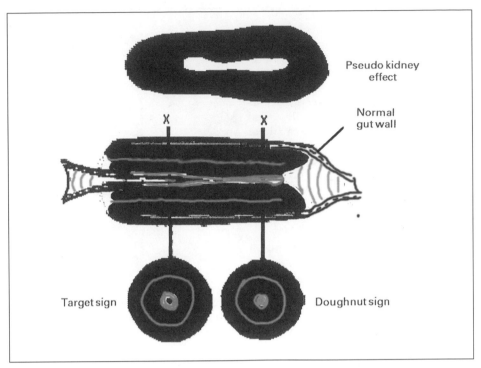

FIGURE 28-4. Intussusception. The small bowel has prolapsed into the large bowel due to peristalsis, causing an obstructing mass that can look like a kidney. A transverse section near the end of the obstructing gut shows an echopenic center. This is known as the "doughnut sign." A transverse section at a more proximal site will show the lumen of the inner segment of the bowel, forming a "target sign."

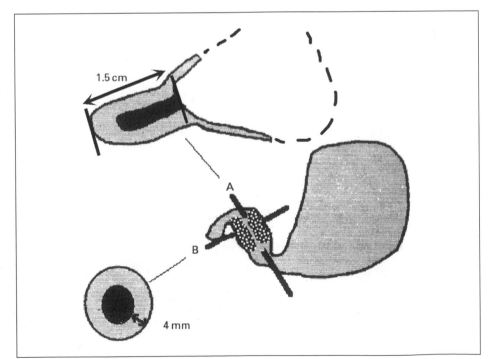

FIGURE 28-5. Pyloric stenosis. The antral region of the stomach resembles a cervix. To make a diagnosis of pyloric stenosis, the antrum should be more than 1.5 cm long and the wall of the pylorus at least 4 mm thick. The axis that shows length is indicated by line A. The axis that shows wall thickness is indicated by line B.

Wilms' Tumor

Wilms' tumor occurs in the 1-to-6-year-old age group. This malignant tumor is evenly echogenic at first, but later develops sonolucent areas that are probably caused by areas of necrosis (Fig. 28-6). This cancer often causes secondary hydronephrosis. Although usually unilateral, Wilms' tumor is bilateral in 10 percent of cases. A more benign but rare variant (mesoblastic nephroma) is seen in the first year of life. The echo pattern is more variable, and the tumor may be partially cystic.

Neuroblastoma

Neuroblastoma, a malignant tumor, generally occurs in the age group from birth to 5 years old. Although neuroblastoma usually originates in the adrenal gland, it can arise elsewhere; for example, it may be paraspinous. The echogenic texture is much more heterogeneous than the texture of a Wilms' tumor, with areas of acoustic shadowing due to calcification (Fig. 28-7). Extension of the cancer beyond the midline is common and affects the staging. Involvement of the major arteries, which precludes operation, should be clearly demonstrated ultrasonically.

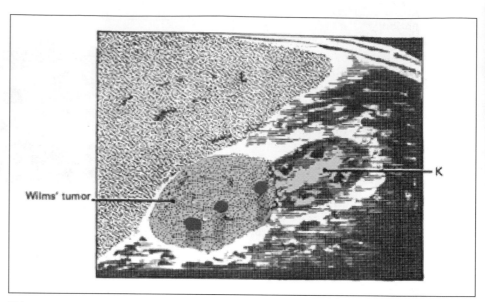

FIGURE 28-6. A Wilms' tumor has an even echogenicity apart from cystic areas that are thought to be due to areas of necrosis.

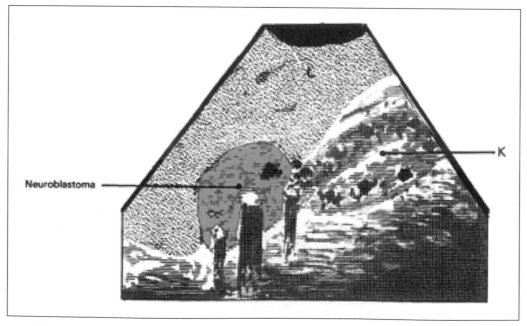

FIGURE 28-7. Neuroblastoma. The echogenicity of the mass is much more heterogeneous than it is in Wilms' tumor, and often shows some areas of calcification that cause acoustic shadowing.

Enteric Duplication

An enteric duplication is a rare congenital lesion. It is either a fluid-filled structure in the mesentery or a mass filled with the usual contents of gut with acoustic shadowing. Most of those recognized ultrasonically are fluid filled.

Mesenteric Cyst

Mesenteric cysts are large, asymptomatic, fluid-filled masses in the mesentery that may be multilocular, but are otherwise echo-free.

Teratoma

Teratomas may contain any of the body's structural elements. Often teratomas contain bone with acoustic shadowing or hair, which may result in an evenly echogenic structure possibly with a fluid-fluid level. At birth, these tumors may be seen arising from the buttocks. Later in childhood, they are usually located in the pelvis or arise from the presacral region, and represent the remnants of a fetal sacrococcygeal tumor (see Chapter 18) that has been incompletely removed. However, teratomas can be seen anywhere in the abdomen, particularly in the region of the adrenals. These tumors may rarely be entirely fluid filled.

Meningocele

Intra-abdominal meningoceles, which are located in the same place as teratomas—anterior to the sacrum—are entirely fluid filled. Correlation with a sacral radiograph may show associated bony changes.

Ovarian Cysts

Ovarian cysts in the neonate are highly variable in position and may occur in the upper abdomen. They may contain septa and echogenic material. The presence of a crescent-shaped echogenic mass or internal acoustic echoes indicates that the cyst has twisted and is infarcted. Echo-free cysts disappear spontaneously.

Ovaries in the neonate or infant are usually very small (under 1 cm in diameter). The uterus is also small. As in the adult, a full bladder is essential for assessment of ovarian size.

Rhabdomyosarcoma

Rhabdomyosarcoma, a sarcomatous lesion, tends to affect the posterior wall of the bladder and can cause adenopathy anywhere in the abdomen.

Hepatoblastoma

Liver tumors in small children are usually single and have variable sonographic appearances, some being echopenic and some echogenic. Occasional tumors have large cystic components. The site of these tumors must be defined with respect to the hepatic veins, because they can be resected if they lie solely within one lobe of the liver (see Chapter 23). Most tumors in the liver in small children are highly vascular on color flow.

Lymphoma

Lymphoma occurs in children and appears similar to adenopathy in adults.

Pancreatitis

Pancreatitis may occur in children and is a cause of unexplained abdominal pain. It has the same features as in adults. The pancreas enlarges and becomes more sonolucent than normal for the pediatric age group. Pancreatic pseudocysts may occur. Pancreatitis is usually caused by trauma or congenital processes such as hyperlipidemia.

PITFALLS

1. *Adrenal hemorrhage vs. tumor.* Do not mistake adrenal hemorrhage for a neoplastic mass. Following the patient for a few days with serial sonograms will show a change in the configuration of a hematoma with development of cystic areas.
2. *Cyst vs. pyramids in kidney.* Do not mistake normal pyramids in the neonate for cystic disease.
3. *Pseudopancreatitis.* Because the pancreas is normally less echogenic in children than in adults, be cautious about making a diagnosis of pancreatitis unless the pancreas appears enlarged.
4. *Echopenic psoas muscle.* The echopenic psoas muscle can be mistaken for a hydronephrotic ureter. When the gain is increased, the subtle muscle texture is brought out.

5. *Apparent hepatosplenomegaly.* Since the liver and spleen are proportionately larger in children, there is a tendency to overdiagnose hepatosplenomegaly.
6. *Fluid-filled stomach.* The stomach, when it is distended with fluid in a small child, can be mistaken for a cyst.
7. *Meconium-filled bowel.* In the neonate, echopenic meconium within bowel can be mistaken for a mass behind the bladder.

 WHERE ELSE TO LOOK

1. If a *Wilms' tumor* is possible, examine:
   a. The second kidney, because this neoplasm may be bilateral
   b. The inferior vena cava and renal vein for clot or tumor; color flow will help
   c. The liver for metastases
   d. The para-aortic area for nodal enlargement
2. If *neuroblastoma* is likely, look for midline spread, with involvement of the aorta and inferior vena cava. It alters the staging. Look for metastatic disease to the liver.
3. If *hydronephrosis* is discovered, examine the pelvis to see if the cause of obstruction is visible—for example, a ureterocele.
4. If a *bladder mass* is found, look elsewhere in the abdomen for evidence of rhabdomyosarcoma.

SELECTED READING

Siegel, M. *Pediatric Sonography.* New York: Raven, 1991.

Teale, R. Ultrasonography of Infants and Children. Philadelphia: Saunders, 1991.

MIDABDOMINAL MASS

Possible Ascites

ROGER C. SANDERS

29

SONOGRAM ABBREVIATIONS

Ab   Abscess
Ao   Aorta

Bl   Bladder

Ca   Celiac artery

GBl Gallbladder

Ia   Iliac artery
Ip   Iliopsoas muscle
IVC Inferior vena cava

K   Kidney

L   Liver

N   Nodes

P   Pancreas
Ps   Psoas muscle

QL   Quadratus lumborum muscle

RA   Rectus abdominis muscle

SMa Superior mesenteric artery
Sp   Spleen

KEY WORDS

Adenopathy. Multiple enlarged lymph nodes in many locations.

Aneurysm. Dilatation of an artery, usually the abdominal aorta. Aneurysms may be true, if they have an intact wall, or false, if the wall has ruptured and only clot prevents hemorrhage into neighboring tissues.

Ascites

Exudative. Free fluid in the peritoneum associated with malignancy or infection; may contain internal echoes.

Transudative. Free fluid in the peritoneum containing little or no protein and associated with heart, kidney, or liver failure.

Bifurcation. The abdominal aorta divides into the iliac arteries at the bifurcation, which is located approximately at the level of the umbilicus.

Crohn's Disease. Inflammatory bowel disease often accompanied by abscesses and associated with bowel wall thickening.

Dissecting Aneurysm. The wall of the aorta is composed of three parts—intima, media, and adventitia. In a dissecting aneurysm the intima separates from the media, so blood can flow through two channels on either side of the intima. The blood usually reenters the aorta at a lower level.

Gutter. Area lateral to the ascending and descending colon where fluid may accumulate ("paracolic gutter").

Haustral Markings. Normal segmentation of the wall of the colon.

Hernia. Protrusion of gut through the abdominal wall into a subcutaneous location. Dangerous because it can lead to obstruction if the bowel is blocked as it passes through the narrow opening. Hernias may be (1) *ventral*—usually midline and associated with previous surgery; (2) *spigelian*—lateral to the rectus muscles; (3) *femoral* or *inguinal*—in the groin.

Intussusception. Obstructed bowel coiled on itself. Seen particularly in children. The walls are thickened (see Chapters 18 and 30).

Ischemic Colitis. Bowel with a very poor blood supply—it has a thickened wall and does not show evidence of peristalsis.

Lymphoma. Malignancy that mainly affects the lymph nodes, spleen, or liver. There are various types (e.g., Hodgkin's, histiocytic, and lymphoblastic lymphoma).

Mechanical Obstruction. When the bowel is blocked by an obstructive process such as a carcinoma. Dilated fluid-filled loops of bowel show much peristalsis unless the obstruction is longstanding.

Mesenteric Sheath (Transverse Mesocolon). A structure within which lie the superior mesenteric artery and the superior mesenteric vein and to which the mesentery that supports the bowel is attached.

Paralytic Ileus. Dilated fluid-filled bowel loops that do not show peristalsis, due to either longstanding mechanical obstruction, poor blood supply, or abnormal metabolic state.

Peristalsis. Rhythmic dilatation and contraction of the gut as food is propelled through it. Visible with ultrasound.

Rectus Muscles. Muscles in the anterior midabdomen that are often the site of hemorrhage. The muscles are paired, one on either side of the midline, and extend the length of the abdomen.

Sandwich Sign. Nodes in the mesentery characteristically form on either side of the mesenteric sheath in two large groups, resulting in an appearance similar to a sandwich.

Valvulae Conniventes. Normal segmentation of the small bowel.

 THE CLINICAL PROBLEM

Many of the masses that apparently lie in the midabdomen arise in the pelvis or upper abdomen and extend into the midabdomen (e.g., splenomegaly, fibroid uterus, pancreatic pseudocyst). Masses of truly midabdominal origin are related to structures in this area, that is, the abdominal wall, the aorta, the gut, and nodes. Air in the gut frequently interferes with sonographic visualization, but fortunately, if a mass is present, the mass itself usually provides an acoustic window and displaces gut.

Aortic Aneurysm

It is useful to look at aneurysms with ultrasound because the true internal and external dimensions of the aneurysm are revealed (Fig. 29-1). An aortogram will show only the blood-filled lumen, not the clot-filled area. Surgeons will appreciate information about how the aneurysm is related to the major aortic branches such as the renal, mesenteric, and iliac arteries because it helps them choose the appropriate graft shape.

If the aneurysm is over 5 cm in width or anteroposterior diameter, operation is usually required. Smaller aneurysms may also be resected or they may be followed up at approximately 6-month intervals. Evidence of expansion between sequential sonograms may indicate the need for surgical intervention.

An aneurysm that is leaking, forming a false aneurysm, is an acute emergency. The walls of a false aneurysm are formed by clot and may give way abruptly.

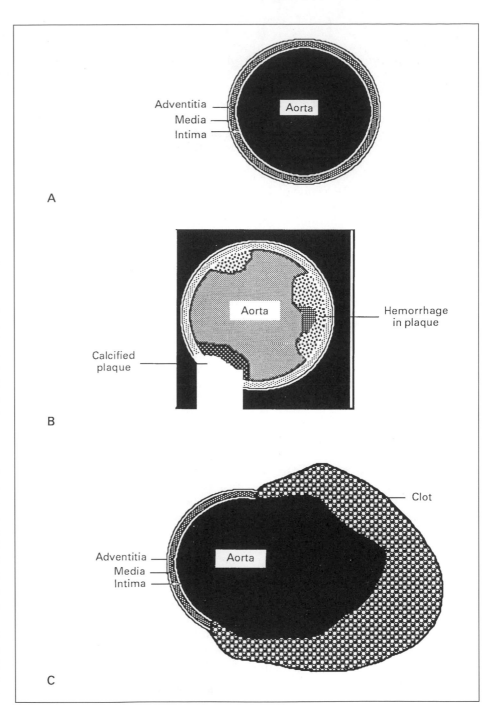

FIGURE 29-1. (**A**) Normal aorta showing the three components of the wall—the intima, media, and adventitia. (**B**) Plaque. Note the echopenic area in the plaque suggesting hemorrhage. Some of the plaque is calcified. (**C**) False aneurysm. The normal components of the wall are absent at the aneurysm site. The clot forms the wall of the blood vessel in a false aneurysm.

Nodes

Initial and follow-up assessment is helpful in dealing with nodal enlargement around the aorta and celiac axis. Such adenopathy is most commonly caused by lymphoma, but may be caused by metastatic nodes from a primary cancer elsewhere. Ultrasound is preferable to lymphography because it shows nodes in locations that cannot be reached by lymphography, such as in the mesentery or around the celiac axis. Detection of minimal nodal enlargement in lymphoma is worthwhile. Planning radiotherapy and chemotherapy for these patients depends on staging, which is based on the extent of lymphomatous spread. Computed tomography (CT) has largely supplanted ultrasound in this area unless the patient is thin.

Lymphoma is staged as follows:

Stage I. Disease limited to one anatomic region.

Stage II. Disease involving two or more anatomic regions on the same side of the diaphragm.

Stage III. Disease on both sides of the diaphragm involving lymph nodes or spleen.

Stage IV. Extranodal involvement such as bone marrow, lung, or liver.

Gut Masses

Masses that arise from gut may be sufficiently large to be palpated by the clinician and may have a typical sonographic appearance—a thick echopenic wall, with an echogenic center.

Although lesions with gut symptoms are investigated by upper GI series or barium enema before an ultrasound examination is requested, some masses are first detected with ultrasound on a study performed for other reasons.

Bowel Obstruction

Another important cause of overall abdominal distention is intestinal obstruction or paralytic ileus. In these conditions the gut is very distended. Dilated gut usually contains a mixture of air and fluid, and not much can be seen with ultrasound. If the bowel is entirely filled with fluid and no air is present, the sonogram can help by showing that the bowel is dilated—a finding that may not be appreciated on a plain radiograph. Sonography is particularly helpful if the obstruction is localized to a small segment of bowel.

With real-time, paralytic ileus can be distinguished from mechanical obstruction. With ileus, there will be no movements within the dilated loop of bowel, whereas with mechanical obstruction—at least early on—the gut will show evidence of marked peristalsis. These two conditions are treated very differently; mechanical obstruction is an indication for surgery and paralytic ileus is treated conservatively.

Ascites

Often the whole abdomen appears enlarged, and the clinical question is whether or not ascites is present. This is assessed relatively easily by sonography; obese people with much subcutaneous fat may be thought clinically to have ascites when none is actually present. Ultrasonic discovery of ascites is important because aspiration of the ascitic fluid often guides patient management. Causes of ascites include congestive heart failure, liver disease such as cirrhosis, the nephrotic syndrome, infections such as tuberculosis and pyogenic peritonitis, malignancy, and blood from, for example, a ruptured aneurysm or trauma.

Abdominal Wall Masses

The nature and presence of masses in the abdominal wall can be usefully clarified by ultrasound. Abscesses may develop in the abdominal wall. A hematocrit drop may be due to a bleed into the rectus muscle.

ANATOMY

See Chapter 21.

Aorta

The aortic wall has three components. The adventitia, media, and intima (see Fig. 29-1) can be separately identified.

As long as the abdomen does not contain much gas, the aorta and the inferior vena cava can be traced as far as the level of the bifurcation. The superior and inferior mesenteric arteries, celiac axis, and renal arteries arise from the aorta. The renal and inferior mesenteric arteries may not be visible because of overlying gas.

There is normally no gap between the spine and the aorta. The iliac arteries sometimes cannot be seen below the level of the sacral promontory because they are hidden by bowel gas (Fig. 29-2).

Mesenteric Sheath (Transverse Mesocolon)

The superior mesenteric artery and superior mesenteric vein run within a structure known as the mesenteric sheath. This fibrous structure is the attachment for the small and large bowels; nodes form on either side of it. It is not visible unless it is surrounded by nodes.

Bowel

Much of the time normal bowel is not recognizable because of gas. However, cross-sectional views through normal empty bowel show an echogenic center with a thin echo-free wall (see Fig. 21-15).

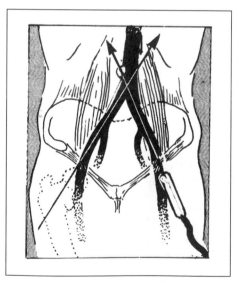

FIGURE 29-2. Attempt to show the iliac arteries by finding the bifurcation of the aorta and the femoral arteries in the groin by palpation. Align the transducer along this axis.

Psoas Muscle

The psoas muscles can be seen on either side of the spine and may be large in muscular individuals (see Fig. 21-17). The psoas muscles join with the iliacus muscles, which coat the anterior aspect of the iliac crest, just above the true pelvis.

Rectus Muscles

The two rectus muscles lie on either side of the midline in the anterior abdominal wall. They are seen well in the upper abdomen but are tendinous and so not readily seen below the umbilicus (see Fig. 21-18).

Abdominal Wall

The abdominal wall may be the site of an abdominal mass. Hence, the various layers of the abdominal wall should be identified anterior to the peritoneal line (see Figs. 21-16 and 21-18). The subcutaneous tissues contain mainly fat and are distinct from the muscular layers.

A strong linear echo represents the peritoneal fascial line. Posterior to this line are the intraperitoneal structures.

◨ TECHNIQUE

Palpation

After feeling an abdominal mass, examine the same area with ultrasound. It should be immediately apparent whether the mass is superficial in the abdominal wall or is located at a deeper level, using the peritoneal fascial line as a landmark (see Fig. 29-13).

Compression

Midabdominal pathology may be obscured by gas. The transducer can be used as a means of pressing away overlying gas and displacing bowel so that pathology is revealed.

Documentation

Once the mass has been found, obtain pictures that demonstrate the relationship of the abdominal wall, the organs, and the vessels to the mass.

Features of a mass at any site that should be documented are the following:

1. How it relates to other organs
2. Whether its borders are rough or smooth
3. Whether it is mobile
4. Its size
5. Its consistency in comparison with a known fluid-filled structure such as the gallbladder or bladder (i.e., whether it is cystic or solid)
6. Vascularity: Are vessels present in the center or only in the periphery? Is flow low or high resistance?

A matched dual linear image may be helpful for documentation. Use a short-focus high-frequency linear array to display abdominal wall pathology.

Aorta

If the mass is clearly aortic in origin (pulsatile with flow within on Doppler), attempt to show both the normal aorta and the aneurysmal segment and to define where the major vessels lie in relation to the aneurysm (Fig. 29-3; see also Fig. 29-2). When there is considerable gas lying over the aorta, pressure with a linear array transducer may displace the gas and perhaps allow visualization. Should pressure prove unsuccessful, placing the patient in the left or right decubitus position will allow partial visualization of the aorta in the area of the kidney (see Chapter 21). Be careful to use optimal gain settings so clot is not missed or invented.

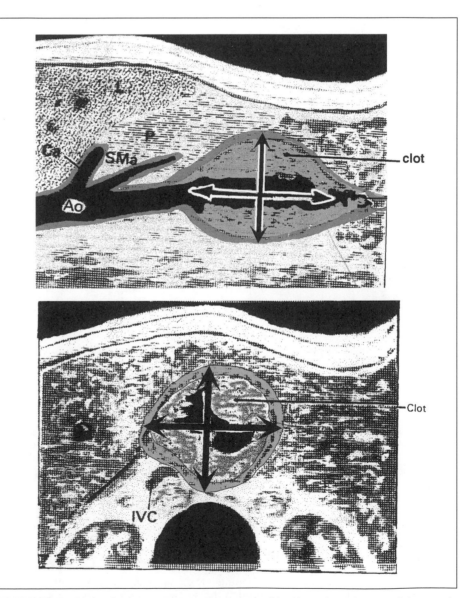

FIGURE 29-3. Abdominal aneurysms are measured to the edge of the wall (arrows). Because they often contain clot, there may be a relatively small patent lumen.

The bifurcation is often best seen with the left-side-up view; this coronal approach allows visualization of both iliac arteries simultaneously. The iliac arteries may also be found with the patient supine by scanning through the small acoustic windows provided by gas-free bowel.

Mesenteric Masses

If the mass is anterior to the aorta within the mesentery, try to show its relationship to the superior mesenteric vein and artery, which lie in the mesenteric sheath.

A left- or right-side-up view looking through the spleen or liver may be needed to see the para-aortic nodes when gas obscures them in a supine position (see Fig. 26-3).

Visualization of peristalsis allows one to decide whether a possible node in the mesentery is gut rather than a node. If a mass has a well-defined margin when examined in two planes at right angles to each other, it is unlikely to be bowel.

Ascites

If the clinical problem is to determine the presence or absence of ascites and it is not immediately obvious that there is fluid surrounding the bowel, examine the pelvis, the subhepatic space, and the paracolic gutters with the patient in a supine position. These are the areas where small amounts of fluid first develop.

If fluid appears to be loculated in one area such as the subhepatic space, place the patient in the right-side-up position and note whether the fluid remains in the same position. If it does not shift, loculated ascites, an abscess, or hematoma should be suspected. Confusion between a pleural effusion and ascites can occur if the diaphragm is not defined (see Fig. 29-14). Pelvic ascites can be distinguished from the bladder by the following:

1. It will outline the uterus by filling the anterior and posterior cul-de-sac.
2. The superior border of the ascites will be irregular; it is indented by gut.
3. The superior border of the bladder will be smooth.

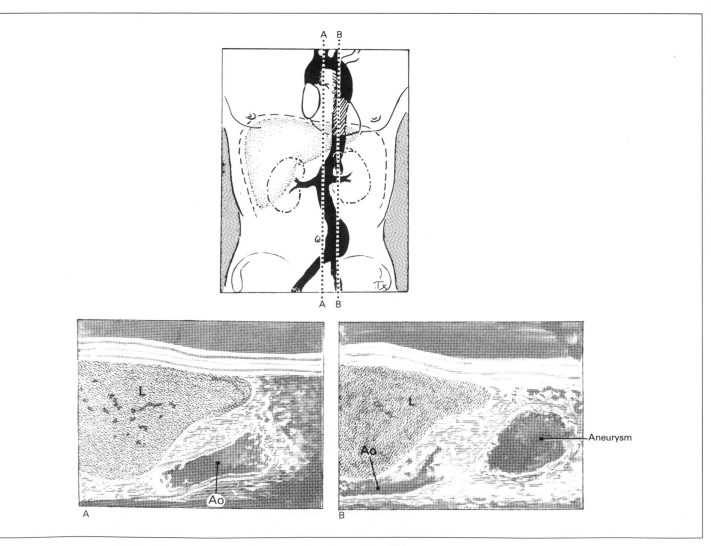

FIGURE 29-4. Because the aneurysmal aorta is often tortuous, complete longitudinal sections through the aorta and the aneurysm may be technically impossible. Line A is drawn through the aorta, where it swings to the right; line B extends through the portion of the aorta where the major vessels arise.

◆ PATHOLOGY

Aneurysm

Aneurysms are pulsatile dilatations of the aorta. Most are found in the midabdomen just above the bifurcation (see Fig. 29-3) and below the origin of the renal arteries.

Midline aneurysms may bulge in either direction, although they generally bulge to the left. It may be hard to align the aneurysm with the normal aorta so that both are shown in a single section (Fig. 29-4; see also Fig. 29-3). A matched linear array view should be attempted. Plaque is often seen in the abdominal aorta (see Chapter 41; see also Figs. 29-1 and 29-3).

Features to Look for in Aneurysms

ILIAC ARTERIES. Lower abdominal aneurysms often involve the iliac arteries. Attempt to show involvement of the iliac arteries by performing an oblique section between the umbilicus and the palpated femoral artery in the groin (see Fig. 29-2).

THROMBUS. Thrombus may be present within the aneurysm. Make sure that reverberation artifacts are not mistaken for an aneurysm, thrombus, or clot (see Figs. 29-1 and 29-3). Conversely, attempts to "clean up" the aorta can prevent visualization of clot or thrombus within the lumen.

Color flow and Doppler greatly simplify decisions about whether or not clot is present. Thrombus may become partially detached from the aneurysm wall and simulate a dissection. This is a dangerous situation because thrombus may detach and cause an embolus in the legs.

INVOLVEMENT OF MAJOR VESSELS. Some aneurysms of the upper abdominal aorta may involve the celiac axis and the superior mesenteric and renal arteries. Make special efforts to image these vessels because surgical management is altered if there is such involvement. The principal renal arteries are almost always located at the level of the superior mesenteric artery.

Use color flow to define the smaller vessels.

DISSECTION. Dissection of an aneurysm is a rare finding in the abdomen. The sonogram will show an echogenic septum that pulsates, obliquely aligned in the middle of an aneurysm (Fig. 29-5). Dissections usually extend from the chest into the abdomen.

LEAKING ANEURYSM. If the aneurysm is leaking, a fluid collection will be seen alongside the aorta, usually to the left of the spine anterior to the kidney. Another common location is at the junction of a graft and the patient's own aorta or iliac artery. The walls of the aneurysm are formed by clot—this constitutes a false aneurysm. Flow between the aneurysmal collection and the aorta may be seen, indicating a surgical emergency.

Color flow may show flow within an aneurysmal "mass" that appears to be solid.

GRAFTS. Grafts can be recognized by the presence of linear parallel echoes within the aorta and iliac vessels. Frequently the grafts are placed within aneurysms, and the aneurysm is left in place. A baseline study following the operation is helpful because any subsequent changes in graft configuration can be detected.

FALSE ANEURYSMS. False aneurysms are aneurysms that do not have a wall but are surrounded by clot. They are usually masses with a large amount of echogenic material within them and a relatively small patent lumen (see Fig. 29-1C).

Color flow may show a mushroom-like appearance within the aneurysm since there will be a small neck at the site of the leak and a larger cavity within the mass.

Lymphadenopathy

Most nodes are lobulated, echo-free masses. Benign nodes have an echogenic center and are bean shaped. Malignant nodes do not have an echogenic center and are of a more random shape.

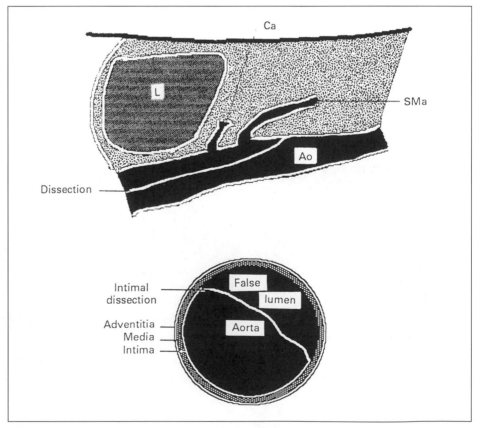

FIGURE 29-5. Longitudinal and transverse sonographic views of a dissecting aneurysm. Note the line from the intima that represents one border of the dissection.

Color flow Doppler analysis of malignant nodes shows a high resistance pattern with a resistive index of .9, whereas benign nodes have a low resistance pattern (a resistive index of less than .5). There are several potential locations for nodes.

Para-aortic Nodes

Para-aortic nodes can be lobulated (Fig. 29-6A) or smooth bordered (Fig. 29-6B). These nodes may surround the aorta so intimately that the wall of the aorta may be invisible (see Fig. 29-6B). The aorta is often displaced anteriorly, and the inferior vena cava is almost always displaced anteriorly. Nodes may be seen between the aorta and the inferior vena cava. A common pattern is a node that lies posterior to the inferior vena cava and anterior to the aorta. Nodes between the aorta and the left kidney are frequent.

Celiac Axis Nodes

Celiac axis nodes are sometimes termed porta hepatis nodes because they extend into the porta hepatis. The main bulk of the nodes lies around the celiac axis posterior and superior to the pancreas. They surround and straighten the celiac axis (Fig. 29-7). The pancreas is displaced anteriorly by such nodes.

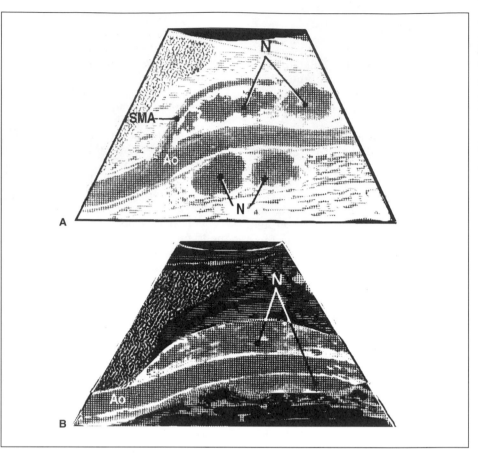

FIGURE 29-6. Para-aortic nodes. (**A**) Lobulated nodes displace the aorta anteriorly and lie between the aorta and the superior mesenteric artery. (**B**) Smooth-bordered nodes silhouetting the aorta make it hard to see the border between the aorta and the nodes (the silhouette sign). Such a group of nodes may be mistaken for an aneurysm.

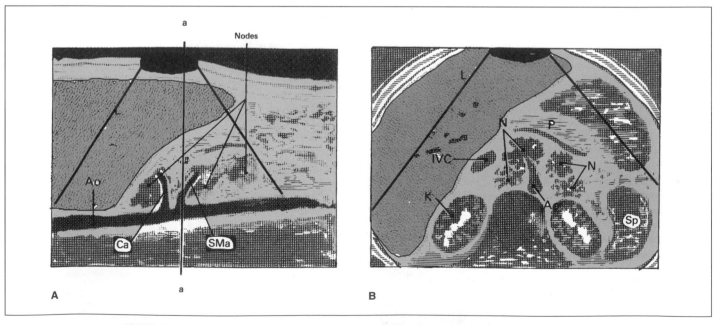

FIGURE 29-7. Nodes straightening and surrounding the celiac axis and the superior mesenteric artery. (**B**) is a transverse scan taken at the level marked "a" in (**A**).

Mesenteric Nodes

Nodes in the mesentery are characteristically placed longitudinally anterior and posterior to the superior mesenteric artery and vein and the mesenteric sheath to form the so-called sandwich sign (Fig. 29-8). Nodes in the mesentery may be mistaken for gut. They have an ovoid shape and are usually echo-free.

Pelvic Nodes

Pelvic nodes coat the lateral walls of the pelvis along the iliopsoas muscles in the region of the vessels. They may compress the bladder (Fig. 29-9).

Inguinal Nodes

Inguinal nodes are not usually large but are easily felt. They lie adjacent to the inguinal ligament in the groin.

Nodes Involving Organs

Any organ can be involved with lymphadenopathy. The nodal mass is usually sonolucent and may be mistaken for a cyst if careful assessment of the degree of through transmission is not made.

Fluid-Filled Loops of Bowel

Bowel loops filled with fluid rather than air are well seen. They form tubular structures and tend to lie in groups (see Fig. 21-15). It is sometimes possible to see the detailed structure of the gut wall (i.e., the valvulae conniventes or the haustral markings). Only a few segments of the dilated bowel loops may be visible because other portions are air filled.

Peristaltic movement indicates a mechanical obstruction. No movement within the dilated loop of bowel indicates that paralytic ileus or longstanding obstruction may be present.

Gut Mass

A palpable mass may originate from the bowel and may show the so-called target or bull's eye sign. In the pathologic segment of bowel, there is a mass consisting of an echogenic center surrounded by a thick sonolucent rim that is more than 4-mm wide (Fig. 29-10). This appearance is generally due to a carcinoma of the stomach or colon. Other causes include a variety of other nonneoplastic conditions in which there is bowel wall thickening such as Crohn's disease, ischemic colitis, and intussusception (see Chapter 30).

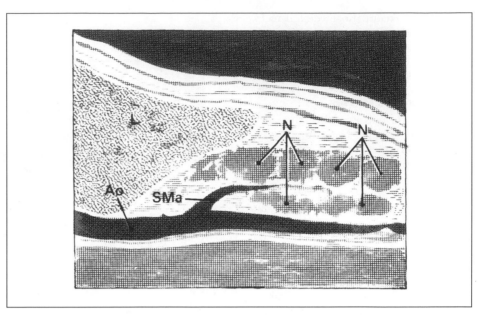

FIGURE 29-8. The sandwich sign. Nodes lie anterior and posterior to the superior mesenteric artery and the mesenteric sheath in the mesentery.

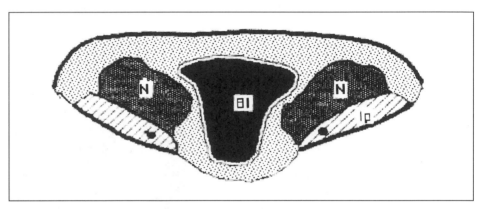

FIGURE 29-9. Typical distribution of nodes in the pelvis lying alongside the iliopsoas muscles compressing the bladder.

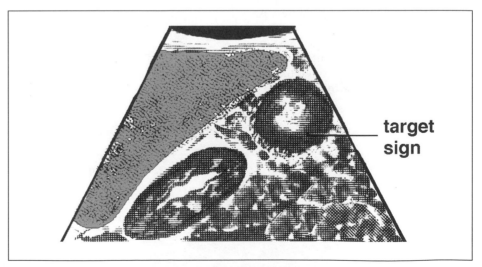

FIGURE 29-10. Target sign of intestinal wall thickening. If the wall is more than 4-mm thick, it is abnormal.

All masses, except those related to ischemic bowel, will show arterial flow on color Doppler. In Crohn's disease and other types of inflammatory bowel disease, color flow will be prominent.

Other Mesenteric Masses

Intramesenteric masses within the peritoneum can usually be distinguished from retroperitoneal masses by the absence of distortion of the psoas muscles, kidneys, or quadratus lumborum muscles. Mesenteric masses can be moved from side to side on palpation. The fat line that runs in front of the retroperitoneal tissues will not be displaced anteriorly by the mass. Other than nodes, most intramesenteric masses are relatively benign, including mesenteric cysts, which are large, fluid-filled, asymptomatic masses that contain septa and are seen mainly in children; and lipomas, which are large, asymptomatic masses that are evenly echogenic.

Ascites

If there is gross ascites, bowel loops surrounded by fluid will be seen. Small amounts of fluid accumulate first in the subhepatic space along the posterior-inferior border of the liver, then in the pelvic cul-de-sac, and finally in the right paracolic gutter, where scanning from a lateral approach is desirable.

It is important to decide whether the ascites is free or loculated. If any segments of bowel are separated from each other or are tethered to the abdominal wall, loculation is present, suggesting malignancy or infection (Fig. 29-11). The presence of ascites may reveal peritoneal metastases that might otherwise be obscured by bowel.

Internal echoes in fluid suggest infection or malignancy. If infection has occurred in the past, a cobweb-like appearance may be seen within the fluid.

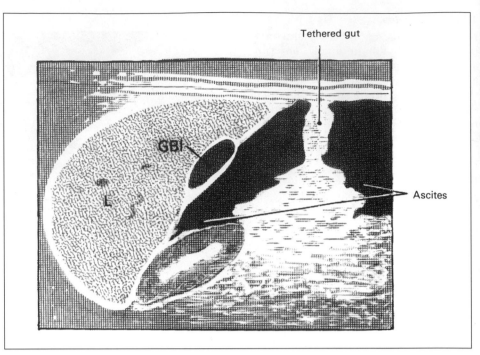

FIGURE 29-11. The usual sites for ascites accumulation are the subhepatic space and the cul-de-sac. In loculated ascites the bowel is tethered to the abdominal wall.

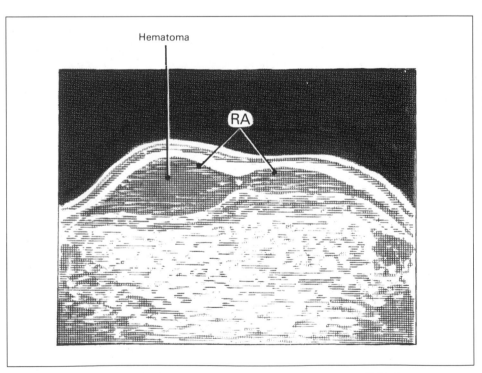

FIGURE 29-12. Widening of the right rectus abdominis muscles (RA) due to a hematoma.

Abdominal Wall Problems

Masses that lie in the abdominal wall are usually easily recognized as superficial by palpation. They remain easily palpable when the patient lifts his or her head. Gain settings, focusing, and transducer selection should be set to concentrate on this superficial area. Abdominal wall masses lie anterior to the fascial/peritoneal echoes (see Fig. 29-13).

Rectus Sheath Hematoma

A rectus sheath hematoma causes enlargement of one of the rectus sheath muscles in the abdominal wall. The other muscle is usually uninvolved (Fig. 29-12). Most rectus sheath hematomas are more echopenic than the normal muscle.

Abscesses

Abscesses do not respect tissue spaces and may involve both the rectus sheath and the area superficial to the muscles (Fig. 29-13). The usual abscess is relatively echopenic with an irregular wall and some internal echoes.

Neoplasm

Neoplastic deposits, like abscesses, also involve muscle, subcutaneous tissue, and intramesenteric areas, but are better demarcated and usually have a more even internal echo structure than abscesses. Color flow will show internal vascularity in the tumor.

Lipoma

Lipomas are benign masses that often occur in the abdominal wall and appear as echogenic structures in the subcutaneous tissues. Lipomatous masses do not break through the tissue planes of the abdominal wall.

Hernia

An intermittently palpable abdominal mass may be caused by a hernia. Ventral hernias are often associated with a previous incision and are found in the midline. Spigelian hernias are found more laterally. Femoral and inguinal hernias are found in the groin. At the site of a hernia, there is an interruption of the peritoneal line between the abdominal wall and the contents of the abdomen. It is common to see an area of acoustic shadowing associated with such a mass because the bowel within the hernia contains gas. The hernia can also contain fluid-filled bowel. Such hernias may be intermittent and become visible with a change in the patient's position and when the patient strains.

★ PITFALLS

1. *Abdominal fat.* In obese people the sonolucent area beneath the peritoneum that is due to fat may be confused with ascites but will not be gravity dependent.
2. *Ovarian cyst.* Ovarian cysts can be huge and may occupy most of the abdomen. They may be confused clinically with ascites because serous fluid will be obtained when a peritoneal tap is performed. The sonographic appearances are quite different because cauliflower-shaped loops of bowel will not be seen within the supposed ascites.
3. *Nodes vs. aneurysm.* Para-aortic nodes may be confused with a partially clot-filled aortic aneurysm. Real-time will show pulsation and on transverse sections the shape of the nodes is usually not like that of an aneurysm. The overall configuration of adenopathy is lobulated, and the nodes extend laterally over the psoas muscles. An aortic aneurysm will be more or less round.
4. *Bowel loops vs. nodes.* Nodes can resemble loops of fluid-filled bowel. Real-time will show evidence of peristalsis in some bowel, and a water enema will clarify some problems in the pelvic region. In other cases a further examination on another day may be required to make sure that there has been no change in shape and that the suspect nodes do not represent bowel.

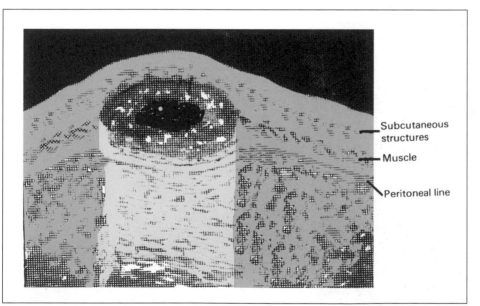

FIGURE 29-13. Abdominal wall abscess. The abscess has expanded and broken through the tissue planes.

Subcutaneous structures
Muscle
Peritoneal line

5. *Ascites vs. peritoneal dialysis.* When ascites is found, make sure that the patient has not had fluid introduced at the time of peritoneal dialysis for renal failure.

6. *Pleural effusion vs. ascites.* Do not mistake pleural effusions for ascites. On a transverse view, ascites lies between the diaphragm and the liver. A pleural effusion lies between the diaphragm and the chest wall (Fig. 29-14).

 WHERE ELSE TO LOOK

1. *Nodes.* If nodes are found, search for splenomegaly. It supports the diagnosis of lymphoma.
2. *Loculated ascites.* If evidence of loculation of ascites is seen, it is worth looking for evidence of peritoneal metastases adherent to the abdominal wall. Remember to shorten your focal zone.
3. *Ascites.* Examine the inferior vena cava and hepatic veins to see if they are unduly dilated as is usual in congestive failure. Study the liver size and shape for any evidence of cirrhosis.
4. *Aneurysm.* If an aneurysm is present, examine the kidneys for secondary hydronephrosis. Try to follow the iliac arteries because they may also be aneurysmal.
5. The presence of a gut mass with a thickened wall suggestive of a gastrointestinal neoplasm such as a carcinoma of the colon should set in motion a look for metastases to the liver and nodes.

SELECTED READING

Choi, M. Y., Lee, J. W., and Jang, K. J. Distinction between benign and malignant causes of cervical, axillary, and inguinal lymphadenopathy: Value of Doppler spectral waveform analysis. *AJR* 165:981–984, 1995.

Lederle, F. A., Walker, J. M., and Reinke, D. B. Selective screening for abdominal aortic aneurysms with physical examination and ultrasound. *Arch Intern Med* 148:1753–1756, 1988.

LeRoy, L. L., et al. Imagery of abdominal aortic aneurysms. *AJR* 152:785–792, 1989.

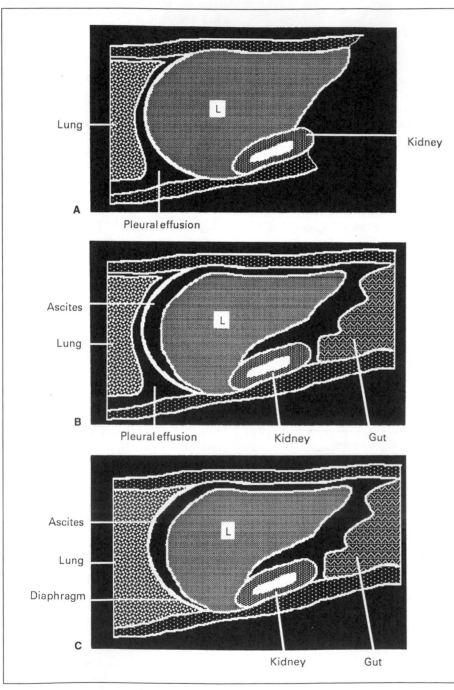

FIGURE 29-14. Pleural effusion and ascites. (**A**) Pleural effusion superior to the diaphragm. (**B**) Pleural effusion and ascites outlining the diaphragm. (**C**) Ascites only. Note the irregular outline to the gut where it is outlined by ascites.

30 RIGHT LOWER QUADRANT PAIN

GRETCHEN M. DIMLING

SONOGRAM ABBREVIATIONS

Ps Psoas muscle

RK Right kidney

KEY WORDS

Adenopathy. Enlarged lymph nodes.

Appendicolith (Fecalith). A calculus which may form around fecal material associated with appendicitis. Sonographically appears as an intraluminal echogenic focus with a varying degree of shadowing.

Bacterial Ileocecitis. Infection of the ileum and cecum.

"Bull's Eye" (Target Sign, Reniform Mass, or Pseudokidney). A characteristic sign of gastrointestinal wall thickening consisting of an echogenic center and a sonolucent rim.

Carcinoid. A yellow, circumscribed tumor occurring in the gastrointestinal tract.

Chronic Intestinal Ischemia. Stenosis or occlusion of the splanchnic (mesentery) arteries. Symptoms may present late in the disease and include upper abdominal pain which intensifies after a meal and weight loss.

Crohn's Disease. A recurrent bowel inflammatory disease usually involving the terminal ileum, but may affect any part of the gastrointestinal tract. Onset usually occurs between the ages of 20 and 40 years.

Diverticulitis. Occurs when a herniated outpouch of the intestinal lining becomes inflamed. May perforate and form an abscess.

Fistula. An abnormal communication between the gastrointestinal tract and other internal organs or to the body surface.

Malabsorption Syndrome. Impaired intestinal absorption of nutrients which results in deficiency of vitamins, electrolytes, iron, calcium, etc.

McBurney's Point. The site of maximum tenderness in the right iliac fossa with appendicitis.

Mesentery. The connective tissue attaching the intestine to the posterior abdominal wall.

Mesoappendix. The layer of connective tissue attaching the appendix to the mesentery of the ileum.

Mesocolon. The layer of connective tissue which attaches the various portions of the colon to the posterior abdominal wall.

Neutropenia. Decreased white blood cell count.

Neutropenic Typhlitis. Inflammation of the cecum that develops in the setting of severe neutropenia when a patient is immunosuppressed.

Peritonitis. Infection of the inner lining of the abdomen.

Rebound Tenderness. Most severe abdominal discomfort when pressure is released quickly rather than when the abdomen is compressed.

Septicemia. Infection involving the bloodstream.

Vasodilation. Increased blood flow in an inflamed organ and the surrounding tissues. Associated with increased heat and redness.

 THE CLINICAL PROBLEM

A number of entities can cause right iliac fossa pain, notably appendicitis. The pathology may be linked to the bowel found in this location (i.e., cecum, terminal ileum, and appendix) or the adjacent organs (i.e., right kidney, right ureter, bladder, ovary, uterus, or gallbladder) (see Fig. 30-3). A rapid and accurate diagnosis can be critical for a patient with acute abdominal pain. Ultrasound is a helpful tool to lead the physician to the correct diagnosis.

Not all intestinal problems require surgery. In approximately 25 percent of appendectomies, a misdiagnosis of appendicitis results in the removal of a normal appendix and a delay of appropriate treatment for the patient. Some conditions, such as bacterial ileocecitis, call for nonsurgical treatments. A thorough history followed by a targeted sonogram will spare the patient unnecessary procedures and point to the proper treatment.

Appendicitis

Although appendicitis is most common in children and young adults, it can occur at any age. The cause of appendicitis is obstruction of the appendix followed by infection. If the obstruction is not relieved spontaneously, inflammation and increased intraluminal pressure cause midabdominal pain which later localizes over the appendix. When surgical intervention is delayed, bacteria may invade the appendical wall and perforation may occur.

At this stage, the patient's life is in danger. When the appendix perforates into the abdominal cavity, peritonitis occurs, followed by abscess formation and occasionally death.

In most cases, the spread of infection is contained by mesentery and intestine in the appendix region. This collection is called an appendical phlegmon or an appendical abscess if there is pus within. An appendical phlegmon may resolve and reabsorb on its own. However, further infections may follow with the development of fistulous tracts to surrounding bowel, the bladder, the skin, or the vagina. If the infection becomes more widespread, death may result from septicemia or peritonitis.

Patients with classic symptoms of appendicitis may go straight to surgery. Atypical cases may be referred to ultrasound to rule out pelvic, renal, or gallbladder pathology. A prompt diagnosis is required to avoid perforation of the appendix.

The presenting symptoms include one or more of the following features:

1. Pain which starts in the periumbilical region then localizes to the right lower quadrant (McBurney's point)
2. Rebound tenderness (tenderness which is most severe when pressure is released)
3. Anorexia, nausea, vomiting, and/or diarrhea
4. Fever
5. Leukocytosis—white blood cell count (WBC) of 10,000 to 18,000/cc

Bacterial Ileocecitis

This is inflammation of the terminal ileum, cecum, and surrounding nodes caused by a bacterial infection. The most common culprits are *Yersinia enterocolitica, Campylobacter jejuni, Salmonella enteritidis,* and rarely *Yersinia pseudotuberculosis* and *Salmonella typhi.* In this condition, the appendix may be affected, but is not obstructed. Therefore, perforation is not a threat and surgery is not indicated.

This entity is often confused with acute appendicitis. A chicken meal in the patient's history may be a clue. Diarrhea may be present and can be bloody.

Crohn's Disease

The cause of this inflammatory process of the gastrointestinal tract is yet unknown. Most patients with Crohn's are young adults. Although this disease may affect any part of the gastrointestinal tract, the terminal ileum is the most common site. The undiagnosed patient may present with the following:

1. A painful mass in the right iliac fossa
2. Crampy abdominal pain
3. Intermittent diarrhea
4. Weakness, fever, increased WBC count, weight loss, or malabsorption syndrome

Crohn's patients are occasionally followed with ultrasound during therapy to monitor bowel wall thickness or abscesses.

Diverticulitis

Clinically similar to appendicitis, although usually on the left, diverticulitis is not often life-threatening. It involves herniated outpouches of large bowel wall, diverticulum, that become infected and inflamed. Similar to appendicitis, the neck of the diverticulum becomes obstructed and infection accumulates within the diverticulum (Fig. 30-1, Stage 1). Usually the pressure builds until the pus is released into the bowel lumen (see Fig. 30-1, Stage 2). Despite the abscess, the bowel often functions normally (see Fig. 30-1, Stage 3). Although not common, perforation may occur followed by fecal peritonitis.

Sigmoid diverticulitis is the most common cause of acute left lower quadrant pain and is referred to as left-sided appendicitis. Cecal diverticulitis can be clinically indiscernible from appendicitis.

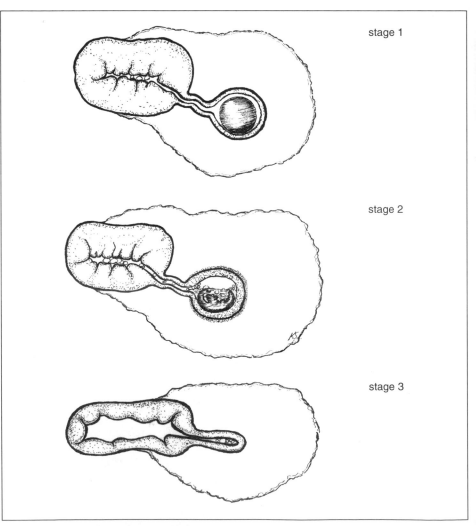

stage 1

stage 2

stage 3

FIGURE 30-1. Illustration demonstrating the stages diverticulitis may follow. (Adapted with permission from J. Puylaert.)

Mesenteric Adenitis

This condition is often the cause of enlarged mesenteric nodes. It is seen mostly in young children. Presenting symptoms are a painful right lower quadrant mass and possibly positive stool cultures.

Intussusception

Patients with intussusception are usually children (see Chapter 28). Most present with a painful abdominal mass, often with vomiting or bloody-mucous diarrhea.

Neutropenic Typhlitis

This disease occurs in immunosuppressed patients. Symptoms include severe neutropenia and right lower quadrant pain. Fever, nausea, vomiting, and bloody diarrhea may also be present.

Intestinal Tumors

Intestinal tumors may be seen at any age. Lymphoma is a disease of young adults. Leiomyosarcoma occurs in the fifth to sixth decades, and most carcinomas are seen in older patients. The clinical signs may include a painful abdominal mass, bloody stool, anorexia, diarrhea, constipation, and weight loss.

ANATOMY

Muscle

The oblique muscles, rectus, and psoas muscles can be visualized in most individuals with high-resolution sonography (Fig. 30-2). These muscles can be the site of abscesses or mistaken for an abdominal mass.

Intestine

The bowel encountered in the right lower quadrant may include the ascending colon, cecum, appendix, and terminal ileum (Fig. 30-3). With the proper technique, the ascending colon and cecum are usually visualized filled with echogenic bowel gas, feces, or hypoechoic fluid. By following the cecum caudally and medially, the terminal ileum may be seen entering the large bowel with active peristalsis. Rarely a normal appendix is identified extending from the cecum. The normal appendix has a diameter of less than 6 mm.

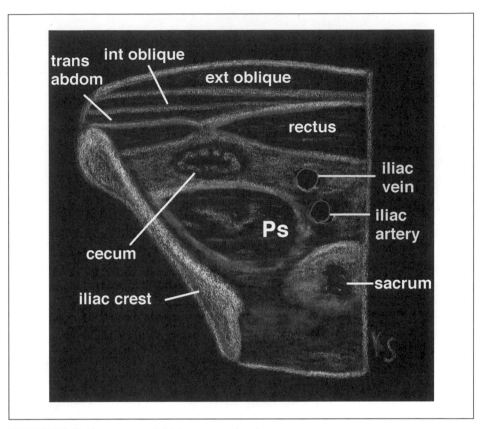

FIGURE 30-2. Transverse right lower quadrant.

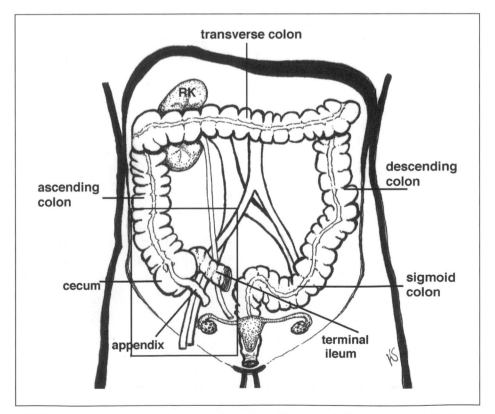

FIGURE 30-3. Diagram of the large intestine. The box delineates the right lower quadrant. Notice the numerous potential origins of right lower quadrant pain: The right ureter, the right ovary, the terminal ilium, cecum, and the appendix.

Histologically, the gastrointestinal wall may be divided into five layers. From the lumen out they are the mucosa, muscularis mucosa, submucosa, muscularis propria, and serosa or fat surrounding the outside of bowel (Fig. 30-4). On ultrasound only three layers are usually discernible—mucosa, submucosa, and muscularis propria. The echogenic echoes of the outer serosa or fat cannot be distinguished from the bright echoes of the surrounding tissue.

Vessels

The external iliac artery and vein should be identified travelling in the medial aspect of the right iliac fossa (see Fig. 30-2). During pregnancy, enlarged uterine vessels may occupy most of the right and left iliac fossas.

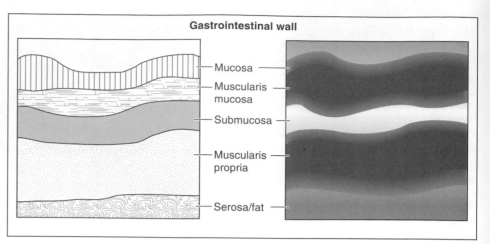

FIGURE 30-4. Diagram showing the components of the intestinal wall with the associated appearance on ultrasound.

◼ TECHNIQUE

To evaluate the right lower quadrant, no patient preparation is necessary; when evaluating gynecologic structures in a female patient, however, a full bladder is needed for a transabdominal approach. For optimal visualization, use a 5- to 7.5-MHz linear transducer. A linear array transducer provides a wide field of view and is best for bowel compression.

Graded Compression

Though first described for acute appendicitis, this technique can be used to evaluate any part of the gastrointestinal tract. As the compression is applied with the transducer, bowel gas and contents are displaced and intra-abdominal structures are brought closer to the transducer and into the focal zone. By applying and releasing pressure gradually, the patient's discomfort is lessened.

1. After obtaining the patient's history, have the supine patient point to the area of maximum tenderness with one finger. Keeping in mind there may be rebound tenderness, carefully palpate the area for masses.
2. Begin the ultrasound examination holding the transducer transversely at a level slightly above the umbilicus. Gradually start to compress the transducer and slowly slide the transducer to the area of interest.

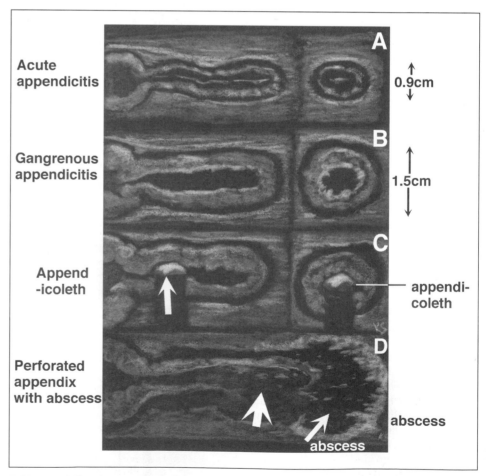

FIGURE 30-5. Illustration demonstrating possible sonographic appearances of appendicitis. (**A**) Acute appendicitis. (**B**) Fluid appears in the lumen. (**C**) An appendicolith (fecolith) may be present, with shadowing. (**D**) The perforation site is shown to attach over a perforated appendix. Abscess is delineated by small arrow.

3. Ask the patient to indicate when the transducer is over the area of maximum tenderness and carefully examine this area. Pathology most likely will be identified under this area. Be sure to release pressure gradually while removing the transducer.

4. After demonstrating the normal and abnormal right lower quadrant anatomy in the transverse plane, place the transducer longitudinally just lateral to the ascending colon and gradually compress. Slowly slide the transducer over the area of interest while moving medially.

5. Repeat this technique in oblique planes if that will best demonstrate the pathology.

 PATHOLOGY

As a rule, bowel inflammation presents with the following features:

1. Noncompressible abdominal mass.
2. The bowel wall may demonstrate three layers, giving a bull's-eye appearance in cross section.
3. Little or no peristalsis.
4. The surrounding tissue (fat and connective tissue) is edematous, with increased echogenicity.
5. Color Doppler will demonstrate vasodilation. Spectral analysis may show decreased arterial resistance and increased velocity. In some cases, the venous flow may be continuous (no respiration phasicity) and even pulsatile.
6. Power Doppler will show increased vascularity.

Appendicitis

Appendicitis diagnosis may be separated into three categories.

Acute Appendicitis

The graded compression technique will reveal a reproducible, noncompressible, sausage-shaped structure without peristalsis originating from the base of the cecal tip at the site of maximal discomfort. The classic bull's-eye sign of gut should be visualized transversely with the total diameter measuring 0.7 to 1.0 cm (Fig. 30-5A). The hyperechoic surrounding edematous connective tissue provides another sonographic sign. Because of this similarity to the homogeneous,

echogenic appearance of the thyroid, this sign is referred to as the "thyroid in the belly." There is usually no fluid within the appendix lumen.

Gangrenous Appendicitis

As the disease progresses, the appendix lumen distends with fluid and an appendicolith may be identified. The inflamed appendix and its fluid-filled lumen will not compress when pressure is applied. An appendicolith is usually calcified so shadowing will be seen originating within the appendix. The transverse diameter ranges from 1.1 to 1.9 cm as the muscular wall thickens (see Fig. 30-5B and C).

Perforated Appendicitis

Because of delay in the diagnosis, the appendicular wall may rupture. An abscess or fluid collection will develop in the right lower quadrant, the pelvis, or both. The appendix may be difficult to identify but if seen it will have asymmetric wall thickening and appear as a hyperechoic, finger-like projection

surrounded by fluid or an abscess (see Fig. 30-5D). Abscesses are usually fluid-filled, possibly loculated, and may have debris within. Inflamed mesenteric nodes may be identified in the adjacent right lower quadrant.

Crohn's Disease

Crohn's disease usually affects the terminal ileum, although other bowel segments may be involved. The inflamed intestinal wall thickens to 0.9 to 1.6 cm and the intestinal lumen is narrowed (Fig. 30-6A). The involved area will have reduced peristalsis but vigorous peristalsis may be seen in the unaffected bowel. There may be many bowel loops involved, congregating together to create a solid abdominal mass. Above the affected area, fluid-filled gut may be seen due to partial obstruction. The affected bowel is noncompressible and lacking haustra. The entire gastrointestinal tract should be evaluated for the above characteristics. Color flow will show much vascular activity in involved loops of bowel.

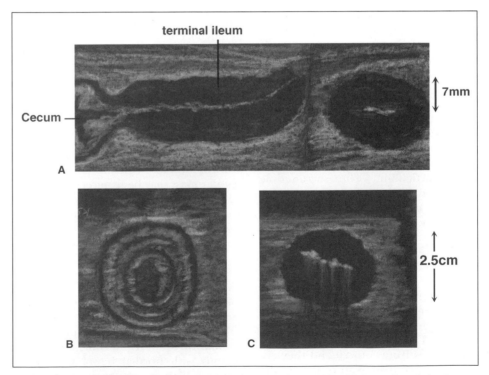

FIGURE 30-6. In Crohn's disease the inflamed bowel wall is thickened and the lumen (arrow) is narrowed. No haustra or peristalsis is evident. (**A**) Diagram illustrating the generally thickened and echopenic wall seen with Crohn's disease. (**B**) The multiple intestinal wall layers seen with intussuception. (**C**) Markedly thickened bowel wall as seen in carcinoma of the colon.

Complications of Crohn's disease include abscess, fistula formation, obstruction, and perforation. Abscesses may be seen adjacent to matted bowel loops and may extend into the psoas or rectus muscles. An abscess will appear as a complex fluid-filled mass. If the muscles are involved, they will appear swollen on ultrasound when compared to the same muscle on the patient's other side and the patient will have discomfort sitting up or with leg movement. Fistulous tracts may form between adjacent loops of bowel, bowel to skin, or bowel to bladder. These are difficult to discern with ultrasound; a 7.5- to 10-MHz transducer may be helpful. With fistulas to the bladder, gas may be seen in the bladder with shadowing. Adenopathy is usually present in these complicated cases.

Ischemic Colitis

In older patients, particularly those who are hypertensive or who have had heart attacks, loss of blood supply to the small bowel or colon can lead to ischemic colitis. The bowel wall will be thickened and the gut inert. Bloody discharge and abdominal pain may develop. Appearances are similar to those seen in Crohn's disease; however, little or no flow will be seen on color flow in the involved segment.

Diverticulitis

Thickened colon wall is seen at the point of tenderness, usually the left lower quadrant. With careful inspection, a fecalith may be seen in the adjacent diverticulum. The surrounding mesocolon will be inflamed and echogenic. In diverticulitis of the cecum, there are fewer but larger diverticula.

Mesenteric Adenitis

An enlarged mesenteric lymph node appears as a sphere with a hypoechoic peripheral zone and a hyperechoic center. The anteroposterior diameter is greater than 0.4 cm and the average dimensions are $1.1 \times 1.3 \times 1.5$ cm. The number of nodes varies from 3 to 20 and they are usually located deep with respect to the oblique or rectus muscles.

Intussusception

Intussusception is described as a section of bowel "telescoping" into the lumen ahead of it. Sonographically, a thick hypoechoic ring surrounding one or more thick hypoechoic rings should be seen on transverse views of the affected bowel (see Fig. 30-6B). An intestinal mass may be found in addition since intussusception in the adult is usually caused by a mass invaginating into the bowel lumen ahead of it.

Color Doppler evaluation is helpful to detect blood flow in all of the layers of the affected bowel. Lack of perfusion indicates bowel gangrene and the need for surgical intervention.

Neutropenic Typhlitis

Limited usually to the terminal ileum, cecum, and ascending colon, neutropenic typhlitis appears on ultrasound as a homogeneously thickened bowel wall ranging from 1.0 to 2.5 cm in the area of abdominal pain.

Intestinal Tumors

Lymphoma

This neoplasm appears sonographically as a hypoechoic, lobulated mass. The intestinal wall may be thickened due to tumor infiltration. Central necrosis is very unusual.

Leiomyosarcoma

Leiomyosarcoma is a large, solid subserosal or intramural mass located in the upper gastrointestinal tract, commonly found in the ileum. This large, irregular mass may be hyperechoic or hypoechoic with anechoic areas that have good through transmission. A central necrotic area may be identified with a fluid level.

Carcinoma

Carcinomas can be located anywhere in the gastrointestinal tract although they are most common in the stomach or colon. Sonographically they appear as a circular or ovoid hypoechoic mass contiguous with normal bowel wall. The center, which is echogenic, may have acoustic shadowing. Depending on the degree of infiltration, the bowel wall thickness can range from 1 to 8 cm (see Fig. 30-6C). Evaluate for enlarged mesenteric nodes and liver metastases.

Carcinoid

This lesion may arise anywhere in the gastrointestinal tract, but usually appears in the appendix, small bowel, or rectum. It usually measures less than 1.5 cm and sonographically appears as a sharply marginated, hypoechoic, lobulated mass with a strong back wall and lack of acoustic enhancement.

⭐ PITFALLS

1. *Nondiagnostic examinations.* In patients with marked tenderness and guarding, excessive gaseous distention, or ascites, or with obese patients, it may be impossible to apply adequate compression to the bowel in order to make a diagnosis of appendicitis or diverticulitis.
2. *False negatives.* An inflamed appendix may not be visualized if it lies behind the gaseous shadows of the cecum.
3. *Appendix vs. terminal ileum.* An inflamed appendix will have a blind end and no peristalsis, whereas an inflamed terminal ileum will widen into small bowel and may have some peristalsis.
4. *Bowel loops.* Fluid-filled loops of bowel can be recognized by watching for peristalsis and by demonstrating compressibility.
5. *Mesenteric nodes.* Nodes should not be mistaken for an inflamed appendix. They will appear as smooth, solid, ovoid structures with an echogenic center. They are not fluid filled.
6. *Blood vessels.* Be careful not to identify the external iliac artery or vein as an inflamed appendix. The transducer should be rotated on any suspicious area. Blood vessels will have an elongated shape and will be pulsatile if an artery or compressible if a vein. Doppler is helpful to demonstrate flow.
7. *Mass mimickers.* Fecal formations and spastic thickening of the bowel wall may appear as intestinal tumors. If uncertain, recheck the suspicious area at a later time to see whether there has been a change. Also be alert to an *ectopic kidney*, which may be mistaken for a mass.

? WHERE ELSE TO LOOK

1. A pelvic ultrasound should be performed on all female patients. Gynecologic pathology often mimics appendicitis symptoms, which is why ovulating women have the highest negative appendectomy rate. The pelvis should be evaluated for infection, ovarian cysts, ovarian torsion, hemorrhagic corpus luteum cysts, endometriosis, ectopic pregnancy, uterine wall rupture, abruptio placentae, and necrotic fibroids.

2. If tumor or adenopathy is found in the right lower quadrant, search the liver and other nodal sites for further disease.

3. If the findings are negative for intestinal pathology, the right upper quadrant should be scanned to rule out biliary obstruction or disease and renal pathology.

4. If a ruptured appendix or abscess is discovered in the right lower quadrant, the pelvis and right and left gutters should be checked for fluid collections.

5. If a mass or abscess is seen, scan through the abdomen for mesenteric nodes.

6. If an intestinal tumor is suspected, the liver and spleen should be scanned for metastasis. Evaluate adjacent organs for infiltration or compression (i.e., hydronephrosis). Scan the gastrointestinal tract for other masses and for indications of bowel obstruction. Check for periaortic nodes.

7. In the case of Crohn's disease, the entire gastrointestinal tract should be scanned for other affected bowel segments, fluid-filled bowel loops, abscesses, or evidence of fistula formation.

Selected Reading

Abu-Yousef, M., Phillips, M., Al-Jurf, A., and Smith, W. Sonography of acute appendicitis: A critical review. *Critical Reviews in Diagnostic Imaging* 29:381–408, 1989.

Gisler, M., Rouse, G., and Delange, M. Sonography of appendicitis: A review. *JDMS* 2:57–60, 1989.

Jeffery, R. B., Laing, F. C., and Lewis, F. R. Acute appendicitis: High-resolution real-time ultrasound findings. *Radiology* 163:11–14, 1987.

Jeffery, R. B., Laing, F. C., and Townsend, R. Acute appendicitis: Sonographic criteria based on 250 cases. *Radiology* 167:327–329, 1988.

Kang, W., Lee, C., and Chou, Y. A clinical evaluation of ultrasonography in the diagnosis of acute appendicitis. *Surgery* 105:154–159, 1989.

Lim, J. H. Colorectal cancer: Sonographic findings. *AJR* 167:45–47, 1996.

Machan, L., Pon, M., Wood, B. J., and Wong, A. The "coffee bean" sign in periappendiceal and peridiverticular abscess. *J Ultrasound in Med* 6:373–375, 1987.

Mittelstaedt, C. *Abdominal Ultrasound.* 2nd ed. New York: Churchill Livingstone, 1995.

Puylaert, J. B. Acute appendicitis: Ultrasound evaluation using graded compression. *Radiology* 158:355–360, 1986.

Puylaert, J. B. Mesenteric adenitis and acute terminal ileitis: Ultrasound evaluation using graded compression. *Radiology* 161:691–695, 1986.

Puylaert, J. B, van der Werf, J., Ulrich, C., and Veldhuizen, R. W. Crohn disease of the ileocecal region: Ultrasound visualization of the appendix. *Radiology* 166:741–743, 1988.

Teefey, S., Montana, M., Goldfogel, G., and Shuman, W. Sonographic diagnosis of neutropenic typhlitis. *Am J Rad* 149:731–733, 1987.

Teefey, S. A., Roarke, M. C., Brink, J. A., Middleton, W. D., Balfe, D. M., Thyssen, E. P., and Hildebolt, C. F. Bowel wall thickening: Differentiation of inflammation from ischemia with color Doppler and duplex US. *Radiology* 198:547–551, 1996.

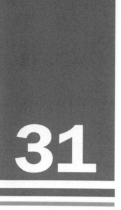

31

RENAL FAILURE

ROGER C. SANDERS, SANDRA L. HUNDLEY

SONOGRAM ABBREVIATIONS

C	Calculus
IVC	Inferior vena cava
K	Kidney
L	Liver
P	Pelvis of the kidney
Ps	Psoas muscle
R	Rib
RRV	Right renal vein
S	Spine
Sp	Spleen

KEY WORDS

Acute Tubular Necrosis (ATN). Acute renal shutdown following an episode of low blood pressure (hypotension). Spontaneous and fairly rapid recovery is usual, but the condition can be fatal.

Anuria. No urine production.

Azotemia. Renal failure.

Benign Prostatic Hypertrophy (BPH). In older men the prostate is enlarged and replaced by glandular tissue. A large prostate may obstruct the urethra.

BUN. Blood urea nitrogen. See *Serum Urea Nitrogen.*

Calyx. A portion of the renal collecting system adjacent to the renal pyramid in which urine collects and that is connected to an infundibulum.

Central Echo Complex (CEC, Sinus Echo Complex). The group of central echoes in the middle of the kidney that are caused by fat and the collecting system.

Column of Bertin. A normal renal variant in which there is enlargement of a portion of the cortex between two pyramids. Can mimic a tumor on pyelography.

Cortex. The more peripheral segment of the kidney tissue. Surrounds medulla and sinus echoes.

Creatinine. See *Serum Creatinine.*

Dehydration. If a patient does not drink enough fluid, the skin becomes lax and the eyes sunken. Hydronephrosis may be present but may be missed sonographically because the kidneys are not producing much urine.

Dialysis. Technique for removing waste products from the blood when the kidneys do not work properly.

> **Hemodialysis.** Used in long-term renal failure. The patient's blood is circulated through tubes outside the body that allow the exchange of fluids and removal of unwanted substances.

> **Peritoneal Dialysis.** A tube is inserted into the abdomen. Fluid containing a number of body constituents is run into the peritoneum, where it exchanges with waste products. A sonogram shows evidence of apparent ascites.

Dysplasia. Condition resulting from obstruction in utero characterized by echogenic kidneys with cysts. Such kidneys function poorly or not at all. Dysplasia is untreatable.

Glomerulonephritis. Medical condition with acute and chronic forms in which the kidneys function poorly owing to inflammation. Usually it is a self-limiting condition if acute, but if chronic, it may require long-term treatment with dialysis or transplantation.

Hydronephrosis. Dilatation of the kidney collecting system due to obstruction at the level of the ureter, bladder, or urethra.

Infundibulum (Major Calyx). A tube connecting the renal pelvis to the calyx.

Medulla. Portion of the kidney adjacent to the calyx; also known as a pyramid. It is less echogenic than the cortex.

Nephrostomy. Tube inserted through the skin into the kidney to drain an obstructed kidney.

Nephrotic Syndrome. Type of medical renal failure, often due to renal vein thrombosis, in which excess protein is excreted by the kidney.

Oliguria. Decreased urine output.

Polyuria. Increased urine output.

Pyelonephritis (Chronic). Repeated infections destroy the kidneys, which become small with some parenchymal areas narrowed by scar formation.

Pyonephrosis. Hydronephrotic collecting system filled with pus.

Pyramids. See *Medulla.*

Serum Creatinine. Waste product that accumulates in the blood when the kidneys are malfunctioning. Levels above approximately 0.6 are abnormal.

Serum Urea Nitrogen (SUN) (Blood Urea Nitrogen [BUN]). Waste products that accumulate in the blood when the kidneys are malfunctioning. Levels above approximately 40 are abnormal.

Sinus Echo Complex. See *Central Echo Complex.*

Staghorn Calculus. Large stone located in the center of the kidney.

Ureterectasia. Dilatation of a ureter.

Ureterocele. Congenital partial obstruction of the ureter at the place where it enters the bladder. A cobra-headed deformity of the lower ureter is seen on a pyelogram.

◆》 THE CLINICAL PROBLEM

Renal failure occurs when the kidneys are unable to remove waste products from the bloodstream. Waste products used as a measure of the severity of renal failure include the serum creatinine level and the serum urea nitrogen (or blood urea nitrogen [BUN]) level. Loss of 60 percent of the functioning parenchyma can exist without elevation of the BUN or creatinine levels.

The onset of renal failure is often insidious. The patient may have the condition for months before seeking medical attention with anemia, nausea, vomiting, and headaches. Other symptoms include increased or decreased urine frequency. Renal failure may be the result of either kidney disease or lower genitourinary tract disease within the ureter, bladder, or urethra with obstruction of urine excretion.

Medical Renal Disease

Kidney disease can be either an acute process or a chronic and irreversible one, which is treatable only by dialysis or transplant. In potentially reversible, short-term renal failure (such as acute tubular necrosis or acute glomerulonephritis), the kidneys are normal in size or large. In patients with longstanding renal failure (such as chronic glomerulonephritis or chronic pyelonephritis),

the kidneys are small. Drugs, particularly the aminoglycoside type of antibiotic, can cause medical renal failure.

Hydronephrosis

By far the most important diagnosis to exclude in patients with renal failure is hydronephrosis. If hydronephrosis is the cause of renal failure, both kidneys are likely to be obstructed unless the patient has some other renal disease coincident with obstruction. If obstruction is the sole cause of renal failure, the level of the obstructive site is probably in the bladder or urethra, because bilateral ureteral obstruction is not common. Once renal obstruction has been documented, a drainage procedure such as bladder catheterization, nephrostomy, or prostatectomy is urgently required to relieve obstruction. If a drainage procedure is not performed and obstruction persists, kidney function will be permanently impaired. Sonography has largely replaced retrograde pyelography as the screening procedure of choice for hydronephrosis in renal failure.

Dysplasia

In children, the kidneys may function poorly as a result of obstruction in utero. Such damaged kidneys are seen with posterior urethral valves or the prune belly syndrome.

ANATOMY

Size and Shape

The normal adult kidney as measured by ultrasound is between 8 and 13 cm in length. The parenchyma is 2.5-cm thick, and the kidney is about 5-cm wide.

The kidneys have a convex lateral edge and a concave medial edge called the hilum. The arteries, veins, and ureter enter the hilum.

Location

The kidneys are located retroperitoneally in the lumbar region, between the 12th thoracic and 3rd lumbar vertebrae. The left kidney lies 1 to 2 cm higher than the right. The kidneys rest on the lower two thirds of the quadratus lumborum muscle, the posterior and medial portion of the psoas muscle, and laterally on the transverse abdominis muscle.

1. The lower pole is more laterally located than the upper pole.
2. The lower pole is more anteriorly located than the upper pole owing to the oblique course of the psoas muscle.
3. The renal hilum is situated in the center of the medial side.

Sinus and Capsular Echoes

The kidney is surrounded by a well-defined echogenic line representing the capsule in the adult (Fig. 31-1). This line may be difficult to see in the infant

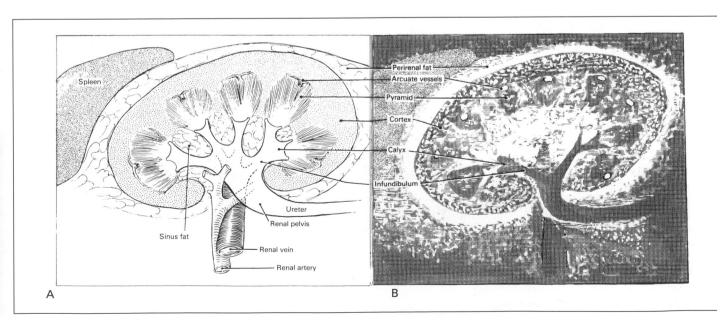

FIGURE 31-1. Major structures of the left kidney. (**A**) Coronal anatomical view. (**B**) Sonogram. The echogenic area at the center of the kidney is due to renal sinus fat. The pyramids are less-echogenic areas adjacent to the sinus. The cortex is slightly more echogenic, and the capsule (perirenal fat) is an echogenic line.

or lean people owing to the sparse amount of perinephric fat. At the center of the kidney are dense echoes (the central sinus echo or sinus echo complex) due to renal sinus fat (see Fig. 31-1). In the infant or emaciated patient these echoes may be virtually absent.

Parenchyma

The renal parenchyma has two components. The centrally located pyramids, or medulla, are surrounded on three sides by the peripherally located cortex. The medullary zone or pyramid is slightly less echogenic than the cortex (see Fig. 31-1). In infants or thin people a differentiation of medulla from cortex may be very obvious, but in other normal adults this separation may be undetectable.

Organ echogenicity from greatest to least in the normal patient is as follows: renal sinus—pancreas—liver—spleen—renal cortex—renal medullary pyramids.

Shape Variants

The spleen may squash the left kidney, causing a flattened outline or distorted outline so that the lateral border bulges, creating what is termed a dromedary hump (see Fig. 32-9). The renal border may show subtle indentations known as fetal lobulations.

Vascular Anatomy

See Figures 31-1, 31-4, and 34-2.

Renal Veins

The renal veins, which are large, connect the inferior vena cava with the kidneys and lie anterior to the renal arteries. The left renal vein has a long course and passes between the superior mesenteric artery and the aorta (see Fig. 21-12).

Renal Arteries

The renal arteries lie posterior to the renal veins. They may be multiple and too small to visualize. (If only one artery is present, visualization is relatively easy.) The right renal artery is longer than the left and passes posterior to the inferior vena cava. The main renal artery gives rise to a dorsal and a ventral branch. These branch first into the lobar arteries and then into the arcuate arteries (see Fig. 34-2). Typical arterial flow patterns in the renal artery are shown in Figure 34-3.

Ureters

See Chapter 33.

Urinary Bladder

See Chapter 33.

 TECHNIQUE

Right Kidney

The right kidney is best examined in the supine position through the liver (Figs. 31-2 to 31-4). Angle the transducer obliquely if the liver is small (see Fig. 31-4). A coronal and lateral approach can

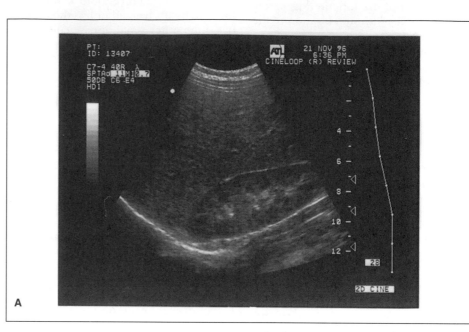

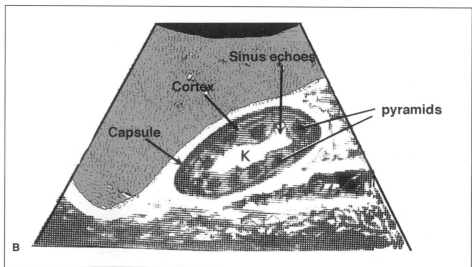

FIGURE 31-2. The normal right kidney demonstrated on supine longitudinal views. The sinus echoes are surrounded by pyramids which are less echogenic than the neighboring cortex.

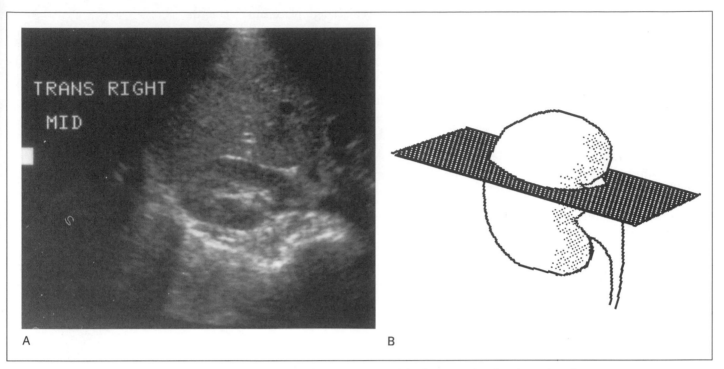

FIGURE 31-3. Transverse view of right kidney with diagram showing how the view was obtained.

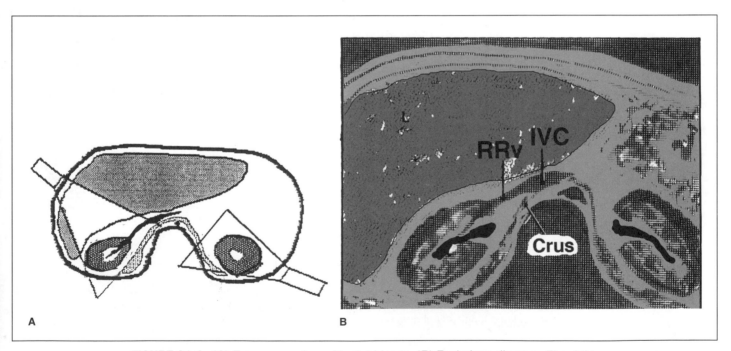

FIGURE 31-4. (**A**) Transverse view of both kidneys. (**B**) Technique diagram. The right kidney is examined with the transducer held obliquely through the liver, which acts as an acoustic window. The left kidney is examined from a posterolateral approach. It may be necessary to put the patient in the left-side-up position for ideal views of the left kidney. The crus (diaphragm) lies behind, posterior to the inferior vena cava and anterior to the aorta.

also be used if the liver is small (Fig. 31-5 and see Fig. 31-4). If bowel gas obscures visualization of the lower pole, it may be necessary to roll the patient into the right-side-up decubitus position and scan from a lateral approach.

Left Kidney

Begin with the patient in the left-side-up position. With the patient's left arm extended over his or her head, and using a coronal approach, scan intercostally through the spleen (Fig. 31-6). Vary the decubitus and oblique positions until you can see the kidney. Suspended inspiration is usually necessary. Use as high a frequency transducer as you can.

If the patient is emaciated, place supportive pillows between the ribs and iliac crest. This will help eliminate the cavity between the ribs and the iliac crest. The prone position gives good results in children, but ribs interfere with this view in adults.

Separate views of the lower and upper poles may be needed. If the lower pole is hidden by the iliac crest, try an expiration view. Erect views may be required for either kidney in patients with high livers or small spleens. Standoff pads are useful in babies or in very thin patients in which the left kidney is too close to the transducer.

Length

Make sure you have found the longest length of the kidney by trying various oblique views to see which yields the largest value (Fig. 31-8).

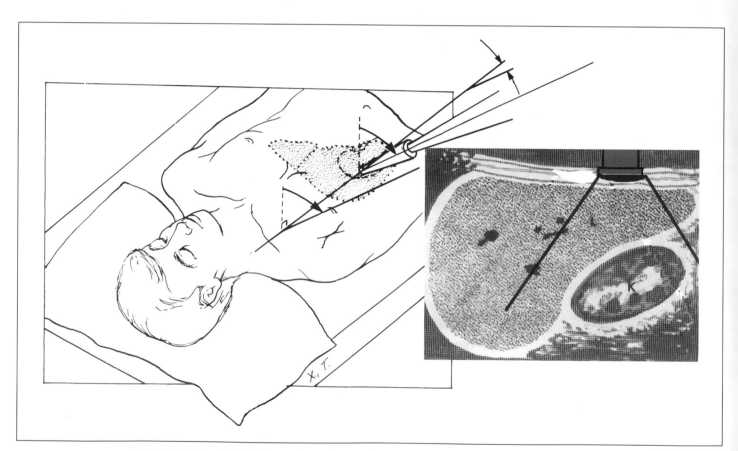

FIGURE 31-5. A helpful technique for viewing the right kidney is to place the transducer on an oblique longitudinal axis but still use the liver as an acoustic window.

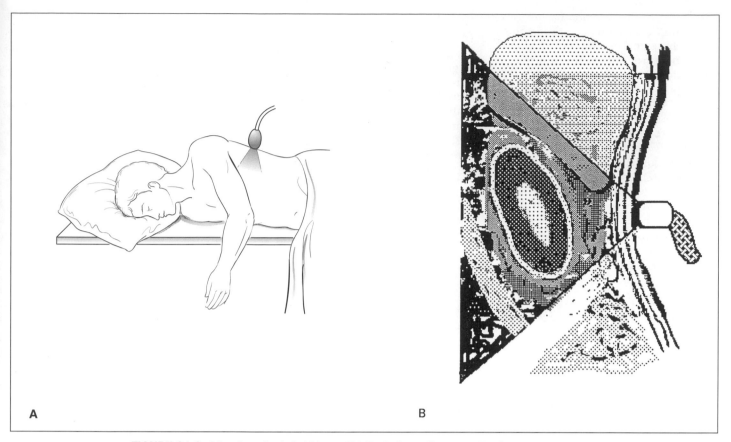

FIGURE 31-6. Viewing the left kidney. (**A**) Technique diagram. (**B**) Sonographic view. The usual technique for viewing the left kidney is to place the patient in the left-side-up (coronal) position using the spleen as a partial window. The same technique can be used on the right.

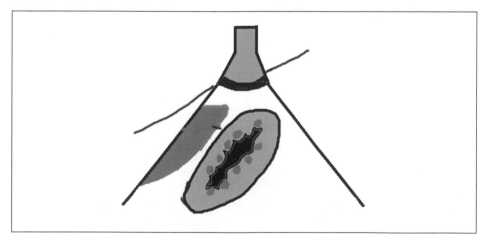

FIGURE 31-7. Oblique position used to obtain length views of the left kidney.

Ideally, there should be an even amount of cortical tissue around the sinus echoes, except on the medial aspect. Be sure not to foreshorten the true kidney length. (Sometimes, the lower pole is obscured by bowel gas; try a more coronal or lateral approach.) For large kidneys, a curved linear array is preferred; the large field of view is needed. It may be necessary to take a rather unsonogenic image in order to be accurate; try angling through the lower pole to the upper pole (Fig. 31-8). This will give you poor detail at the upper pole because the beam is not perpendicular to it, but allows for an accurate measurement without extrapolating. This is especially effective on the left side.

PATHOLOGY

Acute Medical Renal Disease

The kidneys are normal in length or enlarged with acute medical renal disease. Parenchymal echogenicity is generally increased compared with the liver (normally, echogenicity increases from the kidney to the liver to the spleen, with the highest echogenicity in the pancreas). The degree of parenchymal echogenicity can be graded as follows:

Grade I. The renal parenchymal echogenicity equals that of the liver.

Grade II. The renal parenchymal echogenicity is greater than that of the liver.

Grade III. The echogenicity of the renal parenchyma is equal to the renal sinus echoes.

Small End-Stage Kidney (Chronic Medical Renal Disease)

With end-stage kidney disease both kidneys are small, 5 to 8 cm in length, but renal sinus echoes are visible. The amount of renal parenchyma is usually shrunken. Focal loss of parenchyma indicates chronic pyelonephritis or a renal infarct (Fig. 31-9).

The renal parenchyma may show evidence of increased echogenicity. However, if only one kidney is small and diseased (e.g., in recurrent unilateral pyelonephritis), the kidney may be extremely small. In fact, the kidney may be almost impossible to visualize, even though the patient is asymptomatic. Even when an end-stage kidney measures only 2 to 3 cm in length, an echogenic center and some renal parenchyma will still be visible. The parenchyma may show evidence of focal narrowing due to scars (see Fig. 31-9).

Vascular Disease

Renal Artery Occlusion

Bilateral renal artery occlusion can be a cause of renal failure. An infarcted kidney enlarges at first but later shrinks in size. Focal infarcts are usually echopenic at first but may later become echogenic.

Hemorrhagic infarcts may be echogenic. Doppler and color flow are helpful in showing no flow to the involved kidney or area.

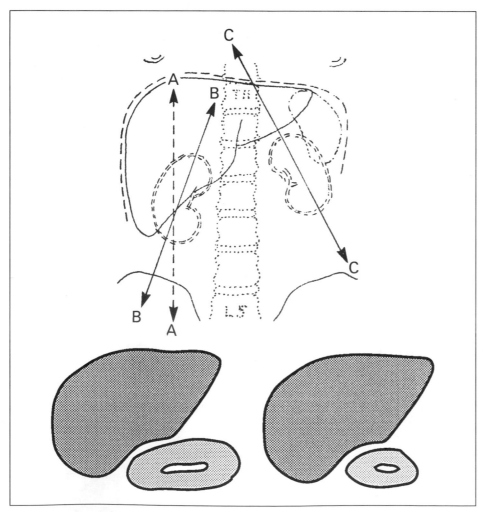

FIGURE 31-8. Renal length. The longest renal length (lines B and C) should be obtained. A length taken along a standard longitudinal view of the kidney (line A) is too short. The kidneys usually have a slightly oblique axis.

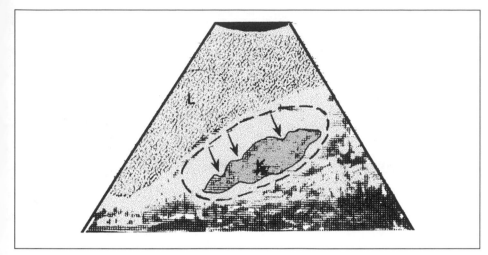

FIGURE 31-9. A small, shrunken, misshapen kidney (arrows) is usually a long-term consequence of chronic pyelonephritis. The dotted lines indicate the original kidney size. L = liver

Renal Artery Stenosis

Drinking fluids for 6 hours prior to a sonogram for renal artery stenosis enhances image quality. Although the arterial narrowing of renal artery stenosis is rarely visible with ultrasound, there may be Doppler evidence of narrowing. At the site of stenosis, there is little or no flow in diastole, much turbulence, and an abnormal systolic/diastolic ratio of over 100. The stenotic site is usually at the junction of the renal artery and the aorta. This area is difficult to see owing to overlying intestinal gas. Distal to the stenotic area, Doppler shows a small peak coupled with a long upswing and slow descent in systole (Fig. 31-10).

The acceleration time—the duration of the ascent segment in systole—is a most sensitive way of assessing renal artery stenosis. Normal is .10, with abnormal values from .12 up (see Fig. 31-10). This pattern is known as the parvus and tardus pattern (see Chapter 5).

Renal Vein Thrombosis

Renal vein thrombosis occurs in both acute and chronic forms. In the acute form, the kidney swells and the central sinus echoes usually become more prominent, although this is a variable phenomenon. Sometimes thrombosis can be visualized within the renal vein. Clot expands the renal vein and inferior vena cava.

Absence of the main renal vein flow may be seen using color Doppler, although all of the clot may be located in the peripheral vessels, so the presence of main renal vein flow does not exclude peripheral vein clot.

In the chronic form, the kidney is small and somewhat echogenic.

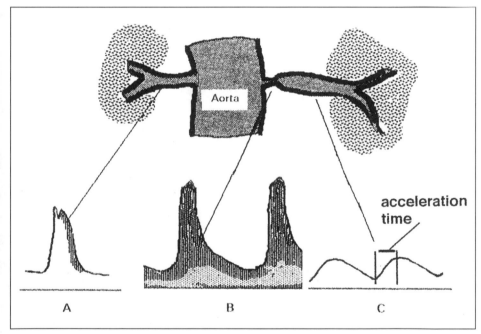

FIGURE 31-10. Doppler flow pattern changes with renal artery stenosis. (**A**) The normal appearance. (**B**) The left main renal artery is narrowed so that there is increased peak systolic flow and much turbulence at the site of stenosis. (**C**) Beyond the stenosis, the systolic peak is lower and longer than normal.

Hydronephrosis

In hydronephrosis the sinus echoes surround a fluid-filled center because the calyces, infundibula, and renal pelvis are dilated. Usually the renal pelvis is more distended than the calyces. The calyces and infundibula can be traced to the pelvis with real-time (Fig. 31-11). The calyces may be so effaced that only a single large sac is seen. However, multiple cystic structures due to dilated calyces may dominate the sonographic picture.

The amount of renal parenchyma may be thinned depending on the severity and duration of hydronephrosis. The normal parenchymal width is about 2.5 cm in the adult.

The ureter can sometimes be traced toward the pelvis or seen behind the bladder, indicating that the obstruction is not at the ureteropelvic junction.

If the hydronephrosis is longstanding, the pelvis and calyces may remain dilated when the obstruction is relieved. It is then difficult to follow recurrent obstruction by the sonographic appearances. Doppler interrogation of the renal arteries is of some help in detecting recurrent obstruction. The resistive index in the renal artery increases when obstruction is present. The normal resistive index is .64. It increases to .72 or more with obstruction.

Ureterocele

On some occasions, the hydronephrosis and renal obstruction is due to a block at the lower end of the ureter in the bladder. Sometimes a stone is impacted at this narrowed site. Alternatively, a ureterocele may be present. A ureterocele is a cobra-headed expansion of the lower ureter as it enters the bladder, which is particularly well seen using the vaginal probe. Sometimes, only the ureter at the entrance to the bladder is dilated. On other occasions, the whole ureter is dilated back into kidney.

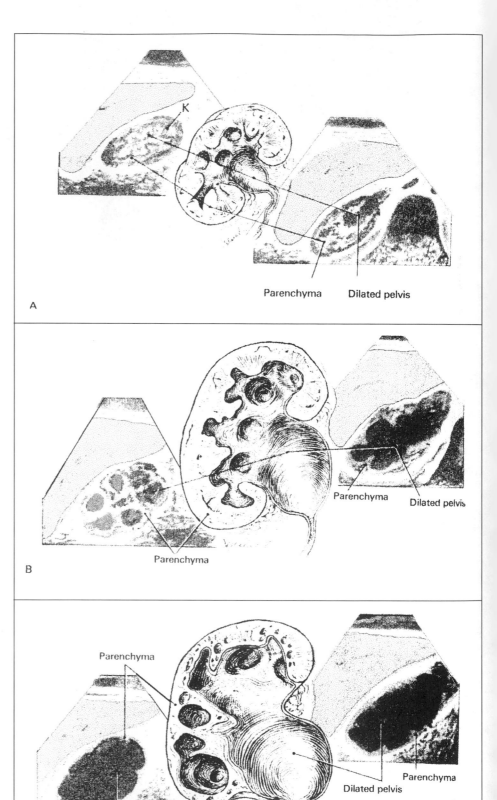

FIGURE 31-11. Varying degrees of dilatation of the renal pelvis due to hydronephrosis. Note the decreased parenchyma as hydronephrosis becomes more severe. The renal parenchyma may shrink to such an extent that only septa are seen between dilated calyces. Note the dominant renal pelvic cystic area in part **C**.

Ureteroceles are often seen in patients with a double collecting system. In this situation, the upper pole of the kidney is obstructed even though the ureter enters inferior to the ureter from the lower segment of the kidney. The lower pole ureter often enters the bladder at a abnormal angle so that reflux occurs and a wide "golf-hole" ureter develops (Fig. 31-12). A similar type of obstruction occurs when the ureter is ectopically inserted into the proximal urethra, rather than the bladder (see Fig. 31-12). The ureter can be traced down lateral to the bladder to a point inferior to its usual insertion into the bladder.

Xanthogranulomatous Pyelonephritis

Xanthogranulomatous pyelonephritis, a rare infection, is associated with renal calculi and hydronephrosis. A large staghorn calculus is usually present with secondary hydronephrosis and echogenic changes in the parenchyma. A rare focal form in which there is a mass lesion with increased echogenicity due to fat may occur. Typically, the renal pelvis is shrunken and contains a stone. The dilated calyces may be seen radiating from the renal pelvis (Fig. 31-13).

Pyonephrosis

A unilateral hydronephrotic kidney filled with stagnant urine may become infected and filled with pus. This life-threatening condition can rapidly lead to death if it is not discovered and treated rapidly. Sometimes a kidney with pyonephrosis is indistinguishable from ordinary noninfected hydronephrosis. More often, low-level echoes occur throughout the pus-filled renal pelvis. A fluid-fluid level may even develop. Percutaneous nephrostomy under ultrasonic control may be lifesaving.

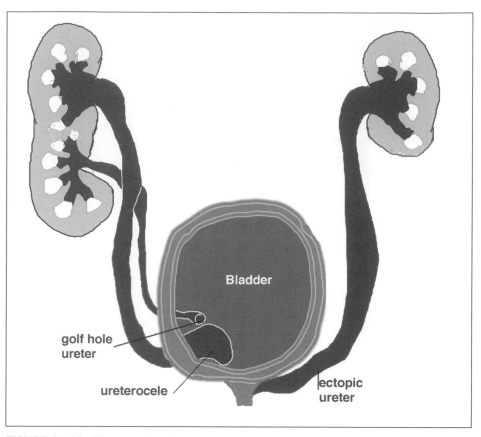

FIGURE 31-12. Diagram showing ureterocele on the right with secondary dilation of the ureter up to the level of the kidney. The lower pole of the kidney in this double collecting system is also dilated because of reflux due to a "golf-hole" ureter. On the left, an ectopic ureter inserts into the proximal urethra, with secondary dilation of the ureter and collecting system.

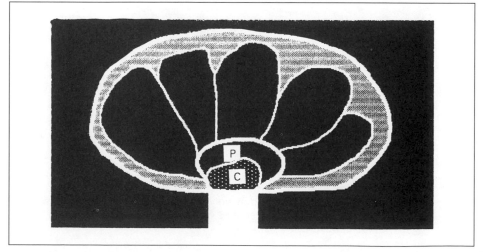

FIGURE 31-13. Xanthogranulomatous pyelonephritis. A stone (c) is present in the center of the pelvis (p) with acoustic shadowing. There are large dilated calyces but the pelvis is small.

Adult Polycystic Kidney

Both kidneys are involved sonographically and are very large (15 to 18 cm) by the time a patient with adult polycystic kidney disease presents with renal failure (usually between the ages of 40 and 50). Multiple cysts with lobulated irregular margins and variable size are present throughout the kidney (Fig. 31-14).

The central sinus echo complex is not easy to see and is markedly distorted by cysts. In areas where no cysts are sonographically apparent, the renal parenchyma will be more echogenic than usual due to cysts that are too small to be demonstrated with current equipment.

Infantile Polycystic Kidney

Infantile polycystic kidney, a congenital condition seen in children, causes bilateral, echogenic, enlarged kidneys. One or two small cysts may be seen. Most of the cysts are too small to be resolved as cystic spaces but are large enough to cause echoes and are most prominent in the medullary area. Increased echoes due to hepatic fibrosis may be noted in the liver parenchyma of older children.

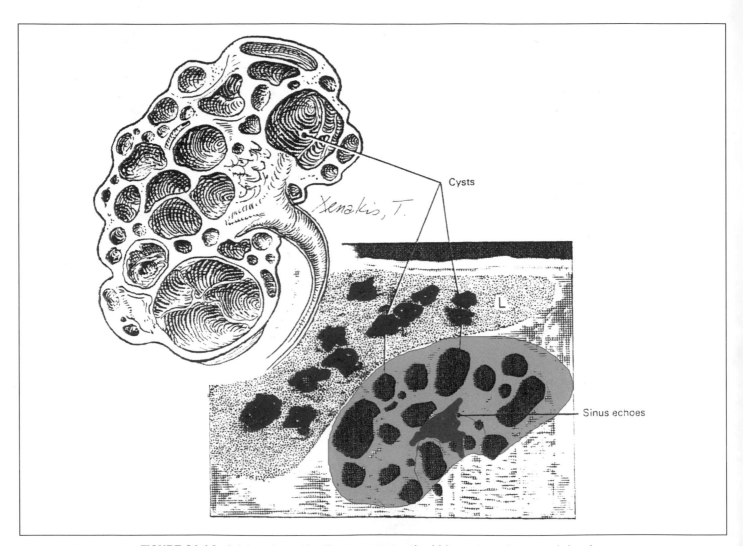

FIGURE 31-14. Adult polycystic disease causes the kidneys to enlarge and develop cysts of differing shapes and sizes. The liver is involved in polycystic disease in 40% of cases.

✦ PITFALLS

1. *Pseudohydronephrosis*
    a. Make sure that the bladder is empty before hydronephrosis is diagnosed definitively. In children and in patients with renal transplants, a full bladder can provoke apparent hydronephrosis, which disappears when the bladder is empty.
    b. Try to ensure that apparent hydronephrosis is not caused by a parapelvic cyst. In general, parapelvic cysts do not have a dense echogenic margin as do dilated calyces. They usually occupy only a portion of the renal sinus echoes.
    c. An extrarenal pelvis may mimic hydronephrosis because it is a large cystic structure at the renal hilum. Dilated infundibula may also be seen normally, but connecting calyces will be delicately cupped (if they can be seen).
    d. The renal vein can be mistaken for a dilated pelvis but can be connected to the inferior vena cava and shows flow on color flow Doppler.
    e. Reflux may be responsible for apparent hydronephrosis; it disappears on standing and changes with voiding.

2. *Possible missed hydronephrosis*
    a. Be cautious about excluding hydronephrosis in the presence of renal calculi, which may obscure dilated calyces.
    b. Make sure that the patient is not dehydrated with lax skin and sunken eyes. Dehydration can mask hydronephrosis. Reexamination when hydrated may be worthwhile.

3. *Calculi.* In the presence of severe hydronephrosis a staghorn calculus can be confused with a normal renal pelvis but will show evidence of shadowing (Fig. 31-15).

4. *Splayed sinus echoes.* Do not overlook relatively mild separation of the renal sinus echoes. The correlation between the severity of hydronephrosis and the degree of separation is not good. Separation of the sinus echoes may be (1) a normal variant due to an extrarenal pelvis; (2) due to a parapelvic cyst; (3) a consequence of overdistention of the bladder; or (4) due to reflux rather than renal obstruction.

5. *Renal parenchyma.* If you are assessing the degree of renal parenchymal echogenicity in comparison with the liver, make sure you think that the liver is normal. Patients with liver disease are prone to renal failure.

6. *Length.* Make sure that you have obtained the longest renal length. Careless technique can make the kidney appear shorter than it really is (see Fig. 31-8).

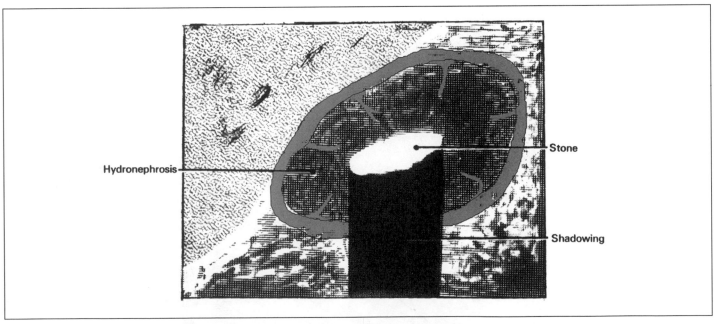

FIGURE 31-15. Gross hydronephrosis with large staghorn stone in the center. The staghorn could be mistaken for the renal pelvis, but note the shadowing. Note that almost no renal parenchyma remains after long-term obstruction.

7. *Sinus fat.* Excess fat within the renal sinus (fibrolipomatosis) can have a confusing sonographic appearance, sometimes appearing more extensive than usual (Fig. 31-16) and at other times appearing less echogenic than normal and mimicking hydronephrosis.

8. *Column of Bertin.* The cortex between pyramids may be unduly large as a normal variant called a column of Bertin. The parenchymal texture will not be altered in the suspect area, which is usually toward the upper pole.

9. *Pseudokidney sign.* Normal empty colon can mimic a kidney, especially if the patient has no kidney. The colon then lies at the site where the kidney usually lies.

10. *Small end-stage kidney.* A very small end-stage kidney can easily be mistaken for the target sign seen with loops of bowel. Conversely, make sure that an apparently small kidney is not a relatively empty colon by a prolonged look with real-time.

❓ WHERE ELSE TO LOOK

The discovery of *hydronephrosis* should prompt an effort to identify the site of obstruction.

1. Look within the kidney and bladder for *renal calculi* (see Chapter 33). Look for an impacted stone at the ureterovesical junction that may be associated with edema of the bladder wall.

2. Look along the course of the ureter as well as in the pelvis for *masses.*

3. Examine the true pelvis to see whether the bladder is distended. If it is, look for evidence of *bladder neoplasm* or *prostatic hypertrophy* (see Chapter 33).

4. Follow the course of the ureter behind the bladder; a *ureterocele* may be present.

5. If *adult polycystic kidney* is present, look in the liver, pancreas, and spleen: 40 percent of patients will have liver cysts, 10 percent (allegedly) will have pancreas cysts, and 1 percent will have spleen cysts.

6. If no kidney is seen in the renal bed, look in the pelvis. They usually lie close to the midline, just above the bladder or uterus.

7. If a congenital anomaly or absence of the kidney is discovered in a female, look for associated uterine anomalies, such as uterus didelphus (see Chapter 7).

SELECTED READING

Bude, R. O., Platt, J. F., Wahl, R. L., Ellis, J. H., and Rubin, J. M. Suspected obstructive pyelocaliectasis: Doppler ultrasonography compared with diuretic renal scintigraphy in proven cases. *Can Assoc Radiol J* 47:101–106, 1996.

Eibenberger, K., Schima, H., Trubel, W., Scherer, R., Dock, W., and Grabenwoger, F. Intrarenal Doppler ultrasonography: Which vessel should be investigated? *J Ultrasound Med* 14:451–455, 1995.

Grafe, D., and Hanson, S. Sonographic detection of renal artery stenosis. *JDMS* 11:67–74, 1995.

Halpern, E. J., Needleman, L., Nack, T. L., and East, S. A. Renal artery stenosis: Should we study the main renal artery or segmental vessels? *Radiology* 195:799–804, 1995.

Kliewer, M. A., Tupler, R. H., Carroll, B. A., Paine, S. S., Kriegshauser, J. S., Hertzberg, B. S., and Svetkey, L. P. Renal artery stenosis: Analysis of Doppler waveform parameters and tardusparvus pattern. *Radiology* 189:779–787, 1993.

Mallek, R., Bankier, A. A., Etele-Hainz, A., Kletter, K., and Mostbeck, G. H. Distinction between obstructive and nonobstructive hydronephrosis: Value of diuresis duplex Doppler sonography. *AJR* 166:113–117, 1996.

Stavros, A. T., Parker, S. H., Yakes, W. F., Chantelois, A. E., Burke, B. J., Meyers, P. R., and Schenck, J. J. Segmental stenosis of the renal artery: Pattern recognition of tardus and parvus abnormalities with duplex sonography. *Radiology* 184:487–492, 1992.

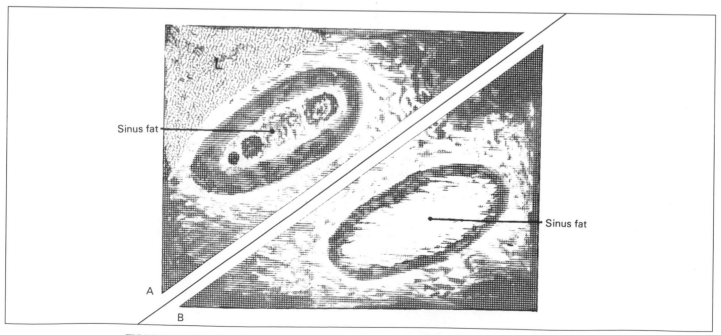

FIGURE 31-16. Fibrolipomatosis. (**A**) The less-echogenic appearances can be mistaken for hydronephrosis or transitional cell cancer. (**B**) Excess fat in the renal sinus usually causes enlargement of the echogenic center of the kidney; on occasion it may look less echogenic as in (**A**).

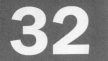

32 POSSIBLE RENAL MASS

ROGER C. SANDERS

SONOGRAM ABBREVIATIONS

Ao Aorta

Bl Bladder

K Kidney

L Liver

Sp Spleen

KEY WORDS

Angiomyolipoma. Rare, benign, fatty tumor of the kidney associated with tuberous sclerosis; usually seen in middle-aged women.

Calyceal Diverticulum. Postinflammatory fluid-filled structure adjacent to a pyramid.

Calyx. A portion of the renal collecting system adjacent to the renal pyramid in which urine collects and that is connected to an infundibulum.

Column of Bertin. Sometimes the calyces and the infundibulum bud from the pelvis in two groups. The intervening parenchyma can raise suspicions of a tumor and is known as a column of Bertin.

Dromedary Hump. A bulge off the lateral margin of the left kidney—a normal variant.

Fibrolipomatosis. Excess fat deposition in the center of the kidney; seen with aging.

Hydronephrosis. Dilatation of the pelvic collecting system due to obstruction.

Hypernephroma, Renal Cell Carcinoma, Grawitz Tumor. Interchangeable terms used for adenocarcinoma of the kidney.

Infundibulum. Funnel-shaped tube connecting the calyx to the renal pelvis. Also known as a major calyx.

Nephroblastoma. Variant form of Wilms' tumor with numerous sites of tumor formation.

Pseudotumor. Overgrowth of a portion of the cortex indenting the sinus echoes and simulating a tumor.

Renal Pelvis. Sac into which the various infundibula drain. The pelvis drains into the ureter.

Transitional Cell Carcinoma. A tumor of the kidney, collecting system, ureter, or bladder lining cells that often recurs in another site in the genitourinary tract after removal.

Tuberous Sclerosis. A disease characterized by skin lesions, epileptic seizures, mental deficiency, and renal angiomyolipoma. Milder forms manifest only one symptom.

Uric Acid Calculus. A renal stone that is invisible on plain radiographs.

Wilms' Tumor. Most common malignant renal lesion seen in children.

THE CLINICAL PROBLEM

Although the intravenous pyelogram (IVP) remains a common method of detecting renal masses, it does not effectively aid in deciding whether such a mass is fluid filled (a cyst) or solid tissue—a decision that can be made with ultrasound. Cysts are managed by cyst puncture or benign neglect, whereas tumors need surgical resection.

In the USA, computed tomography (CT) is often used in the further investigation of renal masses, but the nature of some renal masses may be confusing on CT and may be clarified by ultrasound and Doppler. Clinical symptoms may include pain, fever, pyuria, urinary frequency and urgency, hematuria, a palpable mass, white cells, and protein in the urine. A tumor mass may be clinically silent and discovered incidentally when the study is being performed for other reasons.

ANATOMY

See Chapter 31.

TECHNIQUE

See Chapter 31.

Do not perform a sonogram without first examining the report of the IVP or CT scan if available, so you know you are evaluating the same mass. Doppler is helpful for examining the inferior vena cava and the renal vein to detect tumor involvement. Some stones and their shadowing are visible readily on ultrasound when hard to see with other imaging modalities.

PATHOLOGY

Fluid-Filled Masses

Renal Cysts

Renal cysts are rare in children, gradually becoming more frequent with age. In the elderly, they are very common. They may be single (Fig. 32-1) or multiple (see Fig. 32-3). The sonographic features of a cyst are as follows:

1. Acoustic enhancement (good through transmission with a strong back wall) (see Fig. 32-1)
2. Usually a smooth spherical outline with thin walls
3. Usually fluid filled with no internal echoes

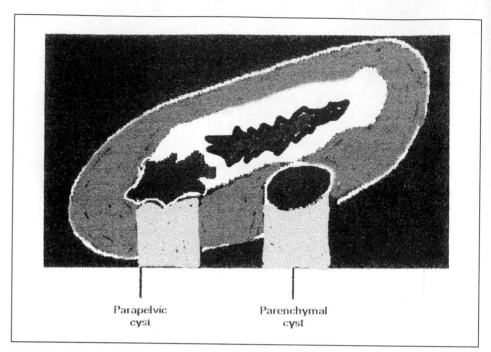

FIGURE 32-1. A parenchymal cyst at the midpole of the kidney shows good through transmission, smooth borders, and absence of internal echoes. A peripelvic cyst at the upper pole has an irregular outline. Peripelvic cysts can be mistaken for dilated calyces.

Unusual cysts may have irregular walls and may contain low-level echoes in a dependent position owing to debris. Debris may be confused with spurious echoes related to the slice thickness artifact (Fig. 32-2); see also Chapter 53.

Septa dividing a cyst into compartments may be seen (see Fig. 32-2). Such septa prove that a cyst is fluid filled but may be difficult to visualize completely and may be mistaken for a mural mass.

Irregular borders, septations, or debris should raise the question of malignancy or necrosis and require further investigation, usually by CT or percutaneous puncture under ultrasound control.

Peripelvic cysts may be centrally located and hard to distinguish from a dilated pelvis or calyx (see Fig. 32-1). Their shape is often irregular.

Adult Polycystic Disease

Renal cysts in patients with polycystic disease usually have an irregular outline and are of markedly varied size (Fig. 32-3A). The background parenchymal echogenicity is often increased in polycystic disease owing to small cysts that are not large enough to be seen as fluid-filled structures but are large enough to cause echoes. This is always a bilateral process, although one side may be more severely affected than the other.

Multiple Simple Cysts

Multiple simple cysts can occur but are fewer in number, more equal in size, and smoother in outline than the cysts seen in polycystic disease (see Fig. 32-3B).

Multicystic Disease

Multicystic disease is a congenital process that involves only one kidney. The entire kidney, which is small, is filled with multiple adjacent cysts (see Chapter 28). In adults, these cysts may develop a calcified shell.

Calyceal Enlargement

Calyceal diverticula and locally obstructed calyces look like cysts but connect with the pelvicalyceal system. They are generally surrounded by an echogenic border owing to sinus fat.

Milk of Calcium

Calyceal diverticula may contain "milk of calcium." An echogenic focus is seen in the region of the calyx. Since it is liquid, it changes shape and forms a fluid-fluid level if the patient is placed in a decubitus or erect position. Usually nonshadowing, it can be mistaken for a small calculus.

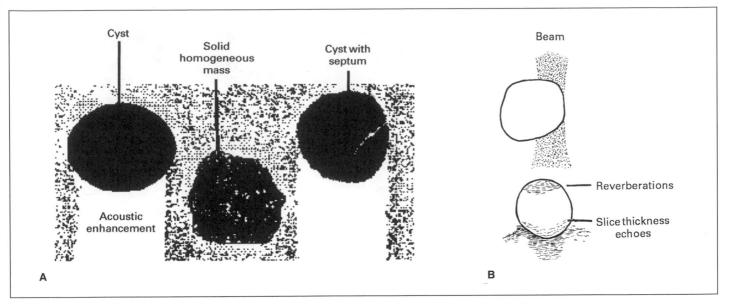

FIGURE 32-2. Cyst versus solid homogeneous mass. (**A**) Diagram showing the difference between a cyst and a solid homogeneous mass. Through transmission beyond a solid homogeneous mass is limited, although there will be a back wall, and there are usually a few internal echoes. Septa within a cyst are incompletely seen unless they are at right angles to the acoustic beam. (**B**) Artifactual echoes due to reverberations and slice thickness effect. (For details of how these artifacts develop, see Chapter 53.)

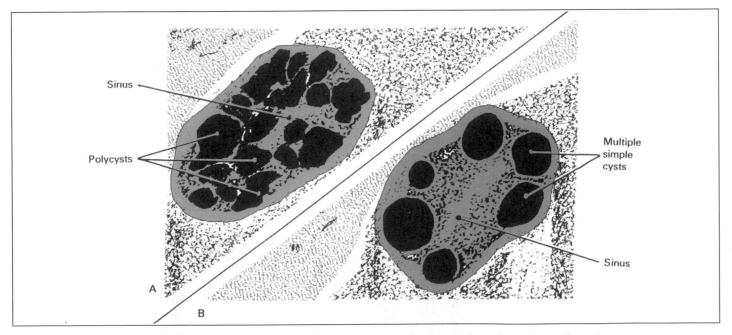

FIGURE 32-3. Multiple cysts. (**A**) Cysts in polycystic disease have irregular walls and are variable in size. They distort the renal sinus echoes. (**B**) Multiple simple cysts have smooth walls, are not nearly as numerous, and vary less in size.

Duplex Collecting System

An upper pole, congenitally duplicated hydronephrotic collecting system may look like a cyst but usually has septa separating the duplicated calyces. Duplication is associated with complete or partial duplication of the ureter. There is often a ureterocele obstructing the upper of the two collecting systems. One may be able to trace the ureter toward the true pelvis. It will lie medial to the lower kidney (see Fig. 31-12).

Abscess and Focal Pyelonephritis

Although abscesses are fluid filled, they are rarely totally echo-free (Fig. 32-4). They may even occasionally contain a number of internal echoes. Local infection without abscess formation causes an area of decreased echoes with swelling and local tenderness. Such local infection is known as focal pyelonephritis or lobar nephronia. One may be unable to distinguish an abscess with drainable pus from an area of inflammation.

Hematoma

Hematomas have a varied sonographic appearance. They may be echo-free or evenly echogenic, or they may contain clumps of echoes. Hematomas usually develop around, rather than within, a kidney. Hematomas are a consequence of trauma, surgical procedure, or abnormal bleeding conditions.

Urinoma

Urinomas may be seen, usually following a surgical procedure. These fluid collections are echo-free. They most often surround the kidney (i.e., they are perirenal).

Renal Artery Aneurysm

A centrally placed cystic structure may represent a renal artery aneurysm. Providing the aneurysm is not clot filled, flow will be seen with color flow Doppler. There is often calcification in the wall of aneurysms.

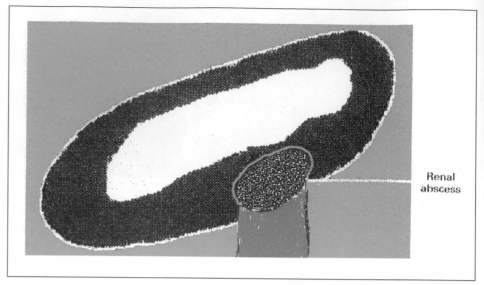

FIGURE 32-4. Abscesses in the kidney tend to have some internal echoes and irregular walls.

Tumor Masses

Adenocarcinoma (Hypernephroma)

Adenocarcinomas or hypernephromas contain internal echoes, do not show good through transmission, and usually have an irregular border that expands the outline of the kidney. Most hypernephromas have the same echogenicity as the adjacent renal parenchyma or a little less (Fig. 32-5) but have one or two dense internal echoes in addition. Some are more echogenic than the remaining kidney. This is the most common renal neoplasm.

Wilms' Tumor (Nephroblastoma)

Wilms' tumor is a malignant lesion affecting children. The tumor is usually unilateral, occupying only part of the kidney. Ten percent are bilateral. They appear as a large, evenly echogenic mass (see Chapter 28 and Fig. 28-6).

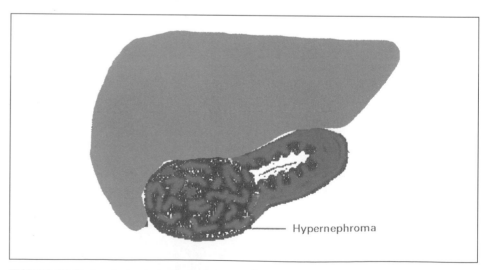

FIGURE 32-5. Large hypernephroma expanding the upper pole of the kidney. Notice that it is slightly more echopenic than the renal parenchyma. Hypernephromas are frequently relatively hypoechoic but show poor through transmission.

Transitional Cell Tumors

Transitional cell carcinomas (Fig. 32-6) occur in the renal pelvis and are difficult to distinguish from fibrolipomatosis. A small, evenly echogenic mass slightly less echogenic than the sinus echoes is seen within the renal sinus. Hematuria often presents clinically when no mass is visible sonographically.

Tumors in Cysts

Tumors may infrequently occur within cysts. There is focal irregularity of the cyst wall at one site. However, the irregularity may be due to a septum. A cyst with an irregular wall and internal echoes is usually subjected to cyst puncture or CT scan to rule out neoplasm.

Lymphoma

Renal lymphoma may have three different appearances in the kidney:

1. A local echopenic mass
2. Diffuse sonolucency of the entire kidney with loss of the sinus echoes
3. Large kidneys that may have reduced echogenicity

Adenoma

Adenomas are small, solid, echogenic tumors that measure less than 1 cm. They are usually located in the renal cortex and may cause a bulging of the renal capsule, but are seldom visible.

Angiomyolipoma

A highly echogenic tumor with a smooth, round outline is suggestive of angiomyolipoma (Fig. 32-7), but may be a hypernephroma.

A CT scan will show fat within an angiomyolipoma. Angiomyolipomas are benign and composed of blood vessels, muscle, and fat. They tend to bleed, causing areas of decreased echogenicity in or around the mass.

Filling Defects in Renal Pelvis (Calculi)

A small filling defect in the renal pelvis on IVP has a number of possible causes, including transitional cell cancer. Some are due to uric acid stones. Stones can be recognized on sonography by an acoustic shadow arising from the renal pelvis echoes (Fig. 32-8).

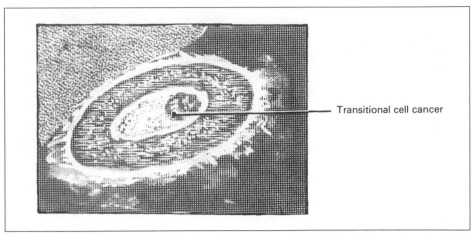

FIGURE 32-6. Transitional cell cancer involving the sinus of the kidney, causing a hypoechoic area.

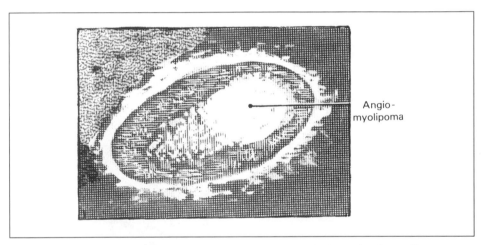

FIGURE 32-7. Angiomyolipoma at the lower pole of the kidney. Angiomyolipomas are almost always densely echogenic.

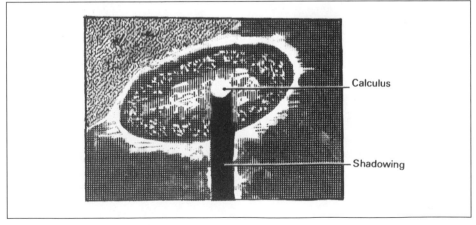

FIGURE 32-8. Renal calculus with acoustic shadowing. Calculi do not cause shadows if they are small (less than about 5 mm).

✳️PITFALLS

Normal Variants
Versus Pseudolesions

Normal variants or congenital abnormalities may create the impression of a mass.

1. An *enlarged spleen or liver* can compress the kidney, causing an apparently abnormal IVP appearance (Fig. 32-9).

2. The left kidney often has a hump on its lateral aspect known as a *dromedary hump* (Fig. 32-10). This is thought to be due to normal renal tissue being compressed by the spleen.

3. A *bifid pelvicalyceal pattern* may suggest a central mass on the IVP. The intervening tissue between the two portions of the collecting system appears sonographically normal (Fig. 32-11). Pseudomasses and the column of Bertin have a similar location and appearance. Angle medially and obtain transverse views to see whether the sinus echoes join at the pelvis. In a bifid pelvicalyceal system, the sinus echoes will join, whereas with a double collecting system, they will be separate.

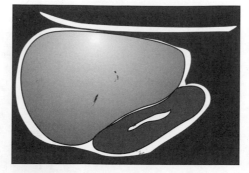

FIGURE 32-9. The left kidney is squashed by an enlarged spleen. Splenomegaly can cause an apparent mass on IVP.

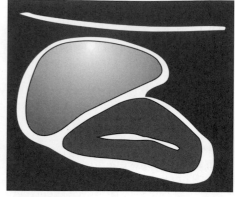

FIGURE 32-10. Bulge at the lateral border of the left kidney shown as a dromedary hump, a normal variant. It is thought to be a consequence of compression by the spleen.

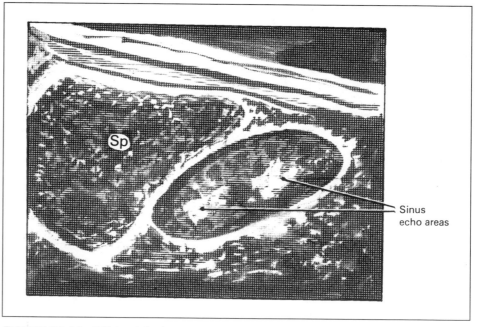

Sinus echo areas

FIGURE 32-11. Bifid pelvicalyceal system; the sinus echoes are separated into two groups. A similar appearance is seen with a double collecting system.

4. *Ectopic renal locations* are common:
   a. A pelvic kidney (Fig. 32-12) is located in the pelvis. Malrotation and pelvic dilatation occur often in pelvic kidneys.
   b. A thoracic kidney, in which the kidney lies partially or completely in the chest, is a rare variant.
   c. In crossed ectopia without fusion, both kidneys are located on one side of the body. The kidney is very long, with two sinus echo groups.
5. *Malrotated kidneys* often look abnormal on IVP but are normal, except for an unusual axis, on the sonogram (Fig. 32-13).
6. *Fibrolipomatosis,* excessive fatty infiltration of the renal pelvis, is often a consequence of aging. The sonographic appearances are variable and include (1) an enlarged central echogenic complex; (2) fat that may be relatively sonolucent, giving the impression of mass lesions or hydronephrosis (use higher gain settings to see low-level echoes); and (3) fat that may be densely echogenic. Confusion with transitional cell carcinoma is possible; transitional cell carcinoma has a more irregular outline and will not be present in the other kidney.

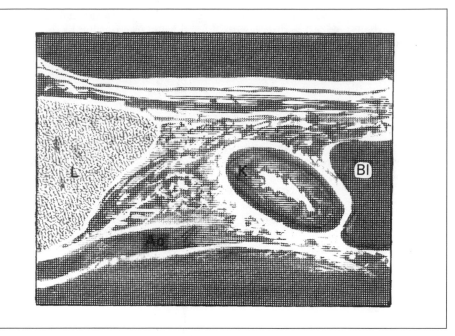

FIGURE 32-12. Pelvic kidney. A sonographically normal kidney is located in the pelvis.

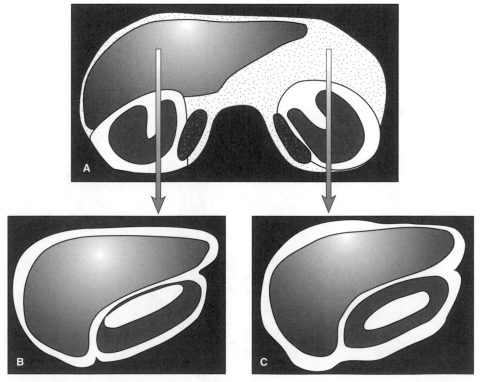

FIGURE 32-13. (**A**) Kidney positions. (**B**) Malrotated kidney. In the right kidney, the axis of the kidney is rotated so that the sinus echoes exit anteriorly. (**C**) Normal kidney position.

7. *Horseshoe kidneys* are bilateral, low-lying, medially placed kidneys with partial or complete fusion, usually of the lower poles, although fusion may occur at the midpoles or upper poles. An isthmus of tissue connects the two kidneys, passing anterior to the aorta and inferior vena cava. The kidneys are often difficult to see on a supine view because of overlying gas (Fig. 32-14). The inferior pole of the kidney is angled medially and may be obscured by gas. A short kidney should precipitate a search for a horseshoe kidney. Use the isthmus as an acoustic window to see the renal pelvis.

8. A *ptotic kidney* is an unusually mobile kidney that descends from its normal location toward the true pelvis.

9. *Persistent fetal lobulation* may result in a lobulated outline to the kidney. It is without pathologic consequence. Indentations separated by an equal distance are seen. The pattern with focal infarcts or scarring is more random.

10. *Supernumerary kidney* is rare. Both a pelvic kidney and two normally placed kidneys are seen.

11. A triangular echogenic area on the anterior superior aspect of the kidney, particularly the right one, is probably a *junctional fusion defect.* This fat-filled area is an embryologic remnant of the site of fusion between the upper and lower components of the kidney.

Cyst Versus Neoplasm

A cyst may be difficult to distinguish from a solid homogeneous mass (see Fig. 32-2). Use of a higher-frequency transducer may help determine whether the lesion is solid. Find the best acoustic window (i.e., through the liver and spleen) and set the focal zone for the center of the cyst. Look at the inner wall of the cyst from different angles so that wall irregularities can be clearly differentiated from artifact. Echoes on the transducer side of the cyst may be due to reverberations, and on the far side, to the "slice thickness" effect (see Fig. 32-2B; see also Chapter 53).

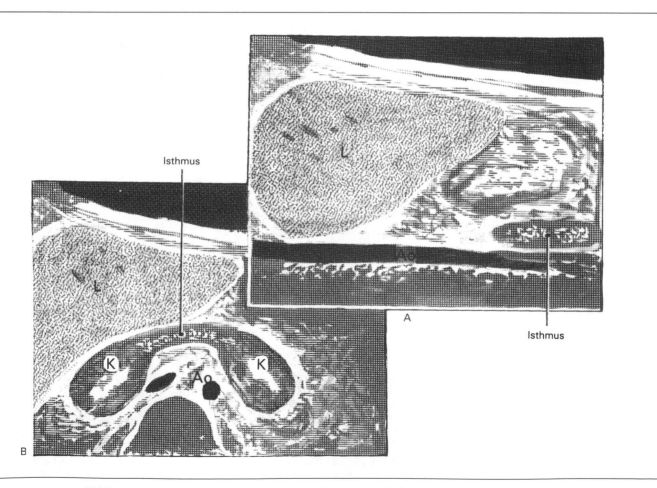

FIGURE 32-14. Horseshoe kidney. (**A**) The isthmus can be mistaken for nodes on longitudinal section. (**B**) Horseshoe kidneys are located more centrally than other kidneys and are connected by an isthmus.

"Blown" Calyx Versus Cyst

Remember to look at the IVP, because a cystic lesion in the kidney might be a focally dilated portion of the renal collecting system.

Subtle textural changes can be enhanced by switching to a higher-frequency transducer and by trying different post-processing features, such as color filters.

Arcuate Vessels

Calcification in the wall of the arcuate vessels may give rise to some subtle acoustic shadowing and mimic the appearance of a stone. Calcified arteries may also occur in the renal sinus echoes. Arteries can usually be distinguished from calculi by the appearance of two walls: two parallel echogenic lines are seen. Check for pulsation with Doppler.

Multicystic and Polycystic Disease Versus Hydronephrosis

Multicystic and polycystic disease are differentiated from hydronephrosis by showing the lack of connection between the cysts.

❓ WHERE ELSE TO LOOK

1. With any *renal tumor,* examine the renal vein and the inferior vena cava for *tumor extension* or *clot.* Look for para-aortic nodes and for liver metastases.

2. With *polycystic disease* of the kidney, examine the liver, pancreas, and spleen for associated cysts. Forty percent of patients with polycystic disease have liver cysts.

3. With a more or less *echo-free mass,* think of *lymphoma* and look for evidence of *splenomegaly* and para-aortic *adenopathy.*

4. With a *tumor in the renal pelvis,* examine the bladder. There may be a synchronous *transitional cell tumor* there as well.

5. With *localized hydronephrosis* of the upper pole of the kidney, look in the bladder for an ectopic *ureterocele* into which the duplicated ureter inserts (Fig. 32-15).

SELECTED READING

Bosniak, M. A. The small (≤ 3.0 cm) renal parenchymal tumor: Detection, diagnosis, and controversies. *Radiology* 179:307–317, 1991.

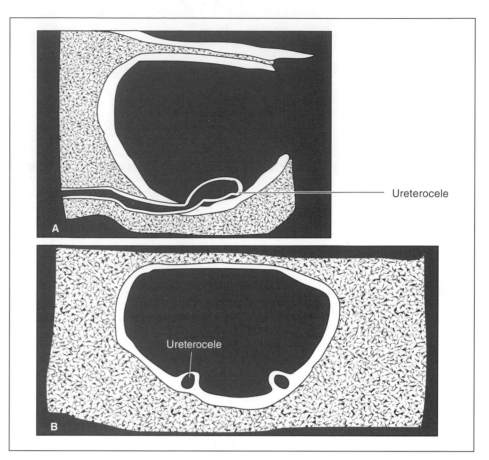

FIGURE 32-15. (**A**) An ectopic ureterocele, a cause of hydronephrosis and ureterectasis, is seen indenting the bladder. This is a congenital condition. (**B**) In this example, bilateral ureteroceles are seen, but they may occur on one side only. (Top: Longitudinal. Bottom: Transverse.)

Einstein, D. M., Herts, B. R., Weaver, R., Obuchowski, N., Zepp, R., and Singer, A. Evaluation of renal masses detected by excretory urography: Cost-effectiveness of sonography versus CT. *AJR* 164:371–375, 1995.

Jamis-Dow, C. A., Choyke, P. L., Jennings, S. B., Linehan, W. M., Thakore, K. N., and Walter, M. M. Small (≤ 3-cm) renal masses: Detection with CT versus US and pathologic correlation. *Radiology* 198:785–788, 1996.

Kier, R., Taylor, K. J. W., Feyock, A. L., and Ramos, I. M. Renal masses: Characterization with Doppler US. *Radiology* 176:703–707, 1990.

Kuijpers, D., Kruyt, R. H., and Oudkerk, M. Renal masses: Value of duplex Doppler ultrasound in the differential diagnosis. *J Urol* 151:326–328, 1994.

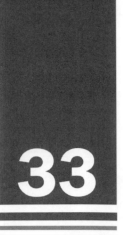

33 HEMATURIA

ROGER C. SANDERS

SONOGRAM ABBREVIATIONS

Bl   Bladder
Pr   Prostate gland

KEY WORDS

Benign Prostatic Hypertrophy. Enlargement of the glandular component of the prostate. The true prostate forms a shell around the enlarged gland.

Cystitis. Infection or inflammation of the wall of the bladder.

Hematuria. Blood in the urine.

Hydroureter. Dilated ureter.

Nephrocalcinosis. Multiple small calculi deposited in the renal pyramids. Found in association with renal tubular acidosis and medullary sponge kidney.

Pyelonephritis. Infection of the kidney without abscess formation.

Pyonephrosis. Pus-filled hydronephrosis.

Staghorn Calculus. A stone that occupies most of the renal pelvis and infundibulum.

Trigone. Base of the bladder. Area between the insertion of the ureters and the urethra.

Urethra. Urinary outflow tract below the bladder.

THE CLINICAL PROBLEM

Hematuria is an important sign of genitourinary tract problems. The abnormality may be located within the kidneys, ureter, bladder, or urethra. Therefore, the segments of the genitourinary tract that can be visualized by ultrasound (i.e., the kidney, upper and lower portions of the ureter, bladder, and upper part of the urethra) should be examined. Although the intravenous pyelogram (IVP) is the primary method of evaluating hematuria, lesions can be found with ultrasound that are not visible on IVP. Because the responsible lesions, such as small calculi or small tumors, are usually relatively minute, good scanning technique is essential.

ANATOMY
Kidneys
See Chapter 31.

Bladder
The bladder has a muscular wall whose thickness can be discerned with ultrasound. It is usually symmetric and is more or less square on transverse section. The base of the bladder where the ureters enter is known as the trigone (Fig. 33-1).

The bladder wall is about 3-mm thick in infants. It is proportionately thicker in infants than in other age groups. The bladder wall is approximately 3-mm thick when distended and 5-mm thick when empty in individuals other than infants.

The normal bladder in an adult contains about 150 to 400 cc and empties completely.

Ureters

The ureters are the small tubes that convey urine from the kidney to the bladder. Each begins where the renal pelvis narrows and travels anterior to the psoas muscle into the true pelvis. They insert into the trigone region, where they can be seen. The ureters are difficult to see with ultrasound under normal conditions since they are small—less than 8-mm wide. In hydroureter, the entire length of the ureter may be seen.

Two small bumps on the posterior aspect of the bladder on either side of the midline represent the ureteric orifices (see Fig. 31-1). As urine squirts into the bladder, the ureteric orifices evert and the jet phenomenon—a series of bubbles coming from the ureteric orifices—may be seen (beautifully demonstrated with color flow). The normal ureter can be seen as a subtle echopenic tube leading obliquely superiorly from the ureteric orifice. It distends with peristalsis (see Fig. 31-1).

Urethra

The urethra is the tube that conveys the urine from the bladder to the tip of the penis. Ultrasound evaluation is limited to the posterior urethra above the external sphincter. In the male, the posterior urethra is surrounded by the prostate. Similar tissue lies around the female urethra (Fig. 33-2) and can easily be mistaken for a mass in the base of the bladder.

Male Anatomy

Posterior to the lower bladder lie the mustache-shaped seminal vesicles (see Fig. 33-1). The prostate lies posterior to the symphysis pubis and inferior to the bladder and seminal vesicles. It is more or less round. Sometimes a line of echoes from the urethra can be seen at its center.

Female Anatomy

In the female the uterus and vagina lie posterior and inferior to the bladder (see Fig. 33-2). The vagina and lower segment of the uterus are normally never separated from the bladder.

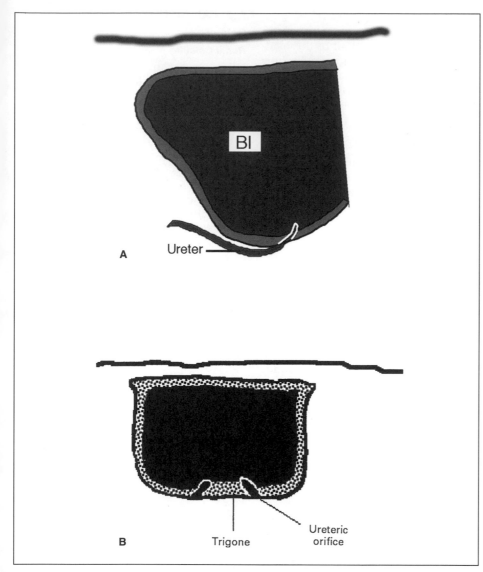

FIGURE 33-1. The ureteric orifices can be seen as two small buds in the trigone. The ureters can be traced through the wall to the ureteric orifice. (**A**) Sagittal. (**B**) Transverse.

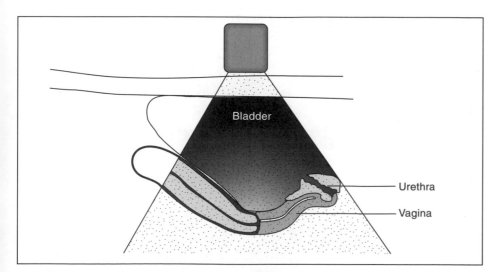

FIGURE 33-2. In the female, the uterus and vagina lie posterior and inferior to the bladder. The posterior urethra is seen as a mass at the inferior aspect of the bladder.

◤ TECHNIQUE

Kidney

The sonographic examination of the kidney is reviewed in Chapter 31.

Bladder

The bladder can be examined only when it is distended. A transducer with a small footprint is pressed, if necessary somewhat vigorously, into a site just above the pubic symphysis and arched superiorly to show the upper portions of the bladder wall. The bladder normally has a smooth curved surface and is surrounded by an echogenic line that represents the wall. The anterior wall of the bladder cannot be seen with a transabdominal approach adequately owing to reverberations unless a water bath technique is used. Some have used the transrectal or endovaginal transducer (see Chapter 35) to examine the anterior bladder wall.

Bladder volume can be calculated by multiplying width, height, and length and halving the result.

Postvoid views should be obtained since residual urine may indicate urethral obstruction or neurological bladder and may result in urinary tract infection.

Ureter

Oblique views along the site of the bump in the posterior wall of the bladder (the trigone) angling laterally show the normal ureter within the bladder wall. The ureteric insertions into the bladder can be well seen with the endovaginal probe.

Catheterization

It may be necessary to insert a catheter to fill the bladder adequately. One cannot perform a satisfactory transabdominal ultrasonic examination of the bladder unless it is well distended. Care must be taken not to introduce air if the patient is catheterized since this will prevent the sound beam from entering the bladder.

Calculi

The highest possible frequency should be used to search for renal calculi because the acoustic shadowing is emphasized by a high frequency, and stones can be subtle.

◆ PATHOLOGY

Calculi

Renal Calculi

Ultrasound can be a more sensitive method of detecting calculi than IVP. Some calculi cannot be seen on IVP because they are not radiopaque or because they are concealed by gas or feces. If they are more than 3 or 4 mm in size, acoustic shadowing can be seen beyond a dense echo (see Figs. 31-15 and 32-8).

Smaller calculi appear as densely echogenic structures within the renal sinus echoes; decreasing the gain makes them stand out more against the background echogenicity of the renal sinus.

In nephrocalcinosis the calculi are often too small to cast shadows but are seen as symmetrically located echogenic areas where the pyramids normally lie (Fig. 33-3).

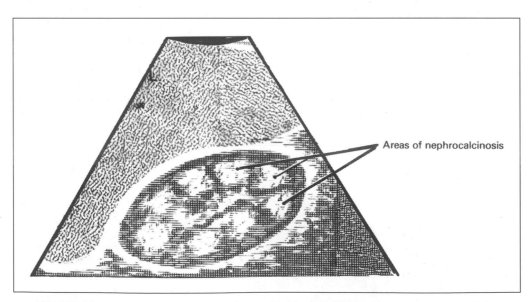

FIGURE 33-3. In nephrocalcinosis the pyramids are filled with small stones. Echogenic areas are seen in the pyramids, although the stones are usually too small to create shadows.

Calculi, whether due to uric acid, cysteine, or calcium mixtures, cause echogenic areas with shadowing if they are large. Smaller calculi may not show shadowing, or shadowing may be seen only fleetingly with real-time. Associated cystic areas adjacent to the calculi may represent dilated calyces. Staghorn calculi in the renal pelvis can be mistaken for the renal sinus echoes.

If there is renal obstruction or hematuria, make a specific effort to see calculi in the distal ureter or within the bladder wall. Usually, the ureter is dilated superior to the calculus; with good technique, shadowing from the calculus can be seen. Subtle calculi may be seen in the distal ureter as it enters the bladder with the rectal or vaginal probe when they cannot be seen with a transabdominal approach.

Bladder Calculi

Bladder calculi may be missed on IVP because they can be confused with phleboliths. They are particularly easy to see with ultrasound because they are surrounded by fluid (Fig. 33-4). Movement of a bladder calculus can be demonstrated by turning the patient to an oblique or decubitus position.

Distal ureteral calculi may be associated with bladder wall edema.

Tumors

Tumors in the kidney and bladder may be seen first with ultrasound and may be responsible for hematuria. Tumor appearances in the kidney are described in Chapter 32. Tumors in the bladder are usually small, relatively echogenic structures adjacent to the bladder wall (Fig. 33-5). The extent of invasion of the bladder wall can be assessed with ultrasound. The echogenic line around the bladder is absent when a tumor has invaded the wall. The degree of bladder wall invasion affects the staging and therefore the therapy of a bladder tumor.

A bladder tumor protruding into the true pelvis through the bladder wall is unresectable; therefore, a cystectomy, the preferred treatment for bladder tumor, cannot be performed.

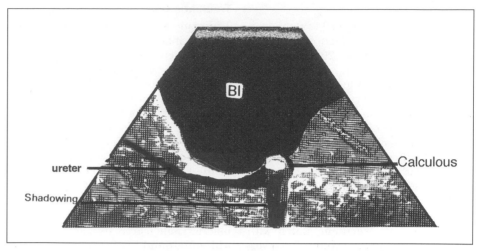

FIGURE 33-4. Bladder calculi usually cause acoustic shadowing.

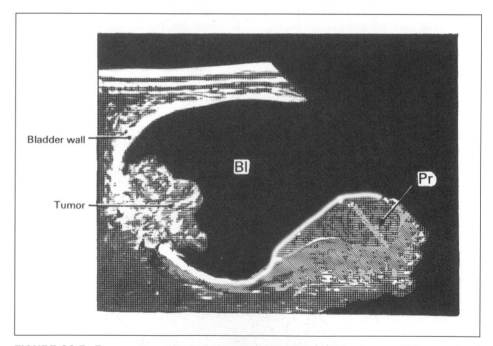

FIGURE 33-5. Tumors are echogenic areas within the bladder lumen. If they extend through the bladder wall, the echogenic line around the bladder is disrupted.

Infection

Infection can be responsible for hematuria. In the kidney, infection looks like an abscess (see Chapter 26) or pyelonephritis. In the bladder, infection may cause generalized or local thickening of the bladder wall (cystitis). If localized, such thickening may be indistinguishable from thickening caused by a tumor.

Infection may occur in association with a diverticulum, a cystic bud arising from a bladder that is chronically obstructed (Fig. 33-6). The neck of a diverticulum is easy to see with ultrasound. To be sure which is the bladder and which is the diverticulum, watch with real-time as the patient voids. The diverticulum will enlarge as the bladder contracts.

Tumors occur more frequently in diverticulum than on the normal bladder wall.

Fluid debris levels may occur due to infection. They change when the patient's position is changed.

Traumatic Changes

Traumatic damage to any site in the genitourinary tract will produce hematuria. When the kidney has suffered trauma, a localized area of altered echogenicity, possibly fluid filled, may indicate a blood clot or a laceration of the kidney. A distorted outline and a line through the kidney may indicate a kidney fracture. A perinephric hematoma will almost certainly develop at the site of the laceration. Bladder trauma is revealed by the presence of a perivesical hematoma—a collection of blood lying outside the bladder. The actual site of a bladder wall tear is usually not visible with ultrasound.

A Foley catheter that has been in place for some time often causes traumatic damage to the superior wall (dome) of the bladder. Local bulging and irregularity are seen at the site of the traumatic cystitis.

Prostatic Hypertrophy

Prostatic hypertrophy may be responsible for hematuria. The engorged veins that run along the surface of an enlarged prostate bleed easily. Enlargement of the prostate is detected by impingement of a prostatic soft tissue mass on the bladder or by extension of the prostate toward the rectum.

The prostate is considered in detail in Chapter 35.

PITFALLS

1. Do not mistake *air* in the kidney or bladder for *calculi*. Air lies in the most superior aspect of the organ being examined even when position is changed.

2. Do not mistake *blood clot* for *tumor* within the bladder. Changing the patient's position usually alters the blood clot configuration and position but does not change tumor appearances.

3. *Renal calculi vs. arterial calcification.* In older patients arterial calcification in the renal sinus is common. Areas of arterial calcification may resemble multiple small calculi in the renal sinus (an unusual site for true small calculi). Calcification may occur in the two walls of an artery and a "tramline" (double) calcification will occur, typical of arterial calcification. It may be impossible to decide whether there is a small calculus or a small arterial calcification if the tramline sign is not seen, but it is worth watching for pulsations in the vessel on a magnified real-time image.

WHERE ELSE TO LOOK

1. If the prostate is found to be enlarged or a mass is found in the bladder, examine the kidneys to be certain there is no secondary hydronephrosis.

2. If a renal calculus is seen, evaluate the bladder for calculi, debris, and wall thickening.

3. If a bladder calculus or tumor is found, look in the kidney for additional calculi or tumor.

4. If an irregular bladder wall is found, look in the patient's chart for a history of infections before dictating a list of differentials.

SELECTED READING

Haddad, M. C., Sharif, H. S., Shahed, M. S., Mutaiery, M. A., Samihan, A. M., Sammak, B. M., Southcombe, L. A., and Crawford, A. D. Renal colic: Diagnosis and outcome. *Radiology* 184:83–88, 1992.

Laing, F. C., Benson, C. B., DiSalvo, D. N., Brown, D. L., Frates, M. C., and Loughlin, K. R. Distal ureteral calculi: Detection with vaginal US. *Radiology* 192:545–548, 1994.

Vrtiska, T. J., Hattery, R. R., King, B. F., Charboneau, J. W., Smith, L. H., Williamson, B., Jr., and Brakke, D. M. Role of ultrasound in medical management of patients with renal stone disease. *Urol Radiol* 114:131–138, 1992.

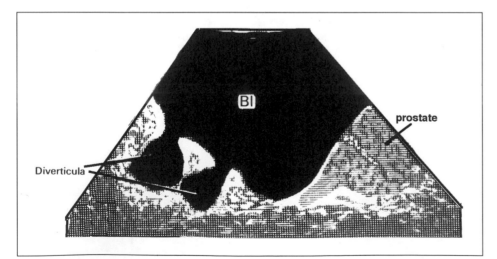

FIGURE 33-6. Bladder diverticula appear as pedunculated extensions to the bladder. They have relatively small necks.

TRANSPLANTS

1. Renal Transplants

OSCAR DEL BARCO, LISA SIMONS, ROGER C. SANDERS

SONOGRAM ABBREVIATIONS

Bl Bladder

D Diastole

K Kidney

R Reversed flow

S Systole

KEY WORDS

Acute Tubular Necrosis. Acute renal shutdown, usually due to abrupt lowering of blood pressure.

Anuria. Total absence of urine production.

Creatinine. A waste product excreted in the urine. Values of more than 1.0 mg/dL indicate that the patient is in renal failure.

Cyclosporine. Drug given to transplant recipients to prevent rejection; may cause a clinical picture resembling rejection.

Iliac Fossa. Area on either side of the lower part of the abdomen. Usual location of a transplanted kidney.

Immunosuppression. Depression of host's immunologic defenses.

Infarct. Occlusion of the blood supply to an organ.

Ischemia. Sudden decrease in blood supply. Prolonged ischemia results in an infarct.

Lymphocele. A collection of lymphatic fluid. Usually a postoperative complication.

Oliguria. Decreased urine production (less than 400 mL per day).

Rejection. Reaction of the body to the presence of a foreign kidney shown by production of antibodies against the transplant.

Steroids. Drugs similar to the hormones produced by the adrenal glands. Steroids lead to a decrease in immunologic response.

Urinoma. A collection of extravasated urine. Usually a postoperative complication.

THE CLINICAL PROBLEM

Renal transplantation has been performed since the 1950s and has become the usual long-term treatment for end-stage chronic renal failure. In the last few years, results have improved considerably with the development of effective immunosuppressive medication and better tissue typing, decreasing the risk of rejection.

The most common indication to examine a renal transplant is worsening renal failure. Possible explanations include obstruction, rejection, acute tubular necrosis (ATN), and vascular problems such as infarct or venous thrombosis. Renal transplant rejection, the usual cause of fever and increasing serum creatinine levels, has a typical although not diagnostic ultrasonic appearance. All of the other causes, notably hydronephrosis, can be diagnosed by ultrasound. Other imaging techniques such as computed tomography (CT) and nuclear medicine are expensive, require patient cooperation, and are not portable.

Another common clinical problem in a renal transplant patient is postoperative fever, which may be due to an infected fluid collection. Types of collections are hematomas, lymphoceles, and urinomas. All these collections are easily localized by ultrasound and can be drained or aspirated under ultrasound guidance. Because transplant patients are immunosuppressed, serious infections may produce few signs and infection may spread rapidly.

Ultrasound is also a useful tool to guide renal biopsy. This procedure is usually done when there is difficulty in distinguishing rejection, acute tubular necrosis, and cyclosporine toxicity.

A donated kidney either from living related donor or a cadaver is rotated and placed in an inverted position in the iliac fossa (Fig. 34-1). The renal artery is attached to either the common or the external iliac artery. The ureter is inserted into the bladder above the ureteral orifice through a submucosal tunnel in the bladder wall. This tunnel creates a valve in the distal end of the ureter to prevent reflux into the renal transplant. Because operative procedures and recipient shape and size vary, the transplanted kidney may have a large renal pelvis or an unusual axis. A baseline ultrasound scan after surgery is therefore worthwhile to document renal size, pelvicalyceal pattern, and any perirenal fluid collection.

ANATOMY

The kidney parenchyma has two main components: the cortex, in which arteries, veins, convoluted tubules, and glomerular capsules are found; and the medulla, which contains the renal pyramids. These are conical masses with papillae projecting into cuplike cavities in the renal pelvis. The main renal artery is located at the hilum, the segmental artery lies adjacent to the medulla, the interlobar artery runs alongside the pyramids, and the arcuate arteries are found at the apex of the pyramids. The veins parallel the arteries. Arterial anatomy must be understood before undertaking Doppler investigation of the kidneys (Fig. 34-2).

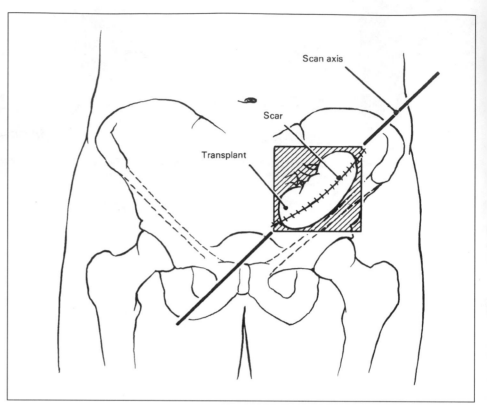

FIGURE 34-1. Diagram showing the usual placement site of the renal transplant. As a rule, the renal transplant is best shown by scans that are parallel to the scar. The transplant can be in either iliac fossa.

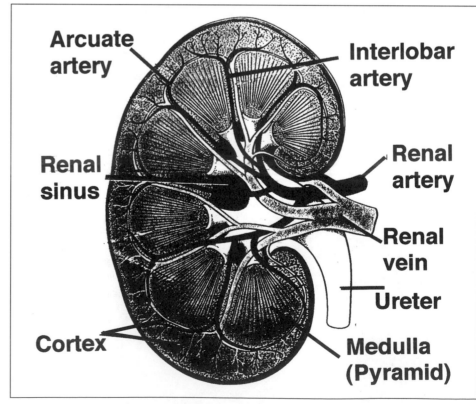

FIGURE 34-2. Diagram showing details of renal arterial flow. Doppler is usually performed at the main renal artery, the interlobar artery, and the arcuate artery.

TECHNIQUE

Perhaps the simplest way of obtaining reproducible sonograms is to scan along the axis of the scar and at right angles to the scar (see Fig. 34-1). The kidney should be measured in both longitudinal and transverse planes (length, height, and width). An accurate measurement is important since size increase is a valuable sign of rejection. Because a transplanted kidney is so superficial, it is too large to fit in the near field of any transducer. The optimal means of obtaining the length measurement is to match two linear array scans side by side, dividing the kidney at an easily reproduced spot (e.g., the middle of a pyramid). If this technique is not available, the second best is to add two measurements, one taken from the upper pole to a given spot, the other taken from that same spot to the lower pole.

The urinary bladder should be scanned; if it is filled with urine the scan should be repeated with an empty bladder. Doppler signals are obtained in the main renal vein and in the main segmental, interlobar, and arcuate arteries (Figs. 34-2, 34-3, and 34-4). Color Doppler is helpful in deter-

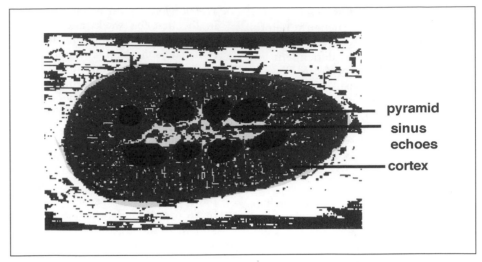

FIGURE 34-3. View of a transplant kidney showing the principle anatomical structures. Doppler signals are obtained from vessels at the sites where the lines end.

mining the best position and angle in which to place the Doppler gate. The resistive index is calculated from the signal as follows:

$$\frac{\text{Systolic height} - \text{Diastolic height}}{\text{Systolic height}}$$

If performing the baseline scan, the incision will be fresh and sterile technique should be used. See Chapter 56 for a discussion of how to scan with a gel-film skin barrier or how to cover the transducer.

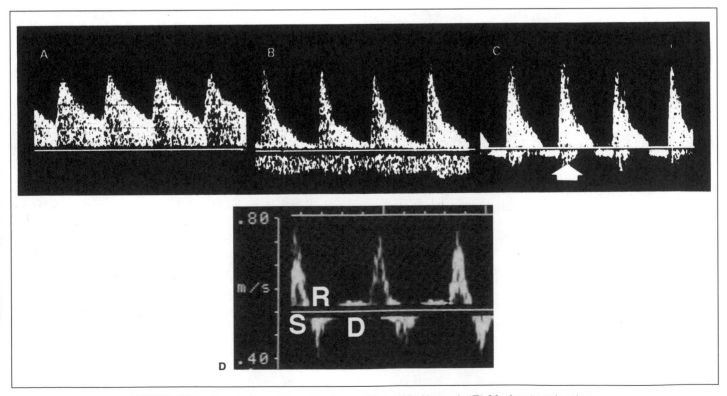

FIGURE 34-4. Renal artery Doppler flow pattern. (**A**) Normal. (**B**) Moderate rejection, little diastolic flow; venous flow also seen below the baseline. (**C**) Severe rejection. Reversal of flow in diastole (white arrow). (**D**) Normal iliac artery showing systolic phase (S), reversal phase (R), and the diastolic phase (D).

Color Doppler Power Imaging

This technology is particularly helpful in the assessment of renal and pancreas transplants. It is less dependent on beam angle and is free from aliasing. Perfusion of the transplant can be assessed so infarcts where there is no flow can be seen. Slower flow can be seen so the venous structures can be investigated.

◆ PATHOLOGY

1. *Acute rejection.* Acute rejection can happen hours, days, or months after transplantation and has a typical sonographic appearance. The kidney is swollen and the pyramids are more prominent and sonolucent than usual; the central sinus echo complex shows a decrease in both size and echogenicity. Volumetric changes in renal size can be followed by using the following formula: length × width × height × 0.5233 (the formula for a prolate ellipse).

    If the Doppler resistive index is greater than 0.75, there is much increased vascular resistance due to swelling of the parenchyma. This generally means rejection but can also be seen with other processes that can cause tissue swelling, such as acute tubular necrosis and cyclosporine administration.

2. *Chronic rejection.* In chronic rejection, the renal parenchyma becomes echogenic and the kidney decreases in size. The vascular resistive index increases. Eventually, the kidney fails.

3. *Acute tubular necrosis.* Acute tubular necrosis is more common than rejection if there has been hypotension and subsequent ischemia; clinically, it is difficult to diagnose since it mimics rejection. There is little sonographic change in the parenchymal pattern but some renal enlargement is seen. The pyramids are generally not enlarged, and the sinus echoes are normal.

4. *Cyclosporine.* Cyclosporine nephrotoxicity occurs when the levels of cyclosporine are elevated, thus compromising renal function. A sonogram usually shows no change in renal size or resistive indices; the only way to diagnose the problem is with renal biopsy.

5. *Hydronephrosis.* Obstruction can occur in the first few weeks after surgery. There are similar symptoms to rejection. The sonographic characteristics of hydronephrosis are discussed in Chapter 31. Obstruction may be due to a fluid collection or a poor-quality ureteral anastomosis. A baseline comparison study is important since some pelvic dilatation may be postoperative. Scans over the bladder may show a dilated ureter due to kinking. If the bladder is full, empty it because apparent hydronephrosis may be caused by an overdistended bladder causing kinking of the ureter.

6. *Vascular problems*
    a. *Renal artery stenosis.* Renal artery stenosis is the most common vascular complication and affects renal function. Scan the main renal artery thoroughly using both duplex and color Doppler. Do not mistake the iliac artery for the main renal artery (flow in the iliacs has high resistance) (see Fig. 34-4). If the renal artery is stenosed, the Doppler signal will show a slow rise in systole with delayed acceleration to peak velocity (see section on renal artery stenosis in Chapter 31). It is helpful to use Doppler to examine other intrarenal arteries in different regions of the kidney.
    b. *Renal artery thrombosis.* Renal artery thrombosis is an unusual complication that sometimes happens in the early postoperative period. Duplex and power Doppler show absent arterial and venous flow within the kidney or a portion of the kidney (an infarct).
    c. *Renal vein thrombosis.* Renal vein thrombosis is a rare complication that usually occurs in the first week after surgery. There will be an enlarged hypoechoic kidney. Both duplex and color Doppler show absent venous flow in the main renal vein and a high-resistance arterial flow with reversed diastolic flow. If the thrombus is in only the peripheral veins, it will not be seen with ultrasound. Sometimes, the renal sinus echoes are more prominent than usual due to hemorrhage.

    d. *Renal vein stenosis.* Renal vein stenosis can be detected with ultrasound if it occurs in the main renal vein. In most cases, the kidney is enlarged and the renal sinus echoes are more prominent than usual. Doppler analysis reveals increased velocity, three to four times greater than that of the prestenotic vein. Color Doppler shows aliasing at the site of stenosis.
    e. *Intrarenal arteriovenous (A/V) fistulas.* Both intrarenal A/V fistulas and pseudoaneurysm complications result from biopsy. These are benign and usually resolve spontaneously. Arteriovenous fistulas are easily detected with duplex and color Doppler. Color shows a localized region of disorganized color that extends outside the normal renal vessels. Doppler shows a high-velocity, turbulent mass with arterial and venous flow within.
    f. *Pseudoaneurysm.* A pseudoaneurysm on gray scale looks like a complex or simple cyst; however, color interrogation of the structure demonstrates arterial flow within the cyst.
    g. *Renal infarcts.* These are usually focal, but may involve all of the kidney. Fresh infarcts present as hypoechoic, wedge-shaped areas within the kidney. Power Doppler shows absent flow in the infarcted areas. Occasionally, there may be a focally echogenic area that relates to hemorrhage into the infarct. Eventually, the infarcts decrease in size and a scar develops at the infarct site.

7. *Fever or local tenderness of renal transplant.* Fever in the postoperative period following a transplant may be due to an abscess, hematoma, or, usually, rejection. Because such patients are treated with steroids, they are immunosuppressed and local tenderness over a collection may be relatively trivial. Whenever hydronephrosis is found, a collection should be sought as its cause.

8. *Fluid collections* (Fig. 34-5)

a. *Hematomas* commonly occur in the postoperative patient and are usually located either in the subcutaneous tissues or around the transplant. The sonographic characteristics vary with age; acute or chronic hematomas are echogenic and typically hard to distinguish from neighboring structures, whereas intermediate ones are complex. The borders are usually well defined. They are often aligned along the renal capsule. Some hematomas are fluid filled and resemble a urinoma.

b. *Abscesses* are suspected when the patient presents with fever and increased white blood count. They can be found in any location and sonographically can vary from an echo-free to a complex echo pattern. They are difficult to distinguish from hematomas by their sonographic appearance.

c. *Lymphoceles* can occur after surgery, especially when there is a blockage or damage of the lymphatic channels. On ultrasound they are usually well-defined, anechoic cystic areas; a majority tend to have septations. Such collections are usually located between the bladder and the kidney. Hydronephrosis due to obstruction by the lymphocele may develop.

d. *Urinoma* is a serious complication and it is most commonly caused by a defect in the ureteropelvic, ureteroureter, or ureterovesical anastomosis. Patients usually present with a decrease in urine output, pain, and swelling around the transplant. This type of collection is usually echo-free. Its location is variable, although it is more commonly seen around the lower pole. As always in the presence of a fluid collection, a percutaneous aspiration can determine the etiology of the collection. Urinomas, however, can be diagnosed by a nuclear medicine study in a noninvasive fashion.

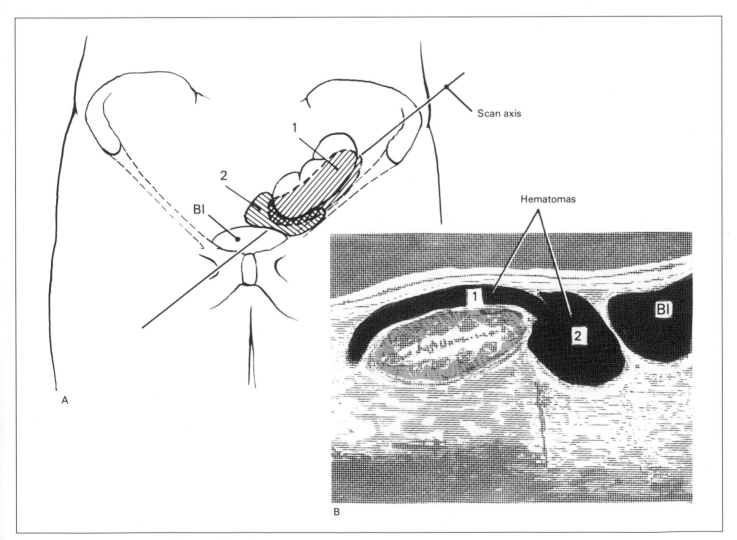

FIGURE 34-5. Collections, generally hematomas, are common with renal transplants. Collection 1 is in the usual site of hematoma accumulation. Collection 2 is in a site where urinomas or lymphoceles commonly occur. The axis along which the "sonogram" was performed is shown in A.

PITFALLS

1. *Pseudohydronephrosis*
   a. *Bladder overdistention.* An erroneous diagnosis of hydronephrosis may be made if the bladder is unduly full. Make sure that a post-void view is obtained if hydronephrosis appears to be present. Sometimes the apparent hydronephrosis disappears when the bladder is empty.
   b. *Baseline sinus distention.* An incorrect diagnosis of hydronephrosis may be made if a baseline study has not been performed because many transplanted kidneys show some apparent renal pelvic fullness.
2. *Time gain compensation problems.* Poor time gain compensation settings may give the appearance of a collection anterior to the kidney or even an anterior infarct if the time gain compensation is too steep (Fig. 34-6).

3. *Echogenic collections.* Hematomas and abscesses may be missed unless their occasional high echogenicity is kept in mind. If bowel is around, look for peristalsis in order to differentiate fluid-filled bowel from an abscess or hematoma.
4. *Bladder vs. collection.* Make sure that an apparent collection below the kidney is not the bladder; ask the patient to void or fill the bladder.
5. *Iliac artery.* Do not confuse the iliac artery with the main renal artery. The iliac artery will be outside the confines of the transplant kidney and will show a high-pressure pattern (see Fig. 34-4D).
6. *Sample gate angle.* Be sure to set the sample gate at a 60-degree angle to the vessel. Patterns suggestive of rejection may be seen if the sample gate is at a wrong angle (i.e., greater than 60 degrees).

7. Because of surgical technique and body habitus, the transplant may be placed in a vertical position, which affects the pulsed and color Doppler signal. One may not be able to examine this type of transplant with ultrasound.

WHERE ELSE TO LOOK

If a patient presents with fever of unknown origin and no collections are found around the transplanted kidney, look at the native kidneys or other areas where abscesses may develop (see Chapter 26). Intrahepatic or perihepatic abscesses may occur. Occasionally, transplant patients develop pancreatitis due to steroid overadministration.

SELECTED READING

Belgrove, N. J., Rouse, G. A., and Williams, D. M. A reevaluation of the use of sonography in the renal transplant. *J Diagn Med Sonographers* 7:339–344, 1991.

Finlay, D. E., Letourneau, J. G., and Longley, D. G. Assessment of vascular complications of renal, hepatic, and pancreatic transplantation. *Radiographics* 12:981–996, 1992.

Kelcz, F., Pozniak, M. A., Pirsch, J. D., et al. Pyramidal appearance and resistive index: Insensitive and nonspecific sonographic indicators of renal transplant rejection. *AJR* 155:531–535, 1990.

Little, A. F., and Dodd, G. D., III. Postoperative sonographic evaluation of the hepatic and renal transplant patient. *Ultrasound Quart* 13:111–119, 1995.

Pozniak, A. M., Dodd, G. D., and Kelcz, F. Ultrasonographic evaluation of renal transplantation. *Radiol Clin North Am* 30:5, 1992.

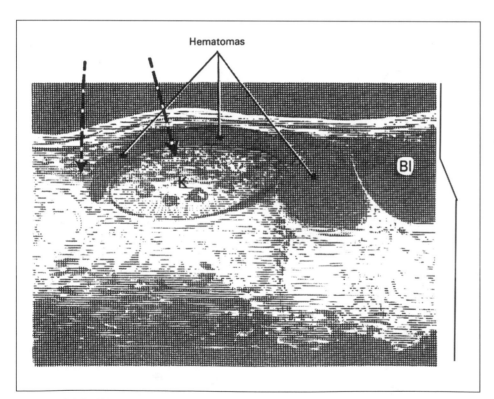

FIGURE 34-6. Unsatisfactory time gain compensation (TGC) settings may prevent assessment of the anterior aspect of the kidney. This hematoma is hard to distinguish from the neighboring tissues because the TGC was too steep (shown on the right side). Broken arrows indicate areas where a TGC artifact is apparent.

2. Liver Transplants

OSCAR DEL BARCO

SONOGRAM ABBREVIATIONS

CBD   Common bile duct

Ha   Hepatic artery

IVC   Inferior vena cava

Pv   Portal vein

KEY WORDS

Allograft. The newly transplanted liver.

Bacteremia. Blood stream infection.

Glucose Homeostasis. Control of the glucose level in the blood.

Ischemia. Impaired blood supply.

Seroma. A fluid collection composed of blood products.

THE CLINICAL PROBLEM

In the last decade, hepatic transplantation has become a successful treatment for many patients with end-stage liver disease. The success rate has increased to about 80 percent with improvements in organ preservation, surgical technique, and immunosuppressive therapy. Common indications for liver transplantation include biliary cirrhosis and chronic hepatitis in adults and extrahepatic biliary atresia and metabolic disorders in children.

Ultrasound is used both in preparation for transplantation and to look for complications after the transplantation has been performed. Typical indications are fever, pain, jaundice, abnormal liver function tests, and vascular complications. Possible pathology seen with ultrasound includes biliary obstruction, liver parenchymal abnormalities, rejection, malignancy, biliary leaks, hematomas, abscesses, and thrombosis or stenosis of the hepatic artery, portal vein, or inferior vena cava.

ANATOMY

The liver transplant takes the place of the native liver. The vascular and biliary tree connections are attached in the way they were prior to the transplant (Fig. 34-7). There is an end-to-end anastomosis of the portal vein and inferior vena cava. The hepatic arteries are sewn together. If the hepatic artery is too small, it is connected directly to the aorta. Either an end-to-end biliary duct anastomosis is performed or the bile duct is connected to the jejunum.

▨ TECHNIQUE

When using ultrasound for screening pretransplant, examine the extrahepatic portal vein with care. If it is severely narrowed or thrombosed, transplantation is not possible.

The liver is examined using the same techniques as described in Chapter 23 using a 3.5-MHz transducer. Particular attention is paid to the following:

1. Defining the biliary and portal structure with pulsed and color Doppler.

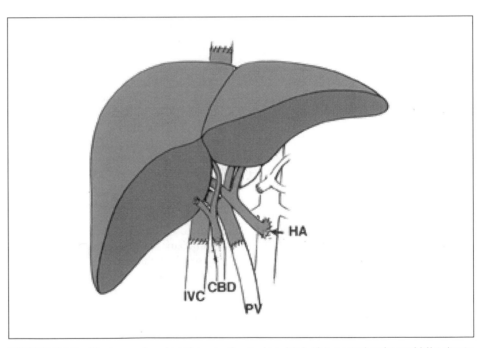

FIGURE 34-7. Diagram showing the usual way in which the portal vein and bile ducts are connected after liver transplant.

2. Carefully examining the anastomosis, looking for any areas of narrowing or irregularity. Doppler will normally show mild to moderate turbulence and an increased flow velocity at the anastomotic site. A normal portal vein should demonstrate flow toward the heart, showing slight variation with breathing. Flow is in the same direction as the intrahepatic artery. The normal inferior vena cava demonstrates variation in flow with the cardiac and respiratory cycles. The hepatic veins also vary flow depending on the cardiac pulsations.

 PATHOLOGY

Rejection

Rejection occurs in approximately 80 percent of liver transplants. With acute rejection, the ultrasonic findings are nonspecific. There may be a heterogeneous echo texture to the liver parenchyma, and an overall decrease in liver echogenicity may be seen. The margins of the hepatic veins may become poorly defined.

In chronic rejection, there may be an increase in periportal echogenicity.

Biliary Complications

Most will occur within 3 months of transplantation. If there is a bile leak, patients usually present with fever, pain, and increasing liver function tests. Leaks occur at the biliary anastomosis most often. Intrahepatic bile ducts may also leak secondary to arterial infarcts or liver biopsy. Typically, fluid collects in the region of the porta hepatis.

Obstruction

Most obstruction relates to a stricture at the anastomosis, but bile duct strictures may also occur when hepatic artery stenosis or thrombosis leads to ischemia. Biliary sludge or stones can occlude the duct system, but are uncommon. Biliary duct dilation to the level of the anastomosis may be seen. Ultrasound is relatively insensitive in the delineation of biliary problems after transplantation, which are usually analyzed using ERCP (endoscopic retrograde cannulation of the pancreatic duct).

Vascular Problems

Thrombosis or stenosis usually takes place within 3 months of transplantation. Patients may be asymptomatic or present with hepatic failure.

HEPATIC ARTERY THROMBOSIS. This is the most common vascular complication. Patients present with infection of the biliary tree or a biliary leak. Typical features of both are abnormal bilirubin, pain, and fever. No arterial signals at the porta hepatis will be detected with color or pulsed Doppler. Power Doppler (CPA) is used to confirm the absence of blood flow in the artery.

Abnormal Doppler waveforms with absence of diastolic flow are commonly seen in the first few days after surgery and usually do not indicate thrombosis or stenosis.

Focal, blotchy, hepatic hypoechoic liver lesions occur. Usually such infarcts are at the liver edge. Eventually, the infarcted area liquefies and becomes cystic.

HEPATIC ARTERY STENOSIS. This usually occurs at an anastomotic site. Thrombus may be a secondary finding. Duplex Doppler shows high-velocity flow that is greater than or equal to 2 meters per second at the anastomosis and turbulence distally (spectral broadening of the waveform). If there is severe stenosis, the parenchyma may be diffusely inhomogeneous, indicating ischemia. Sometimes the stenotic area and the region of the porta hepatis are not visible owing to overlying surgical changes, in which case, the tardus-parvus pattern, with reduced arterial flow amplitude and low acceleration pattern in the hepatic arterial vessels distal to the stenosis, is helpful (see Chapter 31). If normal flow is detected in the right and left hepatic arteries, this is adequate to determine that the main artery is patent.

PORTAL VEIN, IVC THROMBOSIS. The portal vein and inferior vena cava should normally be echo-free postsurgery. The normal portal vein has a luminal diameter of 8 to 12 mm and has flow into the liver in the same direction as the hepatic artery. If the walls are thick, the lumen is small (less than 4 mm), and there are internal echoes, angiography is usually performed. Thrombosis usually causes echogenic material within the vessel lumen. However, thrombus may be isoechoic with blood. CPA is helpful in determining whether blood is flowing in the vein. Venous flow is normally undetectable with color or duplex Doppler, but it may be visible with CPA. After portal vein thrombosis occurs, collaterals develop. Small tubular pulsatile structures develop in the porta hepatis.

PORTAL VEIN, IVC STENOSIS. Focal narrowing of the vessels is seen normally at the anastomosis site. In true stenosis, Doppler assessment will show high-velocity flow and distal turbulence. There will be a loss of the normal pulsation seen in the inferior vena cava. Internal echoes may be seen due to clot.

PSEUDOANEURYSM. This problem occurs at the arterial anastomosis and is most often the result of vascular reconstruction or a complication following a biopsy. A hypoechoic fluid collection in an anastomotic site with arterial flow within a pseudoaneurysm will be seen (see Chapter 29).

Fluid Collections

Distinguishing between the various types of fluid collections often requires a diagnostic puncture which is done under ultrasound control (see Chapter 52).

HEMATOMAS. Hematomas are usually found around the liver, particularly in a subphrenic location, but they may be seen in the abdomen. Very common immediately posttransplant, these collections have varying degrees of echogenicity depending on the amount of liquefaction.

ABSCESSES. Abscesses have varying degrees of echogenicity, similar to hematomas. The patient may or may not be tender or febrile since the patient is immunosuppressed. Some abscesses contain gas (see Chapter 26). They may occur in an intrahepatic or extrahepatic location.

BILOMA. Sonolucent collections of bile seen alongside the biliary tree. Bilomas are a result of a bile leak, usually at the anastomosis, but they may be seen elsewhere since they may be caused by hepatic artery thrombosis and subsequent infarction.

ASCITES. Anechoic free fluid may be seen anywhere in the abdomen or pelvis and is common in the early postoperative course after transplantation.

SEROMAS. Sonolucent collections adjacent to the liver, seromas are common in the early postoperative period.

PITFALLS

1. A slight *narrowing or irregularity of the portal vein or IVC* at the anastomosis is a normal finding in the transplanted liver.
2. *Biliary duct air or sludge* may obscure biliary duct lumen, making determination of biliary dilation difficult; try scanning coronally with the patient supine, or turning the patient.
3. *Respiration.* Doppler may be difficult in these sick patients because of breathing motion. Have the patient suspend respiration when possible.
4. *Bowel gas.* Overlying bowel may obscure anatomy. Rolling the patient into an oblique or decubitus position may be helpful.

WHERE ELSE TO LOOK

1. Scan the patient's left upper quadrant to assess the *spleen.* Occasionally, splenomegaly will persist owing to continued portal hypertension.
2. In the early postoperative period, a *right pleural effusion* is almost always present. Scan above the diaphragm to look for hypoechoic fluid in the chest.
3. *Right adrenal gland.* Liver transplant recipients are at risk for right adrenal hemorrhage, caused by the removal of a portion of the IVC with ligation of the adrenal vein. A suprarenal mass with varying echogenicity, depending on the age of the hemorrhage, will be seen in the right adrenal gland.

Selected Reading

Little, A. F., and Dodd, G. D. Postoperative sonographic evaluation of the hepatic and renal transplant patient. *Ultrasound Quart* 13:111–119, 1995

Morton, M. J., James, E. M., Wiesner, R. H., and Krom, R. A. F. Applications of duplex ultrasonography in the liver transplant patient. *Mayo Clin Proc* 65:360–372, 1990.

Nghiem, H. V., Tran, K., Winter, T. C., III. Schmiedl, U. P., Althaus, S. J., Patel, N. H., and Freeny, P. C. Imaging of complications in liver transplantation. *Radiographics* 16:825–840, 1996.

3. Pancreatic Transplants

LISA SIMONS

SONOGRAM ABBREVIATIONS

Ao   Aorta

Bl   Bladder

IVC Inferior vena cava

KEY WORDS

Glucose Homeostasis. Control of blood glucose levels.

THE CLINICAL PROBLEM

Pancreatic transplantation is used as a treatment for severe (Type I) diabetes. This technique is used when there is multiorgan failure, as occurs in many long-term insulin dependent diabetics, as a means to achieve glucose homeostasis. A pancreas may be transplanted at the same time as a kidney, after a kidney transplant, or alone (in patients without end-stage renal disease).

Many of the complications following pancreatic transplantation may be seen with ultrasound:

1. Pancreatic failure, usually due to rejection. Unfortunately, the ultrasound findings of rejection are usually non-specific.
2. Peripancreatic fluid collections
3. Vascular problems
4. Arteriovenous fistulas
5. Pancreatitis and pseudocysts

ANATOMY

Surgical techniques for pancreatic transplantation are variable. An entire pancreas may be transplanted from a cadaver or a living related donor. Most commonly, a whole cadaver pancreas is removed from the donor along with the duodenum which is then anastomosed to the urinary bladder of the recipient (Fig. 34-8). This allows for direct elimination of pancreatic secretions into the patient's urine. Early diagnosis of rejection by monitoring levels of urinary amylase can then be performed. The arterial supply to the pancreatic transplant is from the donor superior mesenteric artery and celiac artery. Venous drainage is accomplished by anastomosis of the portal vein to the external iliac vein. The pancreas is placed in the iliac fossa. Patients with combination renal and pancreas transplants have the kidney placed on the opposite side.

TECHNIQUE

Standard Scan

1. Find the iliac vessels in the iliac fossa. This can be accomplished simply by using color flow. The transplant allograft is located superficially just medial to the iliac vessels.
2. Examine the texture and the anatomy of the pancreas. The gland is usually fairly well defined with a homogeneous echo texture similar to a native pancreas in the normal location. An anechoic or hypoechoic graft is often seen immediately postoperatively and may be a sign of rejection, of pancreatitis, or of a normally functioning gland. The pancreatic duct should be less than 23 mm in diameter, and the anterior-posterior diameter of the pancreas should measure from 1.5 to 2 cm.
3. The vascular connection to the pancreas may be found by first scanning longitudinally over the iliac vessels, then rotating the transducer to visualize the anastomosis of the celiac axis and superior mesenteric artery to the external iliac artery and the takeoff of the portal vein from its origin at the external iliac vein. The splenic artery and vein are along the posterior portion of the transplant.

Color Flow/Duplex Doppler

Doppler is helpful in identifying anatomy and vascularity in the pancreatic transplant. Color flow Doppler is used to show vascular patency, which is often difficult with conventional Doppler techniques, and to determine whether a vessel is an artery or a vein. Color flow is helpful in determining whether a peripancreatic structure is vascular or is a fluid collection, and to see whether there is adequate flow within the vessels. Duplex Doppler is used to decide whether a vessel is an artery or a vein.

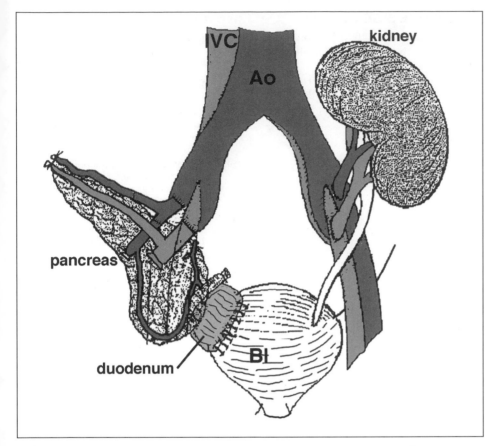

FIGURE 34-8. The usual position of a pancreatic transplant is shown. The pancreas is surgically inserted, so that the head of the pancreas is inverted and lies adjacent to the bladder. The duodenum is anastomosed to the bladder, so the contents of the pancreatic duct can escape into the bladder. The artery and vein supplying the pancreas are anastomosed to the iliac artery and vein.

 PATHOLOGY

Rejection

1. *Acute rejection.* An inhomogeneous parenchyma may be seen with acute rejection. However, this finding is nonspecific.
2. *Chronic rejection.* Sonographic signs may include:
   a. An increase in the parenchymal echogenicity of the pancreas
   b. A decrease in the size of the gland
   c. Calcifications—echogenic foci with posterior acoustic shadowing

Pancreatitis

Findings are similar to pancreatitis in the native gland. These include edema with enlargement, heterogeneous echo texture, and dilatation of the pancreatic duct.

Vascular Complications

GRAFT THROMBOSIS

1. *Clinical presentation.* Patients may present with back, flank, or abdominal pain; increased serum glucose; and decreased urine amylase levels. Graft thrombosis is the most common postoperative vascular complication and usually occurs within the first few days or weeks after surgery.
2. *Ultrasound examination.* Examination shows inhomogeneous echo texture or enlargement of the gland. Documentation of blood flow within the pancreas itself as well as within the vascular pedicle (at the anastomosis site) proves patency of the graft vasculature. Some absence of flow will be seen with graft thrombosis. Knowledge of the vascular construction of a pancreatic transplant is crucial in performing this part of the exam.

PSEUDOANEURYSMS. Pseudoaneurysms are rarely seen with ultrasound. Doppler examination will show arterial flow within a perianastomotic fluid collection.

ANASTOMOTIC STRICTURES. Turbulent color flow suggests a stenosis at the anastomosis site.

Fluid Collections

HEMATOMAS. Usually seen immediately postoperatively in close proximity to the pancreatic transplant. The ultrasound appearance will vary from anechoic to complex.

ABSCESSES. The patient may or may not be tender or febrile. Sonographically, abscesses will appear similar to a hematoma and may require aspiration for differentiation. An abscess may contain gas.

URINOMAS. These collections are usually found at the medial aspect of the pancreas. Urinomas are caused by an anastomotic leak at the duodeno-bladder junction. They appear anechoic unless they contain leaked pancreatic enzymes, in which case they will be complex.

PSEUDOCYSTS. Occasionally associated with pancreatitis, these anechoic to complex collections are found within or adjacent to the pancreas.

ASCITES. Anechoic free fluid may be seen anywhere in the pelvis. Always look for free fluid elsewhere in the patient's abdomen to help confirm the diagnosis of ascites. This free fluid may be related to previous dialysis.

✷ PITFALLS

1. *Obesity.* Blood flow in the transplanted pancreas of an obese patient may be difficult to detect with color flow and duplex Doppler.
2. *Ill-defined borders.* The pancreas may blend in with surrounding bowel, making identification difficult.
3. *Duodenum.* Do not mistake the transplanted duodenum for a complex fluid collection. Watch for peristalsis and use color flow Doppler to rule out vascularity.
4. *Bladder vs. collection.* Do not mistake the patient's urinary bladder for a fluid collection. Ask the patient to void or fill the bladder.
5. *Time gain compensation problems.* Same as for renal transplants.
6. *Echogenic collections.* Same as for renal transplants.

❓ WHERE ELSE TO LOOK

1. If the patient is febrile, look elsewhere in the abdomen for abscesses (see Chapter 26).
2. Scan the native pancreas if there is clinical pancreatitis and the transplant appears normal.

Selected Reading

Letourneau, J. G., Maile, C. W., Sutherland, D. E. R., and Feinberg, S. B. Ultrasound and computed tomography in the evaluation of pancreatic transplantation. *Radiol Clin North Am* 25:345–355, 1987.

Nelson, N. L., Largen, P. S., Stratta, R. J., Taylor, R. J., Grune, M. T., Hapke, M. R., and Radio, S. J. Pancreas allograft rejection: Correlation of transduodenal core biopsy with Doppler resistive index. *Radiology* 200:91–94, 1996.

Patel, B., Markivee, C. R., Mahanta, B., Vas, W., George, E., and Garvin, P. Pancreatic transplantation: Scintigraphy, US, and CT. *Radiology* 167:685–687, 1988.

Patel, B., Wolverson, M. K., and Mahanta, B. Pancreatic transplant rejection: Assessment with duplex US. *Radiology* 173:131–135, 1989.

PROSTATE

Rule Out Prostate Carcinoma; Benign Prostatic Hypertrophy

ROGER C. SANDERS, JOHN CASEY

SONOGRAM ABBREVIATIONS

AFMS Anterior fibromuscular zone

BI Bladder

CZ Central zone

ED Ejaculatory duct

Ip Iliopsoas muscle

NVB Neurovascular bundle

Ob Obturator muscle

Pr Prostate gland
PZ Peripheral zone

SP Symphysis pubis
SV Seminal vesicle

TZ Transitional zone

Ur Urethra

KEY WORDS

Abdominoperineal Resection. An operation that is usually performed for cancer of the colon which includes removal of anus, rectum, and sigmoid colon with the creation of a colostomy.

Anterior Fibromuscular Stroma. Nonglandular region that forms the anterior surface of the prostate.

Apex. Inferior region of the prostate.

Base. Superior region of the prostate.

Benign Prostatic Hypertrophy (BPH). Enlargement of the glandular component of the prostate. The true prostate forms a shell around the enlarged gland.

Central Zone. That portion of the prostate that surrounds the urethra. This area is the site of benign prostatic hypertrophy and is relatively spared by cancer of the prostate.

Corpora Amylacea. Calcification within the central zone of the prostate.

Ejaculatory Ducts. Connect the seminal vesicle and the vas deferens to the urethra at the verumontanum.

Neurovascular Bundle. An echogenic mass composed of nerves, veins, and arteries seen on the postero-lateral aspect of the prostate on transverse images. Damage to this nerve group may render the patient impotent.

Peripheral Zone. The posterior and lateral aspect of the prostate. This is the site of most prostatic cancer. The peripheral zone is larger at the apex (inferior portion of the prostate).

Prostate Specific Antigen (PSA). A protein derived only from the prostate elevated in prostate cancer, prostatic hypertrophy, and prostatitis.

Prostatitis. Inflammation of the prostate.

Seminal Vesicle. Reservoir in which sperm collects that lies superior to the prostate and posterior to the bladder.

Sextant Biopsy. Six biopsies taken from the right and left upper, middle, and lower peripheral zones of the prostate.

TNM. Staging technique for prostate cancer. T = tumor, N = nodes, M = metastasis.

Transitional Zone. Recognized as the third zone of the prostate; comprises approximately 5 percent of the gland. It is located on both sides of the proximal urethra and ends at the level of the verumontanum. It cannot be distinguished from the central zone with ultrasound.

Transurethral Resection of the Prostate (TURP). A knife placed on the end of a cystoscope rotates, removing the prostate surrounding the cystoscope in an apple-coring fashion.

Urethra. Urine is drained from the bladder via this tube that passes through the center of the prostate. The proximal and distal urethra form a 35-degree angle at the verumontanum.

Utricle. Cystic embryologic remnant in the midline within the prostate.

Vas Deferens. The duct linking the testicles and epididymis with the urethra.

Verumontanum. Junction of the ejaculatory ducts with the urethra.

THE CLINICAL PROBLEM

Three common entities involve the prostate: benign prostatic hypertrophy, prostatic cancer, and prostatic infection.

Benign Prostatic Hypertrophy

Benign prostatic hypertrophy (BPH) is common in elderly men who complain of poor urinary stream and frequent urination. Renal failure may occur if urethral obstruction due to the large prostate causes severe renal hydronephrosis. Ultrasound is used to determine the following:

1. The size of the prostate, which dictates the type of treatment
2. The amount of postvoid residual urine
3. Whether any hydronephrosis has developed

Prostate Cancer

Prostate cancer is the second most common cancer in men. It may occur from the age of 40 on, but it is most frequent in the very elderly. PSA (prostate-specific antigen) is a blood test that is usually elevated in the presence of prostate cancer, but may also be elevated by BPH or prostatitis. Many unsuspected cancers are found when a PSA is performed on a screening basis. Ultrasound may identify the site of cancer in a patient with increased PSA and no palpable mass. Ultrasound is used for the following purposes:

1. To confirm clinical suspicion of an intraprostatic mass
2. To aid in the biopsy of patients with increased PSA
3. To attempt to stage periprostatic spread
4. To guide radiotherapy treatment

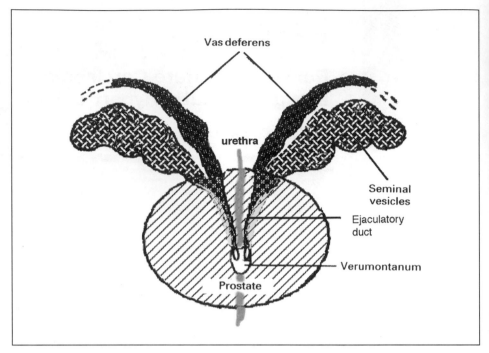

FIGURE 35-1. Diagram showing the relation of the seminal vesicles to the vas deferens. Both structures empty into the ejaculatory duct that ends at the verumontanum.

Prostatitis

In patients with unexplained fever, the cause may occasionally be an intraprostatic abscess. Prostatitis, inflammation of the prostate, has subtle ultrasonic findings. One type of prostatitis (granulomatous) causes an echopenic mass in the prostate. A second form is characterized by echogenic or echopenic areas.

ANATOMY

Seminal Vesicles and Vas Deferens

The seminal vesicles lie posterior to the bladder and superior to the prostate (Fig. 35-1). Usually, they contain internal echoes, but normal cystic components may be seen. The size of the seminal vesicles is variable. A cystic embryologic remnant known as the utricle may be centrally located just inferior to the seminal vesicles in the midline.

The vas deferens, which look similar to the seminal vesicle, lie medial to the seminal vesicle (Fig. 35-1).

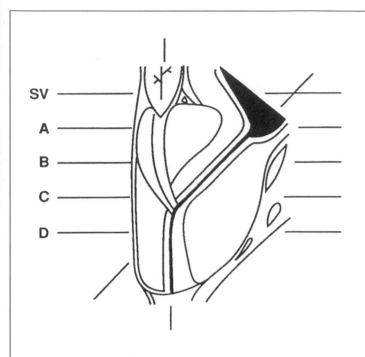

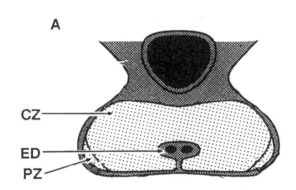

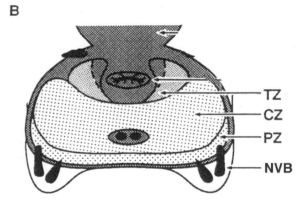

FIGURE 35-2. Diagram of the longitudinal and transverse anatomy of the prostate, showing the location of the central (CZ), transitional (TZ), peripheral (PZ) and fibromuscular zones (AFMS). The neurovascular bundles are seen at the posterolateral aspect (NVB). Adapted from A. Villers, et al. Ultrasound anatomy of the prostate. *J Urol* 143:732–737, 1990, with permission.

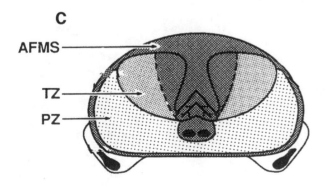

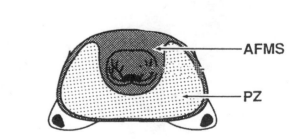

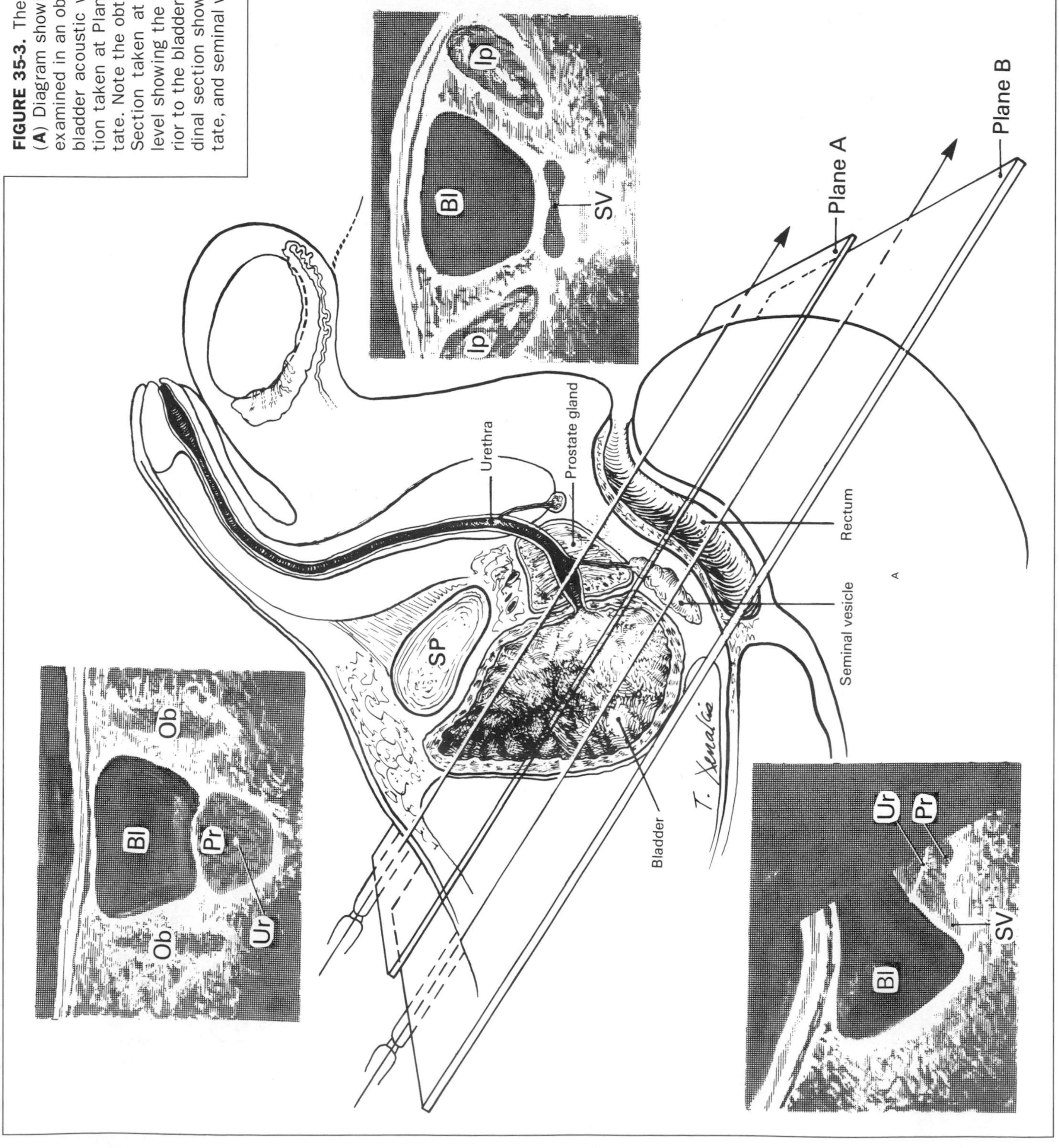

FIGURE 35-3. The prostate and bladder. (A) Diagram showing the prostate being examined in an oblique axis through the bladder acoustic window. Top left: Section taken at Plane A through the prostate. Note the obturator muscles. Right: Section taken at plane B at a higher level showing the seminal vesicle posterior to the bladder. Bottom left: Longitudinal section showing the urethra, prostate, and seminal vesicles.

Prostate

The prostate is more or less a pear-shaped organ. The urethra runs through the center. The end closest to the bladder is known as the base, and the end nearest to the penis is called the apex. At the inferior end of the prostate lies a thin muscular structure, the urogenital diaphragm, dividing the prostate from the penile structures.

The area around the urethra is known as the central and transitional zones. Cupping the central and transitional zones posteriorly is the peripheral zone. The peripheral zone is relatively larger at the apex. Its acoustic texture is different from that of the central and transitional zones.

Ejaculatory Ducts

The ejaculatory ducts run alongside the peripheral zones from the seminal vesicles to the verumontanum and are visible, but subtle (Fig. 35-2; see Fig. 35-1).

Prostate Volume

The prostate volume is normally less than 20 g. The volume is calculated using the formula for a prolate ellipse:

$$\text{Length} \times \text{Width} \times \text{Height} \times 2$$

Since the specific gravity of the prostate is approximately 1, a direct translation to grams can be made.

▰ TECHNIQUE

Transabdominal Approach

The transabdominal technique may be used for estimation of size and radiotherapy planning. The transducer is angled inferiorly under the pubic symphysis. Transverse sections are performed at an angulation of about 15 degrees toward the feet (Fig. 35-3) with the bladder full. Be certain to obtain the longest longitudinal image so the volume can be calculated. This may require suprapubic pressure.

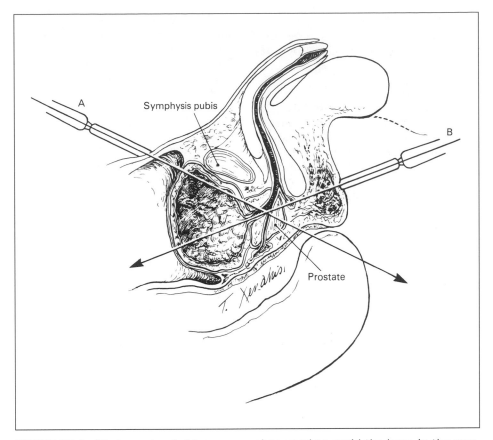

FIGURE 35-4. Diagram showing two approaches used to avoid the bone in the symphysis pubis when scanning the prostate. From an abdominal approach (A) the transducer is tilted toward the feet at an angle of 15 to 30 degrees; the beam passes through the acoustic window of the bladder to the prostate. A second approach (B) uses the perineum as a window for viewing the prostate. The sonographer scans through a site posterior to the scrotum.

Perineal Approach

Imaging the prostate from an abdominal approach may be difficult if the bladder cannot be adequately filled (Fig. 35-4). A perineal approach can be used, scanning between the legs posterior to the scrotum. Both transverse and longitudinal images can be obtained so that the prostate volume can be calculated.

This approach is used for biopsy if the patient has had a surgical removal of the rectum (abdominoperineal resection).

Transrectal Approach

The transrectal approach is necessary if prostate cancer is the diagnostic question (Fig. 35-5).

Probe Preparation

Ultrasound transducers best suited for transrectal visualization are 5- and 7-MHz transducers. To set the transducer off from the rectal wall and to provide good acoustic coupling, the probe may be covered with a water-filled condom or custom-made sheath. This balloon pushes the prostate out of the near field of the transducer. The sheath also functions to protect the transducer against contamination.

Supplies

1. A cup or other suitable container for water
2. A large syringe with extension tubing
3. A stopcock or hemostat to prevent water refluxing into the syringe
4. A 3- to 4-inch-high support to keep the transducer horizontal and to prevent the transducer from poking into the rectal wall. For the sonographer, this provides an armrest as well as a reference for moving the transducer by increments.

Placing the Condom on the Probe

Many endorectal probes can be used with a condom only. Some require water inside the condom to provide an offset for better detail.

Over-the-counter condoms are very thin-walled and tear easily. Two condoms may be used, one inside the other, for double strength and protection. Rinse both condoms with water to remove any powder residue. Fill the first condom with warm water and place it over the end of the probe. Fill the second condom with water and place it on top of the first condom. All of the air bubbles should be squeezed or milked out of the end of the condoms. With the probe pointed toward the ground, wrap a rubber band tightly around two fingers and slide it on the probe, being careful to push all air bubbles and water up the shaft of the probe toward the opening of the condoms. Be sure the rubber band is positioned in the groove on the probe. When all of the air bubbles are out of the secured end, place another rubber band on the shaft of the probe and secure the condoms at their open end to prevent contamination of the probe.

Using the extension tube and stopcock attached to the probe, fill the syringe with warm water and attach it to the stopcock. Draw back on the syringe to withdraw any water still in the inner condom. This will aspirate any air in the extension tube and probe plumbing. Test the water bath for air bubbles by injecting water into the probe. With the probe pointing downward and the water hole inlet at the top or upward, aspirate the last air bubbles. If there are still air bubbles trapped in the outer condom, they should be removed by lifting the rubber band and squeezing them out.

Patient Preparation

Have the patient empty his bladder and bowels if possible. Explain briefly what you are going to do and what is expected of the patient during the exam. Emphasize that this exam is not as uncomfortable as the digital rectal exam that the urologist performed. Then have the patient take off his pants and underwear and lie on the table on his left side (left decubitus) with knees bent up and feet forward.

Probe Insertion

Place a lubricant on the probe and have the patient bear down while you insert the probe. Start by sliding the probe straight in and then angling posteriorly to follow the curve of the rectum. Insert the probe at least until you can see the prostate on the monitor. When the probe is in far enough, there will be a release of back pressure.

Performing the Scan

Transrectal prostate scanning is performed in transverse and longitudinal planes.

TRANSVERSE PLANE. Obtain the transverse images first, since they will show lateral lesions not shown on the longitudinal images. Start above the base of the prostate at the level of the seminal vesicles. Show the symmetry of the seminal vesicles and take multiple images at approximately 5-mm intervals down to the level of the apex of the prostate. Take a transverse measurement midway through the prostate at its widest point. Indicate the approximate distance below the seminal vesicles on the image.

LONGITUDINAL PLANE. Obtain a midline image of the prostate. Use the distal urethra at the apex and the proximal urethra at the base as landmarks. Take a measurement between the two landmarks and another measurement perpendicular to this at the widest anterior-posterior point. Then take multiple images through the right lobe of the prostate to the most lateral aspect. Also take multiple images from the midline through the left lobe. Use a labeling method (e.g., R or L5) to indicate how far lateral the section was obtained.

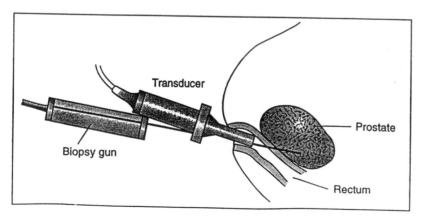

FIGURE 35-5. Transrectal biopsy technique. The needle is inserted alongside the transducer with the transducer inside the rectum.

Problems With Gas

If gas obstructs views of the right lobe of the prostate, take images of the left lobe first. Have the patient roll into the right decubitus (left-side-up) position. The bowel gas should rise to the left side. Views of the right side are usually (in 80 percent of cases) possible. If this approach is unsuccessful, remove the probe, give the patient a Fleet enema, and after stool evacuation, repeat the procedure as before.

Probe Removal

When taking the probe out of the rectum, aspirate all of the water and have the patient bear down and push the probe out. If the water cannot be aspirated, slowly withdraw the probe. The sheath will stretch and the water will trickle out through the anal opening. The sheath will fill up outside the rectum, allowing the retained sheath to be withdrawn.

Probe Care

Pull off the sheath with a gloved hand and invert the sheath to retain any contamination or odor. Soak the probe and flush the internal plumbing of the probe in a suitable disinfectant, such as Cidex (see Chapter 56).

Biopsy

Two methods of prostate biopsy may be used: the transrectal and the transperineal. The transrectal is more popular and less painful but carries a greater risk of infection. The transperineal approach is now only used for radiotherapy seed placement or if the rectum is absent.

Transrectal Technique (see Fig. 35-5)

1. Informed consent is obtained.
2. The patient is prepared by giving an antibiotic such as ciprofloxacin at least 1 hour prior to the performance of the study. Oral pain killers are not helpful and are practically never needed. If necessary, a short-acting intravenous pain killer such as alfentanil 1000 mcg can be given. Using this anesthetic agent requires a pulse oximeter since it depresses respiration.
3. The needle guide is placed alongside the linear transrectal transducer. The guide and the transducer are covered with a sterile condom.
4. The transducer is inserted, and the target site identified. The biopsy guide marks are displayed on the screen.

5. The biopsy device, usually a needle attached to a biopsy gun, is inserted until it can be seen at the rectal edge of the mass. The gun is then fired. Three passes with the obtainment of satisfactory material are made from each suspect site.

Additional random passes are made in the superior central or inferior portion of each side of the gland. This procedure is known as a sextant biopsy.

Transperineal Approach (Fig. 35-6)

1. The patient is placed in the lithotomy position.
2. A linear array transducer is placed within the rectum until the lesion can be seen.
3. The perineal area is cleansed with antiseptic, and local anesthesia is injected. Premedication with Demerol and Valium is useful.
4. When the lesion has been identified and biopsy guide markers have been placed on the screen, a needle is inserted through the perineum. It can readily be seen within the mass.
5. Either an aspiration or biopsy technique for obtaining tissue is used.

Following either procedure, blood pressure and pulse are taken since hemorrhage is a possible complication. Infection on a delayed basis may occur following a transrectal biopsy in about 1 in 400 patients. It is expected that blood will be seen mixed with the stool, urine, or sperm following the procedure for 48 hours. In 2 percent of patients this can continue for up to 4 weeks. Severe bleeds are extremely rare.

◆ PATHOLOGY

Cancer of the Prostate

The typical cancer of the prostate is echopenic and located in the peripheral zone. Echopenic areas in the central zone are common and usually of little significance. Between 10 and 20 percent of echopenic areas in the peripheral zone prove to be carcinoma on biopsy. Cancers can also occur in areas that look normal on ultrasound.

Color flow Doppler shows slightly increased flow in the vicinity of prostatic cancer and in areas of prostatitis.

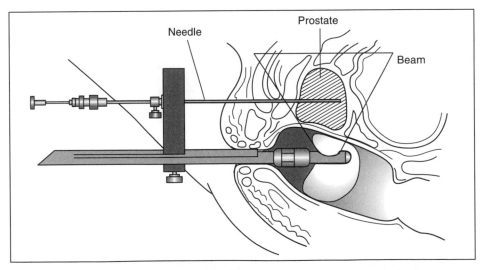

FIGURE 35-6. Transperineal biopsy technique. While the transducer is in the rectum, a device is introduced that allows the needle to penetrate the perineum along a preplanned route so that it ends up in the lesion. If the patient has had the rectum removed, as in an abdoperineal resection, the procedure is performed placing a small footprint transducer on the perineum. A transducer needle guide is used and the biopsy is performed under ultrasound control.

A deformed prostatic outline at the site of the presumed cancer is evidence of capsular invasion. Involvement of the seminal vesicles is much less obvious but more important in predicting inoperability and poor prognosis. Seminal vesicle invasion is likely if the tumor extends to the edge of the seminal vesicle.

Carcinoma of the prostate may spread into pelvic or para-aortic lymph nodes. Enlargement of these nodes can occasionally be seen with ultrasound.

Staging

Staging in carcinoma of the prostate is important in indicating the type of therapy (Fig. 35-7).

Stage A. A cancer incidentally found in the pathologic material obtained during a transurethral resection of the prostate (TURP).

Stage B. A cancer discovered because there is a nodule felt on digital examination. The mass is confined to the prostate.

Stage C. A cancer that has extended through the capsule of the prostate or into the seminal vesicles.

Stage D. A prostate cancer with distant metastases.

Stages C and D cannot be treated with local excision and are treated with chemotherapy or radiotherapy.

The TNM staging techniques are increasingly replacing this staging technique. Staging is by *Tumor*, *Node*, and *Metastasis*. Tumor extent is judged by size and the presence of capsular and terminal vesicle invasion.

Prostatic Calculi (Corpora Amylacea)

High-level echoes in the prostate represent calculi whether or not there is acoustic shadowing. Calculi typically form in a winglike pattern in the area between the central and peripheral zones or along the urethra. Central zone calculi have no clinical significance except that they may resemble a neoplasm on palpation.

Peripheral zone calculi are associated with prostatitis.

Benign Prostatic Hypertrophy

The central zone of the prostate is enlarged in benign prostatic hypertrophy. Typically, the central zone is evenly echogenic, but a very varied texture may be seen.

The gland is spherically enlarged, exceeding a volume of 20 g, possibly reaching a volume of over 100 g. The prostate may protrude into the bladder (middle lobe enlargement); the enlargement may develop toward the rectum. With larger volumes, the urethra is compressed and the bladder enlarges. Obstructive hydronephrosis may develop. Residual urine is present following voiding.

The condition is usually treated by TURP. When a patient has had a TURP, there is a U-shaped defect at the bladder where the urethra enters the prostate.

Transabdominal scanning usually permits volume estimations. If the sagittal length cannot be assessed, a transrectal scan may be needed.

Prostatic Abscess

A cystic area is seen within the central zone that may contain low-level echoes when a prostatic abscess is present.

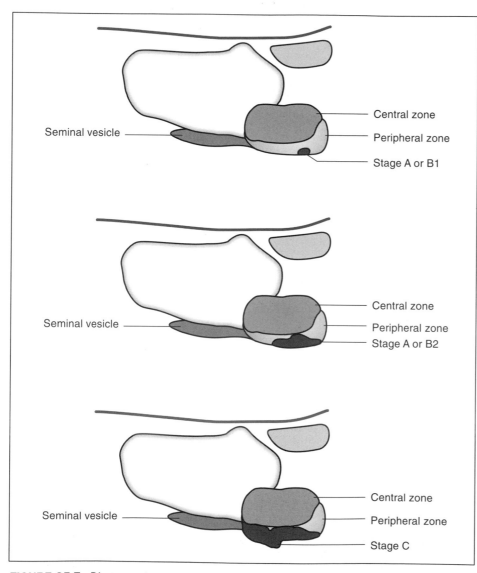

FIGURE 35-7. Diagram showing staging of prostate cancer. Top: Stage A is a cancer incidentally discovered when a transurethral resection of the prostate is performed. Middle: Stage B is a cancer confined to the prostate but palpable. Bottom: In Stage C, there is capsular or seminal vesicle invasion. Stage C lesions have a poor prognosis and are generally not surgically resected.

Prostatitis

With chronic prostatitis there are echogenic areas in the peripheral zone. Sometimes actual calcification is present in the peripheral zone. In acute prostatitis echopenic areas in the peripheral zone are seen. The ejaculatory ducts may be dilated and filled with calculi. Focal prostatitis may cause an area of decreased echoes in the central or peripheral zone that can be mistaken for cancer.

Seminal Vesicle Cyst

A cyst may develop in the seminal vesicles. It is an embryologic remnant and may become infected. Such cysts are often associated with absence of one kidney.

Infertility

Absence of sperm (azoospermia) has various causes. In one form there is blockage of the ejaculating ducts or congenital absence of the seminal vesicles and vas deferens. This deformity is easily seen by transrectal ultrasound.

⭐ PITFALLS

1. The lateral border of the peripheral zone on the dependent side may have an echopenic rim suggestive of neoplasm. When the patient is turned onto the opposite side, this area disappears.
2. A small postero-lateral echopenic area is present adjacent to the peripheral zone on either side. This represents the neurovascular body and is a normal structure (see Fig. 35-2). Color flow will show venous structures within.
3. Too high a gain or reverberation artifact may cause an echopenic neoplasm to be overlooked. Alter the position of the probe in relation to the rectal wall to change the position of the reverberation artifact.
4. Gas can obscure portions of the prostate if there is fecal material present. A repeat study after a Fleet enema is required. Try reinserting the probe first.
5. An echopenic area at the apex may represent smooth muscle. It will disappear if the patient performs a Valsalva maneuver.
6. Seminal vesicle dilation may occur as a normal variant. Look for evidence of obstruction of the ejaculatory ducts or asymmetry between the two seminal vesicles before passing it off as normal.
7. Much peripheral zone calcification can obscure echopenic areas located more centrally.

❓ WHERE ELSE TO LOOK

1. If the prostate is enlarged owing to benign prostatic hypertrophy:
   a. Look at the kidneys to exclude obstructive hydronephrosis.
   b. Check the bladder size before and after voiding and calculate the postvoid residual by using the following formula:

   $$\text{Length} \times \text{Width} \times \text{Height} \times 2$$

2. If carcinoma of the prostate is suspected:
   a. Look for evidence of capsular or seminal vesicle invasion.
   b. Look for pelvic and para-aortic adenopathy.

   In particular, make sure that the mass does not involve the neurovascular bundles since these structures control potency (see Fig. 35-2).

SELECTED READING

Dahnert, W. F., et al. Prostatic evaluation by transrectal sonography with histopathologic correlation: The echopenic appearance of early carcinoma. *Radiology* 158:97–102, 1986.

Littrup, P. J., and Sparschu, R. Transrectal ultrasound and prostate cancer risks. *Cancer* 75:1805–1813, 1995.

Neumaier, C. E., Martinoli, C., Derchi, L. E., Silvestri, E., and Rosenberg, I. Normal prostate gland: Examination with color Doppler US. *Radiology* 196:453–457, 1995.

Sanders, R. C. State of the art in prostate ultrasound. *Ultrasound Quart* 9:171–180, 1991.

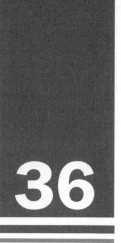
POSSIBLE INVASIVE RECTAL WALL MASS OR ANAL SPHINCTER BREAK

ROGER C. SANDERS

◆≫ THE CLINICAL PROBLEM

The anus and the rectal wall can be seen from a probe inserted into the vagina or rectum. Rectal wall neoplasms may be treated with local resection if a tumor has not invaded beyond the anatomic components of the rectal wall. If a mass invades the perirectal region, however, local excision is no longer possible. Transrectal ultrasound has proved the most reliable way of determining whether the tumor is invasive beyond the intestinal wall. Only tumors arising in the most distal 10 to 12 cm of the rectum close to the anus can be examined. If they lie at a higher level, they cannot be reached with transrectal equipment.

If the muscles that surround the anus are damaged, fecal incontinence ensues. These muscles can be seen well with endovaginal ultrasound. Fistula in ano with abscess development in the perianal area is quite common; both fistula with abscess formation and muscle breaks can be visualized with perianal ultrasound.

ANATOMY

The wall of the rectum consists of five alternating echogenic and echopenic layers and it is only 2 to 3 mm thick (Fig. 36-1).

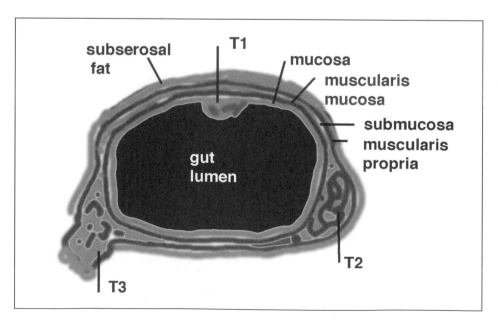

FIGURE 36-1. The five layers of the rectal intestinal wall can be seen. Both the muscularis mucosa and muscularis propria are echopenic. Tumors are staged by their site in relation to the components to the gut wall. T1 tumors are confined to the mucosa and muscularis mucosa. T2 tumors have not breached the muscularis propria and T3 tumors have extended into the subserosal fat. Layer 1, Echogenic—mucosa and transducer main bang; Layer 2, Hypoechoic—mucosa; Layer 3, Hyperechoic—submucosa; Layer 4, Hypoechoic—muscularis propria; Layer 5, Hyperechoic—perirectal fat.

1. The inner echogenic layer represents the *transducer interface* and *mucosa.*
2. An echopenic ring represents the *muscularis mucosa.*
3. A central echogenic layer represents the *submucosa.*
4. An outer echolucent area is the *muscularis propria.*
5. An outer echogenic area is *perirectal fat.*

Landmark information about neighboring structures is difficult using the endorectal probe. If the patient is a male the prostate and seminal vesicle are visible. In the female the cervix and vagina are somewhat useful as landmarks.

Two muscles are seen at the level of the anus. The internal sphincter is a well-defined echopenic ring around the anus and proximal rectum. It is 2 to 3 mm thick. The external sphincter is less well defined with a number of internal echoes. The external sphincter is 5 to 8 mm thick. The external sphincter is the primary muscle of continence control. The puborectalis muscle forms a sling around the anus and blends with the external sphincter. It is located about 2 cm from the anal margin (Fig. 36-2) and connects to the pubis.

▨ TECHNIQUE

Vaginal Approach

In female patients, the anus can be conveniently investigated from the vagina. An end-firing endovaginal probe pointed posteriorly shows the anus and rectum. With the transducer in the transverse axis, the probe is angled acutely toward the anus and gradually moved cranially to see the remainder of the rectum. Sagittal views of the muscles are then obtained.

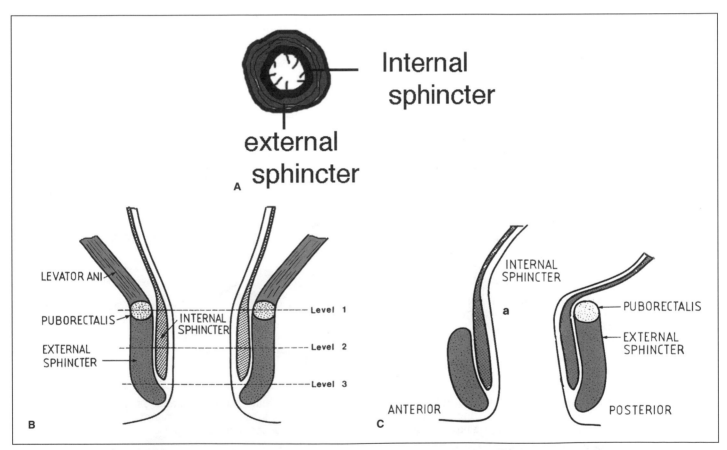

FIGURE 36-2. Internal and external sphincters. (**A**) Transverse view of the anal sphincter. The internal sphincter is a well-defined echopenic structure. The external sphincter has a more streaky appearance. (**B, C**) Coronal and sagittal views of the external and internal sphincters showing the site of the puborectalis muscle.

Rectal Approach

In males, an intrarectal approach is necessary. Ideally, a probe with a 360-degree rotating transducer is used. The sonologist feels the rectum so he or she has an idea where the mass is. The transducer, which should be at a minimum 5 MHz and preferably 7.5 MHz, is covered with a condom (see Chapter 35). The patient is placed in the left-side-down position (left decubitus). A transrectal probe is inserted into the anus. Filling the water bath around the transrectal transducer is worthwhile since the mucosal structures are so superficial. Giving exact information about the level and whether the mass is left or right, anterior or posterior, requires continuous knowledge of where the transducer face is. Most transducers have a groove on the stem which lets you know where the transducer face is. Label images by level in relation to the anus and in a clockwise fashion.

PATHOLOGY

Rectal Approach

CANCER OF THE RECTUM. Tumors are seen as complex, basically echopenic masses. Grading changes management. If the tumor is confined to the mucosa (T1), only the echopenic layer deep to the transducer-mucosa interface will be involved. If the tumor extends through the muscularis mucosa, but is confined by the outer echolucent area, the muscularis propria, it is graded T2 and can be surgically resected. Grading changes again if the tumor extends into the outer echogenic layer, the perirectal fat (T3), or if malignant nodes are present. Confirmatory evidence of malignant invasion is the presence of small malignant nodes. False-positive examinations may occur owing to perirectal inflammation.

Color flow may be helpful in the examination of malignant tumors. A low-resistance Doppler flow pattern has been found in neoplasms, whereas in benign tumors, a high-resistance pattern has been seen.

LYMPH NODES. Small lymph nodes are often seen deep to the mucosa. Neoplastic nodes are echopenic. Inflammatory nodes are echogenic. Benign nodes are oval shaped with an echogenic center.

INFLAMMATION. Inflammatory masses can have a similar appearance to tumors. They can invade through the various layers of the intestinal wall. A marked increase in vascularity will be seen on color flow.

VILLOUS ADENOMA. Villous adenoma are the most common tumors seen in the rectum. They have a similar acoustic appearance to rectal cancer. Most villous adenoma do not invade the muscularis propria even though they may be large. Occasionally, villous adenoma are confusing and cannot be distinguished from malignant tumors.

Anal

ANAL SPHINCTER BREAK. If an anal sphincter break is present, transverse views of the internal anal sphincter will show it to be incomplete with the circle broken at one point (Fig. 36-3). Usually, this is a result of childbirth and delivery trauma. The external sphincter is more important in controlling continence than the internal sphincter. There is usually a break in the external sphincter as well as the internal sphincter. The puborectal muscle may also be lax and deficient when there is incontinence.

FISTULA IN ANO. Fistulas and abscesses in the region of the anus are commonplace and occur particularly in association with underlying diseases such as Crohn's disease, diabetes, and trauma. The tracks related to the abscesses can be seen with ultrasound. A line between the two sphincters or involvement of the sphincter itself is seen. Abscess formation can occur and appears as an echopenic mass with internal echoes and an irregular border.

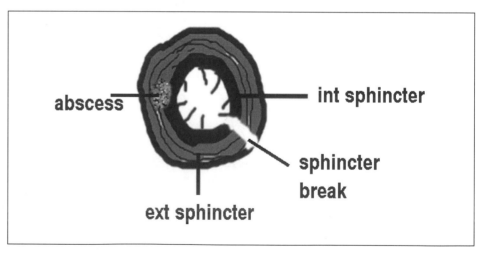

FIGURE 36-3. Transverse view of the anus showing an abscess related to a fistula in ano located between the external and internal sphincters and a break in the external and internal sphincter walls which causes incontinence.

PITFALLS

1. It is easy to get disoriented and not appreciate the level you are viewing with a standard transrectal probe. Without a 360-degree angle probe, tissue can be displaced and it may be hard to be certain whether you are examining a fresh area.

2. It may be difficult to appreciate whether or not the muscularis propria is intact if the tumor is large since the borders may be a good distance from the transducer.

3. Inflammation may give a false impression of tumor spread.

4. When the external sphincter is abnormal, the gap is homogeneous and echogenic, compared with the normal well-structured tissue. Certain normal structures around the sphincters may appear similar, such as the anococcygeal muscle and the anterior perineum.

5. When the patient is in the left lateral decubitus position, structures on the right side may appear asymmetric, compared with those on the left side. This asymmetry is due to the dependent position of the structure. Turning the patient to either the prone or the supine position should cause the asymmetry to disappear.

6. If a stricture is present, it may not be possible to image the rectal wall with an intrarectal probe. A transvaginal probe may well give information in such cases.

7. Gas may interfere with the visualization of right-sided tumors in the rectal wall if the patient is examined in the left-side-down position. Turn the patient into the opposite decubitus position and reexamine if this problem is encountered.

WHERE ELSE TO LOOK

1. If the tumor is extending beyond the rectal wall, a look at the upper abdomen for liver metastases and para-aortic nodes is helpful if it has not already been performed.

2. Consider looking at the abdomen for Crohn's disease (see Chapter 30) if a fistula in ano is present.

Selected Reading

Bachmann Nielsen, M., Pedersen, J. F., Hauge, C., Rasmussen, O. O., and Christiansen, J. Endosonography of the anal sphincter: Findings in healthy volunteers. *AJR* 157:1199–1202, 1991.

Hashimoto, B. E., Kramer, D. J., and Wiitala, L. Applications of ultrasound of the rectum and anus. *Ultrasound Quart* 13:179–196, 1995.

Hussain, S. M., Stoker, J., Schouten, W. R., Hop, W. C. J., and Lameris, J. S. Fistula in ano: Endoanal sonography versus endoanal MR imaging in classification. *Radiology* 200:475–481, 1996.

Joosten, F. B. M., Jansen, J. B. M. J., Joosten, H. J. M., and Rosenbusch, G. Staging of rectal carcinoma using MR double surface coil, MR endorectal coil, and intrarectal ultrasound: Correlation with histopathologic findings. *J Comput Assist Tomog* 19:752–758, 1995.

Rifkin, M. D. Endorectal ultrasound of the rectal wall. *Semin Ultrasound, CT MR* 8:424–431, 1987.

37

UNEXPLAINED HEMATOCRIT DROP

Rule Out Perinephric Hematoma; Possible Perinephric Mass

ROGER C. SANDERS

SONOGRAM ABBREVIATIONS

Ao   Aorta

Du   Duodenum

IVC   Inferior vena cava

K   Kidney

L   Liver

P   Pancreas
Ps   Psoas muscle

QL   Quadratus lumborum muscle

KEY WORDS

Anticoagulant. Drug that increases the time needed for blood to clot; used in treatment of pulmonary emboli and myocardial infarcts. Control of dosage is not always easy, and bleeding may ensue if there is overdosage.

Gerota's Fascia. Tissue plane around the kidney that includes the adrenals and much fat; important in the localization of hematomas and abscesses.

Hematocrit. A measurement of blood concentration; indicates the amount of blood in the body.

Hemophilia. Hereditary bleeding disorder seen in males. Those affected have a particular tendency to bleed into joints and the muscles in the retroperitoneum.

Retroperitoneum. Part of the body posterior to the peritoneum; includes the kidney and the pancreas, as well as many muscles in the paraspinous area.

Urinoma. Collection of urine outside the genitourinary tract.

 THE CLINICAL PROBLEM

The retroperitoneum is a clinically silent area where fluid collections that cannot be diagnosed by conventional radiographic techniques accumulate. Such collections are commonly hematomas, abscesses, or urinomas.

Hematomas

An unexplained hematocrit drop may indicate that a patient has bled internally. Often the site of the bleed is unclear to the clinician. Patients at risk for unexplained hematocrit drop are those who (1) have recently undergone an operation; (2) are taking anticoagulants; (3) have suffered a recent injury in, for example, a road accident or stabbing; or (4) have bleeding or clotting problems, such as hemophiliacs or leukemics.

The following are the most likely sites of asymptomatic hematomas:

1. In the abdominal wall around an incision
2. Deep to an incision
3. In a site where fluid collects adjacent to a surgical site (e.g., in the cul-de-sac, paracolic gutters, or subhepatic space)
4. Around the spleen (perisplenic), liver (perihepatic), or kidney (perinephric)
5. In the retroperitoneum (this site is particularly likely in patients with no previous injury, such as those on anticoagulants or suffering from bleeding problems)
6. In the iliopsoas muscles, particularly in hemophiliacs

Hematomas may develop into abscesses; they are a good culture medium for bacteria. Expansion of a hematoma on subsequent sonograms suggests that the lesion is infected. Normally hematomas slowly retract unless there has been rebleeding.

Urinomas (Uriniferous Pseudocysts)

Urinomas develop mainly in patients who have had trauma, who have passed a renal stone, or who have had operations such as a renal transplant. They may be asymptomatic and may be found years after the original process that caused them occurred. It is useful to follow the progress of urinomas that occur after an operation because they usually resolve spontaneously.

Abscesses

Abscesses quite commonly occur in the retroperitoneum. They may be relatively asymptomatic, particularly in the psoas muscle, presenting with fever rather than with localized symptoms.

ANATOMY

Retroperitoneum

In practice, the retroperitoneum is a term used to describe the area that includes the kidney; the psoas, iliacus, and quadratus lumborum muscles; and the presacral area. Although the pancreas is technically within the retroperitoneum, this organ is not usually included in a retroperitoneal survey (Fig. 37-1).

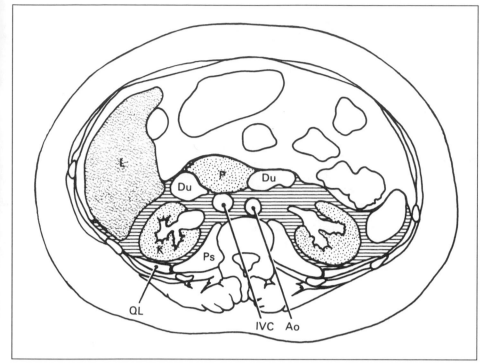

FIGURE 37-1. The cross-hatched area represents the retroperitoneum. Large structures in the retroperitoneum include the psoas muscles, quadratus lumborum muscles, kidneys, and pancreas.

Spaces Around the Kidney

The area around the kidney is traversed by several fibrous sheaths that form natural barriers to the passage of fluid and act as a guide for the site of origin of a collection. The retroperitoneum is divided into the following areas:

1. The *anterior pararenal space*. A space in front of the kidney that communicates with the opposite side around the pancreas.
2. The *perinephric space* within Gerota's fascia. This space may be open-ended inferiorly and encloses the kidneys, fat, and the adrenal glands.
3. The *posterior pararenal space*. This space extends behind the kidney into the lateral aspects of the abdominal wall. The fascial planes can be seen on a good-quality sonogram in an obese patient when they are outlined by fat.
4. The *psoas muscles*. These muscles lie lateral to the spine and widen inferiorly (Fig. 37-2). They eventually join the iliacus muscles that arise on the anterior aspect of the iliac crest to form a joint muscle in the pelvis (see Fig. 37-2).

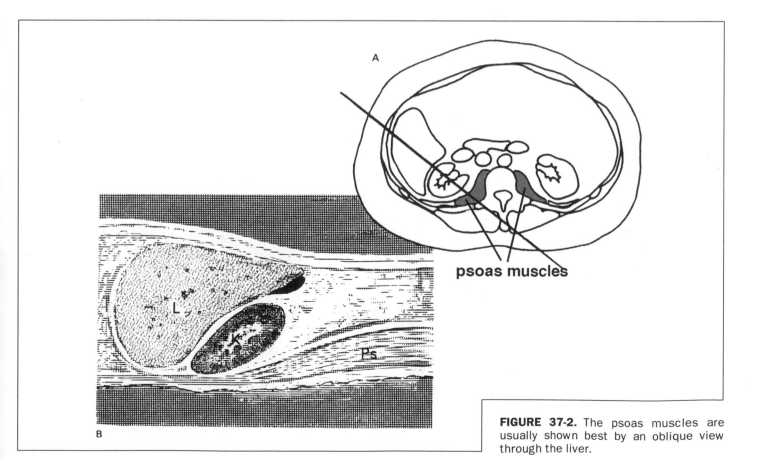

psoas muscles

FIGURE 37-2. The psoas muscles are usually shown best by an oblique view through the liver.

5. The *quadratus lumborum muscles*. These muscles lie posterior to the kidney (see Fig. 37-1) and are often surprisingly sonolucent, giving the impression that a collection is present. If one looks on the opposite side, a similar sonolucent area will be seen.

TECHNIQUE

Perinephric Area

As a rule, the prone or decubitus position gives the best view of the retroperitoneal areas around the kidneys down to the level of the iliac crest.

Psoas Muscles

The psoas and iliacus muscles may be visible on supine and supine oblique views, but gas may obscure the area (see Fig. 37-2). It is usually best to perform a prone oblique decubitus view looking through the kidneys at the psoas muscles and at the area between the aorta and the inferior vena cava. This view is similar to the one used to look at the adrenal glands.

Presacral Area

Visualizing the region anterior to the upper portion of the sacrum can be very difficult. A large bladder may be helpful in the supine position. Deep pressure using a linear array can displace the gut away from this area and allow views of the lower aorta and of the presacral area.

◆ PATHOLOGY

Hematoma

Sonographic Appearances

Most hematomas in this area are sonolucent but may alternatively be evenly echogenic or contain echogenic clumps (Fig. 37-3). Fluid-fluid levels may develop (see Fig. 37-3). If the hematoma occurs following a penetrating injury, there may be visible distortion of an organ, for example, the kidney outline.

Location

SUBCAPSULAR. If the hematoma is adjacent to the kidney in the subcapsular location, it will have circular superior and inferior margins, and the shape of the kidney will be flattened (Fig. 37-4).

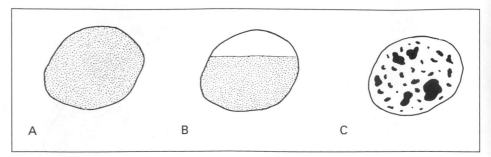

FIGURE 37-3. Patterns of hematoma. Fluid-fluid levels are seen when bleeding occurs into a fluid-filled structure (i.e., a renal or ovarian cyst). Some hematomas are evenly echogenic, while others contain clumps of echoes.

PERINEPHRIC. If the hematoma is in Gerota's fascia, it will usually be located posteromedially and will extend above and well below the level of the kidney.

POSTERIOR PARARENAL. A hematoma in the posterior pararenal space extends up the lateral walls of the abdomen and displaces the kidney anteriorly.

ANTERIOR PARARENAL. Hematomas in the anterior pararenal space lie anterior to the kidney and may extend medially into the region of the pancreas.

INTRAMUSCULAR. A hematoma in the psoas muscle forms an asymmetric bulge within that muscle, displacing the kidney laterally. It tracks down into the pelvis toward the iliacus muscle and the inguinal ligament (Fig. 37-5).

A hematoma secondary to deep cutting trauma (e.g., a stab wound) does not necessarily confine itself to the tissue planes described above. Scan the opposite side to check for symmetry.

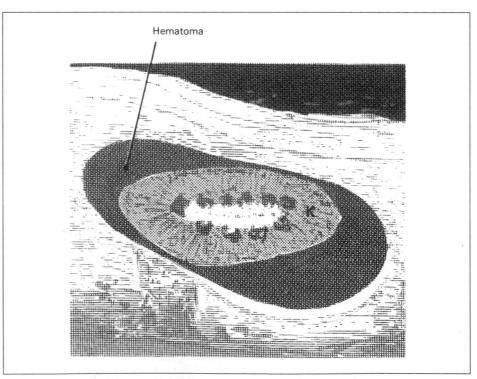

FIGURE 37-4. A subcapsular hematoma may be suggested when the border of the kidney is flattened and the capsular echogenic line is absent.

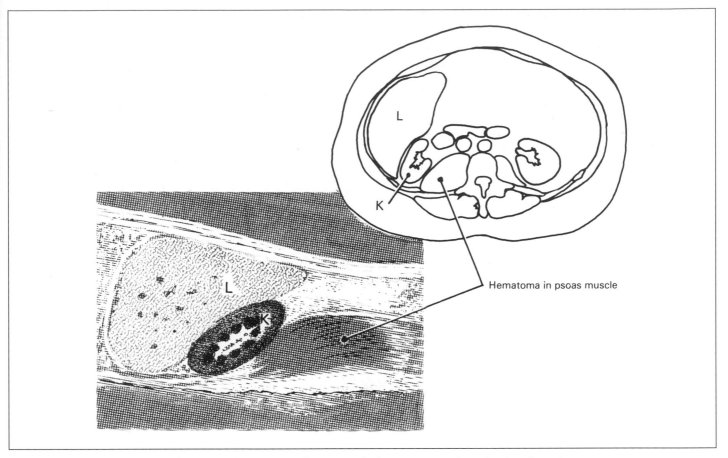

Hematoma in psoas muscle

FIGURE 37-5. Sonolucent area that expands the psoas muscle owing to a hematoma.

Abscesses

Abscesses develop in the same areas as hematomas and are difficult to distinguish from them sonographically. They may bulge more because they are not as well confined by the tissue planes, and evidence of a septum and loculation is more apparent. The borders of abscesses are usually more irregular.

Other Fluid Collections

Urinomas may develop around the kidney, usually within Gerota's fascia. These are echo-free collections.

★ PITFALLS

1. *Collection vs. shadowing.* Particularly in the prone position, it may be hard to distinguish between a true collection and rib shadowing. Attempts to view the suspect area in either the erect or the decubitus position are important. Alteration of the phase of respiration can help to clarify the issue.
2. *Echogenic hematoma.* At some stages in the course of its evolution a hematoma may be markedly echogenic. Do not miss it by scanning at too high a gain.
3. *Quadratus lumborum muscles.* The quadratus lumborum may be much less echogenic than other muscles and may mimic an abscess or hematoma. Comparison with the other side will show its true nature.

4. *Spleen vs. collection.* It may be difficult to distinguish between the spleen and a mass at the upper pole of the left kidney. The interface between these two organs may be seen better with a decubitus view or with the patient in an erect position. Angling up at a different phase of respiration is helpful.
5. *Gut vs. collection.* It is important not to mistake the stomach or colon for a mass in the retroperitoneal pararenal area. Such masses will be fluid filled. Check for peristalsis; if none is seen consider performing a high-water enema to be sure that the mass is not gut.
6. *Duodenum.* The duodenum may lie anterior to the right kidney in the subhepatic space, mimicking a perinephric collection. Real-time will show peristalsis when fluid is administered by mouth.

7. *Malrotated kidney vs. collection.* The pelvis of a malrotated kidney lies anterior to the right kidney and may mimic a collection in the subhepatic space. Careful real-time and color Doppler analysis will show that the renal vein, renal artery, and ureter enter the supposed collection.

8. *Psoas vs. masses.* In young patients or athletes the psoas muscles may be exceptionally prominent and may be mistaken for a mass; they will be symmetrically enlarged.

9. *Perinephric fat vs. mass.* In obese patients considerable perinephric fat may be present, forming a relatively echogenic rim around the kidneys. Do not mistake this for a pathologic process. It will be bilateral.

❓ WHERE ELSE TO LOOK

Psoas abscesses may track along the muscles into the hip (see Fig. 37-5). A subtle collection in the hip may be seen near the femoral head.

SELECTED READING

Hermann, G., Gilbert, M. S., and Abdelwahab, I. F. Hemophilia: Evaluation of musculoskeletal involvement with CT, sonography, and MR imaging. *AJR* 158:119–123, 1992.

King, A. D., Hine, A. L., McDonald, C., and Abrahams, P. The ultrasound appearance of the normal psoas muscle. *Clin Radiol* 48:316–318, 1993.

McClennan, B. L., Lee, J. K. T., and Peterson, R. R. Anatomy of the perirenal area. *Radiology* 158:555–557, 1986.

Molmenti, E. P., Balfe, D. M., Kanterman, R. Y., and Bennett, H. F. Anatomy of the retroperitoneum: Observations of the distribution of pathologic fluid collections. *Radiology* 200:95–103, 1996.

Raptopoulos, V., Kleinman, P. K., Marks, S., Jr., Snyder, M., and Silverman, P. M. Renal fascial pathway: Posterior extension of pancreatic effusions within the anterior pararenal space. *Radiology* 158:367–374, 1986.

POSSIBLE TESTICULAR MASS

Pain in the Testicle

ROGER C. SANDERS

SONOGRAM ABBREVIATIONS

AEp	Appendix epididymis
E, Ep	Epididymis
H	Hydrocele
N	Mass
MT	Mediastinum testis
S	Spermatocele
T	Testis
V	Varicocele

KEY WORDS

Appendix Epididymis. Portion of the epididymis that lies just superior to the testicle and is larger than the remainder of the epididymis.

Cryptorchidism (Undescended Testicle). Condition in which the testicles have not descended and lie either in the abdomen or in the groin. The latter is the site in 95 percent of cases. Such a testicle is more likely to become malignant.

Epididymis. Organ that lies posterior to the testicle in which the spermatozoa accumulate.

Epididymitis. Inflammation of the epididymis.

Hematocele. Blood filling the sac that surrounds the testicle.

Hydrocele. Distention of the sac that encloses the testicle with straw-colored fluid.

Mediastinum Testis. Linear fibrous structure in the center of the testicle.

Pampiniform Plexus. Group of veins that drain the testicle. They dilate and become tortuous when a varicocele is present.

Rete Testis. The tubules at the hilum of the testicle may become so large that they are visible as cysts. This is a normal variant finding.

Scrotum. Sac in which the testicle and epididymis lie.

Seminal Vesicles. Reservoirs for sperm located posterior to the bladder.

Serous. Term used to describe the thin, straw-colored fluid present within a cyst regardless of location (e.g., renal, thyroid, or ovarian cysts or hydrocele).

Spermatic Cyst (Spermatocele). Cyst along the course of the vas deferens containing sperm.

Testicle (Testis). Male gonad enclosed within the scrotum; it produces hormones that induce masculine features and spermatozoa production.

Tunica Albuginea. Membrane surrounding the testicle within the scrotum; may be the source of a cyst or adenoma.

Tunica Vaginalis. Membrane skirting the inner wall of the scrotum. Hydroceles form between the tunica albuginea and tunica vaginalis.

Varicocele. Dilated veins caused by obstruction of the venous return from the testicle. Varicoceles may be associated with infertility or left renal tumor.

Vas Deferens. Tube that connects the epididymis to the seminal vesicle.

THE CLINICAL PROBLEM

Mass

The testicle is superficial and therefore easily examined with high-frequency ultrasound. The detection of a small mass within the testicle is important because such a mass may be a malignancy. However, benign masses in the testicle occur. Although fluid within the scrotal sac is usually easily detected clinically, identification is difficult if the scrotal wall is thickened. An additional mass may be missed on palpation but revealed by ultrasound.

Testicular Pain

Ultrasound helps in the differential diagnosis of acute pain in a testicle. One can differentiate between the common causes: epididymitis, testicular torsion, testicular abscess, or orchitis. Doppler and color flow are particularly useful in making this distinction. Acute epididymitis may be followed by infection of the testicle (orchitis). Infarction of the testicle can occur following severe epididymitis.

Testicular Trauma

Trauma to the testicle is an ultrasonic emergency—rupture of the testicle requiring surgical repair has to be distinguished from a paratesticular hematoma (a hematocele). An unrepaired ruptured testicle atrophies and will not function.

Infertility

A common cause of male infertility is a varicocele. Most varicoceles are palpable, but if a man has unexplained infertility, an ultrasound study to exclude a varicocele that cannot be felt is worthwhile.

Undescended Testicle

Most testicles descend from the abdomen into the scrotum by 28 weeks of fetal life. If descent is arrested in the abdomen or the groin, there is an increased chance of tumor development. Surgeons move the undescended testicle into the scrotum in the first few years of life. Ultrasound can be of help in showing a testicle that cannot be felt within the groin, although those that lie deep in the abdomen cannot be detected with ultrasound.

ANATOMY

Testicle

The testicle is an ovoid, homogeneous, mildly echogenic structure (Fig. 38-1). The adult testicles are normally symmetric and approximately 4 cm × 3 cm in size. A central line within is termed the mediastinum testis.

A series of tubules radiate from the mediastinum testes into the testicle. Sometimes a vague echopenic region is seen. On other occasions visible tubules or even cysts can form in this area as a normal variant, known as "rete testis."

Epididymis

The tubular, slightly sonolucent structure lying posterosuperior to the testicle at the proximal end is termed the epididymis. The body of the epididymis varies in its position and sometimes lies lateral to the testicle. However, on occasions it lies posteriorly. The epididymis expands focally and superiorly to form the appendix epididymis. The testicular artery and the veins of the pampiniform plexus run along the lateral and posterior aspect of the testicle in the region of the epididymis and are not normally visible. The epididymis is an echopenic structure.

Scrotal Wall

The scrotal wall is an echopenic structure that surrounds the testicle and epididymis. The wall thickens with edema and infection. Two membranes called the tunica albuginea and tunica vaginalis form a double layer around the testicle. Fluid can accumulate between the two layers forming a hydrocele. A small amount of fluid is a common normal variant.

TECHNIQUE

A high-frequency linear array transducer gives good results since it shows superficial structures well. The testicle and the scrotum are supported by the examiner's hand or by a towel under the scrotum. Using a towel, the patient can retract the penis. The transducer is moved smoothly and slowly along the anterior aspect of the scrotum, first in the longitudinal axis and then in the transverse axis. Obtain a maximal length in both axes. A coronal view showing both testicles from the side simultaneously is an elegant way of demonstrating anatomy and is helpful in showing differences in echogenicity between the two testicles.

If a mass is palpable it must be identified on the image. This may require placing a finger on the posterior aspect of the mass while performing a scan from an anterior approach. A posterior scanning approach may be necessary with an anterior mass.

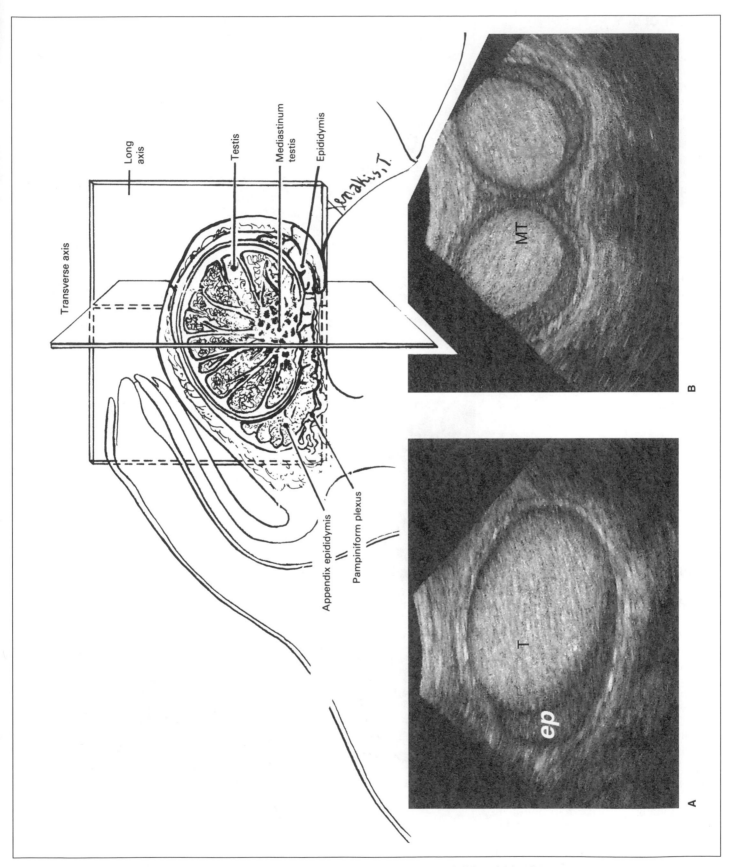

FIGURE 38-1. Diagram showing the normal structures visible within the scrotum. The mediastinum testis is only occasionally seen as an echogenic line. (**A**) Longitudinal axis view. (**B**) Transverse axis view.

PATHOLOGY

Tumors

Normally, the testicle is evenly echogenic. The most common testicular tumor, seminoma, is usually echopenic compared with the remaining testicular parenchyma. The tumor can be as small as 2 to 3 mm (Fig. 38-2). Embryonal cell tumors often show patchy echogenicity.

Teratomas are rare and may be multicystic. Metastases may occur.

Lymphoma, typically echopenic, may persist in the testicle when it has been eliminated elsewhere because chemotherapy often does not reach the testicle.

Benign Testicular Masses

Cysts are quite common within the testicle. Small echopenic masses on the border of the testicle are usually adenomas associated with the tunica. Small, hard, echogenic mobile structures between the tunicae may be palpable but are of no importance. They are scrotal calculi and may show shadowing.

Epididymitis

Acute

The epididymis in acute epididymitis is enlarged and more sonolucent than usual. The epididymis is locally tender.

Chronic

A chronically inflamed epididymis becomes thickened and focally echogenic and may contain calcification (Fig. 38-3).

Orchitis

Orchitis, infection of the testicle, may involve the entire testicle or be focal. The testicle is less echogenic in the involved area. Infarction and some seminomatous tumors may have an identical appearance. The scrotal wall is thickened with epididymitis and orchitis. Color flow shows increased vascularity in many small vessels.

Hydrocele

In hydrocele the testicle and the appendix epididymis are surrounded by fluid, which is usually sonolucent, unless blood (hematocele) is present (Fig. 38-4).

Occasionally hydroceles have a proteinaceous composition and are evenly echogenic. If septa are present and the wall of the fluid-filled area is thickened, the collection may be infected and pus filled (a pyocele). Pyoceles are very tender.

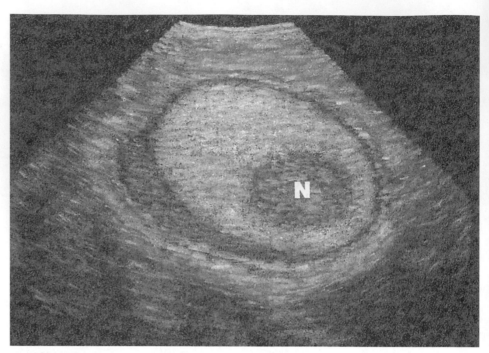

FIGURE 38-2. Intratesticular mass due to seminoma.

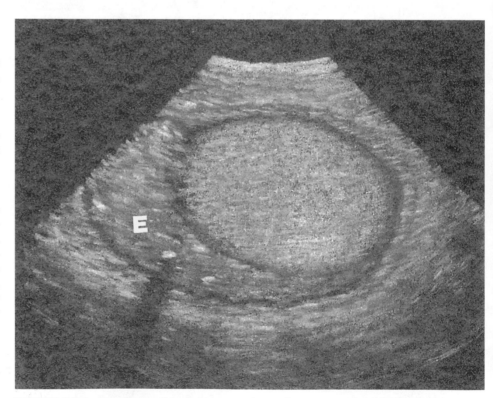

FIGURE 38-3. Enlargement and coarse echogenic texture of epididymis with acute and chronic epididymitis.

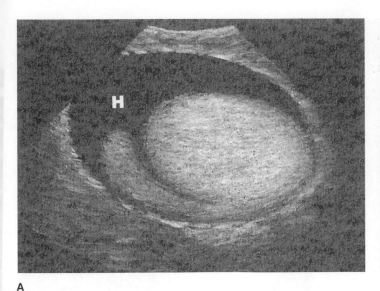

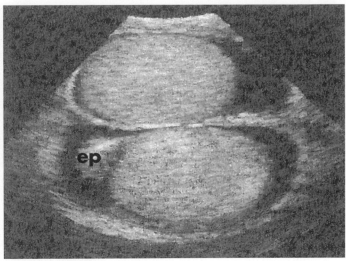

A   B

FIGURE 38-4. Hydrocele. (**A**) The hydrocele outlines the epididymis, which is normally difficult to see. (**B**) Coronal view shows fluid around both testicles and the head of the epididymis (ep).

Varicocele

Varicoceles are numerous tortuous curvilinear venous structures in the region of the epididymis that extend superior to the testicle toward the pubic symphysis (Fig. 38-5). They are always longer on the left than the right. A sizeable right varicocele raises the possibility of a renal tumor.

To demonstrate the dilated veins that form a varicocele, venous pressure must be increased by a Valsalva's maneuver, preferably with the examination performed in the erect position. The veins increase in size with the change in position. Color flow and Doppler show flow which reverses direction when the patient strains, indicating "incompetence" and absence of valves in the vein (see Fig. 38-5).

Testicular Torsion

Acute pain, occurring in the testicles, is most likely either due to twisting or torsion of the testicles or acute infection with epididymitis and orchitis. The distinction between these two problems is important because torsion is relieved by emergency surgery, whereas epididymitis is treated with antibiotics.

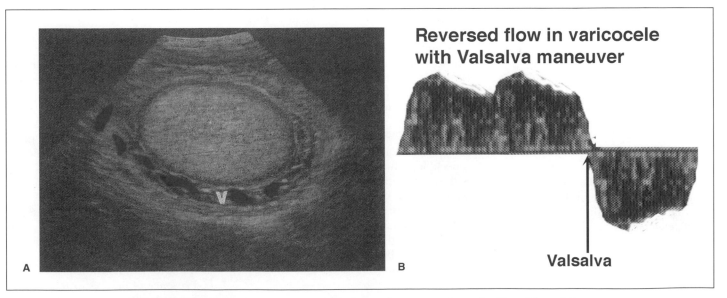

Reversed flow in varicocele with Valsalva maneuver

A   B   **Valsalva**

FIGURE 38-5. Varicocele. (**A**) A varicocele can be seen to be pulsatile with real-time and is composed of numerous veins with a diameter of at least 3 mm. (**B**) Doppler interrogation of the veins shows the venous flow reversing as intra-abdominal pressure increases when the Valsalva maneuver is performed.

Epididymitis and orchitis are treated with antibiotics. The window of opportunity to treat torsion is relatively small (8–12 hours). In acute torsion, the testicle enlarges and develops a mottled texture. As a rule, vascularity is maintained at the periphery, but is decreased or absent in the center. In some instances, torsion is not complete, so vascularity is maintained. In other instances, when there is complete torsion and a 360-degree twist of the cord, all vascularity to the testicle is absent. In this case the diagnosis is easy.

If torsion is untreated (chronic torsion), the texture of the testicle changes, becoming more echopenic and mottled. Secondary enlargement of the epididymis can occur.

Undescended Testicles

During the embryologic development of the genitourinary tract, the testicles descend from the region of the kidneys into a normal location. Arrested development may occur at any point. However, the usual "sticking point" occurs when the testicles are in the region of the inguinal ligament and pubic symphysis in an extra-abdominal location. At this site, undescended testicles can be visualized by ultrasound. They look like normal, malpositioned testicles but can be confused with nodes.

Spermatocele

A cystic structure found along the course of the vas deferens superior to the testicle or in the epididymis, a spermatocele is of little pathologic significance (Fig. 38-6).

Spermatoceles may be multiple. Epididymal cysts may be seen in the epididymis and may also represent sperm collections, but are likewise of no clinical significance.

Atrophic Testicle

An infarcted testicle becomes small and more echogenic. Color flow shows no vascularity within an atrophic testicle. Such testicles are at risk for tumor development.

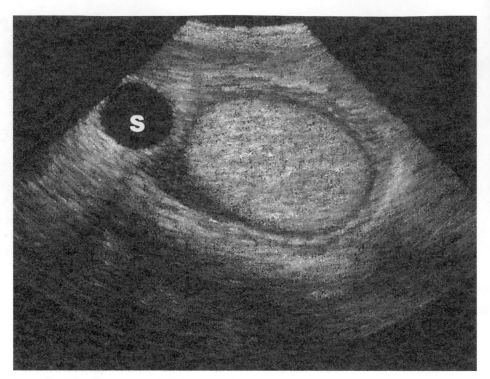

FIGURE 38-6. Spermatocele lying superior to the testicle.

Abscess

Abscesses may develop in the testicle or epididymis and are sonolucent with an echogenic, irregular border.

Hernias

In the fetus there is a connection between the abdomen and the scrotal sac known as the processus vaginalis. This connection may persist, allowing abdominal contents such as gut to descend into the scrotum. Hernias are recognized by the presence of peristalsis on real-time or by shadowing from air in the gut within the apparent mass (Fig. 38-7).

Testicular Trauma

A damaged scrotum almost always contains blood. Blood is generally echogenic with several different patterns. There are usually both echogenic and echo-free areas. The normal testicle has a smooth ovoid border. When the testicle is ruptured, the outline is irregular and there may be echopenic areas within. Sometimes a fracture line divides the testicle (Fig. 38-8).

✴ PITFALLS

1. *Scanning technique.* Scanning the testicle evenly and symmetrically can be difficult. Be sure that an apparent diminution in testicular size is not due to poor scanning technique.
2. *Mediastinum testis vs. echogenic mass.* Do not mistake the mediastinum testis for an echogenic mass.
3. *Node vs. undescended testicle.* It is easy to confuse a benign inflammatory node with an undescended testicle. Benign nodes have an echogenic center due to fat deposition.
4. *Position change for varicocele.* Varicoceles can be overlooked unless the position of the patient is stood up or Valsalva's maneuver is performed. Although varicoceles usually lie superior to the left testicle, they may lie lateral to the testicle.
5. *Hematoma vs. traumatized testicle.* Some blood collections can resemble testicles. Identify the two testicles by noting these features:
   a. Smooth ovoid outline
   b. Presence of mediastinum testis

c. Even echogenic texture. Carefully use the gain control to allow distinction between the testicle and hematoma texture.

d. Subtle vessels in the normal testicle, seen with power Doppler

6. *Infarct vs. focal orchitis vs. seminoma.* All three conditions can look similar. Color flow will show increased vascularity around areas of orchitis. Seminoma may contain flow within the center of the lesion. Infarcts show no flow.

7. *Previous surgery for varicocele.* When previous surgery has been performed, the varicocele does not disappear. However, the reversal of flow seen on Doppler with Valsalva's maneuver is no longer present.

8. *Rete testis.* The tubules that collect at the mediastinum testes may be so dilated that they appear as a group of cysts. This normal variant can be confused with an echopenic tumor if a low-quality system is used.

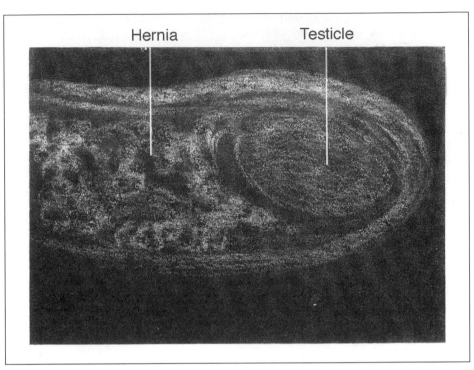

FIGURE 38-7. Hernia. The scrotal sac is almost filled with bowel and has a very unhomogeneous texture. Note the testicle at the inferior aspect of the hernia.

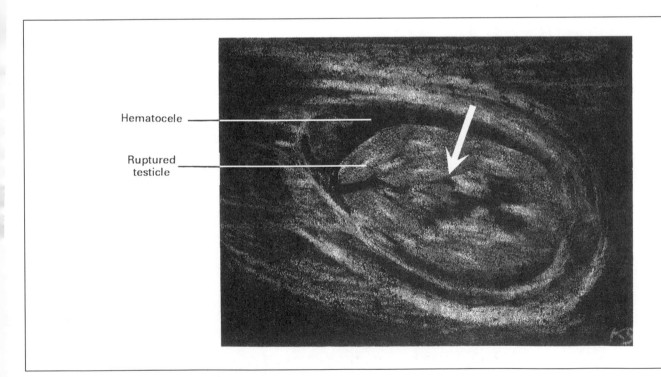

FIGURE 38-8. Fractured testicle following trauma. The arrow points to the fracture. The outline of the testicle is irregular, with tubules visible within the fluid (blood) around the testicle (i.e., a hematocele). The acoustic texture of the hematocele can be varied in echogenicity.

9. *Cleft vs. fracture.* A prominent vessel often normally traverses the testicle. Flow will be evident on real-time. This vessel could be mistaken for a fracture following testicular trauma, and it can cause shadowing over a portion of the testis that could suggest a carcinoma (the "two-tone" testis).

? WHERE ELSE TO LOOK

1. If a testicular tumor is found, look in the abdomen around the region of the renal hilum for possible nodal metastases.
2. If a varicocele is found on the right, look in the kidney for a renal tumor.

SELECTED READING

Dudiak, C. M., Venta, L. A., Olson, M. C., Posniak, H. V., and Salomon, C. G. Ultrasound of the scrotum. *Crit Rev Diagn Imag* 33:369–406, 1992.

Herbener, T. E. Ultrasound in the assessment of the acute scrotum. *J Clin Ultrasound* 24:405–421, 1996.

Langer, J. E. Ultrasound of the scrotum. *Semin Roentgenol* 28:5–18, 1993.

Middleton, W. D, and Bell, M. W. Analysis of intratesticular arterial anatomy with emphasis on transmediastinal arteries. *Radiology* 189:157–160, 1993.

Nicolaou, S., and Cooperberg, P. L. The two-tone testis due to refractive shadowing of the intratesticular artery. *J Ultrasound Med* 14:963–965, 1995.

39 POSSIBLE ADRENAL MASS

IRMA WHEELOCK TOPPER

SONOGRAM ABBREVIATIONS

Ad	Adrenal gland
Ao	Aorta
Ca	Celiac artery
Cr	Crus
IVC	Inferior vena cava
K	Kidney
L	Liver
LRa	Left renal artery
LRv	Left renal vein
Pv	Portal vein
RRa	Right renal artery
RRv	Right renal vein
S	Spine
SMa	Superior mesenteric artery
Sp	Spleen
Spv	Splenic vein

KEY WORDS

Adenoma. Benign tumor of the adrenal cortex seen with Cushing's syndrome; may be bilateral.

Cortex. Portion of adrenal tissue that secretes steroid hormones.

Cushing's Syndrome. Caused by hypersecretion of hormones from the adrenal cortex. An adrenal tumor or excess stimulation of the pituitary may be responsible.

Hyperplasia. Enlargement of adrenal glands.

Medulla. Central tissue of adrenal glands—under the control of the sympathetic nervous system.

Neuroblastoma. Malignant adrenal mass occurring in children.

Pheochromocytoma. Benign adrenal tumor that secretes hormones that elevate blood pressure.

 THE CLINICAL PROBLEM

Conditions that should direct the examiner's attention to the adrenal glands are the following:

1. Intermittent hypertension, flushing, and increased sweating—symptoms of pheochromocytoma.
2. Lung cancer. Thirty percent of lung cancer patients have metastatic disease in the adrenal glands.
3. Abnormal laboratory test results. Some adrenal pathology, such as pheochromocytoma, may be suggested by laboratory studies. Ultrasound can help by determining whether one or both glands are diseased.
4. Neuroblastoma. Children with a neuroblastoma often present with a palpable abdominal mass.

Except in children (whose adrenal glands are more prominent than those of adults) and in thin adults, ultrasound is not the primary imaging modality for suspected adrenal pathology; however, incidental discovery of enlargement of one or both adrenal glands can be a significant contribution to a patient's workup.

ANATOMY

Both glands are normally pyramidal in shape (Fig. 39-1). They are located in the retroperitoneum superior and anteromedial to the upper pole of the kidneys. The right gland lies posterior to the inferior vena cava and anterior to the crus of the diaphragm (Fig. 39-2). The left gland lies between the spleen, the upper pole of the kidney, and the aorta and behind the tail of the pancreas.

Adrenal glands can be found in 80 to 95 percent of neonatal patients, with a lower success rate later in life. Neonatal glands are approximately one third as big as the infant kidney. In the neonate, there is an echogenic center to the gland, which persists to a lesser extent throughout the individual's life. The lack of perinephric fat and the small size of the neonatal patient allow the use of a higher-frequency probe.

◨ TECHNIQUE

Normal adrenal glands are not easy to see. Their small size (approximately 4 cm × 2.5 cm × 0.5 cm) and their acoustic texture make the glands difficult to differentiate from surrounding tissue. Using the liver as an acoustic window with current high-resolution ultrasound equipment, the right adrenal gland can be imaged in 90 percent of patients. The success rate on the left is reduced to approximately 75 percent, owing to the proximity of the stomach and bowel.

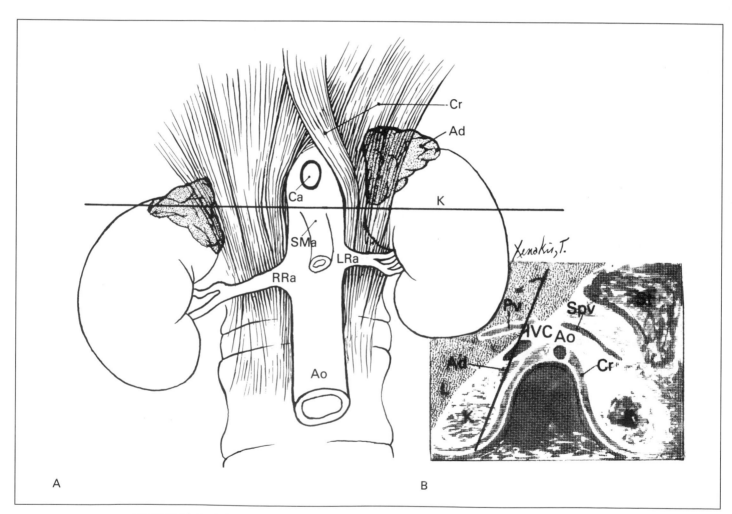

FIGURE 39-1. Adrenal glands. (**A**) The adrenals are pyramidal glands located superior and anteromedial to the kidneys. (**B**) The line illustrates the transducer angle used to show the right adrenal gland through the inferior vena cava.

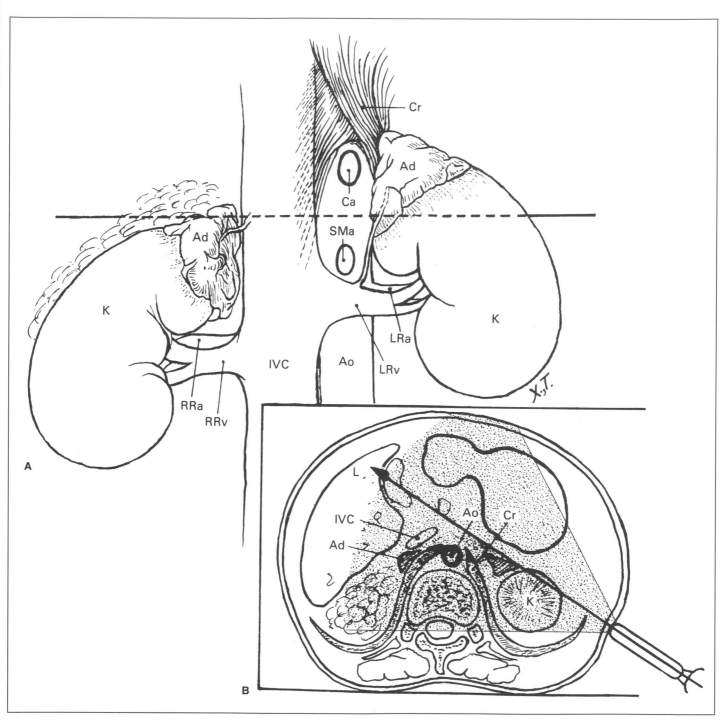

FIGURE 39-2. Right adrenal. (**A**) The right adrenal lies posterior to the inferior vena cava (IVC) and anterolateral to the crus of the diaphragm. (**B**) Transverse view showing the appropriate transducer angle needed to show the left adrenal through the left kidney. Note that the right adrenal vein comes directly off the IVC, while the left adrenal vein takes off from the left renal vein.

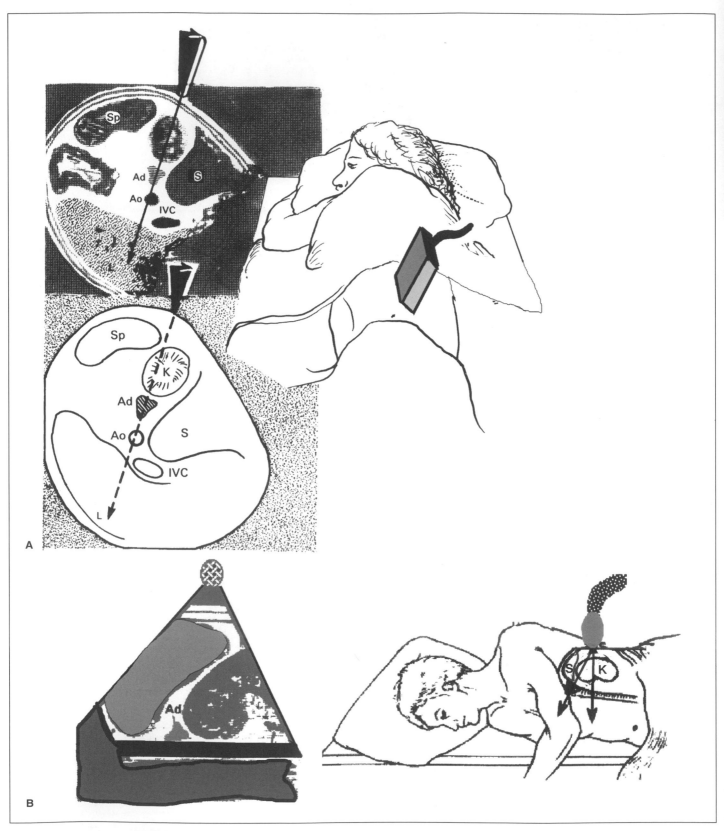

FIGURE 39-3. Demonstrating the left adrenal. (**A**) In a longitudinal axis, adjust the scanning plane to align the upper pole of the left kidney with the long axis of the aorta. (**B**) Then, angle the transducer slightly in an anterior-to-posterior fashion to visualize the left adrenal gland. The resulting longitudinal section should show the adrenal at the junction of the spleen, aorta, and upper pole of the left kidney.

Left Adrenal Gland

The left adrenal is best approached with the patient in the right lateral decubitus (left-side-up) position (Fig. 39-3). Longitudinal views are most helpful.

1. Select the highest-frequency transducer that can be used.
2. Adjust the gain and/or power output controls to obtain good acoustic texture in the spleen. It is extremely important to avoid an overgained image.
3. Scanning longitudinally, locate the intercostal space that allows visualization of the upper pole of the left kidney and the spleen.
4. Maintain that longitudinal orientation and rock the transducer in an anterior-posterior fashion until the aorta can also be viewed longitudinally.
5. The left adrenal should appear as a triangular area where the spleen, the upper pole of the left kidney, and the aorta can be imaged simultaneously. Set the electronic focus at this level. The normal gland has concave or straight margins.

Right Adrenal Gland

The right adrenal can usually be imaged in the traditional transverse and longitudinal views with the patient supine, using the liver as an acoustic window. If this is unsuccessful because of liver size or position, you may reverse the technique described for the left adrenal.

1. Initiate scanning transversely from a right lateromedial approach perpendicular to the medial borders of the liver and kidney and the right margin of the spine (Fig. 39-4).
2. Enlarge the field size to allow visualization of small structures at the level of the adrenal.
3. Select the highest-frequency transducer possible for adequate penetration. Fine resolution is important, but you must be able to penetrate the liver well. Adjust the focal depth of the probe to the level of the adrenal.
4. Adjust the gain or output controls so that liver texture is uniform throughout the field.
5. Start scanning transversely in the region of the middle to upper pole of the kidney. Maintaining the transverse orientation, identify the pertinent normal anatomy (i.e., kidney, liver, crus of the diaphragm). Image the anatomy transversely moving the

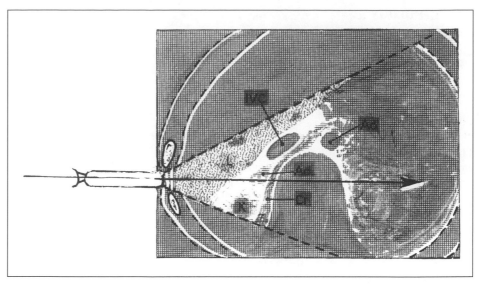

FIGURE 39-4. The right adrenal is most effectively imaged by scanning perpendicular to the right margin of the spine in an area bounded by the inferior vena cava, medial margin of the liver, and crus of the diaphragm. Do not confuse the crus with the adrenal gland.

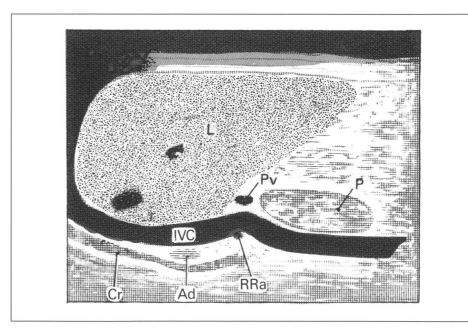

FIGURE 39-5. The right adrenal can be imaged longitudinally in the abdominal midline by using a medial-to-lateral angulation through the inferior vena cava (see also Fig. 39-2).

scan head cephalad until you are just above the right kidney. Be prepared to change to another intercostal space if your ultrasound beam is not perpendicular to the medial liver margin just superior to the kidney.

6. Try to confirm the presence or absence of pathology with longitudinal images. (Transverse scans will probably be more helpful.)

a. Longitudinal sections can be obtained by angling laterally in the midline to show an enlarged adrenal behind the inferior vena cava (Fig. 39-5; see also Fig. 39-1).

b. Longitudinal sections with medial angulation (approximately 30 degrees) aligning the right kidney and IVC may show the adrenal superior to the kidney. This technique is similar to that described for the left adrenal.

PATHOLOGY

Early Signs of Adrenal Enlargement

The normally concave margins of the adrenal gland become convex as the gland enlarges. The larger the gland, the more rounded the outline becomes (Fig. 39-6).

Changes in Position of Adjacent Organs

The changes in position of adjacent organs or structures may assist the sonographer in recognizing the adrenal as the source of a mass.

On the right side, changes caused by an enlarged adrenal include the following:

1. Anterior displacement of the retroperitoneal fat line, which lies in front of the kidneys and adrenal and behind the liver (see Figs. 23-2 and 23-3).
2. Anterior displacement of the inferior vena cava by the mass. It is important to examine this appearance transversely, as a slightly malrotated right kidney may also cause anterior displacement of the inferior vena cava.
3. Posteroinferior displacement of the kidney.
4. Draping of the right renal vein over the mass.

On the left side, changes indicative of an enlarged adrenal include anterior displacement of the splenic vein and posteroinferior displacement of the kidney.

Causes of Enlargement

The following are possible causes of enlargement:

1. *Adenomas.* Smooth, rounded, homogeneous masses. These are often incidentally discovered and are of little clinical consequence as a rule.
2. *Carcinomas.* Predominantly solid, irregular masses that may grow quite large.
3. *Cysts.* Must be distinguished from renal, pancreatic, or splenic cysts. Typical cyst appearances are seen.

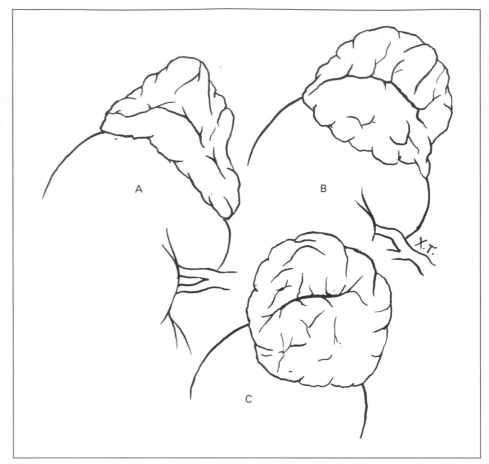

FIGURE 39-6. Progressive signs of adrenal enlargement. (**A**) Normal concave margins. (**B**) Convex margins of the slightly enlarged gland. (**C**) The larger the gland, the more rounded the contour.

4. *Hemorrhage.* Seen in infants. The appearance varies depending on the time elapsed since the bleed. A "fresh" bleed appears echogenic, developing sonolucent areas after a few days. Later the borders may become calcified, causing a mass with very echogenic borders and perhaps shadowing (see Chapter 28).
5. *Metastases.* Relatively common, usually arising from lung carcinoma. They vary in size and echogenicity. These masses may be very large (7 cm).
6. *Neuroblastoma.* A malignant adrenal mass seen in children (see Chapter 28).
7. *Pheochromocytoma.* A mass that causes uncontrollable hypertension and is usually evenly echogenic. These masses may occur in locations other than the adrenal glands.
8. *Myelolipoma.* Densely echogenic adrenal mass. Sound transmission is excellent through this fatty tumor, so the diaphragm may appear posteriorly displaced.

PITFALLS

1. *Mimics of right adrenal:*
   a. *Liver metastases* may be mistaken for adrenal pathology. Note the position of the retroperitoneal fat line, which is displaced posteriorly by liver pathology (see Chapter 23).
   b. The *crus of the diaphragm* may be misread as a normal adrenal. The crus is a tubular muscle that lies medial to the adrenal location.
2. *Mimics of left adrenal.* On the left many structures converge in the vicinity of the adrenal. The *esophagogastric junction,* the *tail of the pancreas, splenic vessels,* the *stomach,* and *lobulations of the spleen or kidney* can all mimic the adrenal. Always identify or rule out a normal structure before deciding that adrenal pathology is present.

? WHERE ELSE TO LOOK

1. If adenocarcinoma is found, examine the liver for possible metastatic lesions.
2. Some adrenal masses produce biochemical and clinical findings that are similar to those of ovarian masses, particularly in small children. If nothing is found in the adrenals, examine the ovaries.
3. If a metastatic lesion is found on one side, examine the opposite side thoroughly. Look for accompanying adenopathy.

Selected Reading

Carroll, B. A. Ultrasound case of the day. *Radiographics* 11:927–928, 1991.

Krebs, C. A., and Rawls, K. Techniques for successful scanning: Positioning strategy for optimal visualization of a left adrenal mass. *JDMS* 5:286–290, 1990.

Middelstaedt, C. M. *Abdominal Ultrasound* (2nd ed.). St. Louis: Mosby, 1994.

Westra, S. J., Zaninovic, A. C., Hall, T. R., Kangarloo, H., and Boechat, M. I. Imaging of the adrenal gland in children. *Radiographics* 14: 1323–1340, 1994.

IMPOTENCE

Penile Problems (Penile Pain and Abnormal Curvature)

JOE ROTHGEB, ROGER C. SANDERS

40

KEY WORDS

Cavernosal Artery. Bilateral arteries centrally placed within the corpus cavernosum. Flow in the artery is measured to detect arterial insufficiency.

Corpora Cavernosum. Two tubular structures in the penis that become filled with blood during an erection.

Corpus Spongiosum. Third tubular structure. The urethra lies in the center of it.

Flaccid. Relaxed and without muscle tone.

Impotence. The inability of the male patient to achieve or maintain erection.

Peyronie's Disease. A painful curvature of the penis during erection due to fibrous plaques.

Prostin. Prostaglandin is a hormone that causes an erection when injected into the penis.

Sonourethrography. Ultrasound of the urethra while injecting fluid into the urethra.

Stricture. The narrowing of a tube or opening, in this case involving the urethra.

Tunica Albuginea. A fibrous coat around the penis that surrounds the corpora cavernosa.

Urethra. The tubular canal that extends from the bladder to the tip of the penis, through which urine passes.

THE CLINICAL PROBLEM

The penis is easy to examine with ultrasound since its internal anatomy is superficial. Four main clinical problems are encountered for which sonography may be of help:

1. *Peyronie's disease.* Calcified or fibrous tissue is deposited in the dorsal portion of the penis so that the organ deviates and is painful when it is erect. The extent of the disease may be defined by ultrasound.
2. *Stricture.* The length of a stricture and the width of the stricture walls may be determined when the urethra is distended with fluid introduced through a catheter while imaging with a linear array transducer over the relevant area.
3. *Impotence due to poor penile arterial flow.* Arterial flow can be calculated using pulsed Doppler studies. An inadequate systolic flow indicates arterial insufficiency.
4. *Impotence due to venous leak.* An inadequate erection occurs because venous blood "leaks" out during attempted erection.

ANATOMY

The penis is considered in correct anatomic position when the dorsum lies against the abdomen, exposing the ventral side (Fig. 40-1). The penile portion of the urethra is midline, ventral, and surrounded by the corpus spongiosum. Posterior and lateral to the urethra are two vascular structures called the corpora cavernosa. All three components are surrounded by fibrous tissue called the tunica albuginea. Contained within each corpora cavernosum is erectile tissue and a cavernosal artery. In the dorsal portion of the penis is the deep dorsal vein and the superficial vein (Fig. 40-2).

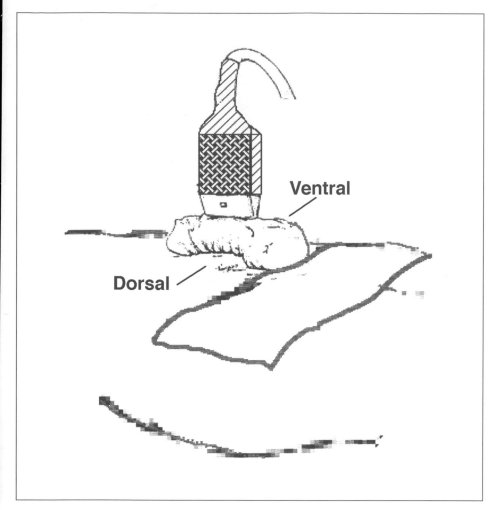

FIGURE 40-1. Position used for examining the penis in penile flow studies. It is also a good position for evaluating the penis for Peyronie's disease. The penis is in the anatomic position.

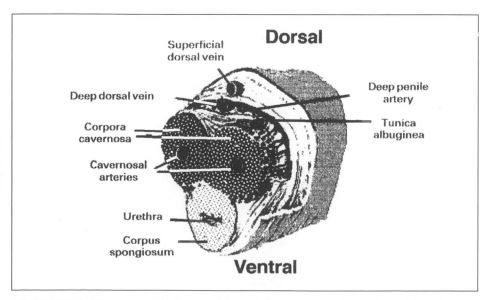

FIGURE 40-2. View showing the position of the cavernosal arteries within the corpora cavernosa and of the urethra within the corpus spongiosum. Note the tunica albuginea surrounding the corpora.

 TECHNIQUE

Evaluation of Peyronie's Disease

Examination of the penis is best performed by two sonographers or one sonographer and a participating patient. One person holds the penis at the distal end against the abdomen, while the other performs the sonogram. Scanning from either dorsal or ventral side is acceptable. Scan from the side opposite to the area of interest. A stand-off pad is helpful. High-frequency linear array (7.5–10 MHz) transducers give the best results.

Evaluation of Stricture

To perform sonourethrography for evaluation of a stricture, a Foley catheter is inserted into the distal urethra. Approximately 2 mL of sterile saline is injected into the balloon to secure the catheter. Longitudinal and transverse views of the urethra are performed while slowly and constantly injecting sterile saline by syringe.

Evaluation of Arterial Flow

To evaluate arterial flow, it is best to scan from the ventral side. First, scan the penis in a flaccid condition. Measure the diameter and flow of the cavernosal arteries. Color flow helps to locate these small arteries, which may not be detectable when the penis is flaccid. Having the patient well hydrated and placing warm compresses along the penis may accentuate these small arteries.

The Doppler angle should be less than 60 degrees and corrected to match the direction of flow. Peak systolic and end-diastolic velocities are measured. Then, Prostin is injected into the corpus cavernosum. At 5, 10, 15, and 20 minutes postinjection, the diameter of the vessels and the Doppler velocities are again obtained until the penis stops being erect. The quality of the erection is assessed.

PATHOLOGY

Peyronie's Disease

Peyronie's disease is an uncommon disease that results in a painful curvature of the penis when it is erect. Fibrous thickening may progress to calcification. These calcifications are usually located in the tunica albuginea on the dorsal aspect. A slightly echogenic fibrous plaque is seen on the uncurved side of the penis. The affected area often contains small foci of calcification. This condition is often associated with impotence and poor arterial flow. Intracavernosal calcification can also be seen in a patient who has repeatedly injected himself with an agent that causes an erection such as papaverine.

Urethral Stricture

Urethral strictures develop following infection (usually gonorrhea) or trauma. The urethra is narrowed, with a markedly thickened wall at the stricture site. The thickness of the stricture wall and the length of the stricture are measured in an ultrasound evaluation (Fig. 40-3).

Impotence

For an erection to occur, arterial blood flows through the cavernosal arteries, filling the erectile tissue in the corpora cavernosa. As this process occurs, the veins are compressed so there is a build-up of blood within the corpora cavernosa with resultant rigidity. Cavernosal systolic arterial velocity greater than 25 m/sec following the injection of Prostin is considered normal. With lower values, poor arterial supply is present. If the end diastolic flow within the cavernosal artery is greater than or equal to 7 m/sec, it is too high and indicative of venous incompetence. The presence of many large collaterals connected to the deep cavernosal artery is abnormal and suggests the diagnosis of venous leak. Venous incompetence is a surgically correctable condition.

To supplement the findings, grading the degree of erection with the Doppler values is helpful. The patient stands when the penis is fully rigid and the angle of the penis with respect to vertical is estimated. If the penile erectile angle is less than 90 degrees, it is considered abnormal.

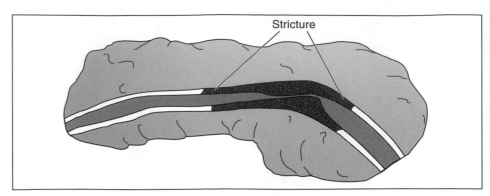

FIGURE 40-3. View of a stricture within the penis. Note that at the narrowed segment the walls are much thicker and the wall thickness extends beyond the narrowed urethral portion. The segment with abnormal wall thickness also needs to be excised surgically.

✳ PITFALLS

1. Excessive near-field gain prevents visualization of Peyronie's plaques. Scanning from the opposite side of the penis or using the stand-off pad may help in showing subtle plaques.

2. The cavernosal arteries can be difficult to find in a flaccid penis. Use the most sensitive settings on Doppler and color flow, with the highest frequency transducer (i.e., 10 MHz). If the machine has the option to lower the dynamic range or lower the Doppler frequency of the transducer, try those options. Warm compresses along the penis may help. The room temperature should not be too cold.

3. The dorsal artery typically has a high-resistance flow pattern. Be careful that you do not scan toward the dorsal aspect of the penis when obtaining the Doppler velocities, which should be obtained from the deep cavernosal artery.

4. If the patient is evaluated too soon after injection and has not reached full rigidity, a low-resistance sonographic pattern may be obtained, producing a false-positive finding. It is best not to wait any longer than 5 minutes postinjection to obtain the initial Doppler velocities. Scanning both sides several times postinjection and documenting the velocities over the next 20 minutes is good technique.

SELECTED READING

Benson, C. B., Aruny, J. E., and Vickers, M. A. Jr., Correlation of duplex sonography with arteriography in patients with erectile dysfunction. *AJR* 160:71–73, 1993.

Broderick, G. A., and Arger, P. Duplex Doppler ultrasonography: Noninvasive assessment of penile anatomy and function. *Semin Roentgenol* 28:43–56, 1993.

Fitzgerald, S. W., Erickson, S. J., Foley, W. D., Lipchik, E. O., and Lawson, T. L. Color Doppler sonography in the evaluation of erectile dysfunction: Patterns of temporal response to papaverine. *AJR* 157:331–336, 1991.

Oates, C. P., Pickard, R. S., Powell, P. H., Murthy, L. N. S., and Whittingham, T. A. W. The use of duplex ultrasound in the assessment of arterial supply to the penis in vasculogenic impotence. *J Urol* 153:354–357, 1995.

Pery, M., Rosenberger, A., Kaftori, J. K., and Vardi, Y. Intracorporeal calcifications after self-injection of papaverine. *Radiology* 176:81–83, 1990.

Schwartz, A. N., Lowe, M., Berger, R. E., Wang, K. Y., Mack, L. A., and Richardson, M. L. Assessment of normal and abnormal erectile function: Color Doppler flow sonography versus conventional techniques. *Radiology* 180:105–109, 1991.

41

NECK MASS

IRMA WHEELOCK TOPPER, ROGER C. SANDERS

KEY WORDS

Adenoma. Benign solid tumor of the thyroid.

Branchial Cleft Cyst. Congenital cystic mass located close to the angle of the mandible.

Cervical Adenopathy. Enlargement of lymph nodes in the neck.

Cold Nodule. A region of the thyroid where radioisotope has not been taken up on a nuclear study. The area of decreased uptake usually corresponds to a palpable mass.

Goiter. Diffuse enlargement of the thyroid gland due to iodine deficiency.

Halo Effect. A sonolucent zone surrounding a mass in the thyroid that is usually found with an adenoma (a benign tumor) but is rarely seen with carcinoma.

Hashimoto's Disease. Inflammatory disease of the thyroid gland usually characterized by diffuse enlargement and echopenic texture.

Major Neurovascular Bundle. A tubular structure that includes the common carotid artery, jugular vein, and vagus nerve.

Minor Neurovascular Bundle. A tubular structure that contains the inferior thyroid artery and the recurrent laryngeal nerve.

Photon-Deficient Area. See *Cold Nodule.*

Thyroglossal Duct Cyst. A developmental fluid-filled space variably extending from the base of the tongue to the isthmus of the thyroid.

Traumatic Pseudocyst. A fluid collection that is a response to damage to the salivary duct.

◆≫ THE CLINICAL PROBLEM

Thyroid Mass

The three most common indications for an ultrasound examination of the neck are as follows:

1. A palpable neck mass
2. A cold nodule or photon-deficient area on a nuclear medicine study
3. Elevated serum calcium levels suggesting parathyroid disease

Thyroid masses are common and are seen in 40 percent of elderly patients. The decision to proceed to biopsy is based on a combination of factors including clinical history, whether the lesion is palpable, physical examination of the neck, and sonographic features. Some patients are sent for a nuclear medicine study.

A cold nodule on a nuclear medicine study indicates a nonfunctioning area within the thyroid gland. Because all cysts and most malignancies do not take up radioisotope, an ultrasound study may then be performed to differentiate a solid from a cystic lesion. Of the lesions that are detected by nuclear scan, approximately 20 percent are cysts, 60 percent are benign, and 20 percent are malignant.

An increasing trend is to go straight to biopsy with or without ultrasound guidance if the mass is felt or revealed by ultrasound.

Clinical management is influenced by the ultrasonic differentiation of cystic from solid lesions. The diagnosis of a cystic lesion is followed by either observation or aspiration of the cyst, whereas the management of a solid mass may involve either a surgical procedure, biopsy, or thyroid medication. If follow-up ultrasound studies or clinical examination show that the lesion continues to enlarge, in spite of administration of thyroid extract to suppress thyroid activity, surgical intervention may be recommended. If no increase in size occurs, a conservative clinical approach may be appropriate (thyroid carcinomas are slow-growing neoplasms).

A high-resolution, high-frequency transducer (7.5–10 MHz) is essential, since its fine resolution will indicate whether multiple rather than single nodules are present. A single solid nodule should be biopsied, preferably under ultrasound guidance, if the lesion is either nonpalpable or difficult to feel. Multiple nodules are usually managed by medical follow-up, since multiple nodules usually carry a benign prognosis.

Neck Mass of Unknown Origin

When a mass is found in the neck, the origin may not be obvious on clinical examination—it may arise from the thyroid, enlarged lymph nodes, salivary glands, or other structures adjacent to the thyroid. Abscess and hematoma are possibilities if fever or trauma are included in the patient's history. Two congenital anomalies, thyroglossal duct cyst and branchial cleft cyst, cause cystic masses outside the thyroid. Recognition of the anatomic structures in the neck and their sonographic appearance is necessary to determine the origin of the neck mass.

Parathyroid Mass

A persistently high blood calcium level may suggest a diagnosis of parathyroid adenoma or cancer even though the gland cannot be felt. Surgery is difficult in this area because of the small size of the abnormal gland and the overlying thyroid; thus the surgeon is greatly assisted by knowing which parathyroid glands are enlarged.

ANATOMY

Thyroid Gland

The thyroid consists of right and left lobes connected by a narrow bridge of tissue anterior to the trachea called the isthmus (Fig. 41-1). The common carotid artery and the internal jugular vein are important landmarks that lie posterior and lateral to the thyroid and define its lateral margins.

The sternocleidomastoid, sternohyoid, and sternothyroid muscles can be imaged anterior and lateral to the more homogeneous texture of the normal thyroid gland (see Fig. 41-1).

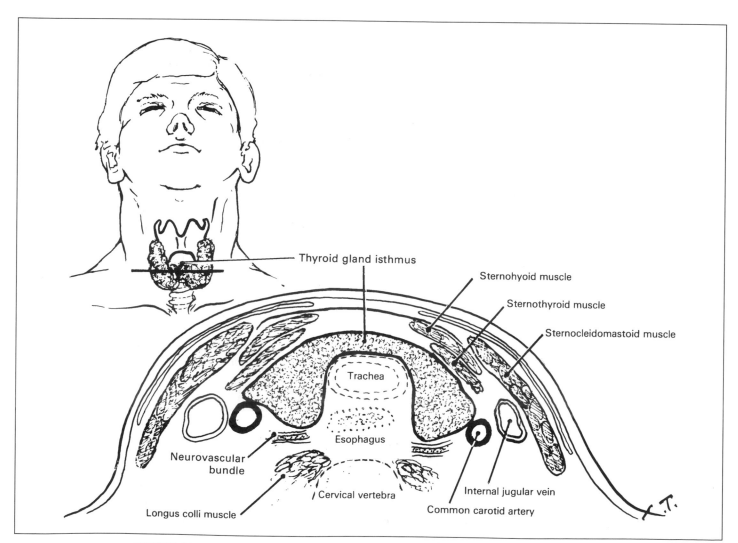

FIGURE 41-1. The thyroid gland consists of right and left lobes joined anteriorly by a narrow band of tissue called the isthmus. The common carotid artery and the internal jugular vein are important landmarks.

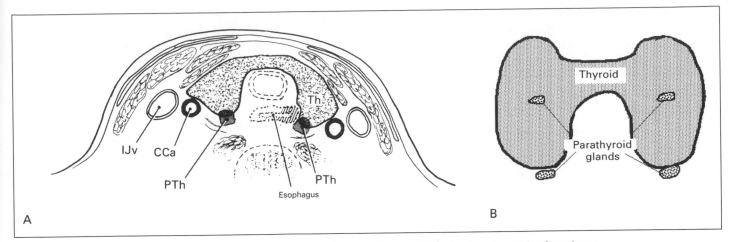

FIGURE 41-2. Parathyroid glands. (**A**) Four tiny parathyroid glands can be found posterior to the thyroid gland at its upper and lower poles. The esophagus often lies a little to the left. It can be mistaken for the parathyroid, but careful observation of the structure as the patient swallows helps to define the anatomy. (**B**) Frontal view showing the location of normal parathyroid glands.

Parathyroid Glands

The parathyroid glands, usually four in number, lie posterior to the thyroid gland (Fig. 41-2), two on each side. The upper glands usually lie posterior to the midportion of the thyroid gland.

The inferior glands lie at the lower border of the thyroid; the left may lie adjacent to the esophagus (Fig. 41-3; see also Fig. 41-2). Variant positions are within the thyroid gland and adjacent to the carotid, lateral to the internal jugular vein (see Fig. 41-3). The minor neurovascular bundle (a combination of the recurrent laryngeal nerve and the inferior thyroid artery) may be mistaken for the gland. The major neurovascular bundle (a combination of the common carotid artery, jugular vein, and vagus nerve) is usually a distinct structure. Parathyroid glands are normally less than 5 mm in size; glands greater than 5 mm should be considered abnormal.

▨ TECHNIQUE

Transducer Choice

If the direct contact method is employed, a 7.5-MHz or higher-frequency transducer with an electronically adjustable focal depth is appropriate. The electronic focus of the transducer must be placed at the level of the thyroid lobes. If a lower-frequency transducer is all that is available, the stand-off pad is necessary. As the distance between the transducer and the area of interest is increased, so must the depth of the focus "caret" be increased.

Patient Position

Place the patient supine with the head extended and a pillow or bolster under the shoulders. A pillowcase or scarf around the patient's hair prevents contamination by the coupling agent.

Scanning Techniques

Neck Palpation

Palpate the patient's neck before beginning the scanning procedure. If the mass is palpable, determine its location and approximate size. The patient may be able to assist you by pointing out a palpable lump or a tender spot. Locating the mass by reviewing the nuclear medicine study can also be helpful. It may be useful to have the patient sit up and swallow as you stand behind, palpating the thyroid.

FIGURE 41-3. Normal parathyroid glands can develop in a number of variant locations. Locate the normal structures (minor neurovascular bundle and longus colli muscle) so that they are not mistaken for normal parathyroid glands.

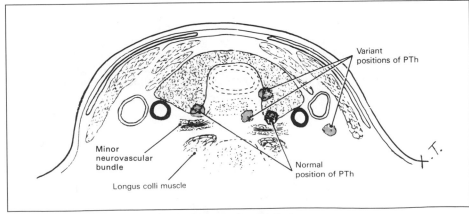

Image Size

The image should be enlarged until the thyroid gland fills the viewing monitor, taking care to include the carotid arteries and jugular veins on the lateral borders.

Scan Direction

TRANSVERSE. Begin scanning transversely in the midportion of the neck until thyroid tissue is identified (use the carotid artery and jugular vein as landmarks) (Fig. 41-4). If the patient's neck contour or the size of the thyroid makes it impossible to image right and left lobes simultaneously in the transverse orientation, they may be examined separately, making sure that the texture is uniform bilaterally. A dual linear format is helpful. Subtle textural differences are more difficult to appreciate if the lobes are imaged independently. Be sure to examine the anteriorly located isthmus, which connects the right and left lobes.

LONGITUDINAL. Longitudinally, first image the carotid artery (palpate if necessary), then carefully slide the transducer medially to view the thyroid gland (usually requires a 10- to 20-degree medial angulation for good contact) (Fig. 41-5). Determining the intrathyroidal or extrathyroidal nature of a neck mass is a good first step toward sorting out its origin. Most extrathyroidal masses displace the carotid artery and jugular vein medially. Mark the site of any palpable mass or textural changes with calipers to draw attention to the changes when the films are reviewed later.

Direct Contact Technique

1. Apply acoustic couplant to the neck. The higher viscosity (thicker) couplants are preferable, since they remain on the skin surface longer.

2. Place the transducer directly on the skin surface in the transverse plane (see Fig. 41-4). Adjust the electronic focus to the level of the thyroid tissue. Additional adjustments in focal depth will probably be needed to image the isthmus adequately. Care must be taken not to obliterate the texture of the isthmus, which may be hidden in near-field reverberations.

3. It is important to be light handed. Excessive pressure on the tissue may make imaging difficult by compressing tissue planes, or it may displace a small lesion from the imaging field.

Stand-off Technique

The stand-off technique incorporates the application of a commercially available polymer pad (usually 1- to 3-cm thick) between the patient's skin surface and the transducer. This technique avoids the problem of scanning over irregular or tender skin surfaces and increases the distance between the transducer surface and the thyroid gland to eliminate near-field reverberation artifacts (Fig. 41-6).

The polymer pad will attenuate a portion of the ultrasound signal, making it necessary to increase gain settings slightly. The greater distance may necessitate using a 5.0-MHz transducer.

A reverberation artifact related to the transducer/polymer pad interface often lies in the middle of the thyroid and makes this technique difficult to use.

Color Flow

Both benign and malignant thyroid lesions are vascular. This technique is of help, however, when the lesion is isoechoic and when one is uncertain whether it is real, since the mass will be outlined with color.

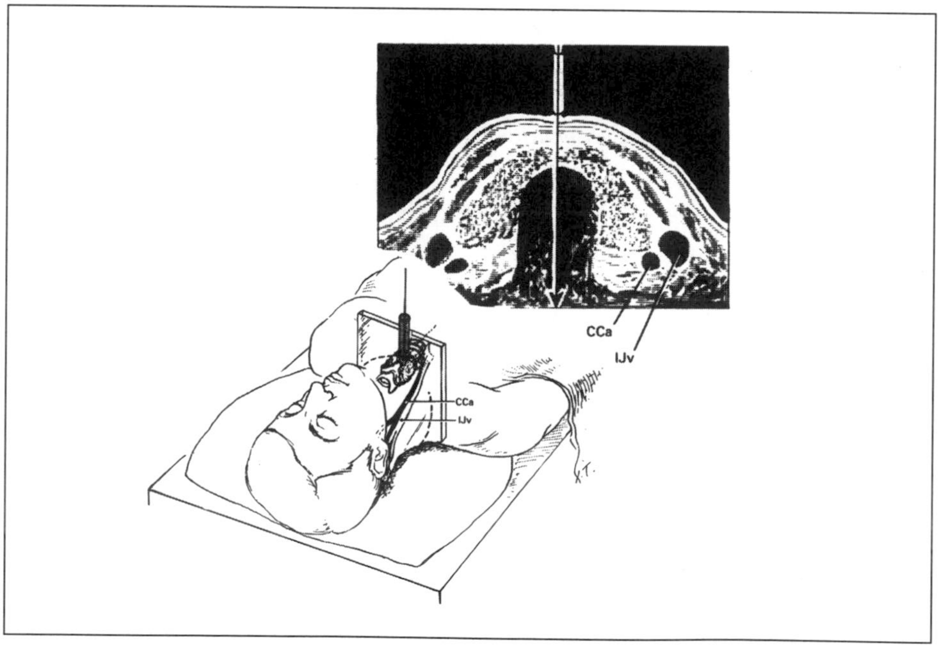

FIGURE 41-4. Occasionally the entire thyroid gland (isthmus, right and left lobes) can be imaged simultaneously in the transverse plane; however, more often the transducer must be placed on the side being imaged, angling 10 to 20 degrees medially. The common carotid artery and the internal jugular vein should be demonstrated on each image.

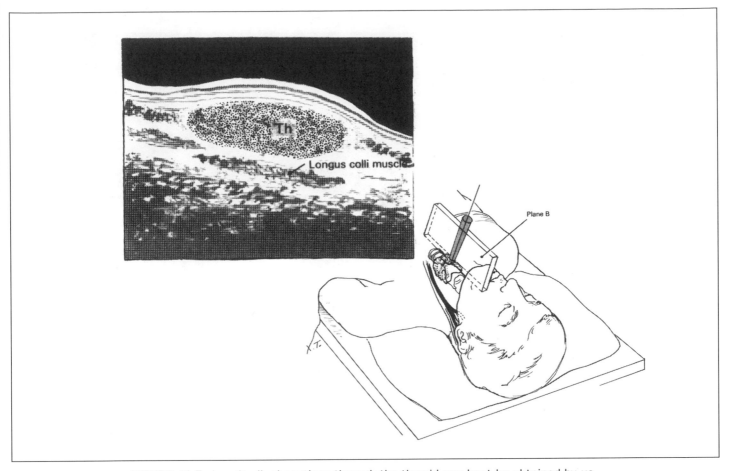

FIGURE 41-5. Longitudinal sections through the thyroid can best be obtained by using a 10- to 20-degree medial angle for maximum contact. Note the longus colli muscle posterior to the thyroid.

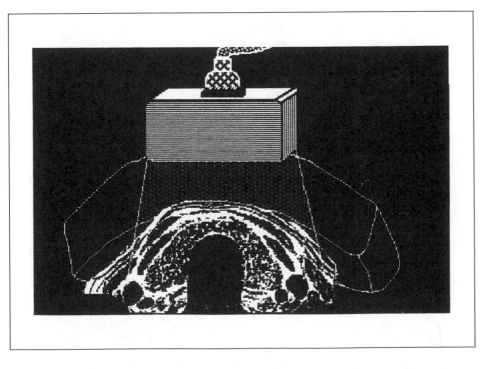

FIGURE 41-6. Both longitudinal and transverse images can be obtained by using a stand-off pad technique. This technique is useful (1) if the neck contour is irregular or painful, making good contact impossible; or (2) to increase the distance between the transducer face and the gland so that the gland falls within the focal range of the transducer.

PATHOLOGY

Intrathyroidal Masses

Cysts

Thyroid cysts resemble those in other parts of the body except that their walls may be irregular and they may contain internal echoes from hemorrhage (Fig. 41-7).

Adenomas

The most common thyroid masses are adenomas. They have several sonographic manifestations. Typical appearances are (1) a halo of echopenic tissue surrounding a more echogenic mass with echoes that are more dense than the remainder of the gland (Fig. 41-8A); (2) a solid homogeneous mass with very few internal echoes that can easily be confused with a cyst; and (3) a densely echogenic lesion. Larger (eggshell) foci of calcification may be seen.

The presence of a comet-tail artifact (see Chapter 53) is a sign that the lesion is benign since the calcific origin of the comet effect is large. Unlike carcinomas, adenomas are almost invariably multiple.

Carcinomas

Carcinomas of the thyroid are suggested by the following features: (1) an echopenic mass with an irregular border (see Fig. 41-8B); (2) tiny foci of calcification (microcalcification); (3) a single nodular lesion; and (4) the development of nodes in neighboring structures.

Peak systolic velocity is increased in malignancy.

Goiters

Goiters are a diffuse, asymmetric expansion of the thyroid with a coarse acoustic texture. Multiple nodules are usually present.

Hashimoto's Thyroiditis

In Hashimoto's thyroiditis, an inflammatory condition, there is diffuse, mild enlargement of the thyroid with multiple small echopenic nodules. Fibrous interfaces between the nodules will be evident.

Hemorrhage

With hemorrhage there is sudden onset of pain with development of a mass associated with intrathyroidal clot. This clot is similar in appearance to clot in other parts of the body.

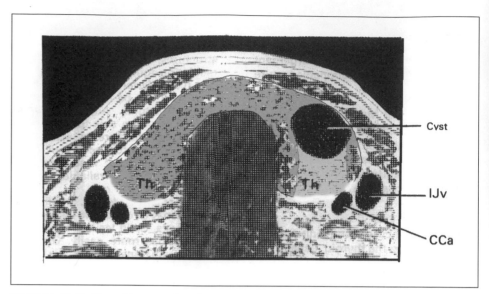

FIGURE 41-7. Thyroid cyst, showing the typical characteristics of smooth borders, lack of internal echoes, and increased through transmission.

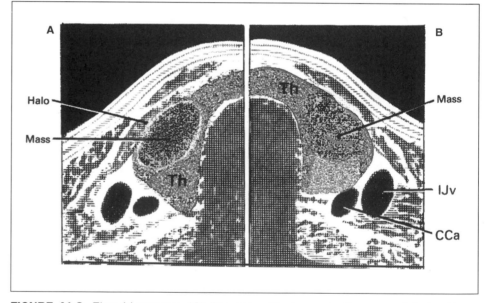

FIGURE 41-8. Thyroid masses. (**A**) The halo effect, most often associated with an adenoma, is typified by an echogenic mass with an echo-free border. (**B**) This solid thyroid mass, a carcinoma, contains echoes and exhibits little through transmission. Note that it is more echogenic than the thyroid.

Subacute Thyroiditis

Subacute thyroiditis is a painful condition exhibiting diffuse, mild enlargement of the thyroid with an echopenic texture but no focal nodules. It may be a prelude to Hashimoto's thyroiditis.

Extrathyroidal Masses

Thyroglossal Duct Cyst

A thyroglossal duct cyst is an embryologic remnant. It has the typical appearance of a cyst and is found in the midline high in the neck above the thyroid.

Branchial Cleft Cyst

Branchial cleft cyst is congenital and is found lateral to the thyroid, usually at a higher level.

Nodes

Enlarged lymph nodes occur quite commonly in the neck and can be difficult to distinguish clinically from the thyroid gland. Sonographically, they lie lateral to the major vessels. Their echo texture is homogeneous, but less echogenic than normal thyroid texture. Most enlarged nodes are benign and have an echogenic center.

Abscess

Abscesses may develop in the neck. They have the typical ultrasonic features of abscesses in other parts of the body and similarly are associated with pain, fever, and focal swelling.

Carcinoma Invasion

Carcinoma (e.g., of the tongue) may invade the neck; the extent of the tumor can be seen with ultrasound.

Parathyroid Enlargement

Enlarged parathyroids can be difficult to distinguish from an intrathyroidal mass or normal anatomy of the neck; they appear as echopenic masses adjacent to the posterior aspect of the thyroid close to the carotid artery. Carefully sort out normal anatomic structures (see Fig. 41-1). A parathyroid gland is considered abnormal if it measures greater than 5 mm in size.

PITFALLS

1. *Cyst vs. solid lesion.* Small solid lesions may be difficult to distinguish from cysts. Solid lesions should fill with echoes more easily. Observe the through transmission.
2. *Identifying the mass.* Small lesions may be displaced by the transducer with a direct scanning technique and may never actually be imaged. Therefore, use very light pressure on the neck while scanning to keep the mass under the transducer. If the mass is palpable, immobilize it with your fingers and scan over the area of interest.
3. *Isthmic mass.* An anterior mass may be overlooked because of near-field artifact (reverberation) and contact problems.
4. *Parathyroid adenoma.* This type of adenoma may be mimicked by the following structures:
   a. The minor neuromuscular bundle. This structure has a longitudinal axis, unlike the ovoid parathyroid (see Fig. 41-3).
   b. The left lateral border of the esophagus. Ask the patient to swallow water drunk through a straw to rule out a normal esophageal structure before calling left parathyroid enlargement (see Fig. 41-2).
   c. The longus colli muscle. This muscle is seen on both sides of the neck.
   d. Intrathyroidal adenoma. It may be impossible to distinguish an intrathyroidal adenoma from parathyroid gland enlargement (see Fig. 41-3). Both are very vascular.

WHERE ELSE TO LOOK

1. If a mass outside the thyroid could represent an enlarged lymph node, look for adenopathy or a primary neoplasm in the abdomen.
2. An enlarged parathyroid gland, usually caused by an adenoma, causes hypercalcemia; check for renal calculi.

SELECTED READING

Ahuja, A., Chick, W., King, W., and Metreweli, C. Clinical significance of the comet-tail artifact in thyroid ultrasound. *J Clin Ultrasound* 24:129–133, 1996.

Gooding, G. A. W. Questions/answers. *AJR* 166: 718–719, 1996.

Kerr, L. High-resolution thyroid ultrasound: The value of color Doppler. *Ultrasound Quart* 12:21–44, 1994.

Vazquez, E., Enriquez, G., Castellote, A., Lucaya, J., Creixell, S., Aso, C., and Regas, J. US, CT, and MR imaging of neck lesions in children. *Radiographics* 15:105–122, 1995.

Yeh, H., Futterweit, W., and Gilbert, P. Micronodulation: Ultrasonographic sign of Hashimoto's thyroiditis. *J Ultrasound Med* 15:813–819, 1996.

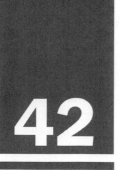

42 CAROTID ARTERY DISEASE

ROGER C. SANDERS, IRMA WHEELOCK TOPPER

SONOGRAM ABBREVIATIONS

Bif	Bifurcation
Cca	Common carotid artery
ECa	External carotid artery
Ica	Internal carotid artery
Subcl	Subclavian artery
Vert	Vertebral artery

KEY WORDS

Aliasing. A Doppler signal is transmitted before the prior returning signal has been received.

Amaurosis Fugax. Transient blindness.

Bruit. Rumbling sound heard over an artery with a stethoscope.

Plaque. Deposit of fibrinous material on the edge of a vessel due to atheroma that may narrow the vessel significantly.

Pulse Repetition Frequency (PRF). The frequency with which an echo signal is sent into and received from the tissue. A limiting factor in the development of Doppler signals.

Sample Volume. The size of the space from which Doppler signals are being obtained.

Spectral Broadening. With flow disturbance, the Doppler signal becomes more varied in pitch, displaying numerous frequencies.

Stroke. Loss of use of a portion of the body due to a brain infarction, hematoma, or embolus.

Subclavian Steal Syndrome. When the subclavian artery is blocked, blood is supplied to the left arm through the left vertebral artery. Flow through the left vertebral artery is thus reversed.

Transient Ischemic Attack (TIA). Transient paralysis of a portion of the body due to temporary interference with blood supply to the brain.

Turbulence. Unusual flow patterns created when an obstructing lesion such as plaque is present within a vessel. The term is incorrect from a physicist's viewpoint—a better term is flow disturbance.

◆》 THE CLINICAL PROBLEM

Neurologic symptoms that suggest the need for a duplex examination of the extracranial cerebral vascular system are the following:

1. *Amaurosis fugax.* The patient experiences the loss of vision in one eye, usually likened to a curtain being drawn before the eye. Since the ophthalmic artery is the first branch from the internal carotid artery, this symptom usually indicates internal carotid artery disease.

2. *Transient ischemic attack.* The patient exhibits the symptoms of stroke but returns to normal within 24 hours. When a patient has a transient ischemic attack, risk of a stroke with permanent neurologic deficit within the next 5 years increases to 17 times that of the symptom-free population. Carotid duplex examination of the carotid arteries can document the extent of disease or rule out carotid disease, suggesting other causes, such as an embolus from a heart lesion.

3. *Stroke.* A condition caused by decreased blood supply to a portion of the brain that results in unconsciousness or unilateral motor or sensory loss for more than 24 hours that is often permanent. If carotid disease is responsible for the stroke, it is located on the side opposite from the paralysis.

4. *A bruit in the region of the carotid bifurcation.* This auditory sign indicates a high-velocity flow of blood through a vessel that is restricted by disease.

5. *A palpable pulsatile mass in the neck.* Such a mass raises the question of carotid artery aneurysm. Often, the mass turns out to be a tortuous subclavian artery that is palpated superior to the clavicle.

Ultrasound is also used to evaluate cerebrovascular flow prior to surgical procedures, such as a cardiac operation, to ensure adequate perfusion of the brain in the event of a drop in blood pressure during anesthesia. There is a 17 percent increase of stroke during surgery in patients with a carotid artery stenosis of 60 percent or greater. The progress of carotid artery disease in the asymptomatic patient can also be followed ultrasonically, since in most institutions surgical intervention is postponed until either the patient becomes symptomatic or the stenosis exceeds 80 percent.

If a carotid sonogram shows a 70% stenosis of the internal carotid artery, surgery is desirable; this is now accepted as adequate presurgical investigation.

Ultrasound is the follow-up technique of choice for patients who have already undergone carotid endarterectomy. Many patients redevelop stenosis within the next 2 years.

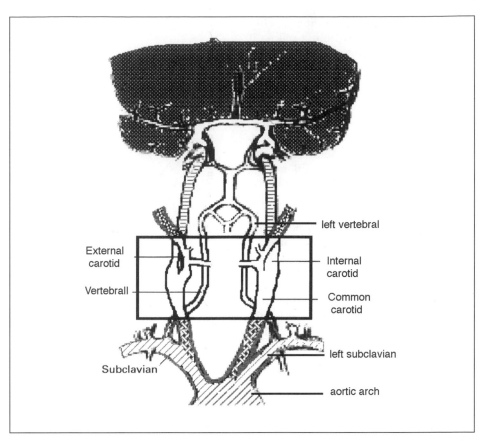

FIGURE 42-1. Diagram of the carotid, vertebral, and subclavian arteries. Only the area within the box can be examined with ultrasound. The vertebral artery arises from the subclavian artery separately from the carotid arteries. The internal carotid arteries are usually medial to the external carotid arteries.

ANATOMY

The blood supply for the brain and facial structures originates from the aortic arch (Fig. 42-1). On the right, the common carotid and the vertebral arteries originate from the subclavian artery, a direct branch from the aortic arch. On the left side, however, both the subclavian artery and the common carotid artery begin directly from the aortic arch. The left vertebral artery arises from the left subclavian artery (see Fig. 42-1).

Both common carotid arteries proceed cranially and bifurcate at about the angle of the mandible into the internal carotid artery, which supplies blood to the brain (usually it takes a posterolateral course), and the external carotid artery, which supplies the facial structures (an anteromedial course). The circle of Willis within the cranium, supplied by both internal carotid arteries and the basilar artery that is formed by the vertebral arteries, provides a communication network of blood vessels that may allow adequate blood flow to the brain even when a severe stenosis or total occlusion exists in one of the extracranial carotid arteries (see Chapter 43).

 TECHNIQUE

Imaging Technique

The sonographer sits at the head of the patient with the equipment oriented so that the controls are within easy reach. Rest the forearm on the stretcher so that tiny changes in transducer position can be made with simple finger and wrist movements. A good-quality Doppler tracing requires that the operator exert light pressure only on the patient's neck and that the operator remain motionless to keep the Doppler sample volume within the vessel wall boundaries.

1. Select a high-frequency transducer (5, 7.5, or 10 MHz). A linear array shows more of the course of the artery but is not as easy to use if the carotid artery bifurcates at or above the mandible.

2. Place the patient supine with the chin extended (usually without a pillow, if the patient can tolerate that position). Turn the patient's head away from the side being examined. This allows easy transducer access and makes it more likely that the internal and external carotid arteries can be imaged at the same time. A 20- to 30-degree lateral-to-medial transducer angle helps you use the sternocleidomastoid muscle as an acoustic "stand-off." You may need to adjust the position of the patient's head from medial to lateral to "open up" the bifurcation of the internal and external carotid arteries (Fig. 42-2).

3. Begin imaging in the long axis at the level of the clavicle to evaluate the origin of the common carotid artery from the subclavian artery on the right or the aortic arch on the left (Fig. 42-3 and see Figs. 42-1 and 42-2).

4. Image the common carotid artery, moving cranially in the longitudinal plane until it widens at the bulb (bifurcation) into the internal carotid and the external carotid arteries. Keeping the distal portion of the bulb in view at the inferior edge of the image, sweep from medial to lateral in very tiny increments to observe the takeoff of the internal carotid artery. Then, angle the transducer anteriorly and look medially to locate the external carotid artery. The course of these branches is often tortuous. Sampling with pulsed Doppler allows identification of the low-resistance flow of the internal carotid artery and the high-resistance flow of the external carotid artery.

5. Transverse imaging may help determine the ideal long axis by showing internal and external carotid arteries as they branch from the bulb.

6. Imaging the common carotid artery, bulb, and internal and external carotid arteries simultaneously is optimal, but this is only possible in a minority of patients.

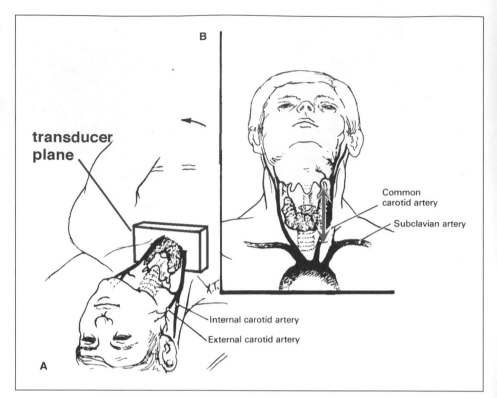

FIGURE 42-2. Diagram showing the normal arteries in the neck with the appropriate transducer angulation. (**A**) Box. (**B**) Gray arrow.

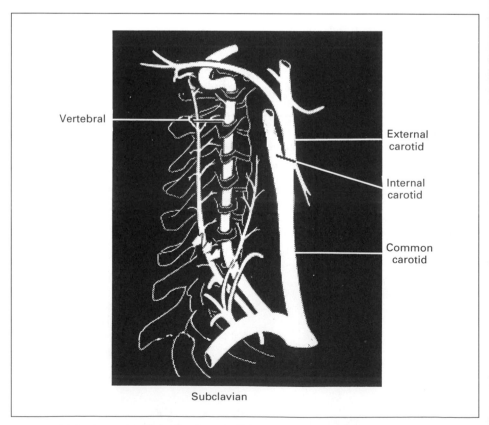

FIGURE 42-3. Diagram showing the relationship of the vertebral artery to the spine and to the carotid artery. (Reprinted with permission from Zweibel, W. J. *Introduction to Vascular Sonography.* New York: Grune & Stratton, 1996.)

7. Look for these features:
   a. Intimal thickening (Figs. 42-4 and 42-5).
   b. Wall irregularities. The wall of the carotid is thicker than usual.
   c. Plaque (soft or calcified). Image areas of plaque transversely so the percentage of narrowing of the vessel can be calculated. Use caution when employing this measurement since diameter reduction can easily be underestimated or overestimated. Area calculation, taken from the transverse view, is more accurate (see Fig. 42-4).
   d. Ulceration of the plaque (see Fig. 42-5). (The diagnostic accuracy for the detection of ulceration in the plaque by ultrasound is low.) The dynamic range with modern ultrasound equipment ranges from 40 to 60 db. As the dynamic range increases, low-level gray shades are detectable, allowing one to visualize soft plaque.

Try to make the exam relatively speedy. A quick exam limits the ultrasound exposure to the patient, since the power output levels for pulsed Doppler are higher than those for imaging alone. Second, most patients are elderly and become uncomfortable or unable to cooperate if they are restricted to lying flat for a long time. Finally, technologist fatigue may compromise concentration and exam quality. Initially allow 60 to 90 minutes to complete the bilateral carotid artery interrogation, but try to refine the examination time to 30 minutes.

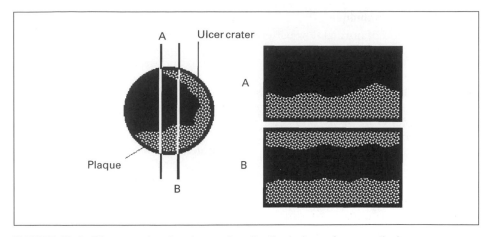

FIGURE 42-4. Diagram showing how a longitudinal view of a vessel plaque can suggest a greater or lesser degree of stenosis than is actually the case. Section A is taken through the center of the vessel and section B through the plaque. Area calculations of the patent versus plaque-filled lumen can be obtained on transverse images such as this, and are more likely to be accurate than diameter calculations obtained from a longitudinal projection.

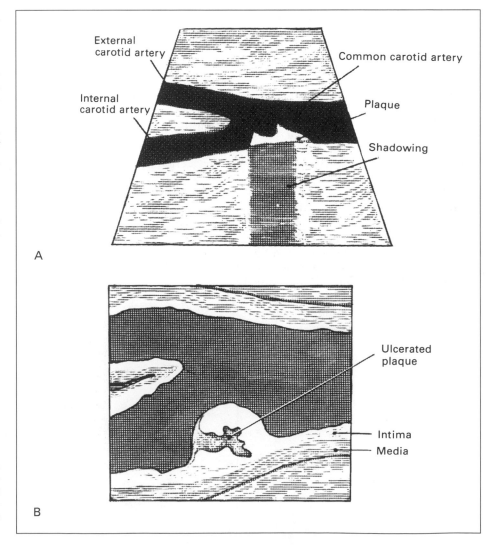

FIGURE 42-5. Atheromatous plaques. (**A**) Sonogram of a partially calcifed carotid artery plaque. Shadowing is seen behind the calcified segment. (**B**) Diagram showing the pathologic appearance of an ulcerated atheromatous plaque.

Pulsed Doppler Technique

For a description of normal flow pattern at different sites, see Figure 42-11.

Spectral Analysis

Locate the vessels using the imaging technique described above. Adjust the pulsed Doppler controls as follows for a standard carotid flow study:

1. *Wall filter.* Settings vary between 50 and 200 Hz, with the higher values indicating significant filtration. The 100-Hz setting reduces the "noise" from pulsed Doppler without filtering much diagnostic information. If a diseased vessel shows no Doppler flow signal, reduce the wall filter to 50 Hz and reexamine the vessel distal to the occlusion in an attempt to detect any preocclusive flow. Much artifact within the signal may indicate the need for a higher filter setting.

2. *Doppler baseline.* The baseline should be located slightly below the center of the monitor. Usually, the forward flow velocities are higher than the reverse flow, which will be shown below the baseline (Fig. 42-6).

3. *Pulse repetition frequency (PRF)* (velocity). The PRF should be set at a range that will allow a velocity measurement of approximately 120 cm/sec to be displayed. If the Doppler flow velocities exceed 120 cm/sec, the PRF will need to be decreased until the entire spectral trace is displayed without aliasing (see Pitfalls).

4. *Sample volume size.* Ideally the sample volume should be between 1.5 and 2 mm. This small sample volume size increases the likelihood of obtaining good center vessel laminar flow information without including the slower-flowing signals from blood near the vessel wall, which produce spurious spectral broadening.

Color Flow

Color Doppler is computer-processed pulsed Doppler; thus, it has the same strengths and weaknesses as pulsed Doppler. Observations can be made about the direction of flow, approximate speed of flow, and presence of turbulence within the vessel. Quantitative (absolute speed of flow) information cannot be measured accurately with color Doppler imaging, since it is currently impossible to angle-correct within the color box. (To obtain quantitative flow information, the system must know the angle of the Doppler beam with respect to the flow direction. The operator must provide this information at a particular sampling site.)

The normal change in direction of the blood flow caused by the tortuosity of the vessel and the division of the internal and external branches can be quickly appreciated within the larger sampling of the color box. Color in an artery can change from red to blue, depending on the vessel direction in relation to the Doppler beam. At sites of vessel narrowing, the blood flow increases in velocity and color flow shows an aliased color signal, usually converting from red or blue to white.

Color flow has several advantages:

1. With color, it is possible to visualize small amounts of flow in unexpected areas since Doppler signals are strong at angles (0 to 60 degrees to flow) where imaging (60 to 90 degrees) is very weak.

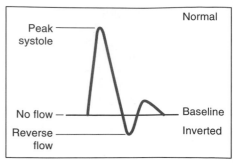

FIGURE 42-6. Diagram showing the components of the Doppler pulse. A quick upswing in systole is plotted above the baseline, while a possible reversal of flow in diastole would be plotted as a signal below the baseline. Constant forward flow would be displayed as a signal that remains above the baseline throughout the cardiac cycle.

2. Vessel identification is rapid.
3. Flow can be visualized on transverse views.
4. The site of critical stenosis can be visualized and the Doppler sample gate placed at the appropriate angle to correspond with the flow.
5. Visualization of good color from wall to wall within the vessel eliminates the need to perform a spectral analysis at many locations, while moving the sample volume throughout the length of the vessel.

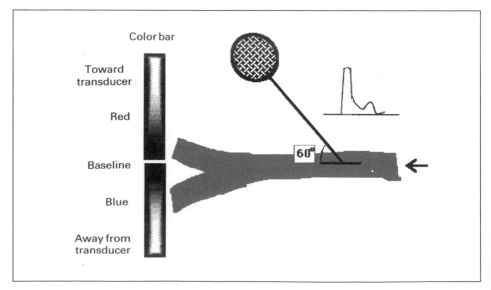

FIGURE 42-7. Diagram showing a good Doppler angle for examination of the common carotid artery with an associated color display.

Technique Protocol

To begin the carotid artery pulsed Doppler examination follow these steps:

1. Locate the proximal common carotid artery with two-dimensional imaging.
2. Activate the Doppler mode.
3. Place the Doppler sample volume in the center of the vessel to be interrogated at an angle to flow of 40 to 60 degrees for the strongest Doppler signal. The Doppler angle should be no more than 60 degrees.
4. If you do not have color Doppler capabilities, move the sample gate along the vessel from wall to wall, proceeding toward the bifurcation. Listen to the Doppler frequency shift and its signal in multiple locations. Flow may be normal to disturbed at the bifurcation point. Be sure that you notice high-velocity signals, which will have a higher pitch, indicating vessel lumen narrowing. If the velocity signals of the spectral waveform cannot be completely displayed (i.e., the peak systolic portion of the spectral waveform extends beyond the top of the viewing monitor), increase the PRF or lower the spectral baseline toward the bottom of the viewing monitor until the aliasing is eliminated. If color is available, note the high-velocity flow by changes in the color assignment. Then place a sample volume at the location of the highest-velocity color signal at an angle to the blood flow of 40 to 60 degrees (Fig. 42-7) to obtain a spectral analysis signal. (The highest-velocity signal could be near the wall if the vessel is tortuous or there is plaque.)
5. Proceed up the common carotid artery to the bifurcation, adjusting the sample volume placement and angle to correspond with the vessel course (Figs. 42-8 and 42-9, and see Fig. 42-7). When the Doppler angle follows the direction of flow, it may be necessary to invert the spectral display so that the peak systolic measurement is displayed toward the top of the display. If using color Doppler, also invert the color bar so the carotid artery continues to be displayed in the red hue.

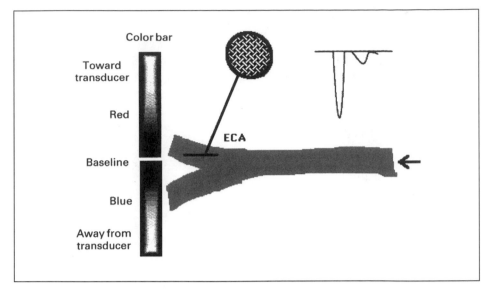

FIGURE 42-8. Diagram showing the correct angle to examine the external carotid artery with the color Doppler signal. The ECa would now be displayed in a blue hue with the spectral display below the baseline because of the change in the interrogation angle. It is considered convention in peripheral vascular exams to invert the color scale to display arteries in red whenever possible. The spectral display is customarily inverted to display the peak flow toward the top of the display.

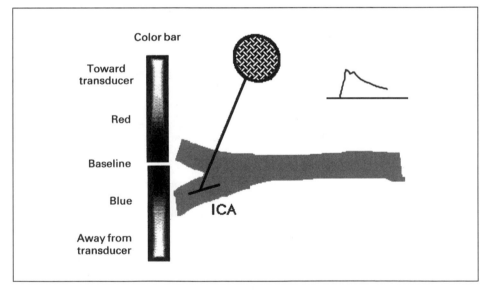

FIGURE 42-9. Diagram showing the correct angle to examine the internal carotid artery with the color Doppler signal. See explanation for Fig. 42-8.

Documentation

Both the imaging and the pulsed Doppler information can be documented with the use of a diagram of the cerebrovascular anatomy, as seen in Figure 42-10. The location and extent of plaque formation should be documented on the diagram. Place the Doppler values at the appropriate site as listed below.

Spectral Analysis

Documentation of the spectral analysis from the pulsed Doppler interrogation can be displayed in either frequency shift (kHz) or velocity (cm/sec). Most of the initial research on the classification of carotid artery disease was done using frequency shift. This method requires a Doppler interrogation angle 60 degrees to the flow and the use of a 5-MHz Doppler frequency (Table 42-1). If another Doppler frequency is used, a different chart for disease classification is required. Velocity measurements are independent of transducer frequency, but require the user to input the Doppler angle to flow with the angle-correct option (see Fig. 42-7) in order to obtain an accurate velocity number in centimeters per second. Documentation should accompany the imaging at the following levels:

1. *Proximal carotid artery.* Expect turbulence; flow changes direction from the subclavian artery to the common carotid artery. A high-velocity Doppler shift indicates an obstructive process at the takeoff of the common carotid artery from the subclavian artery.
2. *Mid common carotid artery* (at a location where you can obtain a Doppler-beam-to-flow angle of 60 degrees or less). Observe the diastolic flow signal in the mid common carotid artery. No diastolic flow should alert you to a probable internal carotid artery occlusion. Make a note of the common carotid artery peak velocity (frequency shift) for calculation of the ICa/CCa (internal carotid artery/common carotid artery) ratio. This number is helpful, particularly in patients with high or low cardiac output (see Table 42-1).

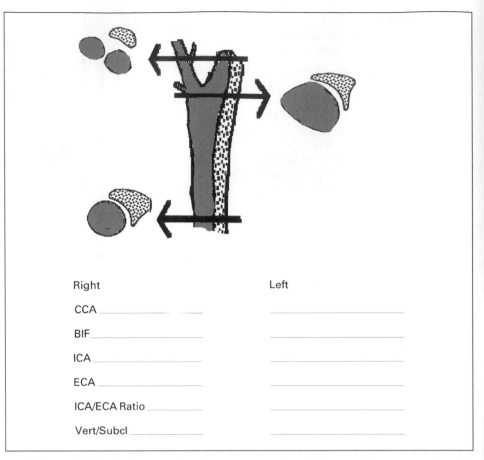

FIGURE 42-10. Worksheet used to document results of the carotid sonogram in a diagrammatic fashion.

3. *Bifurcation area.* Again, expect turbulent flow because flow is dividing into the internal and external carotid arteries. Listen for a high-velocity signal to prepare yourself for the need to adjust the sample volume location in a search for the precise location of the highest-velocity flow (jet). Increase the PRF as needed to display the entire high-velocity signal on the spectral analysis waveform.

4. *External carotid artery.* Flow in the external carotid artery is not considered to be as important as that in the internal carotid artery, since the latter supplies the brain. The normal external carotid artery exhibits a high-resistance waveform (i.e., quick systolic peak with flow nearly to the baseline in diastole). Flow patterns in the external carotid artery may resemble those of the internal carotid artery when internal carotid artery occlusion is present. In internal carotid artery occlusion, the blood supply to the brain follows a collateral pathway through the external carotid artery and the ophthalmic artery into the circle of Willis; thus the external carotid artery may develop a low-resistance signal.

TABLE 42-1. DOPPLER SPECTRUM ANALYSIS: CAROTID ARTERY DISEASE—DIAGNOSTIC PARAMETERS

Diameter stenosis (Classification)	Peak systole (ICA/stenosis)	Peak diastole (ICA/stenosis)	Systolic velocity ratio[1]	Diastolic velocity ratio[2]	Flow character (ICA/stenosis)
0–39% Normal–mild	<3.5 kHz <110 cm/s	<1.5 kHz <45 cm/s	<1.8	<2.6	Normal—mild spectral broadening
40–59% Moderate	3.5–5.0 kHz 110–150 cm/s	<1.5 kHz <45 cm/s	<1.8	<2.6	Mild–moderate spectral broadening
60–79% Severe	5.0–8.0 kHz 150–250 cm/s	1.5–4.5 kHz 45–140 cm/s	1.8–3.7	2.6–5.5	Moderate–severe spectral broadening
80–99% Critical	8.0–20.0 kHz 250–615 cm/s	>4.5 kHz >140 cm/s	>3.7	>5.5	Severe spectral broadening
99% Critical	Extremely low	N/A	N/A	N/A	Highly turbulent Loss of normal cardiac cycle
100% Total occlusion	N/A (CCa diastolic flow is zero.)	N/A	N/A	N/A	N/A

[1]Highest systolic velocity obtained in ICa or site of stenosis/Nonstenotic systolic CCa velocity.

[2]End diastolic velocity in ICa or site of stenosis/Nonstenotic diastolic CCa velocity.

Clinical source: Brian L. Thiele, M.D., et al. Data research and compilation: Chris Walker and Jim Brown, ATL, Inc.

Note: Low cardiac output, cardiac arrhythmias and/or anatomic variations may produce invalid measurements.

All kilohertz statistics based on equipment using a 5-MHz pulsed Doppler carrier frequency with a 1.5 mm cubed sample volume at a 60 degree flow angle.

5. *Internal carotid artery.* The bulb and the origin of the internal carotid artery are the usual sites for plaque formation resulting from flow disturbances. Obtain a Doppler spectral tracing from the proximal and distal internal carotid artery, even if no plaque is observed—plaque may be sonolucent. If plaque is identified, obtain a spectral tracing from the narrowed vessel lumen, repositioning the Doppler sample volume to locate the highest-velocity (kHz shift) signal. High velocities are seen in systole and diastole. A high-velocity jet of blood may be very small, but makes a characteristic audible hissing sound. If this sound is heard, increase the PRF to display the entire high-velocity waveform.

Power Doppler may display a tiny path that is still open through arterial plaque that cannot be seen with conventional color flow.

6. *Internal carotid artery (distal).* Move higher on the patient's neck to obtain a spectral display from a point distal to the narrowing. The flow may remain disturbed (high velocity) or turbulent (above and below the baseline), but not necessarily with a high velocity.

Suspected Occlusion

To confirm a suspected occlusion in the carotid arteries, use this technique, following the routine interrogation procedure described above:

1. Increase the sample size to survey a large area.
2. Increase the Doppler gain, which will introduce some noise but will provide a better opportunity to hear a weak Doppler signal.
3. Use continuous wave. This is more sensitive in picking up subtle signals.
4. Use color and power Doppler since color shows subtle flow in unexpected areas, although it is not as sensitive as continuous wave.
5. Perform analysis in the low, middle, and high points in the common and internal carotid arteries. Listen for (or observe) the blunted signals of flow hitting an obstruction and reversing—a thudlike sound can be heard when there is obstruction not far beyond the site being sampled.

6. Listen for a low-velocity Doppler signal if a near-total occlusion is expected (see Table 42-1) and no high-velocity signal is located. Flow in the vessel lowers from the very high-velocity "jet" to a trickle just before occlusion. Total occlusion of the vessel is an inoperable condition, while any flow detection *is* operable.

Interpretation

Percent Stenosis

The percent stenosis measurement is calculated by comparing the measurement on a transverse image of the outer vessel wall to the vessel lumen at the site of disease (see Fig. 42-4). Obtaining the image at an oblique measurement angle (not at 90 degrees) to the vessel walls will result in an inaccurate measurement.

Diameter reduction can be calculated in the longitudinal plane, comparing the diameter of the outer wall of the vessel with the lumen at the site of disease. This method of quantifying the stenosis is even more risky than calculating percent stenosis as above, since disease is imaged only along two walls (see Fig. 42-4).

The pulsed Doppler spectral analysis reveals information that is compared with the accompanying table (Figs. 42-11 to 42-13 and see Table 42-1).

Spectral Broadening

Spectral broadening may be seen as increased echoes in the "spectral window" caused by irregular movement (varying velocities) of the red blood cells within the lumen of a vessel. This appearance can occur in the presence of turbulent flow or if the sample volume is placed near the vessel wall, where the flow will be less laminar (unidirectional) because of friction of the red blood cells with the vessel wall.

Spectral broadening may be caused by flow disturbance, inaccurate sample volume placement, excessive pressure on the vessel, or excessive gain.

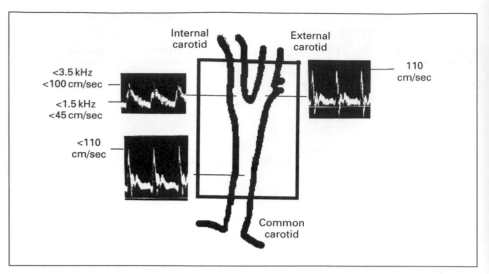

FIGURE 42-11. Diagram showing normal Doppler signal at the standard sites.

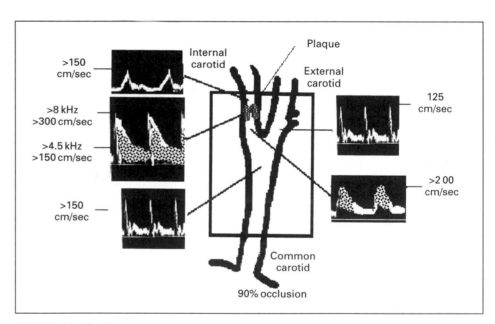

FIGURE 42-12. Diagram showing results of a severe stenosis (90 percent) in the internal carotid artery and the consequences to the Doppler signal at multiple sampling locations within the ipsilateral extracranial carotid circulation.

FIGURE 42-13. Diagram showing the changes that occur in the systolic and diastolic Doppler flow pattern with varying degrees of narrowing of the internal carotid artery.

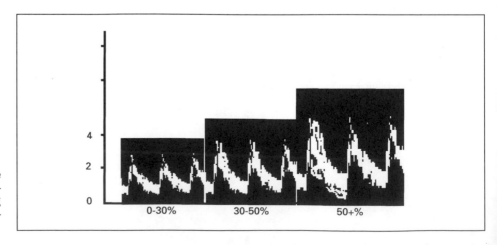

Criteria for Significant Flow Disturbance

The following five criteria are useful in determining a 50 percent or greater diameter reduction:

1. *ICa/CCa ratio.* The internal carotid artery peak systolic measurement is performed at the location of the tightest stenosis and should be compared with the peak systolic velocity (frequency shift) in a nonstenotic portion of the common carotid artery. An ICa/CCa velocity ratio below 0.8:1 indicates no stenosis. A ratio of 1.5:1 or greater indicates severe stenosis.
2. *Turbulence.* An internal carotid artery velocity with a spectral width of 40 cm/sec or more indicates worrisome spectral broadening and significant stenosis.
3. *Velocity.* Maximal internal carotid artery systolic velocity of 110 cm/sec or more indicates significant vessel narrowing.
4. *No flow.* Inability to detect internal carotid artery flow with complete occlusion.
5. *Plaque.* Visible plaque producing a cross-sectional area of 50 percent or less. Some plaque is sonolucent, so there may be a much larger narrowing than you can image although it will be visible on color flow.

Some Special Situations

1. *Stenosis at the carotid origin* (Fig. 42-14). Stenosis at the carotid origin outside the field of view of the carotid sonogram results in weak signals on the involved side. A distinction can be made from low cardiac output by the asymmetry of the low signal.
2. *Stenosis in the distal carotid arteries.* Stenosis that is not visible in the distal carotid artery beyond the highest visible level (Fig. 42-15) may be identified by seeing a high-velocity signal in systole and low-velocity in diastole (i.e., a pattern like the external carotid artery seen in the internal carotid artery).

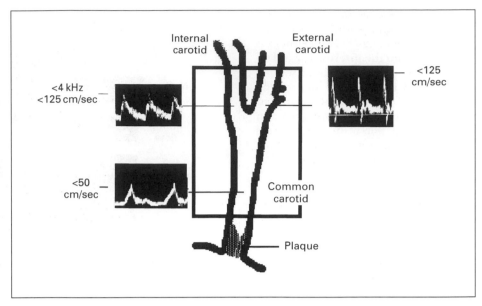

FIGURE 42-14. Diagram showing the consequences of plaque causing a near occlusion at the origin of the common carotid artery to the signals in the vessels higher up in the neck.

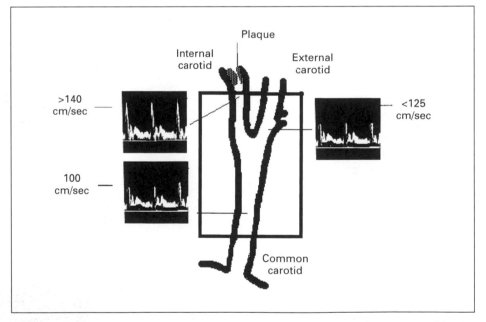

FIGURE 42-15. Diagram showing stenosis of the internal carotid artery outside the field of view and the consequences to the carotid artery flow. Temporal auscultation (see Fig. 42-17) will help in identifying the actual ECA. Flow patterns with any cerebrovascular stenosis will alter if there is significant disease in the contralateral side.

3. *Occluded internal carotid artery.* An occluded internal carotid artery may be confusing (Fig. 42-16). Since there is no flow within the internal carotid artery, you may not be able to see the vessel, and may mistake one of the branches of the external carotid artery for the internal carotid artery. In ICa occlusion, flow within the external carotid may have a low-resistance appearance because the collateral flow will be supplying the brain through the ophthalmic and the external carotid artery. The internal carotid artery may be visible as a sonolucent tube without plaque within, but there will be no flow on Doppler. Gently tapping the temporal artery should cause a response in the diastolic portion of the spectral waveform, verifying that ECa is being examined. Also note the absent or dampened diastolic flow in the common carotid Doppler spectral waveform (Fig. 42-17).

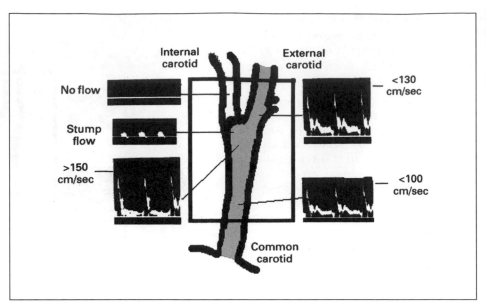

FIGURE 42-16. Diagram showing a complete occlusion of the internal carotid artery. Note that the external carotid artery may now display a low-resistance pattern. Significant disease on the contralateral side as well as the patency of the circle of Willis will also alter the signals on the side being examined.

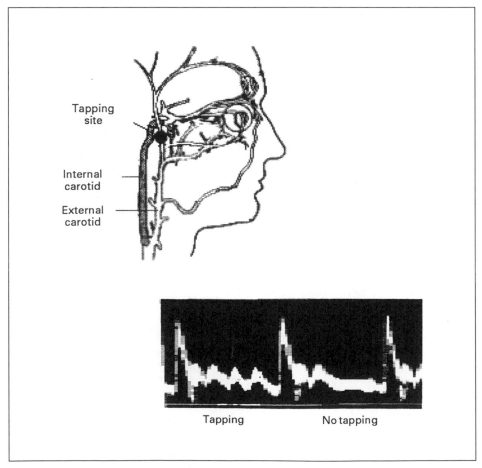

FIGURE 42-17. Top: Diagram showing the site where tapping of the temporal artery branch off the external carotid artery will cause changes in the diastolic flow pattern in the external carotid artery. **Bottom:** Diagram showing the effects on the external carotid artery diastolic signal while tapping the temporal artery.

Vertebral Artery

Examination of the vertebral artery is very limited because its course from the subclavian artery to the basilar artery in the posterior brain circulation (see Fig. 42-3) passes through foramina in the transverse processes of the cervical vertebrae.

It is useful to examine the vertebral arteries bilaterally at a level about 3 cm above the origin from the subclavian arteries. The flow should be in the same direction as that in the common carotid artery and should have similar velocity on the right and left sides.

If flow is reversed in the vertebral artery (it will usually be the left vertebral artery), there is a subclavian steal syndrome (see Fig. 43-11). Blockage of the subclavian artery proximal to the take-off of the vertebral artery (see Fig. 42-1) causes flow in the left vertebral artery to reverse so that the flow demand for the left arm (especially following exercise) is fulfilled. Flow to the left vertebral artery takes place through the circle of Willis from the right vertebral artery and carotid arteries.

 PITFALLS

1. *Aliasing.* If the time elapsed from the initial Doppler signal pulse to return from a target vessel exceeds the PRF (pulse repetition frequency) (i.e., the time before another signal is emitted), the peak Doppler signal will not be shown at the top of the display and may appear on the low side of the baseline. This phenomenon occurs when very high velocity flow states are present or a low PRF is used (Fig. 42-18). To eliminate aliasing, use a lower PRF and/or lower the baseline on the spectral display to enable a higher-velocity waveform to be displayed without aliasing.

2. *External vs. internal carotid artery confusion.* If the internal carotid artery pressure is increased by the presence of plaque and stenosis, the Doppler pattern in the external carotid artery may resemble that in an internal carotid artery, since the external carotid artery will then, through collateral circulation, supply blood to the brain. The absence of vessels branching from the internal carotid artery helps in recognition of this situation. Also, quickly tapping on the temporal artery (anterior to the pinna of the ear) while listening to the Doppler and observing spectral display will cause momentary alterations in the diastolic flow of the external carotid artery (see Fig. 42-17).

3. *Absence of internal carotid artery flow.* If the internal carotid artery is occluded, a branch of the external carotid artery may be confused with the internal carotid artery. This branch would be considerably smaller. Usually, the occluded internal carotid artery can be recognized and no flow can be detected within it with Doppler. Look for confirmatory signs:
   a. No diastolic flow in the spectral waveform in the common carotid artery.
   b. Blunted flow with reversal at the obstruction site.

4. *Tortuosity.* Both the internal and external carotid arteries can be very tortuous, making it easy to confuse the course of the two vessels, especially if both have a high-resistance pattern. The absence of vessels arising from the internal carotid artery (no branches) should be helpful. Tapping the temporal region will result in changes in the diastolic portion of the external carotid artery flow pattern, but not in the internal carotid artery (see Fig. 42-17). In a tortuous vessel, the velocity will be focally elevated as the blood rounds vessel bends, even in disease-free vessels. Color Doppler imaging makes the task of following the course of tortuous vessels much simpler.

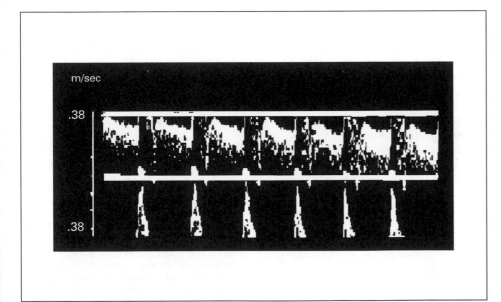

FIGURE 42-18. Diagram showing aliasing. Much of the flow is now below the baseline. To eliminate aliasing move the spectral baseline toward the bottom of the display and/or decrease the PRF to show the entire waveform.

5. *Low flow volume and velocity.* If the flow volume and velocity are lower than expected in the common carotid or internal carotid artery, there may be occlusion distal to the examined site. If the occlusion is beyond the angle of the jaw, it can be an especially difficult diagnosis, since it is out of the range of the ultrasound transducer. Be sure to include ICa/CCa ratios from both right and left carotid arteries. This will eliminate low cardiac output as the cause of the low flow question (see Fig. 42-14). Also note that immediately prior to a total occlusion, the flow in the poststenotic ICa will be very low (see Table 42-1).

6. *Mirror image.* A mirror image of the Doppler spectral information can be caused by excessive Doppler gain (Fig. 42-19) or poor Doppler-interrogation-to-flow angle. Reduce the Doppler gain until the strongest signal persists. An error in the interpretation of flow direction and underestimation of the velocity of the signal will occur if the mirrored signal is measured. If the mirrored signal is the same intensity as the forward flow signal, poor Doppler-to-flow angle is the likely cause. Ad-

just the Doppler angle to achieve a 30- to 60-degree angle to flow, resulting in a more unidirectional Doppler spectral display.

7. *Suboptimal Doppler angle.* A poor Doppler interrogation angle (70 to 90 degrees to flow) will cause a poor-quality spectral display with evidence of signal both above and below the baseline. It will also give inaccurate flow information. Adjust the scan angle to obtain a better Doppler angle to flow for more precise spectral information. If color Doppler imaging is available, its use will speed the localization of flow and flow direction in a patient with extensive disease in the carotid. A poor angle will make it difficult to obtain adequate color filling in a vessel (color is also pulsed Doppler).

8. *High wall filter settings.* Loss of the diastolic component of the spectral display or inability to display low venous flow may be the result of a wall filter setting that is too high. Check the wall filter level—if the spectral signal is missing near the baseline, lower the wall filter to 50 Hz or its lowest setting before diagnosing a no-flow state.

9. *Large sample size.* Spectral broadening can be created by using a sample volume that is too large (more than 2 mm) or by placing the sample volume adjacent to the vessel wall. Both errors will record many velocities because of slower flow along the vessel wall, giving a false impression of turbulent flow.

10. *Difficulty identifying a vessel when calcification obscures the vessel lumen.* Pulsed Doppler spectral signals and the color Doppler do not pass through calcification. Look for Doppler shift information by randomly adjusting the sample volume placement and listening for Doppler sounds around and above the calcified plaque formation or color flow adjacent to the area of calcification. Try using Doppler even if there is no hint of a vessel by imaging techniques. Remember, Doppler signals are strongest parallel to the flow, whereas imaging is strongest at 90 degrees to the vessel. This may enable you to obtain a flow signal when imaging is poor.

SELECTED READING

Bude, R. O., Rubin, J. M., Platt, J. F., Fechner, K. P., and Adler, R. S. Pulsus tardus: Its cause and potential limitations in detection of arterial stenosis. *Radiology* 190:779–784, 1994.

Derdeyn, C. P., Powers, W. J., Moran, C. J., Cross, D. T., III, and Allen, B. T. Role of Doppler US in screening for carotid atherosclerotic disease. *Radiology* 197:635–643, 1995.

Fox, A. J. How to measure carotid stenosis. *Radiology* 186:316–318, 1993.

Kirsch, J. D., Wagner, L. R., James, E. M., Charboneau, J. W., Nichols, D. A., Meyer, F. B., and Hallett, J. W. Carotid artery occlusion: Positive predictive value of duplex sonography compared with arteriography. *J Vasc Surg* 19:642–649, 1994.

Kotval, P. S. Doppler waveform parvus and tardus. *J Ultrasound Med* 8:435–440, 1989.

Middleton, W. D., and Melson, G. L. The carotid ghost: A color Doppler ultrasound duplication artifact. *J Ultrasound Med* 9:487–493, 1990.

Moneta, G. I., Edwards, J. M., Papanicolan, G., et al. Screening for asymptomatic internal carotid artery stenosis. Duplex criteria for documenting 60% to 90% stenosis. *J Vasc Surg* 21:989–994, 1995.

Polak, J. F., Kalina, P., Donaldson, M. C., O'Leary, D. H., Whittemore, A. D., and Mannick, J. A. Carotid endarterectomy: Preoperative evaluation of candidates with combined Doppler sonography and MR angiography. *Radiology* 186:333–338, 1993.

Zweibel, W. J. *Introduction to Vascular Sonography.* New York: Grune & Stratton, 1992.

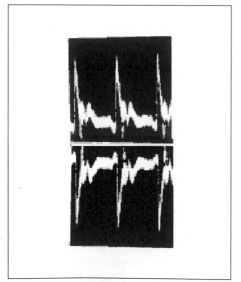

FIGURE 42-19. Diagram showing the mirror effect. When this appearance is noted, reduce the Doppler gain until the strongest signal persists. If the signals above and below the baseline are of equal intensity, reposition the Doppler sample volume to improve the Doppler angle to flow (40–60 degrees).

43

INTRACRANIAL VASCULAR PROBLEMS

GAIL SANDAGER

SONOGRAM ABBREVIATIONS

A Arch	Aortic arch
Aca	Anterior cerebral artery
Acoa	Anterior communicating artery
AW	Anterior window
Ba	Basilar artery
ICa	Internal carotid artery
INNa	Innominate artery
LACa	Left anterior cerebral artery
LCCa	Left common carotid artery
LICa	Left internal carotid artery
LMCa	Left middle cerebral artery
MCa	Middle carotid artery
MW	Middle window
Oa	Opthalmic artery
Pca	Posterior cerebral artery
PW	Posterior window
RACa	Right anterior cerebral artery
RCCa	Right common carotid artery
RECa	Right external carotid artery
RICa	Right internal carotid artery
Rva	Right vertebral artery
Sa	Subclavian artery
Va	Vertebral artery

KEY WORDS

Arteriovenous Malformation (AVM). An abnormal communication between arteries and veins.

Basal Intracranial Arteries. Large vessels at the base of the brain.

Butterfly Pattern. The characteristic Doppler velocity spectra seen at the normal middle cerebral artery/anterior cerebral artery bifurcation, displaying the middle cerebral artery flow above the baseline directed toward the probe and the anterior cerebral artery flow below the baseline moving away from the probe. This is a major reference point used for vessel identification.

Collateral Circulation. An alternate circulatory route that is evoked when the normal circulatory pathways are obstructed.

Critical Stenosis (Hemodynamically Significant). A narrowing of the vessel lumen that results in a decrease in pressure and flow.

Endarterectomy. Surgical technique in which a diseased portion of the carotid artery is removed and replaced with a vein.

Foramen. Natural passage or opening.

Genu. Acute bend of the carotid in the brain.

Hyperdynamic Flow. Increased volume of flow gives rise to increased velocities.

Hyperostosis. Bone hypertrophy (overgrowth).

Parasellar. Close to the sella turcica in the region of the pituitary gland.

Range Ambiguity. If a large Doppler sample site is used, a variety of signals will be received giving a wide range of results.

Supraclinoid. Above the clinoid process, close to the pituitary.

Vasospasm. Constriction or narrowing of the arteries usually occurring after a subarachnoid hemorrhage; velocities become markedly elevated in the presence of vasospasm.

 THE CLINICAL PROBLEM

Ultrasonic evaluation of the basal intracranial arteries was in the past limited by inability to penetrate the skull with ultrasound. Angiography was, until recently, the only method available for evaluation of intracranial arteries. However, angiography only provides anatomic information with limited functional information. It is too risky and invasive to use as a screening examination. Transcranial Doppler (TCD) is a noninvasive method of examining the intracranial arteries that provides both anatomic and hemodynamic flow information.

Assessment of the major basal intracranial arteries is important in a variety of clinical conditions. The presenting symptoms or clinical indications will vary depending on the problem.

Clinical indications for TCD include the following:

1. Detection of major basal intracranial artery critical stenoses
2. Detection of vertebrobasilar insufficiency
3. Evaluation of cerebral artery vasospasm: onset, location, severity, and course over time. This usually occurs after a subarachnoid hemorrhage from a ruptured cerebral artery aneurysm.
4. Assessment of patterns and extent of collateral circulation
5. Extension of carotid exam to determine intracranial blood flow velocity in the presence of severe extracranial carotid artery disease
6. Detection of arteriovenous malformation (AVM)

7. Determining the state of circulation in patients with suspected brain death
8. Intraoperative monitoring of cerebral hemodynamics during cerebrovascular or cardiovascular surgery
9. Evaluation of patients posttreatment—success of embolization of arteriovenous malformations
10. Determining the effect of subclavian steal on intracranial hemodynamics

ANATOMY

The major basal intracranial arteries form the circle of Willis. The circle of Willis is comprised of an anterior segment and a posterior segment with a right and left side. The anterior portion of the circle of Willis circulation arises from the right and left internal carotid arteries (Ica), whereas the posterior circulation arises from the vertebrobasilar arteries (Fig. 43-1).

Anterior Circulation of the Circle of Willis

The extracranial (neck) segment of the ICa begins at the common carotid bifurcation and ends where the ICa enters the skull. At this point it becomes the intracranial ICa. The intracranial ICa then courses cephalad to the carotid siphon region. At the carotid siphon, the ICa forms an S-like configuration as it first runs anterior, then medial, and then posterior. This segment of the ICa will normally display different flow directions depending on which segment is insonated (Fig. 43-2). This tortuous segment of ICa gives rise to the ophthalmic artery (Oa), which provides blood supply to the eye. Just beyond the Oa, the ICa branches into the anterior cerebral artery (ACa) and the middle cerebral artery (MCa). These vessels form the anterior circulation of the circle of Willis. The right and left sides of the anterior circulation are connected by the anterior communicating artery (ACoa). This completes the right and left sides of the anterior portion of the circle of Willis (Fig. 43-3).

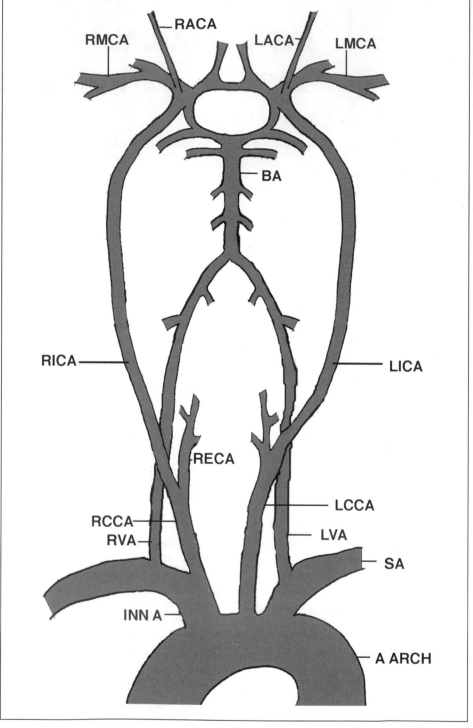

FIGURE 43-1. Diagram showing normal intracranial anatomy. A Arch = aortic arch. INNa = innominate artery. Sa = subclavian artery. LVa = left vertebral artery. LCCa = left common carotid artery. LICa = left internal carotid artery. LMCa = left middle cerebral artery. LACa = left anterior cerebral artery. RACa = right anterior cerebral artery. RMCa = right middle cerebral artery. Ba = basilar artery. RICa = right internal carotid artery. RECa = right external carotid artery. RCCa = right common carotid artery. RVa = right vertebral artery.

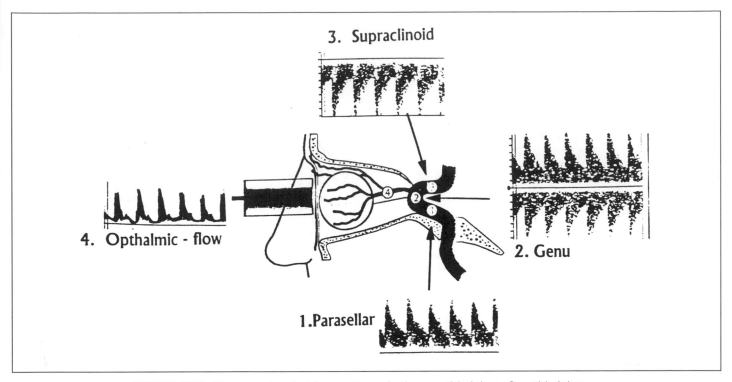

FIGURE 43-2. Diagram showing flow patterns in the carotid siphon. Carotid siphon—lateral view; 1. Parasellar—flow toward the probe; 2. Genu—bidirectional flow; 3. Supraclinoid—flow away; 4. Ophthalmic—flow toward.

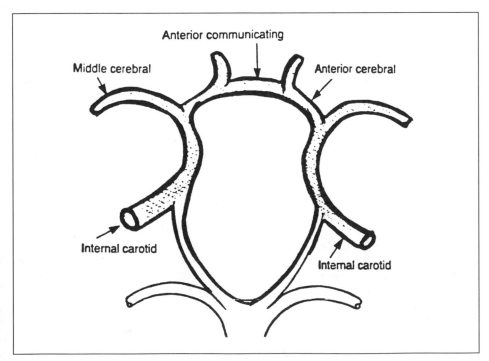

FIGURE 43-3. Anterior portion of the circle of Willis.

Posterior Circulation

The vertebrobasilar arteries give rise to the posterior portion of the circle of Willis.

The right and left vertebral arteries originate as the first branch of the subclavian arteries and course superoposterior through the cervical vertebrae. The vertebral artery (Va) then passes through the foramen magnum and becomes the intracranial portion of the Va. The right and left intracranial vertebral arteries join to form the basilar artery (Ba). The Ba is about 3- to 4-cm long and branches into the right and left posterior cerebral arteries. The anterior and posterior segments of the circle of Willis are then joined via the posterior communicating arteries. These vessels make up the posterior portion of the circle of Willis (Fig. 43-4).

Anatomic variants of the intracranial cerebral circulation are common and reported to occur in up to 50 percent of the population. Vessel size, course, location, and origin can all be varied. The most frequently observed variants include an incomplete circle of Willis, absent communicating arteries, and asymmetry of the Va size.

◼ TECHNIQUE

Preparation

Place the patient in a comfortable position supine with the head flat or slightly elevated. The technologist sits at the head of the patient positioned to maintain stability of the hand with the transducer. A steady hand is essential since slight movement or variation in transducer position may compromise the exam results. Place the equipment within easy reach as frequent adjustments are required throughout the exam; a foot pedal is helpful. Headphones are required to optimize the quality of the audio signal which is a crucial part of the exam.

The status of the extracranial carotid circulation must be known as obstructive lesions of the extracranial carotid vessels may affect the intracerebral circulation and impact on the TCD findings.

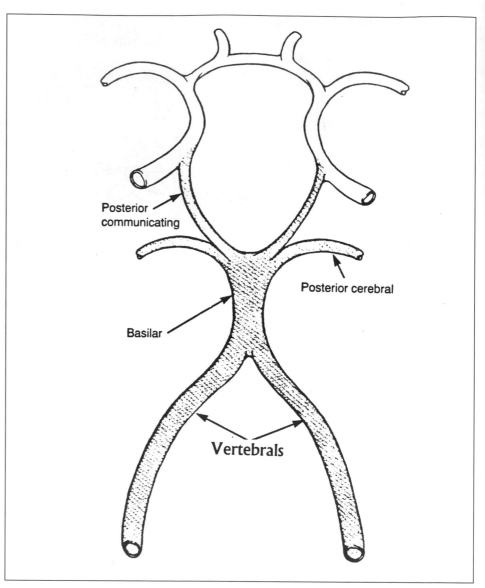

FIGURE 43-4. Posterior portion of the circle of Willis.

Equipment

Instrumentation requirements include (1) a 2- to 3-MHz range gated pulsed Doppler with enhanced power levels to penetrate areas of the skull that are naturally thin; and (2) online spectral analysis that provides time-averaged velocity measurements including peak systole, mean velocity, and pulsatility index.

Currently there are two ways for performing TCD. These include a nonimaging, hand-held probe that provides online spectral analysis; and color duplex imaging that includes a real-time B-mode image, color Doppler, and pulsed Doppler spectral analysis.

Although several different techniques are used, the only currently available diagnostic criteria are based on Doppler velocity calculations from a 2-MHz, hand-held pulsed Doppler. Color duplex imaging provides additional information that can be used in combination with the Doppler-derived velocity calculations from the hand-held Doppler.

Vessel Identification Criteria

Vessel identification is based on several observations that should agree to ensure accuracy:

1. Direction of blood flow relative to the transducer
2. Relationship to the acoustic window used—probe orientation
3. Depth of vessel
4. Traceability—distance that the course of the vessel can be followed
5. Spatial relationships to other vessels
6. Response to common carotid artery (CCa) compression
7. Bony landmarks (used only for imaging studies)

Acoustic Windows

There are four ultrasonic windows used to obtain a complete TCD examination. The four windows are the transtemporal, transorbital, transoccipital, and the submandibular approach. Each window provides information regarding specific vessels of the circle of Willis (Figs. 43-5 and 43-6).

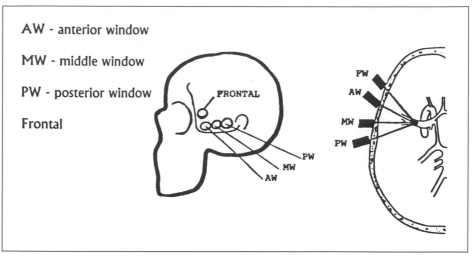

AW - anterior window

MW - middle window

PW - posterior window

Frontal

FIGURE 43-5. Ultrasonic windows from the transtemporal approach.

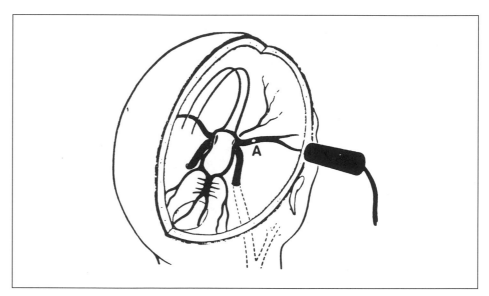

FIGURE 43-6. Transtemporal approach.

The Transtemporal Window

A routine exam begins with the transtemporal window on either the right or the left side. This window is over the temporal bone immediately superior to the zygomatic arch. The window has four parts, the anterior, middle, posterior, and frontal (see Fig. 43-5). The best window will vary from patient to patient; you may find and only use one or you may use a combination of windows. It is important to find the window that provides the highest-quality signal. The vessels evaluated routinely from this approach include the MCa, the ACa, the posterior cerebral artery (PCa), and the terminal portion of the intracranial ICa (t-ICa). The anterior and posterior communicating arteries are examined using this approach but are not routinely identified owing to size and low flow states under normal conditions. The ACoa and the posterior communicating artery (PCoa) act as collateral pathways that enlarge and may be identified. Normal values in each location are shown in Table 43-1.

The Transorbital Window

This window is located directly through the eyelid (as opposed to supraorbital) and provides access to the Oa and the intracranial portion of the ICa/carotid siphon. Decrease power levels to 5 to 10 percent of the maximum power output to minimize ultrasound exposure to the retina since signal attenuation is low when using this window.

The Suboccipital Window— Transforaminal

This acoustic window is created by the natural opening found at the base of the skull called the foramen magnum (Fig. 43-7). Using this approach, the intracranial portions of the right and left vertebral arteries and the Ba can be insonated. The patient's position is changed to provide access to the posterior portion of the base of the skull. The patient can turn onto either the right or left side with the head flexed forward to create a larger opening between the atlas and the base of the skull. If this position is not comfortable for the patient, almost any position is acceptable that allows forward flexion of the head and adequate space for the transducer.

Doppler Only—Standard Technique

Place the transducer over the temporal bone slightly superior to the zygomatic arch. Start with the sample volume set at 55 mm. Slide the probe across the four windows until an arterial signal is detected. After optimization of the arterial signal locate the MCa and trace it throughout its course. The MCa runs from depths of 30 to 60 mm with flow directed toward the transducer. The characteristic waveform patterns are low resistance, low pulsatility, with forward flow throughout diastole. Normal mean velocities are 55 ± 12 cm/sec (Fig. 43-8).

Complete the evaluation of the MCa then locate the MCa/ACa bifurcation. This is identified by moving the sample volume to a depth of 55 to 65 mm and angling superior and anterior until bidirectional flow is displayed. The large sample volume size (5 mm) causes insonation of both the MCa and ACa at their bifurcation. This pattern is referred to as the "butterfly" pattern and is an important reference point for spatial relationships of other intracranial arteries.

The ACa can be traced from depths of 60 to 80 mm by aiming the ultrasound beam slightly superior and anterior. Flow direction of the normal ACa is away from the transducer with normal mean velocities of 50 ± 11 cm/sec. Once the sample volume depth is moved beyond the MCa/ACa bifurcation, the MCa signal will disappear. After complete investigation of the entire ACa, trace the Doppler signal back to the MCa/ACa bifurcation; this is always the reference point one returns to for tracking the other vessels.

Evaluate the terminal portion of the intracranial ICa by angling the ultrasound beam inferior from the MCa/ACa bifurcation. The sample volume depth remains unchanged. Flow direction is toward the transducer with a normal mean velocity of 39 ± 9 cm/sec. This is generally the only segment of the distal ICa identified.

TABLE 43-1. NORMAL INTRACRANIAL ARTERIAL VELOCITY VALUES

Artery	Acoustic Window	Depth of Sample Volume	Normal Mean Velocity	Color Coding Flow Direction	Normal Direction of Flow
MCa	Transtemporal	35–60 mm	55 +/− 12 cm/sec	Red	Toward the probe
ACa	Transtemporal	60–80 mm	50 +/− 11 cm/sec	Blue	Away from the probe
PCa(P1)	Transtemporal	60–70 mm	39 +/− 10 cm/sec	Red	Toward the probe
PCa(P2)	Transtemporal	60–70 mm	39 +/− 10 cm/sec	Blue	Away from the probe
t ICa	Transtemporal	55–65 mm	39 +/− 9 cm/sec	Red	Toward the probe
Oa	Transorbital	40–60 mm	21 +/− 5 cm/sec	Not used for the Oa	Toward the probe
Supraclinoid, Genu, Parasellar	Transorbital	60–75 mm	40 +/− 11 na 47 +/− 14 cm/sec	Not used for the carotid siphon	Away from the probe Bidirectional Toward the probe
Va	Transforaminal	65–90 mm	40 +/− 10 cm/sec	Blue	Away from the probe
Ba	Transforaminal	80–120 mm	40 +/− 10 cm/sec	Blue	Away from the probe

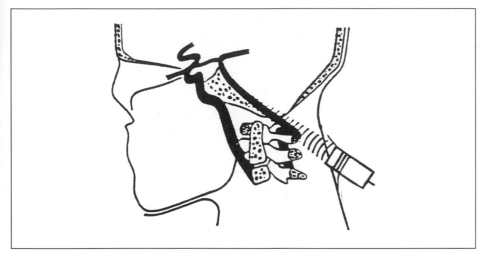

FIGURE 43-7. Transoccipital approach for evaluation of the vertebrobasilar arteries.

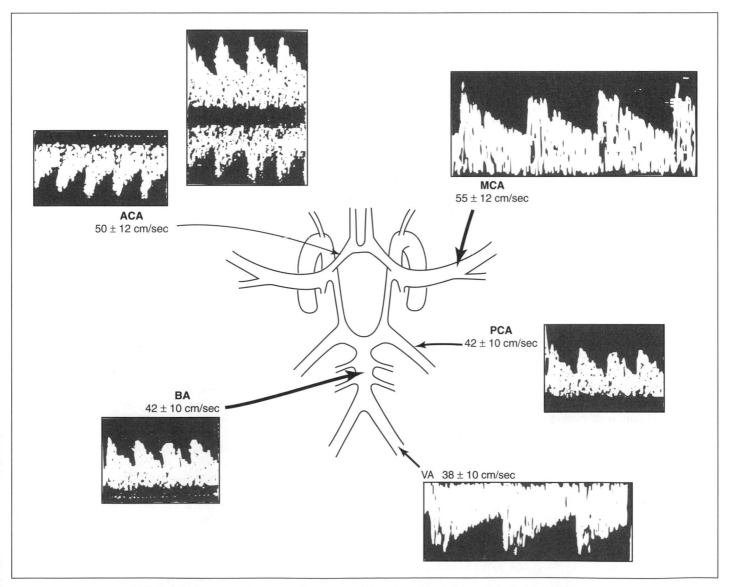

FIGURE 43-8. Normal mean velocities and Doppler signals from the circle of Willis.

The PCa is located by directing the ultrasound beam posterior and inferior from the MCa/ACa bifurcation. If the near (P1) PCa precommunicating segment is insonated, the flow is toward the transducer, whereas the contralateral (P2) PCa postcommunicating signal is away from the transducer. The sample volume depth is between 60 to 80 mm with a normal mean velocity of 39 ± 10 cm/sec (see Fig. 43-8).

Common Carotid Artery Compression Maneuvers

After completion of the transtemporal evaluation, CCa compression maneuvers may be used to confirm vessel identification. These maneuvers are used only if needed to provide more information regarding confirming vessel identification and the presence of collateral pathways. Before initiating compression, the status of the extracranial carotid arteries must be known. Carotid compression maneuvers are *contraindicated in the presence of severe carotid artery disease, low carotid bifurcation, and unstable carotid plaque.* The decision is made by the appropriate medical personnel; medical supervision should be available during this part of the examination since there is some risk.

Common carotid artery compression is performed by palpating the carotid artery in the neck and slowly applying pressure until the pulse disappears. This is done while insonating the intracranial vessel in question. Pressure is applied for only a few seconds, or two to three cardiac cycles; in the presence of an intact circle of Willis, compression of the right CCa will cause the right MCa to shrink and flow will be obliterated. The right ACa exhibits either reversal of flow or diminished or obliterated flow. Compression of the left CCa should not affect the contralateral intracerebral vessels unless collateral pathways (cross-filling) has occurred.

Transorbital Approach

The transducer is placed over the closed eyelid with coupling gel. The transducer beam is angled medial with the sample volume depth between 40 and 60 mm. The probe is moved slightly until an arterial signal is located; this is the Oa. The flow direction is toward the probe with normal mean velocities of 21 ± 5 cm/sec. The normal waveform pattern is higher resistance than the other intracerebral vessels. Trace the Oa distal to approximately 65 mm to locate the carotid siphon.

The course of the carotid siphon–intracranial ICa forms an S-like configuration (see Fig. 43-2). There are three components to the carotid siphon that forms the "S," the parasellar, the genu, and the supraclinoid. All three segments are evaluated by tilting the probe from inferior to superior at depths of 60 to 70 mm.

The proximal parasellar segment is inferior with flow directed toward the transducer. The genu is slightly superior to the parasellar portion with flow seen both above and below the baseline due to range ambiguity from the large sample volume. The most superior segment is the supraclinoid with flow moving away from the transducer. Although flow direction changes owing to the course of the vessel, all segments are located at approximately the same depth of 60 to 75 mm. The mean velocities detected are the supraclinoid segment at 40 ± 11 cm/sec and the parasellar segment at 47 ± 14 cm/sec. The waveform configuration is low resistance with low pulsatility.

Submandibular Approach

Narrowing of the vessel lumen and increased flow volume both increase the velocities of the major basal intracranial arteries. To differentiate narrowing from increased flow volume, a hemispheric ratio is used. The hemispheric ratio is the peak systolic velocities of the MCa divided by the peak systolic velocities of the ICa (MCa/ICa). Vessel narrowing causes increased velocities at the site of narrowing where an increased volume of flow (hyperdynamic flow) causes increased velocities in both vessels. A hemispheric ratio of less than 3 is consistent with hyperdynamic flow, whereas a ratio of over 3 is compatible with vasospasm.

Velocity measurements of the extracranial ICa are obtained using the submandibular approach. The 2-MHz probe is placed at the angle of the jaw and angled posterior and medial. The power levels are decreased to 5 percent. The transducer is rotated until a low-resistance ICa signal is located. To assure proper vessel identification, rock the transducer slightly anterior to listen to the external carotid artery and compare the Doppler signals. By rocking back and forth between vessels, you can distinguish the ICa from the external carotid artery by the latter's characteristic high-pitched Doppler signals and vessel location. Optimize the ICa Doppler signal and then obtain the appropriate Doppler measurements.

The Suboccipital Window

The right and left vertebral arteries enter the base of the skull through the foramen magnum, which provides a natural window to evaluate the vertebrobasilar arteries. Change the patient's position so that he or she is lying on either the right or left side with the head flexed forward. This position opens up the window at the base of the skull to facilitate transducer placement.

The probe is placed midline just below the base of the skull with a sample volume depth of 75 mm. The ultrasound beam is aimed toward the patient's nose. Owing to wide variations in the course and location of the right and left vertebral arteries, the transducer may need to be moved right and left of midline with the same beam direction until an arterial signal is identified.

Two distinct vessels should be located by rocking the transducer back and forth from right to left and locating two separate arterial signals. Each Va is tracked from depths of 60 to 90 mm with flow moving away from the transducer (see Fig. 43-8). The normal mean velocities are 40 ± 10 cm/sec with a low-resistance, low-pulsatility waveform. A second arterial signal may be encountered at depths of 60 to 70 cm, displaying flow in the opposite direction. This is a main branch of the Va, called the posterior inferior cerebellar artery. Owing to its course, the signal will disappear when the sample volume depth is moved either in front of or behind the vessel's origin.

Continuing along the course of the Va is the Ba, where the right and left vertebral arteries converge at a depth of 80 to 90 mm with flow continuing away from the probe. The Ba is about 3- to 4-cm long. The normal mean velocities are 42 ± 10 cm/sec, approaching the Va (see Fig. 43-8).

Color Doppler Imaging Technique

Color Doppler imaging is used in combination with the standard nonimaging exam. Color Doppler imaging adds the following: (1) more efficient and confident vessel identification; (2) quicker recognition of anatomic variants; and (3) easier location of flow abnormalities.

Using any commercially available scanner, select the dedicated TCD set-up. The two-dimensional B-mode image depth of field is set to 8 cm. Place the transducer over the temporal bone in a transverse oblique orientation, so that anterior is located on the left side of the screen and posterior is on the right side, with lateral along the top of the image and medial at the bottom.

Using only the gray scale image, move the probe until an adequate window is found. Optimize the window by aligning the bony and soft tissue landmarks. The temporal window landmarks are the sphenoid wing and petrous portion of the temporal bone, the anterior clinoid process, the foramen lacerum, and the mesencephalic brain stem (Fig. 43-9). Align the sphenoid wing, petrous ridge, and foramen lacerum then turn on the color.

Vessels examined from this approach are the MCa, ACa, and PCa. Aiming the beam inferiorly, the intracranial ICa is seen just superior to the foramen lacerum; the foramen lacerum will appear as a small anechoic circle with flow toward the transducer coded in red. With this landmark, angle superior to locate the intracranial basal arteries. The MCa is seen running parallel to the sphenoid wing; flow is toward the transducer and coded in red. Occasionally branches of the MCa are visualized; this is a normal finding.

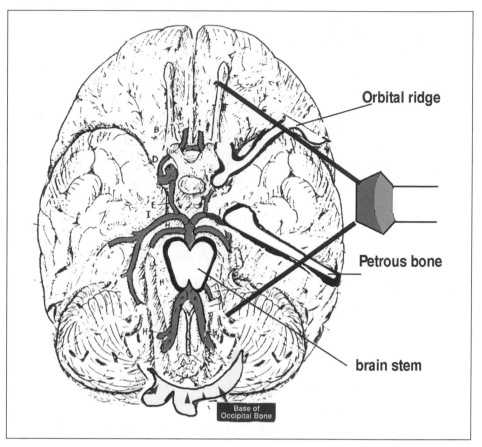

FIGURE 43-9. Diagram showing the bony window to the intracranial arteries. The heart-shaped structure is the mesencephalon in the brain stem, which is an obvious landmark.

Since direction of flow is vital to vessel identification, color coding is not changed during the exam. The standard set-up displays red toward and blue away from the transducer. The pulsed Doppler information is obtained by tracking the course of the MCa while recording the standard information. Angle correction with color imaging is controversial at this time. Whatever protocol is used, angle-correction measurements or an assumed angle of zero, be consistent and standardize the procedure.

Trace the course of the MCa with the Doppler until the MCa/ACa bifurcation (butterfly pattern) is located. The ACa will be coded in blue with flow moving away from the transducer. Follow the ACa with the Doppler recording the necessary calculations, always monitoring all the variables for vessel identification. At depths of 70 mm or more, the contralateral ACa is sometimes visualized and will be displayed in red with flow toward the transducer. To investigate the vessels of the opposite hemisphere, the contralateral temporal window is used.

To locate the PCa, optimize the image at the MCa/ACa bifurcation and then angle posterior and inferior. The PCa has the lowest velocities normally and gain settings or velocity controls may need to be reset to aid color filling. The mesencephalon portion of the brain stem is the major landmark for the PCa. The mesencephalon is a posterior hypoechoic structure (see Fig. 43-9). The PCa courses around the mesencephalon. The P1 segment is coded red and the P2 in blue. Doppler recordings are taken throughout the entire course of the vessel.

Transforaminal Approach— Transoccipital

This window is used to evaluate the intracranial vertebrobasilar arteries. The probe is oriented in a transverse oblique plane and positioned in the back of the head just below the base of the skull. The probe is angled superiorly toward the patient's nose. Color settings may need to be adjusted for the lower velocities normally seen in the vertebrobasilar arteries. The depth of field is set at approximately 8 cm. Using the B-mode image, locate the foramen magnum, which is circular in appearance with low-level echoes in the center. The right and left vertebral arteries appear to course around the foramen magnum, with flow directed away from the transducer and coded in blue. If the right and left vertebral arteries are not seen in the same plane, move the transducer to the right and left of midline until a vessel is detected.

The vertebral arteries join together to form the Ba at approximately 8.5 cm. To follow the course of the Ba, the transducer may need to be rotated and angled superior. In many cases only the proximal portion of the Ba can be identified.

Transorbital Window

This approach is not currently used with color Doppler because of the high ultrasonic dose required.

 PATHOLOGY

Vasospasm

The diagnosis of vasospasm is the most widely accepted use of TCD today. Vasospasm is usually seen after a subarachnoid hemorrhage (SAH), with a predictable course between days 4 and 14 after the SAH. TCD provides information regarding the location, onset, duration, and severity of the vasospasm. Vasospasm causes narrowing of the arterial lumen which will increase the mean velocities. The increase in velocity is related to the narrowing; the more severe the narrowing, the higher increase in mean velocities. There are three categories of vasospasm:

Mild: 120 to 140 cm/sec

Moderate: 140 to 200 cm/sec

Severe: >200 cm/sec

There is also a strong correlation between the patient's clinical status and the daily changes in TCD findings. Mean velocities of greater than 250 cm/sec daily are associated with a poor outcome.

Arteriovenous Malformation (AVM)

1. Diagnostic criteria for large and medium-size AVMs include changes that occur from the feeding artery to the AVM and within the AVM. The amount of change is dependent upon the size and number of vessels involved and communicating with the AVM.
2. In the feeding artery, both systolic and diastolic flow velocity increases are seen with decreased pulsatility. Peak systolic velocity is usually greater than 180 cm/sec with an end-diastolic volume of greater than 140 cm/sec. The pulsatility index can be as low as 0.26.
3. The flow within the AVM is turbulent and chaotic.
4. The velocities between the right and left hemispheres are asymmetric.
5. AVM treatment is to embolize the malformation. TCD is performed pretreatment to obtain baseline values, and then again postembolization to determine the success of therapy. The goal is to embolize and obliterate the AVM.

Brain Death

TCD is a useful tool for documentation of cerebral circulatory arrest and brain death. However, it is not a definitive exam and is only used as a screening tool. Since it is noninvasive and portable, it can help select those patients that may need more invasive studies for which transport is required. Brain death is associated with the absence of cerebral perfusion. This cessation of intracranial flow causes a characteristic Doppler signal that exhibits "to-and-fro flow," forward flow in cardiac systole and equal net retrograde flow during cardiac diastole. This is associated with an increase in intracranial pressure which causes increased vascular resistance. The Doppler signal varies at different stages of cerebral circulatory arrest (Fig. 43-10); therefore repeat examinations are performed at various intervals to confirm the findings and the diagnosis.

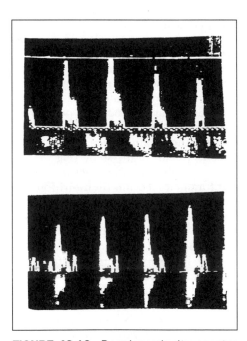

FIGURE 43-10. Doppler velocity spectra from the middle cerebral artery consistent with cerebral circulatory arrest, demonstrating increased vascular resistance and a "to-and-fro flow" pattern.

Intracranial Cerebral Artery Stenoses

Flow-reducing lesions of the intracranial cerebral arteries cause a focal increase in velocity with associated turbulence or disturbed flow beyond the stenosis. Other associated findings may include decreased velocities proximal or distal to the area, delayed systolic upstroke, and abnormal pulsatility index.

Extracranial Carotid Artery Stenoses or Occlusions

TCD is an extension of the extracranial carotid duplex exam. It provides information regarding blood flow velocity of the intracranial vessels in the presence of extracranial occlusive disease. Associated findings in the presence of extracranial carotid disease will depend on the amount and extent of disease and the ability of the intracranial vessels to collateralize. Changes observed include decreased blood flow velocity, change in direction of flow, delayed systolic upstroke, decreased pulsatility, and turbulence.

Subclavian Steal

Subclavian steal is caused by a stenosis or occlusion that occurs in the subclavian arteries, or right innominate artery, proximal to the origins of the Va. These lesions can cause a pressure gradient between the Va circulation and the distal subclavian artery. This pressure gradient causes the subclavian artery beyond the origin of the Va to steal flow from the vertebral circulation; flow direction then reverses in the Va. If flow reversal occurs up through the Ba, it can cause brain stem ischemia (Fig. 43-11).

Examining the patient for subclavian steal includes extracranial duplex exam of the Va (see Chapter 42) with TCD evaluation of the Va, Ba, and posterior cerebral arteries. Diagnostic criteria are based on blood flow velocity calculations, direction of flow, and waveform configuration.

Intraoperative TCD Monitoring

Intraoperative TCD is used to monitor cerebral blood flow during carotid endarterectomy and cardiac surgery while on cardiopulmonary bypass. This procedure is done via the transtemporal window with the standard nonimaging probe secured onto a headset. This allows for continuous monitoring throughout the surgical procedure. The MCa is the vessel used for monitoring, as it is an end vessel that can be reliably insonated.

During carotid endarterectomy when the carotid artery is clamped, TCD is done to assess the patient's response to carotid clamping. A drop in mean blood flow velocity in the ipsilateral MCa of more than 65 percent from the preclamp value or a drop to zero is consistent with inadequate collateral flow. These findings help to identify those patients that need a carotid shunt during the endarterectomy.

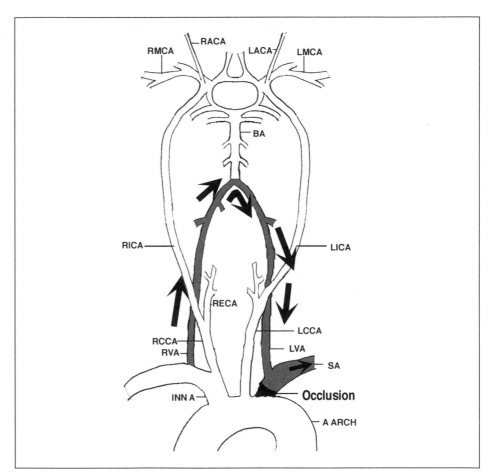

FIGURE 43-11. Subclavian steal—proximal left subclavian artery occlusion with reversed flow in the left vertebral artery.

★ PITFALLS

1. *Temporal window abnormality.* Absence of a temporal window occurs in up to 15 percent of the population, with age, race, and sex being major factors. The most difficult patients to access include older women and African-American patients. Lack of a temporal window may only be unilateral; therefore always examine both sides.

2. *Occlusion vs. technical difficulty.* If a vessel is not identified, a total occlusion cannot be ruled out, although the cause may be technical difficulty.

3. *Operator dependence.* The examination is extremely operator dependent, with a significant learning curve. A number of exams need to be performed in conjunction with an experienced sonographer to correlate findings before working independently.

4. *Lack of patient cooperation.* If the patient is uncooperative or cannot hold still, the exam maybe incomplete and nondiagnostic. If possible, the exam should be repeated when optimum positioning can be obtained.

5. *Aliasing.* Aliasing may be a factor when extremely high velocities are encountered with severe vasospasm or critical stenoses (see Chapter 42).

6. *Other factors.* Variables that may affect exam findings include age, hematocrit, hyperventilation or hypoventilation, cardiac output, and the presence of extracranial carotid disease.

7. *Anatomic variants.* Anatomic variants occur frequently, in up to 50% of the population, with the most common variations including vessel course, size, and origin.

8. *Eye surgery.* If the patient has had recent eye surgery, the orbital portion of the exam may be contraindicated. Approval for the procedure should be given by the ophthalmologist.

9. *Color allocation.* Confusion can arise if color allocations are changed in the course of the study, so that red is substituted for blue.

SELECTED READING

Aaslid, R., Huber, P., and Nornes, H. A transcranial Doppler method in the evaluation of cerebrovascular spasm. *Neuroradiology* 28:11–16, 1986.

Aaslid, R., Markwalder, T. M., and Nornes, H. Noninvasive transcranial Doppler ultrasound recording of flow velocity in basal cerebral arteries. *J Neurosurg* 57:769–774, 1982.

Bogdahn, U., Becker, G., Winkler, J., Greiner, K., Perez, J., and Meurers, B. Transcranial color-coded real-time sonography in adults. *Stroke* 21(12):1680–1688, 1990.

Diethrich, E. B. Normal cerebrovascular anatomy and collateral pathways. In Zwiebel, W. F. (Ed.). *Introduction to Vascular Ultrasonography.* Philadelphia: Saunders, 1986.

Fujioka, K. A., and Douville, C. M. Anatomy and freehand techniques. In Newell, D. A., and Aaslid, R. (Eds.). *Transcranial Doppler.* New York: Raven Press, 1992.

Fujioka, K. A., Gates, D. T., and Spencer, M. P. A comparison of transcranial color Doppler imaging and standard static pulsed wave Doppler in the assessment of intracranial hemodynamics. *J Vasc Tech* 18(1): 29–35, 1994.

Hashimoto, B. E., and Hattrick, C. W. New method of adult transcranial Doppler. *J Ultrasound Med* 10:349–353, 1991.

Lindegaard, K. F., Grolimund, P., Aaslid, R., and Nornes, H. Evaluation of cerebral AVMs using transcranial Doppler ultrasound. *J Neurosurg* 65:335–344, 1986.

Newell, D. W., Gradys, M. S., Sirotta, P., and Winn, H. R. Evaluation of brain death using transcranial Doppler. *Neurosurg* 24:509–513, 1989.

Shoning, M., and Walter, J. Evaluation of the vertebrobasilar-posterior system by transcranial color duplex sonography in adults. *Stroke* 23(9):1280–1286, 1992.

44 BREAST

ROGER C. SANDERS

KEY WORDS

Areola. Pink or brown area around the nipple.

Cooper's Suspensory Ligaments. Fibrous strands forming a lobular network within the breast.

Cystosarcoma Phyllodes (Giant Myxoma). Huge mass similar in nature to a fibroadenoma; occasionally malignant.

Fibroadenoma. Benign mobile breast mass seen in young women; commonly called a "breast mouse."

Fibrocystic Disease. Multiple small cysts with fibrosis are common in young women. This condition is benign but is not necessarily easy to distinguish clinically from carcinoma.

Galactocele. Milk collection within the breast.

Galactorrhea. Milky discharge from nipple not associated with pregnancy.

Invasive Ductal Carcinoma. Most common neoplasm in the breast. Certain sonographic features can suggest this diagnosis.

Medullary Cancer. Unusual type of breast cancer that has a sonographic appearance resembling a fibroadenoma.

Sclerosing Adenosis. Benign condition affecting much of the glandular portion of the breast; occurs in menstruating women.

 THE CLINICAL PROBLEM

Ultrasound is a useful adjunct to mammography and digital palpation in the investigation of breast masses. Some consider ultrasound preferable to mammography as a follow-up to a digital examination showing a palpable mass.

Any palpable mass can be accurately categorized as cystic or solid, and to some extent, benign solid masses can be distinguished from malignant ones. Ultrasound is of particular value in (1) examining young glandular breasts for which mammography is less valuable; (2) confirming the presence of a possible mass found by palpation or seen on mammography; (3) separating cysts from solid lesions; (4) directing puncture and biopsy procedures of breast masses; and (5) diagnosing rupture in breast implants.

Ultrasound may also be used in conjunction with mammography as a follow-up examination for patients who are at increased risk for breast cancer, such as those with a maternal family history of breast cancer or a previous cancer in the other breast.

ANATOMY

The breast undergoes fatty replacement with age, and after menopause the breast is virtually all echopenic fat. This type of breast is not easy to examine with ultrasound, in contrast to mammography. On the other hand, in the menstruating woman, the breast consists of a large, somewhat echogenic central glandular element with a small fatty component in a subcutaneous location. These patients are easy to examine ultrasonically but difficult to evaluate with mammography.

Much anatomic information can be obtained with ultrasound. Some of the ducts leading to the nipple can be visualized. The rib cage and muscles beneath the breast are visible with ultrasound. Cooper's ligaments (echogenic fibrous strands) are sometimes delineated by echopenic fat (Fig. 44-1).

Breast implants consist of single bag or, more recently, double-layered bags containing silicone. The silicone is echofree but conducts sound at a faster speed than normal soft tissues. The breast and chest wall tissue behind an implant may appear a little depressed due to the speed of sound difference. A strong reverberation echo is usually seen just deep to the anterior surface of the bag. A variant form of bag is the expander type in which there is a silicone exterior bag and a saline interior bag which can be topped up when necessary. The central insert is difficult to see and may be missed; one or two small linear echoes are all that is seen in the implant. The port through which additional injections are made is seen at one side of the implant as a set of parallel lines. The more posterior line is slightly curved.

◧ TECHNIQUE

Prior to any breast ultrasonic examination, examine the breasts to get a clear idea of where the mass is and obtain a clinical history. If a mammogram is available, locate the suspect mass on the films prior to the ultrasound exam. Inquire about the rapidity of onset, any recent pregnancy, whether the lesion is painful, and whether there has been any nipple discharge.

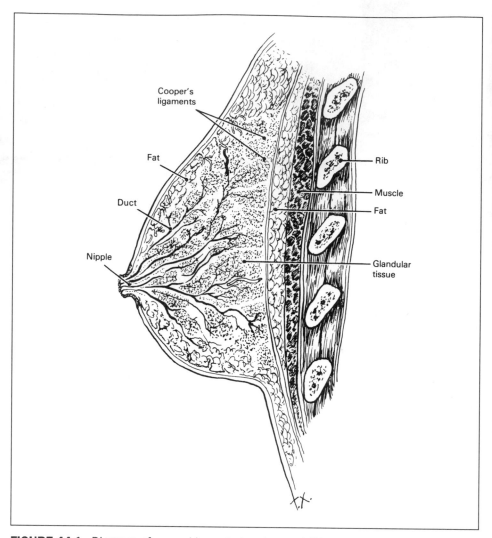

FIGURE 44-1. Diagram of normal breast structures visible on a sonogram.

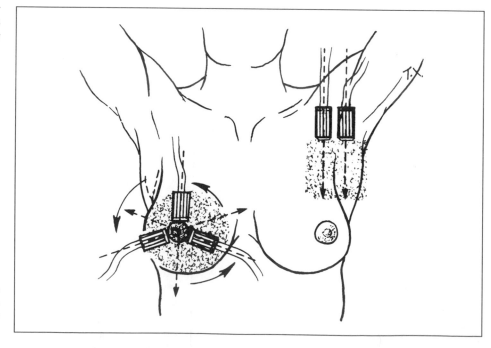

FIGURE 44-2. Diagram showing technique for examining the breast with real-time using a clockwise approach for the breast and parallel views for the axilla.

Linear Array Real-Time

A linear or curved array real-time system with a 5-, 7.5-, or 10-MHz transducer is usually used. A high-frequency transducer is desirable to obtain detailed views of the mass. The mass is palpated and fixed between the fingers while the patient is examined. The erect position helps to immobilize large breasts. With smaller breasts, the use of a stand-off pad may be helpful in defining the near field anatomy.

Limited Mammogram Correlation

Sometimes the ultrasound exam is limited to examination of a mass already imaged by mammography. While it is still necessary to sweep through the rest of the breast, documentation is not usually expected of any region except the mass. These are usually cyst-versus-solid determinations.

Comprehensive Scanning Routine

If ultrasound is the primary imaging tool, as is sometimes done with very young women, both breasts must be imaged—not just the worrisome side. A clockwise approach is employed, using the nipple as a reference point (Fig. 44-2). The patient is supine with her arm raised on the side being scanned; if the breast is large and tends to fall laterally, it helps to oblique the patient slightly away from the side in question. Ask her to raise her knee and let it fall medially to help confine the rotation to the lower body.

The Breast

Label the top right of the screen "nipple," then be consistent with all of your images as you document each "hour" of the clock. 12:00 is from the nipple toward the clavicle in the center of the breast, 6:00 is from the nipple down, and so forth. After documenting these 12 views, go back and take a view across the nipple, or angle slightly to see under it if there is a lot of shadowing. Remember to keep the transducer perpendicular to the skin, so that a suspicious area can be reproduced. There are no orienting landmarks in the breast!

The Axilla

Always sweep through the axilla (see Fig. 44-2) to look for enlarged nodes. Palpate the area first; it may be helpful to lower the arm slightly.

Compression

If a mass or even just a suggestion of a mass is seen, compression with the transducer can clarify the area. If the patient has fibrocystic disease the scan may be ordered to take place just before her period. This can be the best time to see cysts; it is also when the breasts are exquisitely tender. Be gentle.

◆ PATHOLOGY

Cysts

Cysts are common in menstruating women and may resemble a solid mass on mammography. They have the sonographic features of cysts elsewhere in the body (i.e., smooth walls, enhanced through transmission, and absence of internal echoes). They may be multiple or septated. Calcification in a cyst wall may prevent through transmission. Proteinaceous debris within a cyst may cause internal echoes. A thickened cyst wall, mural nodules, and papillary fronds are worrying features that may be due to cancer. Aspiration under ultrasound control is often performed if these features are seen. Typical greenish-black or tan fluid can be discarded. Bloody fluid should be sent for cytopathologic review. If there is concern for a mural nodule, pneumocystography can be performed following aspiration. In this technique, a small amount of air (0.5–2 cc, depending on the size of the cyst) is injected into the drained cyst cavity and a mammogram is obtained. Injection of air also decreases the recurrence rate of cysts.

Fibroadenomas

Fibroadenomas are usually ovoid in shape with uniform low-level internal echoes and a smooth, round, or mildly lobulated border (Fig. 44-3). In a minority of cases, the internal echoes are isoechoic or hyperechoic. Cystosarcoma phyllodes has a similar appearance, but the mass is much larger and multiple cystic spaces within the mass are often seen. Most pathologists just use the term "phyllodes" tumor rather than cystosarcoma since these tumors vary from low malignant potential to high malignant potential. They tend to recur.

Benign features in a mass are as follows:

1. *Hyperechogenic.* Markedly hyperechogenic tissue which is well circumscribed corresponds to normal stromal fibrous tissue. It can form a ridge or a localized mass.
2. *Ellipsoid shape.* Benign tumors expand transversely along tissue planes, and so develop an ellipsoid pattern.
3. *Gentle lobulations.* Two or three lobulations are an acceptable normal finding.
4. *Thin capsule.* A thin echogenic capsule is often seen around benign lesions.
5. *Compressibility.* Benign tumors are more easily compressed than malignant masses.

FIGURE 44-3. Relatively smooth-bordered mass with a few internal echoes and some shadowing—a fibroadenoma.

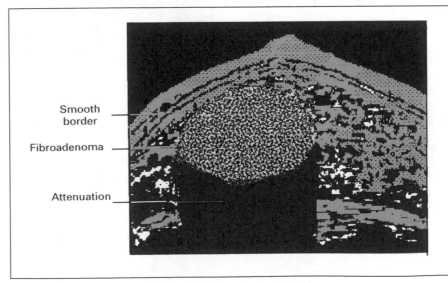

Smooth border

Fibroadenoma

Attenuation

6. *Acoustic shadowing.* Shadowing is even and less marked in benign lesions.
7. *Calcification.* Calcifications are larger and more discrete in benign lesions.

Invasive Ductal (Squamous) Carcinomas

A number of sonographic signs of invasive carcinoma (Fig. 44-4) have been described:

1. *Spiculated outline.* Alternating echopenic and echogenic straight lines radiate from the surface of the mass. When the nodule is surrounded by echogenic fibrous tissue, the strands appear hypoechoic. In an echopenic fatty breast, the nodular strands appear relatively hyperechoic.
2. *Taller than wide.* Typically, benign masses spread in a horizontal direction because they are limited by the tissue planes. Cancers are not confined by tissue planes and therefore often spread vertically and become "taller than they are wide."
3. *Shadowing.* Hypercellular stromal tissue in cancers tends to provoke shadowing. The shadowing is accentuated by the upright position and the use of a sector or curved linear transducer.
4. *Calcifications.* If punctate areas of calcification are seen within a mass, the likelihood of malignancy is increased.
5. *Duct extension pattern.* Cancers tend to expand toward the nipple within ducts.
6. *Microlobulation.* Multiple small lobulations on the border of a mass increase the likelihood of cancer.

Ductal Carcinomas

Ductal carcinomas lead to an increase in duct size. Dilated ducts can be traced to the site of the mass. However, the mass itself may be quite small (Fig. 44-5). Dilated ducts may be seen as a normal variant not related to obstruction.

Medullary Carcinomas

Medullary carcinomas are hard to distinguish from fibroadenomas, but it is said that medullary carcinomas have a few more internal echoes and a slightly more irregular border.

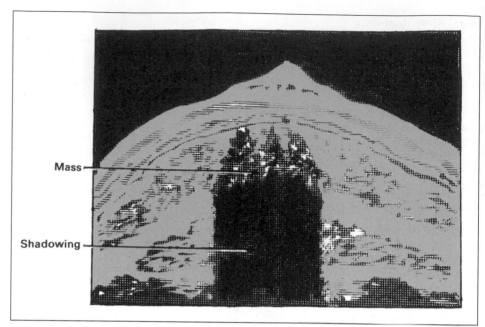

FIGURE 44-4. An infiltrating ductal (squamous) carcinoma with an irregular outline and acoustic shadowing. Note that it is taller than it is wide.

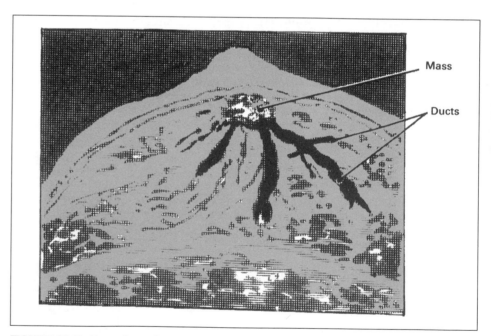

FIGURE 44-5. Ductal carcinoma with dilated ducts distal to a relatively small mass.

Abscesses

Abscesses are fluid filled and usually contain some internal echoes. They have a well-defined border, which is thick and irregular, and tend to occur in the periareolar area. They are very tender and the breast is red and hot over the mass.

Fat Necrosis

Fat necrosis can closely mimic a cancer in the older patient. It exhibits poor through transmission and a ragged border.

Galactoceles

A galactocele is a rare milk collection seen as a poorly outlined, relatively echo-free area with a few internal echoes.

Intramammary Lymph Node

Benign intrabreast nodes are found in the upper outer quadrant of the breast and are well-defined rounded, oval, or kidney-shaped masses with an echogenic fatty center typical of benign lymph nodes elsewhere. Loss of the fatty hilus can be seen in inflammatory and neoplastic conditions.

Implant Problems

Although implants are not as popular as they were, numerous silicone implants are still in place and are still being inserted. Older implants have a single lining while newer implants are double-lined with an inner silicone bag and an outer bag filled with a small amount of saline. A normal implant is echo-free apart from a prominent reverberation echo parallel to the anterior implant surface. Small linear echoes near the borders of the bag represent bag folds. The excellent through transmission and increased speed of sound through silicone lead to apparent posterior displacement of the posterior bag wall.

Implant Rupture

The silicone gel is surrounded by a bag with a single or double layer which may rupture. Ultrasound has proved a good way of assessing implant rupture, though MRI is more reliable.

EXTRACAPSULAR RUPTURE. In most implant ruptures, the gel is confined by the fibrous scar or "capsule." Implant rupture with gross silicone spread most often occurs with single-layered bags, and is therefore becoming less common. An echopenic mass is seen alongside the implant. The echopenic mass is usually surrounded by a highly echogenic area with no acoustic transmission—an area of noise called the "snowstorm" appearance.

INTRACAPSULAR BAG RUPTURE. Several findings are associated with intracapsular bag rupture:

1. There are multiple parallel horizontal echogenic lines within the bag which form a so-called "*stepladder*" pattern. This sign represents the layers of collapsed bag.
2. *Areas of increased echogenicity* develop within the implant. This is a relatively nonspecific sign of implant rupture; the diagnosis depends on how many echoes are seen in the bag.
3. *Globules of silicone* may visibly line the edge of the bag. These represent silicone which has escaped from the bag and now surrounds it.
4. *A contour bulge* may indicate rupture.

MASSES IN ADDITION TO THE IMPLANT. Masses that develop in the breast outside the implant are difficult to detect with mammography owing to the substantial proportion of tissue obscured by the implant and fear of implant rupture when compression is used. They are readily seen with ultrasound and have the appearances described above if they are cancerous. Biopsy with ultrasound guidance is performed so puncture of the implant can be avoided.

⭐ PITFALLS

1. Large, floppy breasts are difficult to examine, and the mass may get lost if the breast is not immobilized. Examining a lesion in the erect position with real-time so that the breast tissue can be swept in front of the transducer may be helpful.
2. Lactating breasts normally contain large tubular structures corresponding to milk-filled ducts.
3. Interpretation of a breast sonogram is difficult and requires considerable experience. Pseudolesions can be easily invented.
4. Apparent posterior placement of the chest wall behind an implant may be mistaken for pathology.
5. Strong reverberation artifacts in a breast implant may be mistaken for implant rupture.
6. Small normal folds in an implant may raise the question of rupture.

SELECTED READING

Berg, W. A., Caskey, C. I., Hamper, U. M., Kuhlman, J. E., Anderson, N. D., Chang, B. W., Sheth, S., and Zerhouni, E. A. Single- and double-lumen silicone breast implant integrity: Prospective evaluation of MR and US criteria. *Radiology* 197:45–52, 1995.

Jackson, V. P. The current role of ultrasonography in breast imaging. *Radiol Clin North Am* 33:1161–1170, 1995.

Mendelson, E. B., and Tobin, C. E. Critical pathways in using breast US. *RadioGraphics* 15:935–945, 1995.

Nelsen, D. J., Rouse, G. A., and DeLange, M. Sonographic evaluation of solid breast masses. *JDMS* 10:312–316, 1994.

Schepps, B., Scola, F. H., and Frates, R. E. Benign circumscribed breast masses. *Obstet Gynecol Clin North Am* 21:519–537, 1994.

Skene, A. I., Collins, C. D., Barr, L., and Cosgrove, D. O. Technical note: Appearances on ultrasound of impalpable injection port in a double chamber breast prosthesis. *Br J Radiol* 66:1050–1051, 1993.

Venta, L. A., Dudiak, C. M., Salomon, C. G., and Flisak, M. E. Sonographic evaluation of the breast. *RadioGraphics* 14:29–50, 1994.

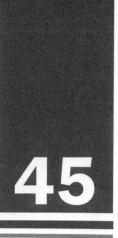

45

PAIN AND SWELLING IN THE LOWER LIMBS

ROGER C. SANDERS

KEY WORDS

Achilles Tendon. Tendon connecting the calf muscles to the calcaneus bone. It lies at the back of the ankle. It tends to be broken by jumping from a height.

Amyloid. Abnormal tissue deposited in body organs when infection and arthritis are prolonged.

Baker's Cyst (Popliteal Cyst). Synovial fluid collection adjacent and posterior to the knee joint due to trauma or rheumatoid arthritis.

Bursa. Inflammatory fluid collection, limited by a capsule, forming adjacent to a joint.

Cellulitis. Inflammation of the soft tissues of the limbs characterized by swelling, hyperemia, and increased echogenicity.

Deep Vein Thrombosis (DVT). Clot in the deep leg veins; causes swelling of the calf and thigh pain.

Gout. Chronic arthritis affecting feet and hands particularly.

Homans' Sign. Pain in the calves on flexing the toes backward. A clinical sign of deep vein thrombosis.

Metaphysis. Portion of the long bone adjacent to the epiphysis where no growth takes place.

Popliteum. Area posterior to the knee joints.

Rheumatoid Arthritis. Chronic arthritis affecting many joints, particularly the hands and knees, in which there is an exuberant overgrowth of the synovial surrounding of the joint. This is known as pannus.

Synovium. The lining of the joint. It produces the fluid that occupies the joint space and a Baker's cyst.

Tenosynovitis. Inflammation of the synovial membrane that surrounds a tendon. Fluid develops around the tendon causing a target appearance on ultrasound.

 THE CLINICAL PROBLEM

Two common causes of pain and swelling in the legs are blood clot in a deep vein (deep vein thrombosis) and a burst knee joint space with extravasation of synovial fluid into the surrounding soft tissue (Baker's cyst).

Deep vein thromboses are common in patients who have recently undergone an operation or who are immobilized in bed. Diagnosis and treatment are important because venous thromboses commonly give rise to emboli that break off from the clot and end up in the lungs. Such pulmonary emboli can be lethal. Deep vein thromboses in the arm occasionally occur due to trauma to the upper arm.

The superficial veins of the leg are not of much sonographic interest. Local clot formation may give rise to pain and redness, but the danger of emboli is minimal. The superficial veins may be used for vessel grafts elsewhere in the body, and the sonographer may be asked to track their course.

Long-term dialysis patients are at risk for complications related to their arteriovenous shunts. In these patients a communication between the main artery and the vein is created, usually in the arm, through which dialysis is performed. Either the vein shuts down due to clots, or arterial plaque develops.

Masses or collections in limbs are easy to demonstrate with ultrasound. Those located near the knee joint are especially confusing clinically, but well seen with ultrasound. Baker's cysts are synovial fluid collections that develop posterior to the knee joint and can extend down into the calf. They are common in people with rheumatoid arthritis, and when they rupture they can mimic the clinical features of deep vein thrombosis. Popliteal artery aneurysms occur in the same location. Clinically, other confusing masses such as abscesses, hematomas, and tumors, recognizable by ultrasound, may occur around the knee joint or at any other site in the limbs.

Limb pain, related to infection, can be difficult to analyze. Ultrasound can distinguish between an abscess which needs to be drained, cellulitis (a soft tissue infection without abscess formation), and acute osteomyelitis (bone infection). The latter requires early antibiotic treatment or long-term refractory infection may develop.

Traumatic limb injuries can be examined with ultrasound. Tendon problems are particularly well seen. Distinguishing between a tendon break and a tendon bruise is clinically important. Foreign bodies in the hands or feet can be detected with ultrasound. Muscle tears and muscle injuries are well seen.

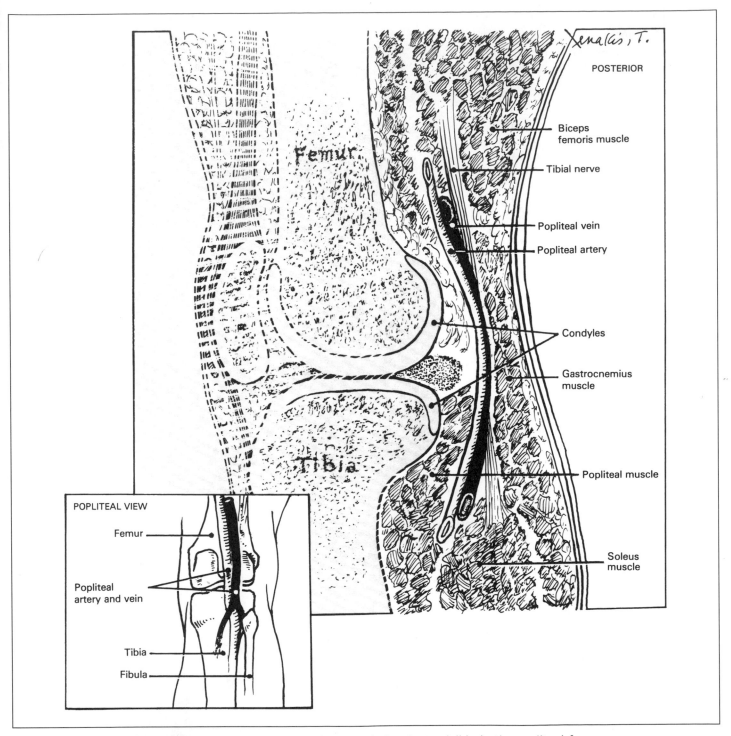

FIGURE 45-1. Diagram showing the normal structures visible in the popliteal fossa and the course of the popliteal artery and vein in relation to the knee joint.

ANATOMY

Vascular System

The femoral artery and vein can be found in the inguinal region in the groin lateral to the pubic symphysis. The vein lies medial to the artery (Fig. 45-2). Major branches, the greater saphenous vein and the deep femoral vein, join just below the groin. The femoral vein can be traced along the medial aspect of the upper leg as it gradually approaches the popliteal fossa and becomes the popliteal vein. At this point the vein lies posterior to the artery.

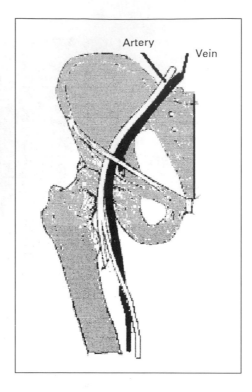

FIGURE 45-2. The femoral vein is medial to the artery in the groin but is lateral to the artery in the popliteal region.

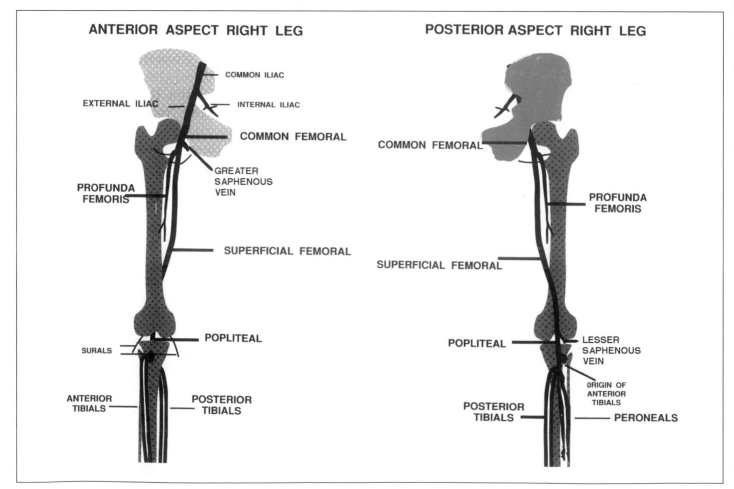

FIGURE 45-3. Anterior and posterior views of the legs showing the deep veins that drain the leg.

The popliteal artery runs posterior to the knee joint (see Fig. 45-1); the popliteal vein runs lateral to the artery. The lesser saphenous vein joins the popliteal vein behind the knee joint. The popliteal vein splits into three veins, the anterior and posterior tibial and the perineal veins which supply the calf (Figs. 45-3 and 45-4), commonly known as the trifurcation. The bones around the knee joint can be recognized posterior to the popliteal artery. Groups of muscles are seen in the adjacent lower thigh and upper calf.

The saphenous vein follows a similar course, but is much more superficial. Duplication of the common femoral vein and the popliteal vein is quite common.

Muscles

The muscles of the thigh and calf can be individually visualized by the alignment of muscle fibers. Muscles are separated by an echogenic line due to connective tissue. As the limb is moved, the muscles move and the individual muscle groups can be distinguished.

Bone

Because bone reflects almost the entire ultrasound beam, only the surface of bone can be seen. Tendons are well analyzed with ultrasound. Tendons have a distinct structure: two echogenic lines outline a series of strongly echogenic linear structures.

◢ TECHNIQUE

A linear array with 7- to 10-MHz frequency is preferred. Whenever there is concern about a questionable appearance, the contralateral side should be examined.

Deep Vein Thrombosis Versus Baker's Cyst

The usual study is performed in the supine position with the affected limb mildly flexed and turned laterally. This allows the upper and middle portion of the thigh and the popliteal and calf veins to be examined without moving the patient. If a Baker's cyst is suspected, place the patient prone and examine the calf.

Vein Recognition

Identify the takeoff of the saphenous vein and the deep femoral vein (see Fig. 45-6). The saphenous vein, although superficial, can be mistaken for the deep femoral vein.

Evaluating Deep Vein Thrombosis

1. Find the femoral vein by locating the femoral artery with palpation and looking along the medial aspect. Do not confuse the saphenous, which is superficial, and the profunda femoris vein, which is deep, with the femoral vein.

2. At each vein intersection with the popliteal vein, take images of the vein at right angles both at rest and with compression so that propagation of any clot can be followed. Typical sites are the greater saphenous vein, the deep femoral vein, the lesser saphenous vein, and the trifurcation. Take sagittal views in between.

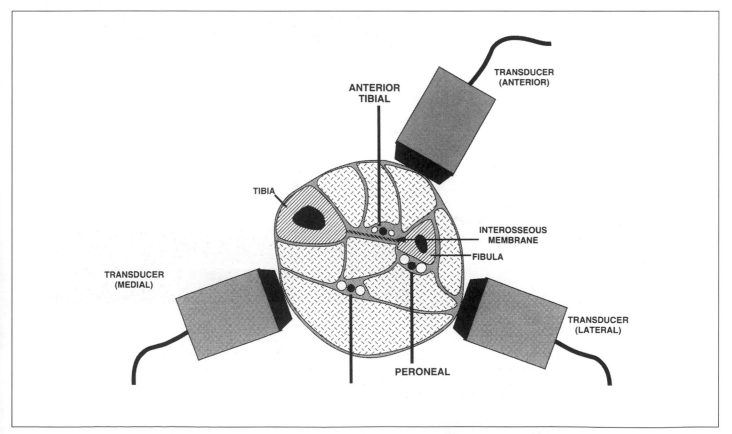

FIGURE 45-4. Diagram showing the approach required to demonstrate the calf veins.

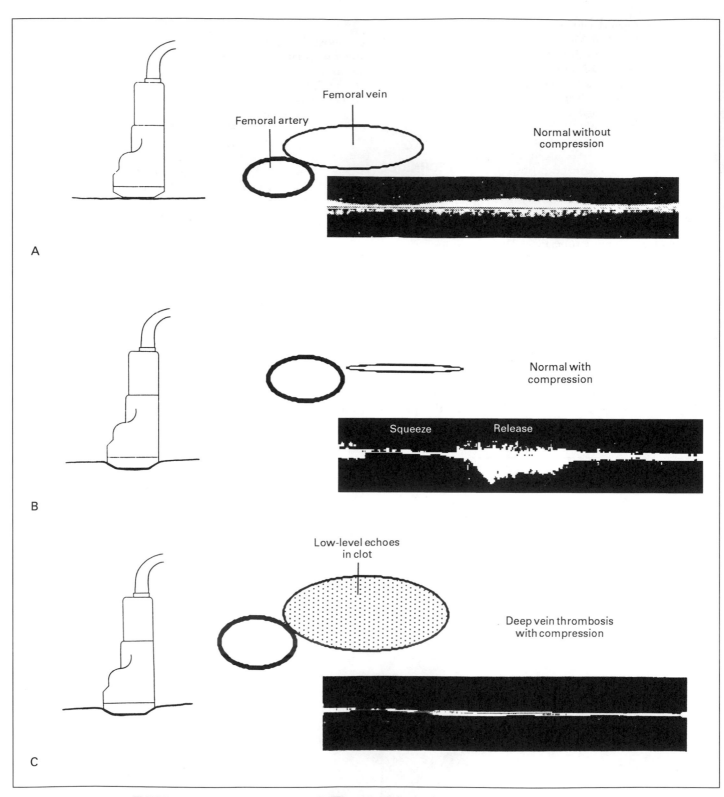

FIGURE 45-5. The femoral vein. (**A**) The normal femoral vein shows good venous flow without compression. (**B**) With compression, the femoral vein collapses, and there is no flow. On release, flow will be seen. (**C**) With deep vein thrombosis, the vein will not compress. There is no flow, and low-level echoes can be seen within the clot.

3. Compress the vein with the transducer in a transverse position and see whether it changes. A normal vein will flatten, whereas a clot-filled vein will not change (Fig. 45-5). Compression is most readily demonstrated on the transverse view; if the compression is performed solely in a sagittal fashion, the transducer may slip off the clot. Comparison with the other leg's femoral vein (as long as it is normal) helps.

4. Place the Doppler cursor within the femoral vein and listen for the typical low-pitched phasic signal of a vein. Since there is not much flow in veins, it may be normal for no signal to occur.

5. Ask the patient to perform Valsalva's maneuver. The patient takes in a full inspiration, holds it, and contracts his or her abdominal muscles. As the patient lets his or her breath go, there should normally be a venous signal.

6. With the transducer on the vein, squeeze the thigh over its medial aspect. Flow should occur in the vein when this "augmentation procedure" is performed. Perform the comparison test at several sites.

7. Attempt to follow the vein along the medial aspect of the leg to the popliteal fossa to look for clot.

Evaluating the Popliteal Vein

1. The popliteal vein is found behind the medial aspect of the knee joint. Look for clot within the vein; compress it with the transducer to see whether it changes shape in a normal fashion. Use Doppler to show flow.

2. Compress the thigh with the transducer over the popliteal vein. As compression is released, a large venous signal normally occurs.

3. Compress the calf. As compression (augmentation) is performed, a Doppler signal is normally evoked.

Track the popliteal vein into the calf. In the usual examination position, the posterior tibial vein is the easiest of the three veins to follow. Take multiple images and videotape the exam if clot is found. Resolution or worsening of a clot on serial ultrasound studies determines therapy so consistent, repeatable views should be taken.

Saphenous Vein Mapping for Vein Graft Procedures

Track the superficial saphenous vein from the popliteal fossa along the medial anterior aspect of the leg (Fig. 45-6). Mark the skin with a grease pencil where the vein is seen. A 10-MHz linear array transducer with color flow is needed for this difficult study. This vein is removed and placed in other body locations if a vein graft is needed.

Evaluating Dialysis Grafts

1. Use a high-frequency transducer, preferably a linear array. A sector scanner with a stand-off pad is an alternative.

2. Use Doppler to see whether there is flow.

3. Examine the wall to make sure there are no small, narrowing plaques. The walls of dialysis grafts are made of Teflon, so they are normally thick and smooth.

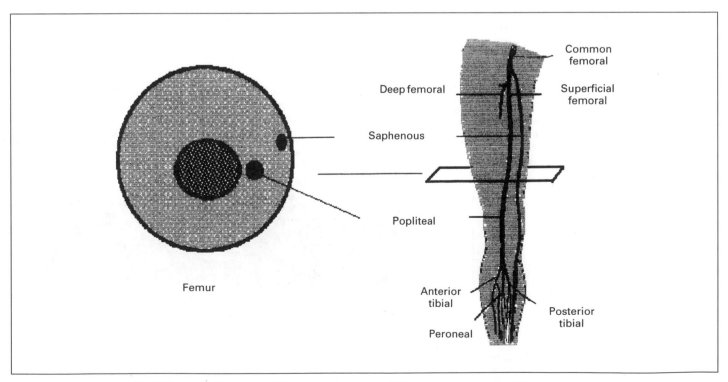

FIGURE 45-6. Diagram of the normal course of the saphenous vein. The saphenous vein is superficial, whereas the popliteal vein is deep.

Tendons

For tendon analysis, a high-frequency linear array gives best results. An offset pad may be helpful, but modern transducers are designed in a fashion that makes offset pads unnecessary. It is important to keep the linear array in the axis of the tendon; slight obliquity will prevent the typical appearances from being seen. Putting tension on the tendon should allow distinction from large nerves, which have, at rest, a similar appearance. Only in the wrist region do they lie in a similar location.

Inflammation

Inflammation most commonly affects joints. Lateral or anterior views of the hip joint may reveal fluid that would not otherwise be seen. Views from a lateral or posterior axis of the knee joint are also helpful in showing unexpected bursa or joint fluid. Color flow is helpful in delineating inflammatory problems because vascularity increases if inflammation is present. Both arthritis and infection give rise to increased vascularity.

 PATHOLOGY

Baker's Cyst

A Baker's cyst is a fluid-filled collection posterior to the knee joint that may extend into the calf or, rarely, into the thigh. The collection may contain internal echoes or have an irregular outline (Fig. 45-7).

Popliteal Aneurysm

A focal expansion of the popliteal artery that shows pulsation on real-time and may contain clot is a popliteal aneurysm. The walls may be partially calcified (Fig. 45-8).

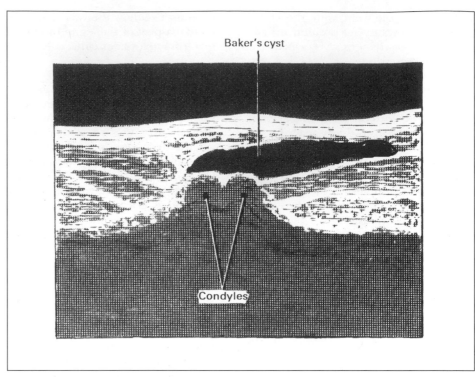

FIGURE 45-7. A Baker's cyst is a fluid-filled structure extending into the calf that usually communicates with the knee joint.

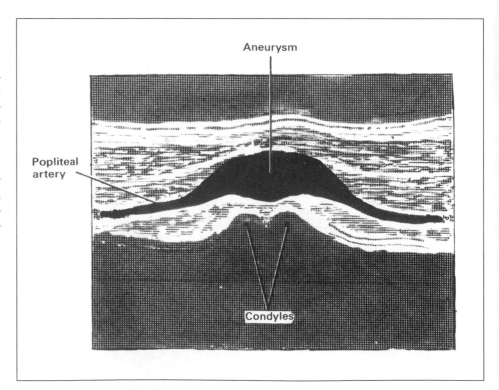

FIGURE 45-8. A popliteal artery aneurysm expands the popliteal artery posterior to the knee joint.

Pseudoaneurysm

Following trauma, particularly femoral vein catheterization, an echogenic collection may be seen alongside the the artery. Sometimes, these hematomas contain an irregularly shaped echo-free area that shows flow on Doppler, representing a pseudoaneurysm (false aneurysm; see Chapter 29). Clot forms the wall of the aneurysm. Flow may be detected in such false aneurysms, even though no echo-free area can be seen. These lesions, which require prompt surgical attention, are elegantly demonstrated by color flow Doppler; a mushroom-like appearance is seen. After a pseudoaneurysm has been localized with ultrasound, persistent compression (for at least 10 minutes) may cause the aneurysm to clot.

Muscles

Hematomas in muscles can either be the result of tearing of the muscles or of a blunt damage to the limb. If there is a complete muscle tear, the two segments of the muscle are separated by a hematoma, which forms an echopenic area. Older hematomas may be echogenic (see Chapter 37). Localized bruising can produce a fluid collection within the muscle or it can diffusely enlarge the muscle without altering the underlying muscle organization. The muscle should be compared to the contralateral muscle.

Rhabdomyolysis is a rare condition occurring typically in drug addicts who have stayed in the same position with the muscle contracted for hours. An echopenic mass area will be seen within the muscles at the point of tenderness. Normal muscle fibers run through the affected area. The muscles have been partially dissolved by enzymes during the period when they were contracted. Eventually, healing with calcification may take place.

Tendons

Injuries to the Achilles tendon in the ankle are the most common. (Other tendons have a similar appearance—this discussion will focus on the Achilles tendon.) Achilles tendon injuries often occur following a fall or a jump from a high level.

Normally the tendon runs from the posterior calf muscles to the posterior aspect of the ankle. With rupture, the tendon retracts upward and bloody fluid fills in the intervening tissue. With partial rupture, there is discontinuity of the longitudinal fibers within the tendon. If the tendon is bruised, an echogenic hematoma will be interspersed with the tendon fibers. Sometimes pain from the Achilles tendon relates to a bursa deep to the tendon. This can become enlarged and inflamed. Ultrasound is useful in this area because of the following:

1. Pain not related to the Achilles tendon will show normal tendon appearances.
2. A thickened or nodular tendon is seen with tendonitis.
3. Partial discontinuity of the Achilles tendon may be seen.
4. Neglected Achilles tendon rupture can be clinically confusing.

Other tendons where the same approach can be used include the posterior tibial, distal biceps, and quadriceps tendons.

Deep Vein Thrombosis

Acute Deep Vein Thrombosis

1. A deep vein thrombosis is suspected when there is fever, leg swelling, and pain, particularly on dorsiflexion of the foot. The leg vein clot may be anywhere along the course of the deep veins, but is usually in the thigh, where there is a single deep vein.
2. A typical acute clot expands the vein, which is filled with low-level echoes. The vein will not be compressible.
3. Either there will be no flow with color flow and Doppler or a small channel will be present.
4. "Acute" deep vein thrombosis may persist for a number of weeks.
5. There are several deep veins in the calf that cannot be seen by ultrasound. Usually, indirect signs (described under Technique) suggest clot in the calf, although clot may not actually be seen.
6. If clot is found in the femoral veins, look at the iliac veins and inferior vena cava; the clot may propagate into these veins. There will be no or less flow by Doppler, and low-level echoes will be seen in the lumen.

7. The iliac veins can be seen on either side of the pelvis with the bladder full.
8. Normally a phasic variation in flow is seen. If this is absent, deep vein thrombosis can be suspected.

Chronic Deep Vein Thrombosis

A chronic thrombus increases in echogenicity and decreases in size. The affected vein has a normal caliber although it still contains echogenic clot which partially blocks the vein. Lateral veins will form alongside the larger veins which will diminish in size once they are partially clot filled.

Inflammation

Early signs of inflammation in limbs result in the development of fluid, whether in a joint, a bursa, or alongside bone.

Osteomyelitis (Bone Infection)

Acute

In the initial phase, anechoic fluid is seen adjacent to the bony periosteum in the metaphysial region. Ultrasound precedes other imaging techniques in detecting early signs of osteomyelitis. Aspiration of the fluid can be aided by ultrasound guidance.

Chronic

In chronic osteomyelitis, a dip in the bony outline will be seen and calcification will form in a sequestrum at the site of the infection. These signs may be seen while the infection is inactive. Signs that an infection has been reactivated include the development of local abscesses and sinus tracks.

Cellulitis

This infection follows soft tissue cuts or trauma. Diffuse thickening of soft tissues occurs with increased vascularity. Tissue borders become more echogenic. No fluid collection is seen.

Abscess

Well-defined fluid collections occur with irregular echopenic borders in the center of an inflamed area. A sinus track may be demonstrable. Appearances can be confused with a tumor. If an abscess is demonstrated, drainage under ultrasound control is often initiated.

Septic Tenosynovitis

If an infection develops within the tendon, a target appearance develops due to fluid within the synovial sheath. A central echogenic area will be surrounded by more echopenic fluid still within the confining connective tissue that surrounds the tendon.

Arthritis

The sonographic appearances of arthritis are somewhat similar to inflammation due to infection. Simple effusions are seen in gout, and periarticular fluid collections, such as bursa, develop. Proliferative synovitis appears in rheumatoid arthritis. Thick synovial walls develop within the joint effusion, known as pannus. These masses can achieve a large size and are moderately echogenic. Solid echopenic bumps, particularly in the elbow region, are seen with rheumatoid arthritis, amyloid, and gout. Baker's cysts are more common with rheumatoid arthritis (see earlier discussion).

Foreign Bodies

Suspected foreign bodies in the hands or feet can be usefully assessed with ultrasound. The painful area is examined in a variety of positions to see whether there is shadowing. All types of foreign bodies, including wood, elicit shadowing. Plastic and wood are less reflective, however, than metal or glass. Surgical excision is greatly facilitated if foreign body localization by ultrasound is used to help choose the exploratory incision approach.

☆ PITFALLS

1. *Leg extension with Baker's cyst.* Undue extension of the leg obliterates a Baker's cyst that communicates with the knee joint because the fluid returns into the knee joint proper.
2. *Anechoic thrombus.* Venous thrombus may not contain echoes and may be recognized only with compression or with the use of color flow Doppler.
3. *False aneurysm.* False aneurysms may be echo filled as if they were a solid mass. Doppler will show flow.
4. *Saphenous vs. femoral vein.* The saphenous vein may be confused with the femoral vein. It is small and superficial.

5. *Problems with compression.* If compression views are not obtained in a transverse fashion the clot may be missed because the transducer slips off the clot (Fig. 45-9).
6. *Acute vs. chronic deep vein thrombosis.* Acute appearances can persist in a vein for a number of weeks. Problems have arisen when a report suggested that a clot is acute when acute appearances are actually longstanding.
7. *Tendon vs. nerve.* Tendons and nerves can look similar. However, tendons change as the tendon is shortened, whereas nerves have an unchanged position and appearance.

❓ WHERE ELSE TO LOOK

1. If a popliteal aneurysm is found, the aorta and the opposite popliteal artery should be examined; abdominal aortic aneurysms are often present in association with popliteal artery aneurysms.
2. If a deep vein thrombus is found in the leg, look in the iliac veins and in the inferior vena cava.
3. Multiple venous thromboses are said to be associated with carcinoma of the pancreas. Look in the pancreas if there has been more than one episode.

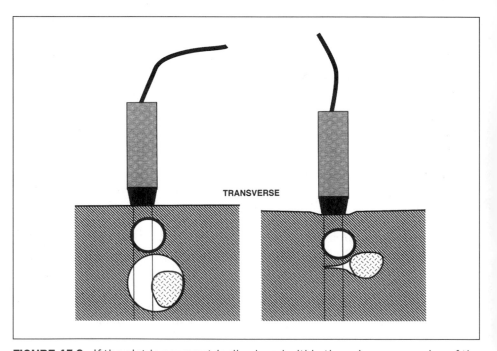

FIGURE 45-9. If the clot is asymmetrically placed within the vein, compression of the site which is free of clot may give an erroneous impression that there is no clot within the vein. It is better to use a transverse position, rather than a longitudinal compression to compress the veins.

SELECTED READING

Abiri, M. M., Kirpekar, M., and Ablow, R. C. Osteomyelitis: Detection with US. *Radiology* 172: 509–511, 1989.

Aspelin, P., Pettersson, H., Sigurjonsson, S., and Nilsson, I. M. Ultrasonographic examinations of muscle hematomas in hemophiliacs. *Acta Radiol Diagn* 25:513–516, 1984.

Bianchi, S., Zwass, A., Abdelwahab, I. F., and Banderali, A. Diagnosis of tears of the quadriceps tendon of the knee: Value of sonography. *AJR* 162:1137–1140, 1994.

Chhem, R. K., Kaplan, P. A., and Dussault, R. G. Ultrasonography of the musculoskeletal system. *Radiol Clin North Am* 32:275–289, 1994.

Cleveland, T. J., and Peck, R. J. Case report: Chronic osteomyelitis demonstrated by high resolution ultrasonography. *Clin Radiol* 49: 429–431, 1994.

Fornage, B. D. Achilles tendon: US examination. *Radiology* 159:759–764, 1986.

Fornage, B. D. The hypoechoic normal tendon: A pitfall. *J Ultrasound Med* 6:19–22, 1987.

Fornage, B. D., and Nerot, C. Sonographic diagnosis of rhabdomyolysis. *J Clin Ultrasound* 14:389–392, 1986.

Fornage, B. D., and Schernberg, F. L. Sonographic diagnosis of foreign bodies of the distal extremities. *AJR* 147:567–569, 1986.

Lozano, V., and Alonso, P. Sonographic detection of the distal biceps tendon rupture. *J Ultrasound Med* 14:389–391, 1995.

Nazarian, L. N., Rawool, N. M., Martin, C. E., and Schweitzer, M. E. Synovial fluid in the hindfoot and ankle: Detection of amount and distribution with US. *Radiology* 197:275–278, 1995.

Newman, J. S., Adler, R. S., Bude, R. O., and Rubin, J. M. Detection of soft-tissue hyperemia: Value of power Doppler sonography. *AJR* 163:385–389, 1994.

Nypaver, T. J., Shepard, A. D., Kiell, C. S., McPharlin, M., Fenn, N., and Ernst, C. B. Outpatient duplex scanning for deep vein thrombosis: Parameters predictive of a negative study result. *J Vasc Surg* 18:821–826, 1993.

Polak, J. F. *Peripheral Vascular Sonography: A Practical Guide.* Baltimore: Williams & Wilkins, 1992.

Silverstri, E., Martinoli, C., Derchi, L. E., Bertolotto, M., Chiaramondia, M., and Rosenberg, I. Echotexture of peripheral nerves: Correlation between US and histologic findings and criteria to differentiate tendons. *Radiology* 197:291–296, 1995.

Wright, D. J., Shepard, A. D., McPharlin, M., and Ernst, C. B. Pitfalls in lower extremity venous duplex scanning. *J Vasc Surg* 11:675–679, 1990.

ARTERIAL PROBLEMS IN THE LIMBS

GAIL SANDAGER

SONOGRAM ABBREVIATIONS

ABI	Ankle brachial index
ATa	Anterior tibial artery
Bif	Bifurcation
CFa	Common femoral artery
CFv	Common femoral vein
CIa	Common iliac artery
DPa	Dorsalis pedis artery
EIa	External iliac artery
GSV	Greater saphenous vein
IIa	Internal iliac artery
PERa	Peroneal artery
PFa	Profunda femoris artery
POPa	Popliteal artery
POPv	Popliteal vein
PSV	Peak systolic velocity
PTa	Posterior tibial artery
PVD	Peripheral vascular disease
SFa	Superficial femoral artery
SFv	Superficial femoral vein
TB	Tibioperoneal trunk

Key Words

Abduct. To move a leg away from the other leg.

Ankle Brachial Index. A ratio of Doppler-derived ankle systolic pressure to Doppler-derived brachial artery systolic pressure (ABI = ankle pressure/highest brachial pressure). The index is an indicator of arterial insufficiency. The normal ABI is greater than 1.0. As the severity of peripheral vascular disease (PVD) increases, the ABI will decrease.

Antecubital Fossa. The anterior aspect of the elbow joint.

Gangrene. Tissue death that can result from inadequate blood supply. Gangrene from peripheral vascular disease (PVD) is identified by its typical distal location on the toes or forefoot.

Geniculate Artery. Small tributary to the popliteal artery in the popliteal fossa.

Hunter's Canal. Arterial pathway on the medial aspect of the thigh, just above the knee. The artery is deep within the muscle at this point and difficult to see.

Intermittent Claudication. Means "to limp"; symptoms of leg pain experienced during exercise and relieved with rest. The symptoms are produced by arterial insufficiency.

Laminar. Normal pattern of blood flow in a vessel; the flow in the center of the vessel is faster than at the walls.

Rest Pain. Due to insufficient arterial supply causing ischemia to the tissues that results in pain at rest in the toes and forefoot.

Spectral Broadening. Echo fill-in of the spectral window proportional to the severity of the vessel stenosis (see Fig. 5-7). It may also result from poor technique, with too much gain or too large a sample volume.

Sural Arteries. Small branches of the popliteal artery in the popliteal fossa.

◆⟩⟩ THE CLINICAL PROBLEM

Lower extremity arterial color duplex sonography is useful to identify, localize, and grade the severity of arterial lumen narrowing from peripheral vascular occlusive disease. The most common cause of PVD is atherosclerosis. Other problems that affect peripheral circulation are thrombosis, embolism, trauma, and aneurysms. Clinical indications for performing peripheral arterial color duplex imaging are intermittent claudication, limb rest pain, abnormal peripheral pulses, gangrene or tissue necrosis, blue toe syndrome, and arterial trauma, as well as to follow-up therapeutic intervention.

Intermittent Claudication

Claudication is manifested by pain in the various muscle groups of the legs brought on by exercise. The muscle groups that elicit pain are related to the location of the arterial obstruction. Muscle cramping or a tired, aching feeling is experienced during exercise; these symptoms are due to the inability of the arterial blood supply to meet the increased oxygen and nutritive demands of exercise. Since this is a fixed lesion that does not change, without treatment the symptoms always recur. A predictable pattern occurs with respect to the onset of pain, location of pain, and resolution of pain with a brief rest or cessation of exercise. This is the classic presentation of vascular claudication—exercise-pain-rest-relief—and the cycle repeats.

Neurospinal compression patients present with a similar description of pain that can mimic true vascular claudication. Neurogenic claudication can be differentiated by a thorough history. Neurogenic claudication is not repeatable; symptoms are brought on by a variety of circumstances not related to a specific situation or exercise. Patients' symptoms vary, with good and bad days, and no relief from cessation of exercise.

Rest Pain

The patient complains of pain or numbness of the toes or forefoot. This most often occurs at night, causing the patient to awaken from sleep. Rest pain results from the inability of the circulation to meet the demands at rest. Symptoms are pronounced with elevation and will improve with the limb dependent. Patients will often say they have to hang their leg over the bedside to relieve the symptoms.

Tissue Necrosis/Gangrene

These lesions are seen distally on the toes and forefoot and represent tissue loss associated with loss of vascular nutritive supply.

ANATOMY

The lower extremity arteries are the common femoral, profunda femoris, superficial femoral, popliteal, anterior tibial, tibioperoneal trunk, posterior tibial, and peroneal artery (Fig. 46-1).

The Femoral Arteries

The common femoral artery (CFa) starts at the level of the inguinal ligament and courses lateral to the common femoral vein (CFv) (see Fig. 46-3). The CFa is approximately 3- to 5-cm long and bifurcates into the superficial femoral artery (SFa) and profunda femoris artery (PFa). This arterial bifurcation is just proximal to the confluence of the superficial femoral and profunda femoris veins.

The SFa is anterior to the PFa and medial to the femur; the SFa is the most common site for atherosclerosis. The SFa and superficial femoral vein (SFv) run parallel to each other in the thigh, coursing distally to the adductor canal (Hunter's canal). The SFa terminates at the adductor canal, becoming the popliteal artery (POPa). The PFa courses lateral from its origin going deep into the thigh; only the first few centimeters can be visualized by ultrasound.

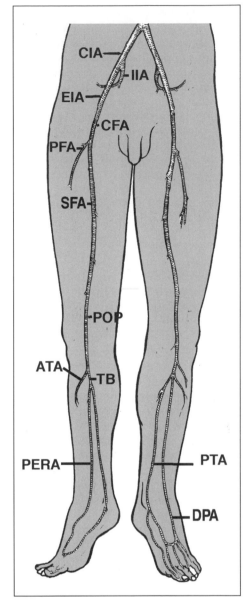

FIGURE 46-1. Normal arterial anatomy of the leg. CIa—common iliac artery. IIa—internal iliac artery. EIa—external iliac artery. PFa—proximal femoral artery. CFa—common femoral artery. SFa—superficial femoral artery. POPa—popliteal artery. ATa—anterior tibial artery. TB—tibioperoneal trunk. PERa—peroneal artery. PTa—posterior tibial artery. DPa—dorsalis pedis artery.

Popliteal Artery

The POPa begins above the knee at the adductor canal and continues inferiorly through the popliteal fossa and into the proximal calf. The POPa has numerous sural branches and geniculate arteries that are a major collateral route in the presence of arterial obstructions (Fig. 46-2). The geniculate arteries supply blood flow to the muscles around the knee and the sural branches supply the gastrocnemius muscle. At the level of the anterior tibial tubercle, the POPa divides into the anterior tibial artery (ATa) and the tibioperoneal trunk.

Trifurcation Vessels

The ATa is the first tibial artery arising from the POPa. The ATa enters the anterior compartment of the leg between the tibia and the fibula and runs inferior along the lateral aspect of the calf down into the foot where it becomes the DPa.

The tibioperoneal trunk has a variable length of a few centimeters before dividing into the posterior tibial artery (PTa) and the peroneal artery (PERa). These tibial arteries are located in the posterior compartment of the calf.

The PTa courses along the medial aspect of the lower leg to the medial malleolus. At the level of the ankle the PTa branches into the plantar arteries.

The PERa runs posterolateral through the posterior compartment to a few centimeters above the ankle. At the ankle the PERa terminates into branches communicating with the anterior tibial and dorsalis pedis arteries.

▨ TECHNIQUE

The patient is positioned supine with the head slightly elevated for comfort. The leg being examined is abducted and externally rotated with the knee flexed. Acoustic coupling gel is applied from the groin to the knee medial to the femur. A 5-MHz (or similar frequency) linear array transducer is used with corresponding Doppler frequency. The exam is performed using both transverse and longitudinal views.

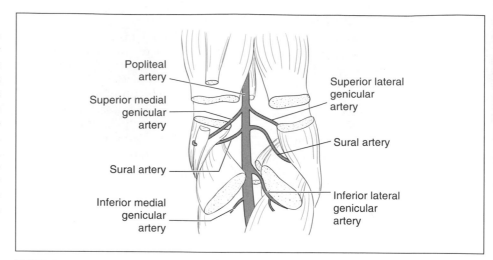

FIGURE 46-2. Popliteal artery anatomy.

Upper Leg

The transducer is placed in the groin using a transverse orientation. The vessels visualized are the CFa and CFv (Fig. 46-3). The CFa is lateral to the vein with obvious pulsations seen. Compression of the CFv can be performed to distinguish it accurately from the CFa. After correct identification of the CFa, the probe is angled superiorly to visualize the origin or most proximal segment of the vessel at the inguinal ligament.

Move the transducer inferior until the CFa bifurcates into the SFa and the PFa just below the level of the groin. The SFa is the more anterior vessel, whereas the PFa courses lateral and posterior. Generally only the first few centimeters of the PFa will be visualized before moving out of the field of view.

Just below the arterial bifurcation is the confluence of the SFv and the profunda femoris vein. The SFv is used as a landmark to identify the SFa, as they run parallel to each other throughout the thigh. Using this landmark, follow the SFa/vein distal. The SFa appears anterior to the vein in the B-mode image. These vessels run medial to the femur in the thigh and can be followed to the adductor canal. At the level of the adductor canal, the SFa will move deeper. At this point the image quality may be limited owing to the depth of the vessel and the poor penetration through the fascia.

Popliteal Fossa

Because of the anatomic position of the proximal POPa, it is best imaged from a posterior approach. Maintaining a transverse orientation, place the transducer in the popliteal fossa; both the POPa and the popliteal vein (POPv) are seen, with the artery positioned deeper than the vein. To assess the above-knee portion of the POPa, move the probe superiorly along the posterior thigh until the entire artery has been evaluated. Trace the entire artery back to the SFa, as short-segment occlusions are common at this site. Tendons frequently encountered from a transverse approach may limit its usefulness, as the large footprint linear array probe may slide off the tendons. A longitudinal view may provide better image quality. After complete evaluation of the proximal POPa, follow the artery back to and through the popliteal fossa, until its termination below the knee.

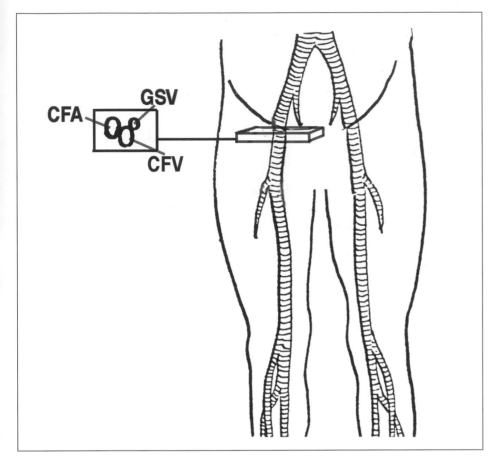

FIGURE 46-3. In the groin, the common femoral vein (CFv) lies medial to the common femoral artery (CFa). The greater saphenous vein (GSv) arises from the femoral vein in the groin.

The Lower Leg

The branches arising from the POPa are visualized from a posterior approach and should not be mistaken for the ATa. The POPa divides into the ATa and the tibioperoneal trunk below the knee. The ATa is the first tibial artery branch arising from the POPa and will course posterior and lateral from the POPa.

Anterior Tibial Artery

The ATa runs along the lateral aspect of the calf accompanied by the paired anterior tibial veins. The veins and artery run together throughout their course in the calf. If the ATa is difficult to track from its proximal segment, move to the distal segment just above the ankle and scan back to the proximal ATa.

Tibioperoneal and Posterior Tibial Artery

The tibioperoneal trunk is difficult to visualize owing to its anatomic location and is only adequately visualized in approximately 70 percent of the population. From the posterior approach it is the more anterior vessel at the ATa/tibioperoneal trunk division. The tibioperoneal trunk is relatively short before dividing into the PTa and the PERa. At this point only one artery can be examined; it does not matter which vessel is scanned first. The PTa runs medial and anterior from the PERa. The vessel origins are difficult to track and can be scanned from the distal segment at the ankle back to their origins. This provides easier and more rapid vessel identification. The PTa is examined by placing the probe just above the medial malleolus; the PTa is medial to the tibia and courses superior with the paired posterior tibial veins.

Peroneal Artery

The PERa can be imaged from either a medial or lateral approach as it runs down the center of the leg. From either approach it is approximately 3- to 4-cm deep, surrounded by the two peroneal veins, and is next to the fibula. The PERa is the most difficult tibial artery to visualize completely owing to its deep anatomic location in the posterior compartment of the calf. Successful visualization depends upon the size of the patient's calf.

The B-mode imaging technique is performed uniformly throughout the lower-extremity arterial tree. Both transverse and sagittal views are performed. The sagittal view is used in conjunction with the pulsed Doppler evaluation. The B-mode image is used to evaluate the quality of the vessel, intraluminal defects, plaque, size, collateral pathways, and anatomic location.

DISEASE DISTRIBUTION

Peripheral arterial occlusive disease is most commonly found at arterial bifurcations and distal segments of vessels. The distal SFa is the most prevalent area of disease. However, the disease distribution is different in diabetic patients, with an increased incidence below the knee in the infrapopliteal arteries. In the nondiabetic patient, disease occurs more often in the iliac and the SFa, whereas the younger patient with claudication will have a higher incidence of iliac artery disease.

Peripheral arterial aneurysms commonly occur in the POPa and the femoral arteries and are often bilateral or multiple. If an aneurysm is detected, all other sites are routinely examined (see Chapter 45).

PULSED DOPPLER TECHNIQUE

The entire length of the vessel is examined with Doppler. At a longitudinal view, the pulsed Doppler sample volume (2 mm) is placed center stream or center to a flow jet using an angle of 60 degrees or less. Angles above 60 degrees give erroneous results. The Doppler waveforms are assessed for direction of flow, peak systolic velocity (PSV), spectral broadening, and waveform configuration. End diastolic velocities are not routinely measured unless there is greater than 50 percent stenosis.

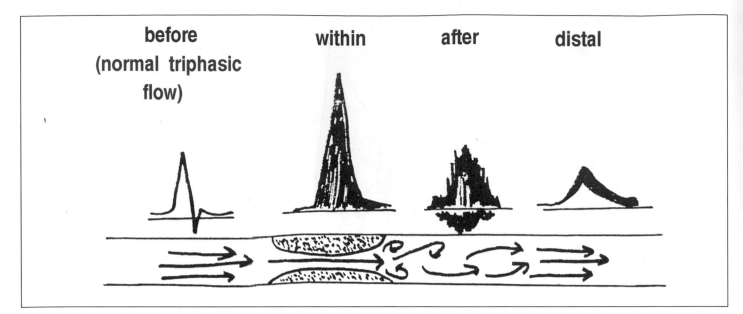

FIGURE 46-4. Doppler spectral changes in the presence of a hemodynamically significant stenosis.

Record all Doppler calculations at proximal, mid, and distal artery segments. All changes in Doppler velocity spectra are recorded with calculations displayed at the area of change and immediately proximal and distal to the change (Fig. 46-4). If B-mode image abnormalities are detected without a change in Doppler velocity, this is recorded, showing the image abnormality and the corresponding Doppler waveform. All abnormal Doppler findings are repeated from several views to avoid an error in calculations.

The normal lower extremity arterial waveform is triphasic with a marked systolic upstroke, early diastolic reverse flow, and end diastolic forward flow (Fig. 46-5). The third phase of diastolic forward flow exhibits low velocities and may be obliterated if the wall filter is set too high. Wall filters of 50 to 100 Hz are recommended for normal peripheral arterial profiles. Peak systolic velocity diminishes as the examination moves toward the feet.

EXAM PROTOCOL

Both anatomic and physiologic testing are used to determine the degree of peripheral vascular occlusive disease. The standard examination for peripheral arterial disease includes ankle brachial index (ABI) measurement in conjunction with color Doppler sonography.

Ankle Brachial Index

ABIs are an initial screening assessment as an indicator of the absence or presence of PVD. Blood pressures are taken at multiple sites in the leg and compared to the arm. Arterial narrowing decreases flow with a resultant pressure drop distal to the stenosis.

Equipment

1. An 8- to 10-MHz continuous wave Doppler and acoustic coupling gel
2. Appropriate-sized pressure cuffs for the arms and ankles; cuff sizes will vary depending on patient size
3. A standard sphygmomanometer

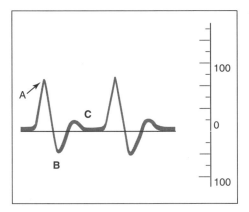

FIGURE 46-5. Normal triphasic waveform. (**A**) Systolic upstroke. (**B**) Early diastolic reverse flow. (**C**) Diastolic forward flow.

Procedure

The patient is placed supine and at rest for 10 minutes before starting. The pressure cuffs are placed on the upper arms and ankles bilaterally and connected to the sphygmomanometer. Using Doppler, obtain the best-quality signal in the antecubital fossa then inflate the cuff. The pressure in the cuff is inflated to 20 mm Hg above the systolic blood pressure. Deflate the cuff slowly until the first audible arterial signal is detected and record this as the brachial systolic pressure. Repeat this on the opposite arm. The same procedure is performed at the ankle for the dorsalis pedis artery (DPa) and the PTa. The DPa is located on the top of the foot lateral to the bone, whereas the PTa is just posterior to the medial malleolus (Fig. 46-6).

The ABI is calculated by taking the ankle pressure and dividing it by the highest brachial pressure. This is done for both the DPa and the PTa on both sides. A normal ABI is greater than 1.0.

Color/Duplex Imaging

PATIENT SELECTION. The procedure can be used for any patients that have abnormal ABIs and require direct visualization of the arteries. Patients with normal ankle brachial indices and no significant clinical history are not routinely examined. A significant clinical history in the presence of normal ABIs includes prominent peripheral pulses suspicious for aneurysm, trauma near to major arteries, or postreconstructive evaluation.

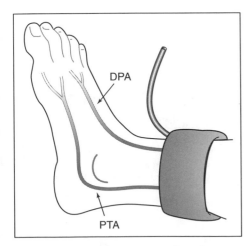

FIGURE 46-6. Cuff position for ABI

PATIENT PREPARATION. The examination begins in the groin of the leg being examined after the patient has rested supine for 10 minutes. If the patient has intermittent claudication and has been active prior to examination, the initial recordings will be erroneous; therefore a 10-minute rest before examination is essential. A brief history is taken to define symptoms, previous surgery, and relevant risk factors. The routine examination includes evaluation of the CFa down to the tibioperoneal trunk. Diagnostic parameters and good B-scan information are limited for the tibial arteries, which are therefore not routinely imaged.

B-SCAN IMAGING. The leg is slightly flexed, abducted, and externally rotated so that all of the major arteries can be examined. The CFa is examined with standard gray-scale B-scan imaging in a transverse orientation. The proximal CFa to the bifurcation of the SFa/PFa is imaged first to evaluate the anatomic course and location of the vessels. After correct vessel identification, record the anatomic information, displaying each vessel and its relationship to the vein. All bifurcations are included in the corresponding documentation. This technique is performed throughout the thigh, popliteal fossa, and below the knee to the tibioperoneal trunk.

DOPPLER IMAGING. Repeat the exam using color, pulsed Doppler, and a longitudinal view. Obtain sagittal views of the CFA and place the Doppler sample volume at 60 degrees and in the center of the vessel or center to the flow stream in the presence of disease. Move the sample site throughout the vessel segment being examined. Determine the most accurate representation of the Doppler waveform and record both the image showing the sample site location and the Doppler velocity waveform. Display and record all the necessary Doppler calculations. This technique is repeated and recorded from all segments of the peripheral arterial system.

DOCUMENTATION. Documentation of abnormal stenotic or occluded areas anywhere in the periphery includes the following:

Doppler velocity calculations

Proximal, within, and distal to the area of stenosis (see Fig. 46-5)

Number of lesions

Location and length of lesions

Vessel measurements are recorded when the exam is performed for aneurysms. The artery is measured from a transverse view with anterior-posterior and medial and lateral external diameter measurements. If an aneurysm is present, measurements are taken from both transverse and sagittal views measuring both the diameter and length. In the presence of an aneurysm the vessel diameter immediately proximal to the aneurysm is recorded, along with measurements of the aneurysm in both transverse and sagittal views.

Diagnostic Criteria

Normal PSV Criteria	PSV (cm/sec)	Vessel Diameter (mm)
CFa	114.1 +/− 24.9	7–10
Prox. SFa	90.8 +/− 13.6	6–9
Dis SFa	93.6 +/− 14.1	6–9
POPa	68.8 +/− 13.5	5–8

Categories of Per Cent Stenosis

DIAGNOSTIC CRITERIA USING PSV RATIOS (KOHLER, 1987)

1% to 19% diameter reduction

Triphasic waveform

No appreciable spectral broadening

Less than 30% focal PSV increase from proximal segment of vessel

Normal PSV and waveform distal to plaque

B-mode image—minimal plaque

20% to 49% diameter reduction

Triphasic waveform

Spectral broadening

Focal PSV increase 30% to 100% from proximal segment

Proximal and distal waveforms remain normal

Visible plaque

50% to 99% diameter reduction

Waveform loss of reverse flow component

Focal PSV increase greater than 100% from proximal segment

Distal waveform monophasic with decreased PSV

Spectral broadening

Poststenotic turbulence

Visible plaque

Occlusion: no detectable Doppler flow from the arterial segment involved

Proximal signal will vary depending on collateralization

Monophasic low-velocity waveform distal to occlusion

Diffuse intraluminal echoes

DIAGNOSTIC CRITERIA USING ABSOLUTE PSV

	PSV	Velocity Ratio*
Normal	<150 cm/sec	<1.5:1
30%–49%	150–200 cm/sec	1.5:1–2:1
50%–75%	200–400 cm/sec	2:1–4:1
>75%	>400 cm/sec	>4:1
Occlusion	No detectable color or Doppler flow	

*Velocity ratio PSV at stenosis to PSV proximal artery. (Cossman et al. 1989)

ANKLE BRACHIAL INDEX CATEGORIES

Greater than 0.95: Normal

0.80 to 0.95: Mild disease

0.50 to 0.80: Moderate disease (claudication range)

Less than 0.50: Severe disease

Less than 0.30: Severe disease associated with ischemia

DIAGNOSTIC PARAMETERS
FOR PERIPHERAL ANEURYSM

Measurements of an artery are consistent with an aneurysm when the external diameter of the aneurysm is 2 cm greater than the diameter of the proximal artery.

Diagnostic Interpretation

The diagnostic parameters for percent stenosis include the PSV ratios, the degree of spectral broadening, absence or presence of turbulence, and loss of reverse flow component. The shape of the waveform should be used as an additional tool to support the direct findings. The waveform shape changes immediately distal to a critical stenosis, becoming dampened and monophasic. If a normal, patent CFa is visualized with no evidence of plaque but there is a low-velocity, monophasic waveform with delayed systolic upstroke, one should suspect proximal aortoiliac disease causing compromised flow distal to the stenosis. However, a short focal stenosis greater than 50 percent can return to normal laminar flow a few centimeters distal to the stenosis. This is why spot checking with Doppler has a low accuracy.

⭐ PITFALLS

1. *Proximal aortoiliac artery stenoses or occlusions.* A hemodynamically significant lesion in the aortoiliac arteries can alter flow distally by decreasing pulse amplitude and reducing systolic acceleration. These alterations may be very subtle or extremely obvious. With any question of proximal disease, the aorta and iliac arteries should be investigated to avoid this pitfall.

2. *Short segment occlusions.* A well-collateralized short segment arterial occlusion can be missed, especially in areas of the adductor canal where image resolution is poor. To avoid this problem always check the relationship of the artery to the vein; any variance should be evaluated. Any distinct change in waveform configuration from level to level calls for reevaluation of the vessel. The only way to detect these changes with a high degree of accuracy is to always be consistent with the Doppler sampling process.

3. *Arterial wall calcification.* Medial wall calcification is not uncommon in the U.S. patient population. Such calcification can cause problems with vessel imaging and obtaining correct Doppler information. This problem has no real solution except to attempt imaging from all possible windows and

clearly document the limitation on the record. Arterial calcification also limits the use of the ABI since an accurate blood pressure cannot be determined. In such a case, cuff pressure can exceed 200 mm Hg without causing arterial compression; this is like trying to take a blood pressure on a bathroom pipe.

4. *Previous vascular surgery.* Patients may present with a history of previous vascular reconstruction; information on the nature of the surgery may not be available to the sonographer. Detecting the exact problem is then complicated, as patients do not necessarily return to normal after vascular intervention.

5. *Tandem or multiple lesions.* A hemodynamically significant proximal lesion causes diminished flow distal to the lesion. The second more distal lesion may not display the true PSV increase; flow is already decreased from the proximal lesion. It is important to document this information in the formal report.

6. *Collateral vessels.* Distinction between a collateral and an occluded vessel can be difficult. Collateral vessels are generally smaller in diameter than the native feeding artery.

SELECTED READING

Cossman, D. V., Ellison, J. E., Wagner, W. H., et al. Comparison of contrast arteriography to arterial mapping with color-flow duplex imaging in the lower extremities. *J Vasc Surg* 10(5):522–529, 1989.

Hatsukami, T. S., Primozich, J. F., Zierler, R. E., Harley, J. D., and Strandness, D. E. Color Doppler imaging of infrainguinal arterial occlusive disease. *J Vasc Surg* 16(4):527–533, 1992.

Jager, K. A., Ricketts, K. A., and Strandness, D. E. Duplex scanning for the evaluation of lower limb arterial disease. In Bernstein, E. F. *Noninvasive Diagnostic Techniques in Vascular Disease* (3rd ed.). St. Louis: , 19xx.

Kohler, T. R., et al. Duplex scanning for diagnosis of aortoiliac and femoropopliteal disease. *Circulation* 76:1074, 1987.

Moneta, G. L., Yeager, R. A., Lee, R. W., and Porter, J. M. Noninvasive localization of arterial occlusive disease: A comparison of segmental pressures and arterial duplex imaging. *J Vasc Surg* 17(3):578–582, 1993.

47

RULE OUT PLEURAL EFFUSION AND CHEST MASS

NANCY SMITH MINER

SONOGRAM ABBREVIATIONS

Ao Aorta

D Diaphragm

K Kidney

L Liver

S Spine

Sp Spleen

KEY WORDS

Atelectasis (Collapsed Lung). Segmental collapse of the lung due to volume loss; caused by either an extrinsic compression by pneumothorax or pleural effusion, or by an intrinsic obstruction of a central bronchus.

Consolidation. An infected segment of the lung filled mainly with fluid instead of air.

Empyema. Pus in the pleural cavity.

Hemothorax. Blood in the pleural cavity.

Paradoxical Motion. Downward motion of the diaphragm with expiration and upward motion on inspiration due to hemidiaphragm paralysis.

Pleura. A serous membrane that lines the thorax and diaphragm and surrounds the lungs.

　Parietal (Costal) Pleura. Extends from the inferior aspect of the lungs and covers the sides of the pericardium to the chest wall and backward to the spine.

　Visceral Pleura. Lines the lungs and the interlobar fissures; it is loose at the borders to allow for lung expansion.

Pleural Cavity. The space between the layers of the pleura.

Pleural Fibrosis. Fibrous tissue thickening the pleura; results from chronic inflammatory diseases of the lungs such as tuberculosis.

Pneumothorax. Air within the pleural cavity outside the lung—a possible complication of thoracentesis.

Subpulmonic. Inferior to the lungs, above the diaphragm.

Thoracentesis. Puncture of the chest to obtain pleural fluid.

◆》 THE CLINICAL PROBLEM

Because of the air in the lungs, chest sonography is limited to assessing pathology adjacent to the pleura. Fluid accumulates in the pleural space as a reaction to underlying pulmonary or upper abdominal disease, or as a consequence of systemic disease such as heart failure. Effusions are usually detected by chest radiography. Free fluid falls to the base of the chest; however, loculated fluid, which is the result of adhesions or malignancy, does not layer on chest radiograph. The distinction is easily made using ultrasound, providing the pocket lies adjacent to the ribs.

Obtaining a fluid sample can be important for diagnostic purposes or may be a palliative measure to alleviate shortness of breath. Clinicians customarily localize for thoracentesis in the patient's room by percussing the chest and listening for dullness. In obese or muscular patients, clinical localization may fail. In cases like these, ultrasound is helpful in guiding thoracentesis. Ultrasound is also helpful in determining the nature of an opaque hemithorax on the chest radiograph. Such an opacification may indicate tumor, fluid, collapsed lung, or a combination of these entities.

Diaphragmatic movement can be shown in the presence of pleural fluid. This demonstration is especially helpful in ruling out paradoxical motion in patients who cannot be transported to the radiology department.

ANATOMY
Normal Chest

When no fluid or mass is present, the tissues within the chest do not conduct sound. There are alternating bands of echogenicity due to reverberations from air and the rounded, bright reflectors seen due to the bone. Between the skin and ribs are subcutaneous fat and muscles; the soft tissue between ribs is mostly muscle. Because the intercostal vessels lie under the lower lip of each rib, they are poorly seen; however, remember their location when deciding on needle placement.

The pleural space is that potential space between the parietal and visceral pleura, which normally contains only a few millimeters of a lubricating secretion. The surface of the lung can be seen moving up and down with respiration, and the ventilated portion produces a comet-tail artifact in the intercostal spaces (Fig. 47-1).

Diaphragm

The diaphragm is seen as an echogenic, curved line above the liver and spleen. The diaphragm can be difficult to demonstrate, especially on the left, because it lies along virtually the same axis as the ultrasonic beam. The spleen provides less of a window to angle through than does the liver.

TECHNIQUE

For masses or loculated effusions, position the patient so the pathology site is easily accessible and so he or she is comfortable enough not to move during the procedure.

Pleural Effusion

Pleural effusions (see Fig. 47-1) usually pool above the diaphragm along the posterior chest wall. It is sometimes necessary to scan along the axillary line to check for fluid laterally. Loculated effusions can be found in any location. Plan the search by examining the chest radiograph.

The patient is scanned upright, sitting on a stool without a back, thus affording ready access from all sides (see Fig. 47-1). If looking in the posterior chest, the area behind the scapulae can be better visualized by having the patient cross his or her arms, rotating the scapulae outward. Scanning in the supraclavicular fossa will allow access to the superior sulcus to look for loculated effusions or apical tumors. Subpulmonic masses or empyema may be best seen by scanning from the abdomen.

A 3.5- to 5-MHz transducer is usually an appropriate frequency to display the chest wall and the distance to the lung. A curved linear transducer with a wide footprint is best for the initial search, whereas changing to a smaller sector is helpful in evaluating deeper structures, where the near field is less important.

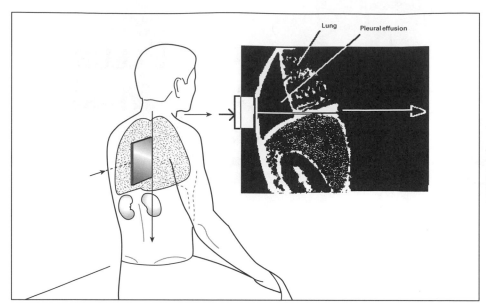

FIGURE 47-1. Diagram of the usual position used when scanning a pleural effusion. The ultrasonic appearance of a pleural effusion and lung are shown in the inset. Note the alternating pattern of reverberations from the air and absent transmission from bone in the lung area.

The diaphragm must be shown well. This can be difficult, especially on the left side where there is no liver to act as an acoustic window; angling up through the liver and spleen helps to show the diaphragm. The spleen may be mistaken for an effusion if the diaphragm is not demonstrated, so find the upper pole of the left kidney if necessary to localize the spleen and diaphragm.

Supine Views

Right-sided pleural effusions can be easily assessed on a supine view looking through the diaphragm and liver (Fig. 47-2). Effusions on the left are more difficult to see in the supine position but can sometimes be seen with an oblique scan through the spleen.

The upright position is not necessary if no fluid shift is seen on a decubitus radiograph. Patients with loculated effusions can be examined in any position.

Pleurocentesis (Pleural Effusion Aspiration) or Chest Mass Aspiration

Obtaining fluid by percutaneous puncture may be necessary either to determine the nature of the fluid or as a therapeutic maneuver to relieve shortness of breath. Thoracentesis, when not performed in the ultrasound suite, is customarily done in the patient's room. A site is chosen after percussing the chest and listening for dullness. A short needle is routinely used.

Pleurocentesis without ultrasonic guidance has potential pitfalls. The effusion may be in a location different from the one that was percussed or may not be present at all. In an obese or muscular patient, a deeper penetration than is possible by a short needle is often required. If a tap is unsuccessful when attempted "blindly," the patient is often referred to ultrasound so that the puncture can be attempted again with the aid of ultrasound.

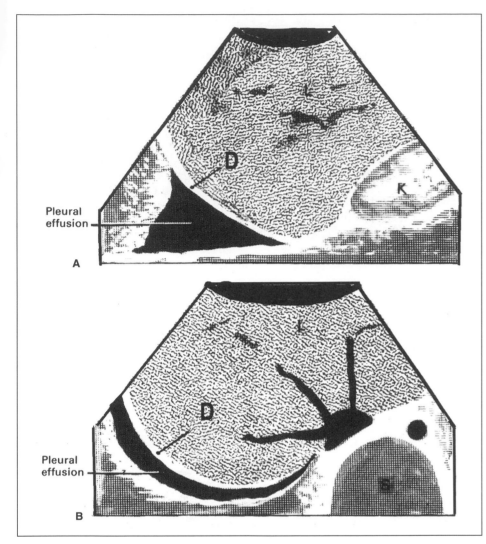

FIGURE 47-2. Pleural effusion above the diaphragm (D) on a supine longitudinal view (**A**), and supine transverse view (**B**). Note that the fluid extends to the spine on transverse views.

Initial Localization of Pathology

Look at the most recent chest radiograph to see whether the fluid is mobile or loculated. If the fluid is free-flowing, a blunted costophrenic angle means there are at least 200 cc of fluid present. If it is loculated, a computed tomography scan may be better for characterizing the position of the loculations. Often ultrasound alone may be all that is necessary, but sometimes, loculated fluid in a fissure (pseudotumor) is impossible to detect on ultrasound because it is obscured by air; however, this will be readily detectable on a chest x-ray film.

Fluid in the pleural space, as opposed to pleural thickening, will change shape with respiration. This can be characterized by a "flash" of color on color Doppler. Serous fluid may also exhibit thin septations that will float gently on respiration.

1. *Free-moving fluid.* Free-moving fluid will flow to a dependent site in the chest, just above the diaphragm, if the patient is upright, which is the preferred position for aspirating free collections. The best sites are usually along the posterior chest wall or in the axial line. Look for the biggest pocket. Identify the diaphragm by finding the kidneys and moving superiorly.

2. *Loculated fluid.* A lateral chest radiograph will help decide whether fluid is anterior or posterior. Scan the entire chest, including the anterior chest wall, before ruling out a loculated effusion. Collections in the left anterior chest may be cardiac in origin, such as pericardial effusions or pericardial cysts. If the loculation contains septa, measure out more than one depth for needle insertion to take samples from different pockets with the same needle stick.

3. *Tumor.* If a solid mass is adjacent to the diaphragm, its texture may be similar to that of liver or spleen. Careful localization of the diaphragm is imperative. Some mediastinal masses are localized with ultrasound for core biopsy.

Patient Position

The patient should be sitting and leaning against a support such as a bedside table or raised head of a stretcher. If it is necessary to keep one of the patient's arms raised throughout the procedure, pull up the edge of the hospital gown to form a kind of sling that will keep the patient from getting tired.

Localization of Pathology and Aspiration

In order to visualize the pleura, use a transducer with a low enough frequency (usually 3.5 MHz) to penetrate the patient's chest wall and the pathology to visualize the pleura. Although a linear array gives a "picket-fence" appearance from shadowing ribs that may obscure a small collection, it can be preferable to a small footprint transducer because its larger field of view makes diaphragmatic and pleural effusion movements easier to see, and more of the superficial tissues can be seen.

A small footprint transducer will fit well between the ribs, but the angle must be carefully calculated because the slightest angulation of the transducer throws the beam into an entirely different plane. Biopsy guides are difficult to use in the chest because of rib interference.

The aspiration may be performed either (1) after localization with ultrasound if the pocket is large; or (2) after bagging the transducer with a sterile bag and performing the puncture alongside the transducer, if the pocket is small.

1. *Premedicate the patient.* If a tube is being placed in the chest for drainage, premedicating the patient helps to ensure cooperation and comfort.
2. *Demonstrate the diaphragm.* This is particularly important on the left side where the spleen can look cystic, and the upper pole of the left kidney can simulate a curved diaphragm in a large patient.
3. *Watch respiration.* If the pocket is small, watch on real-time to see which phase of respiration best shows the effusion; have the patient practice holding his or her breath at that point so he or she can reproduce it for the needle insertion.
4. *Use a needle stop.* This is especially important in the chest. If the needle enters too deeply, the lung may be pierced and pneumothorax may result. Document the needle site with a Polaroid or paper print for the chart if the puncture is to be performed elsewhere. Use a 20-gauge needle unless the patient has abnormal blood coagulation tests. Even better may be an 18-gauge sheathed needle, such as an angiocath, to prevent laceration as the fluid is removed and the lung reexpands. Larger gauges may be necessary if the fluid is thick.
5. *Prepare for laboratory tests.* The most commonly ordered laboratory tests for pleural effusions require the following fluid containers: tubes, cytopathology tubes, heparinized tubes (if the tap is bloody), anaerobic culture bottle (one can use a sealed syringe instead).
6. *Use a vacuum bottle.* If a large amount of fluid is being removed for therapeutic purposes, it is much faster to use a large vacuum bottle attached to a length of tubing. This tubing may collapse if used with a 22-gauge needle owing to the vacuum. Place the bottle on the floor, making sure the tubing is attached to the needle end first so the bottle does not fill quickly with air. Generally, no more than 2 L is removed at one time. A postprocedure expiration chest radiograph should be obtained to exclude pneumothorax.

◆ PATHOLOGY

Pleural Effusion

Pleural effusions (see Figs. 47-1 and 47-2) are usually echo-free, wedge-shaped areas that lie along the posterolateral inferior aspect of the lung. Occasionally they contain internal echoes, sometimes indicating the presence of a neoplasm. These echoes may be due to blood or pus (empyema), especially when the collection is loculated. Loculated effusions do not necessarily lie adjacent to the diaphragm and may be located anywhere on the chest wall. Subpulmonic effusions lie between the lung and the diaphragm.

Pleural Fibrosis

Pleural fibrosis can be confused with pleural fluid on a radiograph. There are some subtle sonographic differences between the two (Fig. 47-3):

1. A simple effusion is echo-free, whereas pleural fibrosis should contain low-level echoes.
2. Free fluid appears wedge-shaped as it fits between the lung base and the diaphragm (see Fig. 47-1).
3. Pleural fluid changes shape when the patient breathes, and usually flashes on color; pleural fibrosis does not (see Pitfalls).

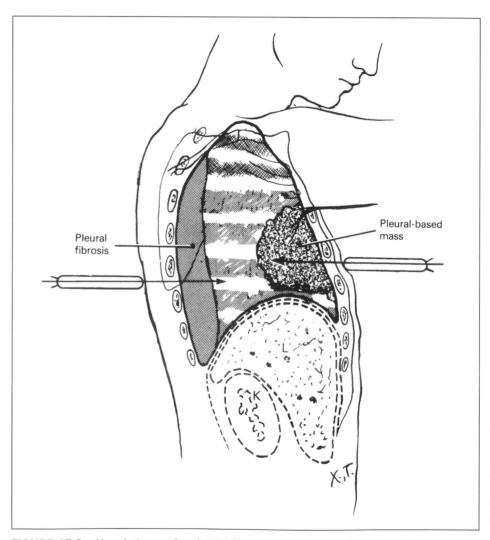

FIGURE 47-3. Usual shape of a pleural fibrosis (posterior lesion). There will be some internal echoes. A pleura-based solid mass is shown on the anterior aspect of the chest.

4. Pleural effusions taper sharply at the upper end, whereas pleural fibrosis tends to be the same width throughout (see Fig. 47-3).
5. Fluid exhibits more through transmission than fibrosis, but this is difficult to assess; the air-filled lung forms a strong interface, whether it be fluid or fibrosis.

Solid Mass

If a lesion seen on x-ray film touches the pleura, ultrasound is a good place to continue the work-up. If there are numerous internal echoes within a mass when compared with a known fluid-filled structure such as the heart, one can be fairly confident that the lesion is a mass (see Fig. 47-3). Solid homogeneous masses with few internal echoes are more difficult to distinguish from fluid because they simulate a cystic collection. They may have strong back walls and appear to have no echoes at low gain settings. Because the lung lies beyond the lesions and does not conduct sound, through transmission is not easy to evaluate. Mass analysis is greatly simplified if there is a coincidental pleural effusion. Peripheral tumors often obliterate the pleural parenchymal line as they spread into the chest wall.

Pneumothorax

With pneumothorax, the normal comet-tail appearance of aerated lung seen intercostally is missing; also absent is the usual gliding of the visceral pleura under the parietal pleura during respiration. Instead, there is only the bright, specular reflection of air in the pleural cavity, which does not move. Although this is usually a radiographic diagnosis, understanding this appearance can be helpful when scanning a patient too ill to be moved from the intensive care or oncology unit, or when using ultrasound as an adjunct to an invasive procedure that could result in a pneumothorax.

Consolidation

A consolidated lung contains a lot of fluid and may conduct sound, even though there will be a number of internal echoes with a radiating linear pattern due to small pockets of air in bronchi. The appearance of consolidated lung can be similar to that of liver or spleen. Coincident pleural effusion is often present and makes the diagnosis much more simple.

Passive Atelectasis

If pleural effusion is present, a wedge-shaped mass is seen. An increase in the size of the mass on inspiration may be seen if bronchial obstruction is incomplete. With complete lung collapse, no change with inspiration will be seen and there will be no echogenic air bronchogram pattern within the mass. Tubular vascular structures will be seen with color flow with both veins and arteries visible.

⭐ PITFALLS

1. *Reverberation vs. effusion.* At times there may be doubt about whether an "effusion" is real on decubitus or supine views, or just a mirror artifact (Fig. 47-4; see also Chapter 53). Place the patient in a sitting position when scanning for fluid to change the angle of the transducer to the area in question and eliminate this artifact.

2. *Spleen vs. effusion.* The spleen may be mistaken for an effusion in a large patient if the position of the kidney in relation to the spleen is not documented and the diaphragm is not seen adequately.
3. *Mass vs. effusion.* A solid mass may be mistaken for a loculated effusion if the contents of the mass are particularly homogeneous. Watch for the fluid to change shape on respiration. Usually soft tissue masses adjacent to the pleura do contain internal echoes.
4. *Consolidation vs. liver or spleen.* Consolidation can be confused with liver or spleen. In consolidation there will be a linear pattern to the bronchi with small pockets of air; just make sure the area of concern is superior to the diaphragm.
5. *False-positive fluid color sign.* It is possible to have color signals appear in areas adjacent to an anechoic fluid collection, or even potentially in hypoechoic pleural thickening, if the color gain is set inappropriately high or the wall filter is set inappropriately low.

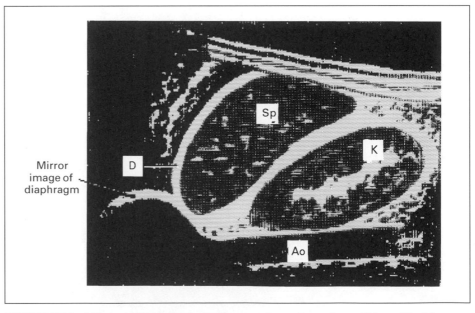

FIGURE 47-4. Mirror artifact of the diaphragm above the spleen. This artifact is seen when the patient is scanned from an oblique axis through the spleen.

SELECTED READING

Civardi, G., Fornari, F., Cavanna, L., Di Stasi, M., Sbolli, G., Rossi, S., Buscarini, E., and Buscarini, L. Vascular signals from pleura-based lung lesions studied with pulsed Doppler ultrasonography. *J Clin Ultrasound* 21:617–622, 1993.

Dodd, G. D., III, Esola, C. C., Memel, D. S., Ghiatas, A. A., Chintapalli, K. N., Paulson, E. K., Nelson, R. C., Ferris, J. V., and Baron, R. L. Sonography: The undiscovered jewel of interventional radiology. *Radiographics* 16:1271–1288, 1996.

Ferrari, F. S., Cozza, S., Guazzi, G., Sala, L. D., and Stefani, P. Ultrasound evaluation of chest opacities. *Ultrasound Internat* 1:68–74, 1995.

Lichtenstein, D. A., and Menu, Y. A bedside ultrasound sign ruling out pneumothorax in the critically ill. *Chest* 108:1345–1348, 1995.

Lomas, D. J., Padley, S. G., and Flower, C. D. R. The sonographic appearances of pleural fluid. *Br J Radiol* 66:619–624, 1993.

Marchbank, N. D. P., Wilson, A. G., and Joseph, A. E. A. Ultrasound features of folded lung. *Clin Radiol* 51:433–437, 1996.

Sistrom, C. L., et al. Ultrasound for diagnosis and intervention in thoracic diseases. *Postgraduate Radiology* 14:21–49, 1994.

Targhetta, R., Bourgeois, J. M., Chavagneux, R., Coste, E., Amy, D., Balmes, P., and Pourcelot, L. Ultrasonic signs of pneumothorax: Preliminary work. *J Clin Ultrasound* 21:245–250, 1993.

Targhetta, R., Chavagneux, R., Bourgeois, J. M., Dauzat, M., Balmes, P., and Pourcelot, L. Sonographic approach to diagnosing pulmonary consolidation. *J Ultrasound Med* 11:667–672, 1992.

Versluis, P. J., and Lamers, R. J. S. Lobar pneumonia: An ultrasound diagnosis. *Pediatr Radiol* 23:561–562, 1993.

Wu, R., et al. "Fluid color" sign: A useful indicator for discrimination between pleural thickening and pleural effusion. *J Ultrasound Med* 14:767–769, 1995.

Yu, C. J., Yang, P. C., Chang, D. B., and Luh, K. T. Diagnostic and therapeutic use of chest sonography: Value in critically ill patients. *AJR* 159:695–701, 1992.

48 INFANT HIP DISLOCATION

SANDY STEGER

KEY WORDS

Acetabular Dysplasia. Abnormal development of the acetabulum tissue.

Acetabular Labrum (Limbus Cartilage). Cartilaginous ring surrounding the periphery of the acetabulum that aids in stabilizing the femoral head within the acetabulum.

Acetabulum. Cup-shaped bony structure formed by the ilium, ischium, and pubis that articulates with the femoral head.

Congenital Hip Dislocation. Displacement of the hip joint existing from or before birth.

Dislocatable Hip. The femoral head displaces from the acetabulum during certain stress maneuvers of the leg, but returns to its normal position spontaneously once the pressure is released.

Fovea. Indentation (pit) on the femoral head which provides attachment for the ligamentum teres.

Gluteus Medius Muscle. Originates from the ilium and inserts at the greater trochanter acting to stabilize the hip.

Greater Trochanter. Bony process at the superolateral portion of the proximal femoral shaft.

Ilium. Forms the superior portion of the acetabulum.

Intertrochanteric Crest. Prominent ridge between the greater and lesser trochanters on the posterior portion of the proximal femoral shaft.

Ischium. Forms the inferoposterior portion of the acetabulum.

Lesser Trochanter. Bony process at the posteromedial portion of the proximal femoral shaft.

Ligamentum Teres. Extends from the edges of the fovea on the femoral head to the edges of the acetabular notch and contains the branch of the obturator artery.

Ossific Nucleus. Bony formation appearing as early as 4 weeks of age in the center of the femoral head.

Pavlik Harness. Corrective harness that supports the hips in flexion and abduction without force.

Pubis. Forms the inferoanterior portion of the acetabulum.

Subluxation. Incomplete displacement of the femoral head from the acetabulum during certain stress maneuvers of the leg.

Triradiate Cartilage. Connects the ilium, ischium, and pubis of the acetabulum.

◆》 THE CLINICAL PROBLEM

Ultrasound is widely used to detect developmental displacement of the hip in the neonate. Ultrasound is used to evaluate the neonatal hip in the following circumstances:

1. When the clinical examination is indeterminate
2. To confirm a clinical impression of dislocation and to quantitate severity
3. As follow-up to show proper migration of the femoral head with treatment

Although radiography is the diagnostic modality used most often with congenital hip dislocation, it cannot image the cartilaginous structures of the hip. Since only ossified portions of the neonatal hip can be visualized, measurements are subject to some guesswork. This coupled with the difficulty of placing and maintaining the infant in the proper position can easily lead to an inaccurate diagnosis. Arthrography is another modality that demonstrates hip anatomy, but it is little used because the neonate must be sedated or given general anesthesia. Contrast media must be injected into the joint space, and, like radiography, it subjects the infant to radiation exposure. Computed tomography is helpful in infants confined to a cast, but it is not routinely used in diagnosing congenital hip dislocation since it is nondynamic, results in gonadal radiation exposure, and also requires sedation. Magnetic resonance imaging provides exquisite anatomic detail of the soft tissue, cartilage, and bony structures with no radiation exposure, but requires sedation, has a long scanning time, is expensive, and is not dynamic.

Ultrasound, on the other hand, can safely and effectively visualize the nonossified or cartilaginous structures of the neonatal hip in a short amount of time without the use of radiation, a sedative, or contrast agent. Ultrasound can visualize the neonatal hip dynamically in three dimensions, and an exam can be performed with the infant confined to a corrective device such as traction, a cast, or a Pavlik harness.

Although the cause of congenital dislocation of the hip is unknown, certain associated factors are known:

1. Females are affected substantially more frequently than males (4:1).
2. The left hip is more often involved than the right hip or both hips.
3. Breech presentations are associated with higher incidence of congenital hip dislocation, which is thought to be due to extension of the fetal knees and hyperflexion of the fetal hip while in the breech position.
4. Hip dislocation is more common when there has been oligohydramnios.
5. Dislocation is more common in children with a family history of congenital dislocation of the hip (e.g., parent or sibling).
6. Firstborns are affected more often.
7. Neuromuscular abnormalities (e.g., spina bifida and arthrogryposis), congenital torticollis, and certain congenital foot deformities have a higher incidence of congenital hip dislocation.
8. Caucasians, certain Native American tribes, Scandinavians, and people from some regions of Japan appear to have a higher incidence of congenital dislocation of the hip as compared to people of African or Asian descent.

The clinical examination remains the principal screening tool for detection of congenital dislocation of the hip and is most valuable when done by experienced hands with a passive infant. The clinical examination usually consists of the Ortolani (reduction) test and the Barlow (dislocation) test. The infant is placed supine on a firm surface and must be relaxed. The legs are examined one at a time with the hip and knee flexed to 90 degrees.

The examiner holds the infant's thigh and positions his or her middle finger over the greater trochanter.

1. The Ortolani test is performed by abducting and lifting the thigh to bring the femoral head into the acetabulum. The examiner will sense reduction by a palpable "click" if the hip was in fact dislocated.

2. The Barlow test is performed by abducting the hip with gentle downward pressure. Dislocation is palpable as the femoral head slips out of the acetabulum. The diagnosis can be confirmed with the Ortolani test.

Certain ancillary signs may be seen with congenital dislocation of the hip, although they are not conclusive:

1. Asymmetric gluteal skin folds
2. Limited abduction of less than 45 to 60 degrees
3. Poor movement of affected limb
4. Limb maintaining a position of outward rotation
5. Shortening of the femur

Early diagnosis and treatment of congenital hip dislocation is essential for proper development of the hip joint.

The most favorable time for sonographic screening evaluation appears to be between 4 and 6 weeks of age, for the following reasons:

1. Newborns may have minimal subluxation which corrects itself without intervention by 4 weeks of age.
2. Orthopedic surgeons like to begin treatment by 2 months of age.
3. Some dysplasia may not occur until after the newborn period.

ANATOMY

Acetabulum

The acetabulum is a cup-shaped structure that articulates with the femoral head. The articular surface in the acetabulum is horseshoe shaped and smaller than the articular surface of the femur. The acetabulum is formed by three bones. The ilium forms the superior portion; the ischium forms the inferoposterior portion; and the pubis, which is the smallest of the three bones, forms the inferoanterior portion of the acetabulum. Sonographically, these bony segments appear echogenic and cast an acoustic shadow.

The triradiate cartilage is a useful landmark that connects the ilium, ischium, and pubis (Figs. 48-1 and 48-2). It is not ossified at birth. Sonographically, it appears hypoechoic and allows penetration of the sound beam. The triradiate cartilage becomes ossified in adulthood and fuses with the ilium, ischium, and pubis to form one bone.

The acetabular labrum, sometimes called the limbus cartilage, is a cartilaginous ring that surrounds the periphery of the acetabulum and forms an extension of the acetabular roof. The labrum narrows the acetabulum and increases its depth, thus supporting and stabilizing the femoral head within the acetabulum. The labrum is best seen in the coronal view as a triangular structure adjacent to the ilium and superolateral to the femoral head. The acetabular labrum is composed of hyaline cartilage with a fibrocartilaginous tip; sonographically, it appears mainly hypoechoic except for the echogenic fibrocartilaginous tip.

Femur

The femoral head, femoral neck, and greater and lesser trochanters are cartilaginous in the neonate and can be well visualized by ultrasound. The femoral head appears as a hypoechoic circle with smooth borders containing numerous tiny echoes. The fovea (pit) of the femoral head provides attachment for the ligamentum teres. The ligamentum teres runs from the edges of the fovea on the femoral head to the edges of the acetabular notch. It contains the branch of the obturator artery which supplies blood to the femoral head. The echopenic femoral neck angles medially, superiorly, and anteriorly as it tapers toward the femoral head. The greater and lesser trochanters are seen as echopenic areas at the base of the femoral neck protruding from the proximal femoral shaft. The greater trochanter is superolateral, and the lesser trochanter projects off the posteromedial portion of the proximal femoral shaft. The intertrochanteric crest of the femur is the area found between the greater and lesser trochanters at the base of the neck on the posterior portion of the proximal femoral shaft. The femoral shaft is ossified at birth, appearing echogenic and casting an acoustic shadow.

The ossific nucleus is a bony formation that appears in the center of the femoral head. It is seen as early as 4 weeks after birth and appears as an echogenic focus that gradually increases in size with age. If large enough, the ossific nucleus may cast an acoustic shadow.

◢ TECHNIQUE

The ultrasonic features of both hips should be compared using a 5- or 7.5-MHz real-time linear array transducer. Sector and curved transducers are less desirable because they slightly distort anatomy. It is desirable that the sonologist be present or that the examination be videotaped, since observing movement of the femoral head in relation to the acetabulum is crucial.

The infant is examined in the supine or lateral position, although flexion-stress views are best done in the supine position. The infant's hips may need to be elevated so they are more accessible. A second person should be present to assist in immobilizing the infant. A lateral approach is used to obtain transverse and coronal views. Both views are obtained with the infant's legs first in a neutral position (approximately 15 to 20 degrees of flexion) and then in a flexed position (hip and knee in 90 degrees of flexion). The infant must be relaxed for the dynamic and stress maneuvers of the examination.

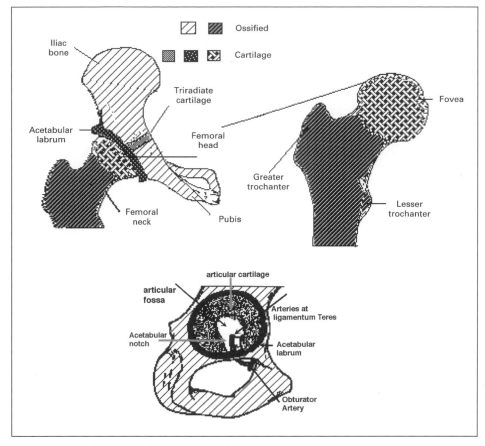

FIGURE 48-1. Anatomic drawing of acetabulum and femur.

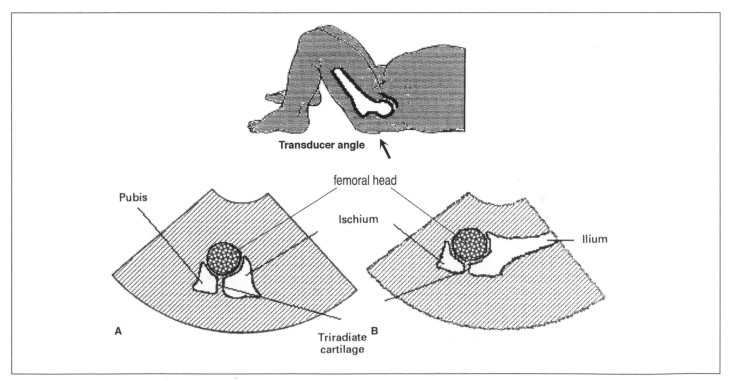

FIGURE 48-2. Sketch of an infant, showing the transverse (**A**) and coronal (**B**) approach.

Coronal View

The coronal view is taken in the midacetabular plane and is crucial for assessment of acetabular development.

1. *Neutral position.* Place the transducer on the infant's thigh in the coronal plane, or parallel to the femoral shaft. Using the femoral shaft as a landmark, slide the transducer cephalad until the femoral head is visualized. Adjust the angle of the transducer to align the largest diameter of the femoral head with the deepest portion of the acetabulum. The echogenic ilium or lateral portion of the acetabulum is superior to the femoral head and should lie in a horizontal plane on your image. A horizontal line drawn through the femoral head contiguous with the ilium demonstrates the depth of the acetabulum. The triradiate cartilage is seen at the base of the acetabulum (see Fig. 48-2). The acetabular labrum is seen adjacent to the ilium and superolateral to the femoral head. The gluteus medius muscle of the hip joint can also be visualized superolateral to the femoral head and lateral to the ilium.
2. *Flexion-stress.* Maintaining the transducer in the same plane as the coronal neutral position, flex the infant's hip and knee 90 degrees to bring the femoral shaft perpendicular to the table top. Slide the transducer posteriorly to visualize the posterior portion of the triradiate cartilage. The ilium and ischium border the triradiate cartilage and will have a linear appearance. With the transducer fixed in this plane, gently stress the leg (similar to the Barlow test of the clinical examination). If the femoral head is visualized to any degree in this plane, there is posterior displacement. The amount of displacement varies from minimal subluxation to total dislocation, depending on how much of the femoral head is seen over the posterior portion of the acetabulum.

Transverse View

1. *Neutral position.* Place the transducer on the infant's lateral thigh transversely (perpendicular to the femoral shaft). Slide the transducer cephalad along the femoral shaft until it widens at the intertrochanteric crest. The femoral head can be visualized slightly cephalad. Using slight changes in beam angulation, find the largest diameter of the femoral head as it relates to the acetabulum. The femoral head should sit firmly upon the ischial and pubic portions of the acetabulum and concentrically over the triradiate cartilage (see Fig. 48-2). A vertical line drawn through the femoral head at the junction of the ischium and triradiate cartilage should bisect it into two equal portions.
2. *Flexion stress.* Visualizing the same anatomy as in the transverse view neutral position, flex the infant's hip and knee 90 degrees to bring the femoral shaft perpendicular to the table top. The femoral shaft will now be more anterior to the femoral head. Slight posterior movement of the transducer may be necessary to visualize the anatomy adequately. While viewing the femoral head under real-time, gently push the femur posteriorly while adducting the hip (Barlow test of the clinical examination) to provoke dislocation. If the hip dislocates, reduction of the dislocated hip can be assessed by gently pulling and abducting the femur (Ortolani test of the clinical examination). Stability of the femoral head can be evaluated by gently moving the hip from maximum abduction, which stabilizes the hip, to maximum adduction, which stresses the hip.

In the transverse-flexion view, the echogenic femoral shaft and metaphysis lie adjacent to the femoral head and the echogenic acetabulum surrounds the femoral head posteriorly to produce a "U" configuration (Fig. 48-3). If the hip is dislocated, this U configuration cannot be obtained.

 PATHOLOGY

Dislocation

Dislocation of the neonatal hip is present when the femoral head is completely displaced from the acetabulum. The femoral head most commonly dislocates laterally and superiorly over the posterior acetabular rim onto the iliac wing. Sonographically, there is a loss of normal anatomic landmarks and an empty acetabulum.

Superior dislocation often results in the bony femoral shaft obscuring the acetabulum and triradiate cartilage. On the coronal view, the femoral head will rest against the bony ilium rather than inferior to it.

When dislocation occurs, it is important to visualize the acetabular labrum and show its relationship to the femoral head. If the labrum becomes inverted, it will obstruct the femoral head from relocating into the acetabulum, and surgical correction may be the only management option.

Dislocatable Hip

The hip is said to be dislocatable when the femoral head is properly positioned within the acetabulum, but during the flexion-stress maneuver completely displaces from the acetabulum. Once the pressure is released, the femoral head returns to its normal position within the acetabulum.

Subluxation

Subluxation occurs when the femoral head incompletely displaces from the acetabulum during the flexion-stress maneuver. This is best seen on the transverse view.

Normal newborn hips may show signs of minimal subluxation during the stress maneuver which resolves within the first month of life without intervention.

Acetabular Dysplasia

The bony development of the acetabular roof can be assessed sonographically by determining what portion of the femoral head is covered by the ilium on the coronal view. Acetabular dysplasia should be considered when the ilium covers significantly less than one half of the femoral head. Dysplasia occurs secondary to the abnormal position of the femoral head within the acetabulum.

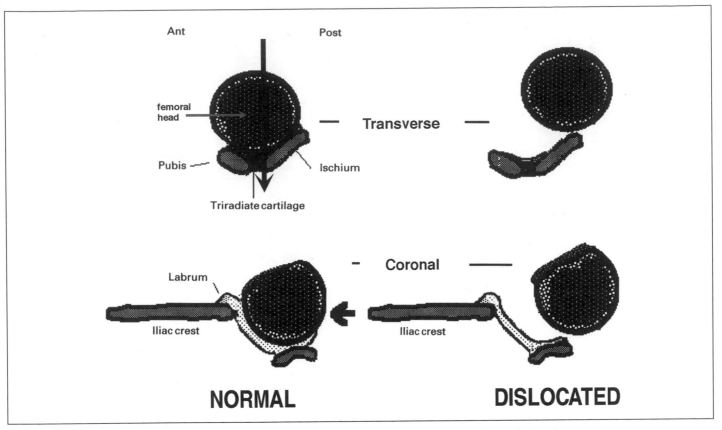

FIGURE 48-3. Top: Normal transverse view with a vertical line through the femoral head at ischial and triradiate cartilage borders. Bottom left: Normal coronal view with a horizontal line through the femoral head from ilium. Bottom right: Transverse and coronal views showing dislocation.

The normal acetabulum is deep with a concave contour and a sharp superolateral margin. The labrum will appear narrow and triangular as it covers the femoral head. An abnormal acetabulum becomes more shallow and flattened, losing its sharp superolateral margin. The labrum also becomes deformed and displaces cranially. With dysplasia, the labrum often becomes fibrotic, causing the hyaline cartilage to become more echogenic.

✴PITFALLS

1. *Ossific nucleus.* Acoustic shadowing produced by the ossific nucleus may be mistaken for the triradiate cartilage or may make the medial acetabulum and triradiate cartilage difficult to identify on the transverse view. The transducer must be angled above or below the ossific nucleus to see the triradiate cartilage medially and avoid false interpretation.

2. *Ossification of the femoral head and acetabulum.* Acoustic shadowing produced by the bony femoral head and acetabulum prohibits visualization of the hip by ultrasound. Ossification of the femoral head and acetabulum occurs at different ages. Radiographic evaluation may replace ultrasound once ossification has occurred.

3. *Neonates confined to a corrective device such as a cast, traction, or Pavlik harness.* A lateral window large enough to accommodate the transducer may be cut from the cast. The window should be cut no larger than necessary and replaced as quickly and securely as possible after the ultrasound examination. When a lateral approach is not possible, an anterior ultrasound examination can be performed through the perineal opening.

4. *Improper alignment of the normal anatomic landmarks.* False-positive results can occur from improper alignment of the femoral head with the acetabulum and triradiate cartilage. Accurate angulation of the sound beam must be attained.

SELECTED READING

Boal, D. K. B., and Schwentker, E. P. Assessment of congenital hip dislocation with real-time ultrasound: A pictorial essay. *Clin Imag* 15:77–90, 1991.

Graf, R. Guide to sonography of the infant hip. New York: Thieme Medical Publishers, 1987.

Harcke, H. T. Screening newborns for developmental dysplasia of the hip: The role of sonography. *AJR* 162:395–397, 1994.

Harcke, H. T., and Grissom, L. E. Infant hip sonography: Current concepts. *Semin Ultrasound, CT, MRI* 15:256–263, 1994.

Keller, M. S., Chawla, H. S., and Weiss, A. A. Real-time sonography of infant hip dislocation. *Radiographics* 6:447–456, 1986.

Novick, G. S. Sonography in pediatric hip disorders. *Radiol Clin North Am* 26:29–53, 1988.

49 SHOULDER PROBLEMS

SANDY STEGER

KEY WORDS

Acromion Process. Spinous projection from the scapula that articulates with the clavicle.

Acute Tendonitis. Rapid onset of inflammation of a tendon; symptoms are severe but the course is short.

Adduction. Movement of a proximal limb toward the body (e.g., moving the arm alongside the chest).

Biceps Tendon. The tendon of the long head of the biceps muscle that arises from the glenoid fossa, arches over the humeral head, and descends through the bicipital groove to insert at the radial tuberosity. The tendon of the short head of the biceps muscle arises from the coracoid process and inserts at the radial tuberosity.

Biceps Tendon Sheath Effusion. Fluid within the dense fibrous sheath covering the biceps tendon.

Biceps Tendonitis. Inflammation of the biceps tendon.

Bicipital or Intertubercular Groove. Deep depression between the greater tuberosity and lesser tuberosity.

Bursa. A small, serous sac between a tendon and a bone.

Calcific Tendonitis. Inflammation and calcification resulting in pain, tenderness, and limited range of motion.

Chronic Tendonitis. Inflammation of a tendon that progresses slowly and has a long duration.

Clavicle. Articulates with the acromion process of the scapula and the upper portion of the sternum to form the anterior portion of the shoulder girdle.

Coracoid Process. Extends from the scapular notch to the upper portion of the neck of the scapula and can be palpated just below and slightly medial to the acromioclavicular junction.

Deltoid Muscle. Originates from the spine and acromion of the scapula and from the lateral one third of the clavicle to insert on the deltoid tuberosity of the humerus.

Deltoid Tuberosity. Ridge on the humerus where the deltoid muscle inserts.

Glenoid Fossa. Oval depression of the scapula that articulates with the head of the humerus.

Greater Tuberosity of the Humerus. Located on the lateral surface of the humerus just below the anatomic neck. Site of insertion for three muscles: supraspinatus, infraspinatus, and teres minor.

Infraspinatus. One of the muscles/tendons comprising the rotator cuff that originates from the infraspinatus fossa of the scapula and inserts on the middle posterior portion of the greater tuberosity of the humerus.

Lesser Tuberosity of the Humerus. Located on the anterior surface of the humerus just below the anatomic neck. Site of insertion for the subscapularis.

Rotator Cuff. Consists of the subscapularis, supraspinatus, infraspinatus, and teres minor muscles and tendons that give support to the glenohumeral joint.

Rotator Cuff Tear. Partial or complete break of one of the four muscles/tendons comprising the rotator cuff.

Scapula. Forms the posterior portion of the shoulder girdle.

Spine of the Scapula. A bony plate projecting from the posterior surface of the scapula.

Subdeltoid Bursa. A bursa located beneath the deltoid muscle that reduces friction in this area.

Subdeltoid Bursitis. Inflammation of the subdeltoid bursa.

Subscapularis. One of the muscles/tendons comprising the rotator cuff that originates from the anterior or costal surface of the scapula to insert at the lesser tuberosity of the humerus.

Supraspinatus. One of the muscles/tendons comprising the rotator cuff that originates from the supraspinatus fossa of the scapula to insert on the highest portion of the greater tuberosity of the humerus.

Synovial Cyst. Accumulation of synovia in a bursa.

Teres Minor. One of the muscles/tendons comprising the rotator cuff that originates from the upper two thirds of the axillary border of the scapula.

◆》 THE CLINICAL PROBLEM

Shoulder arthrography requires injection of contrast material into the joint space, which often causes discomfort and limits the examination to one shoulder per visit. Ultrasound is noninvasive, painless, less expensive, and allows comparison of both shoulders at one visit.

Often the scan is ordered to diagnose a rotator cuff tear; most of these are chronic conditions and occur late in life, but others are acute injuries from overuse. Rotator cuff tears usually present with one or more of the following symptoms:

1. Shoulder pain
2. Dysfunction, with limited range of motion
3. Weakness and pain with elevation or abduction of the arm
4. Pain at rest from rolling onto the affected shoulder

Other conditions that can be evaluated sonographically include tendonitis, bursitis, cysts, and effusion in the shoulder area.

ANATOMY

Rotator Cuff

The rotator cuff consists of four muscles and their corresponding tendons whose major function is to hold the humeral head within the glenoid fossa.

Subscapularis Muscle

The subscapularis muscle originates from the anterior or costal surface of the scapula to insert at the lesser tuberosity of the humerus (see Fig. 49-3). The lesser tuberosity is located on the anterior surface of the humerus just below the anatomic neck. The subscapularis acts as a medial or internal rotator of the shoulder.

Supraspinatus Muscle

The supraspinatus muscle originates from the supraspinatus fossa of the scapula, and its tendon passes beneath the acromion to insert on the highest portion or anterior impression of the greater tuberosity (see Fig. 49-4). The greater tuberosity is on the lateral surface of the humerus just below the anatomic neck. The supraspinatus works with the deltoid muscle to abduct the shoulder.

Infraspinatus Muscle

The infraspinatus muscle originates from the infraspinatus fossa of the scapula and inserts on the middle posterior portion of the greater tuberosity of the humerus (see Fig. 49-5). The infraspinatus acts as a lateral or external rotator of the shoulder.

Teres Minor Muscle

The teres minor muscle originates from the upper two thirds of the axillary borders of the dorsal surface of the scapula and inserts at the posterior lower portion of the greater tuberosity (see Fig. 49-6). The teres minor acts as a lateral or external rotator of the shoulder.

Deltoid Muscle

The deltoid originates from the spine and acromion of the scapula and from the lateral one third of the clavicle to insert on the deltoid tuberosity of the humerus (see Figs. 49-1 to 49-7). The deltoid can extend, flex, abduct, and laterally and medially rotate the shoulder.

Bicipital Groove and Biceps Tendon

The greater and lesser tuberosities of the humeral head are separated by a deep depression called the bicipital or intertubercular groove (see Figs. 49-4, and 49-7). The tendon of the long head of the biceps muscle arises from the upper portion of the glenoid fossa, passes through the capsule of the shoulder joint, and arches over the humeral head as it descends through the bicipital groove. The biceps tendon acts to stabilize the shoulder from superior displacement.

Subdeltoid Bursa

The subdeltoid bursa is located between the deltoid muscle and the rotator cuff, and its purpose is to relieve friction on the tendon of the rotator cuff.

◢ TECHNIQUE

A small-parts linear array transducer, 5 MHz or greater, produces the best images. Both shoulders are examined for comparative purposes. The patient is seated on a low rotating stool so that he or she can easily be positioned. The arm should be adducted as close to the body as possible with the elbow flexed 90 degrees and the patient's hand resting on the contralateral thigh.

Biceps Tendon/Bicipital Groove

Begin the examination by placing the transducer transversely over the bicipital groove (Fig. 49-1). The biceps tendon is seen as an echogenic ovoid structure within the bicipital groove. A small amount of hypoechoic fluid may surround the biceps tendon, representing a normal variant.

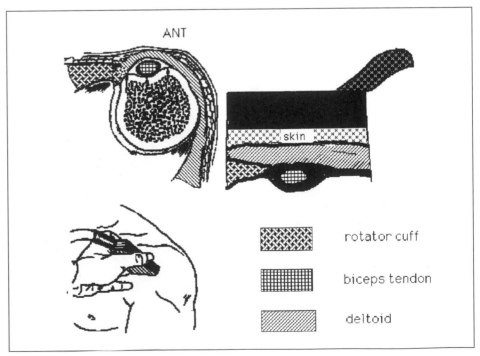

FIGURE 49-1. Transducer position and sonographic image of the biceps tendon as it runs beneath the rotator cuff.

Rotate the transducer 90 degrees (longitudinally) to visualize the biceps tendon parallel to its long axis. The biceps tendon will appear as an echogenic linear structure anterior to the humerus.

Subscapularis

Rotate the transducer transversely or perpendicular to the humerus at the level of the bicipital groove (Fig. 49-3). Move the transducer proximally and medially until the subscapularis is seen at its attachment to the lesser tuberosity. The subscapularis is best imaged in this view parallel to its fibers. Dynamic imaging of the subscapularis using passive internal and external rotation is necessary to visualize the entire tendon. When the arm is internally rotated, a portion of the tendon retracts and is obscured behind the coracoid process, but with external rotation, the tendon is drawn out from beneath the coracoid process. Sweep through the entire tendon while passively rotating the arm, and examine it carefully for any irregularities. Repeat this maneuver, imaging the subscapularis longitudinally or perpendicular to its fibers.

Supraspinatus

With the transducer once again in a transverse orientation, move it posteriorly and laterally from its position over the subscapularis to visualize the supraspinatus, posterior to the biceps tendon (Fig. 49-4). The supraspinatus is seen between the deltoid muscle and the humerus. The echogenicity of the supraspinatus and the rotator cuff tendons is usually greater than the echogenicity of the deltoid muscle, although in older patients the supraspinatus and rotator cuff tendons may be as echogenic or less echogenic than the deltoid. Comparison with the contralateral shoulder shows whether the echogenicity is a normal variant or an indication of a pathologic process. The subdeltoid bursa is visualized between the deltoid and supraspinatus and appears as highly echogenic parallel lines.

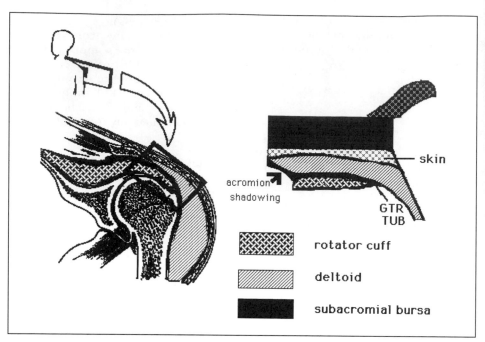

FIGURE 49-2. Transducer position and sonographic image of the rotator cuff and the deltoid.

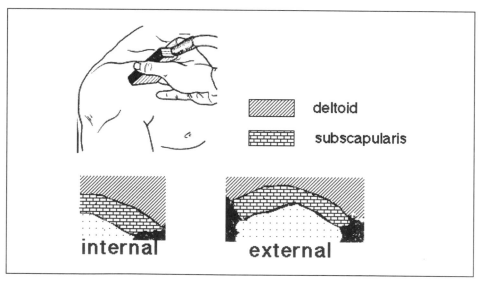

FIGURE 49-3. Transducer position and sonographic image of the subscapularis muscle. Both internal and external rotations should be evaluated.

Rotating the transducer 90 degrees or longitudinally, the supraspinatus is visualized parallel to its long axis. The supraspinatus is seen as a beaklike structure projecting from beneath the acoustic shadowing caused by the acromion. Dynamically visualizing the supraspinatus with passive adduction and abduction of the humerus is important in the detection of pathologic processes within the tendon. With the elbow flexed 90 degrees and extended behind the patient's back, the supraspinatus tendon moves anteriorly, out from under the acromion.

Infraspinatus

With the transducer transversely oriented or perpendicular to the humeral shaft, move posteriorly from the supraspinatus position to visualize the infraspinatus (Fig. 49-5). The infraspinatus muscle appears triangular in shape and tapers to form the infraspinatus tendon, which attaches to the greater tuberosity. The tendon will be visualized parallel to its long axis. Passive internal and external rotation of the arm in adduction enhances visualization of the tendon. Images perpendicular to the infraspinatus tendon should be obtained.

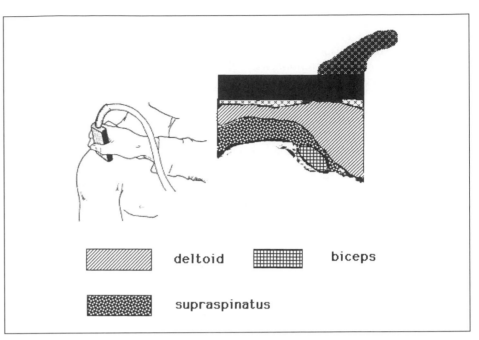

FIGURE 49-4. Transducer position and sonographic image of the supraspinatus muscle.

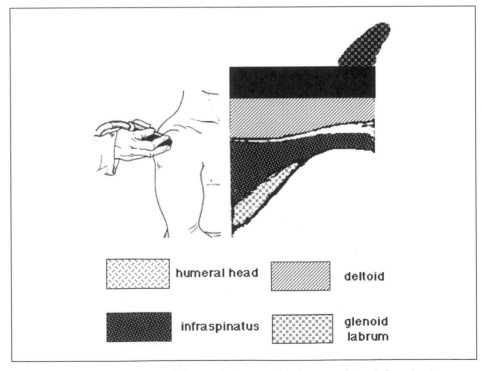

FIGURE 49-5. Transducer position and sonographic image of the infraspinatus muscle and glenoid labrum.

Teres Minor

Moving the transducer distally from its position over the infraspinatus reveals the teres minor muscle and tendon. The teres minor appears rhomboid shaped (Fig. 49-6). Passive internal and external rotation of the arm in adduction also enhances visualization of the teres minor tendon. The teres minor should also be evaluated in both imaging planes for optimal visualization.

 PATHOLOGY

Rotator Cuff Tears

Rotator cuff tears most frequently involve the supraspinatus tendon anterior and lateral to the acromion process, in an area of decreased vascularity which is just proximal to its insertion into the greater tuberosity (Fig. 49-7).

A rotator cuff tear may have one or more of the following features:

1. Focal area or areas of thinning or irregularity of the tendon
2. An entire tendon or a portion of a tendon that cannot be visualized

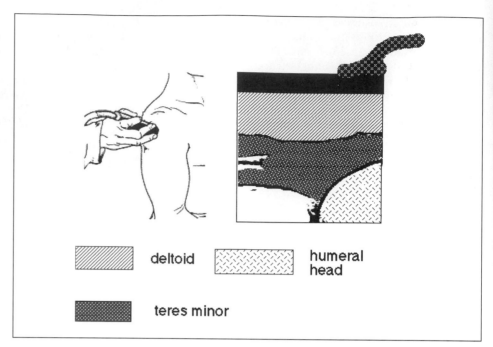

FIGURE 49-6. Transducer position and sonographic image of the teres minor muscle.

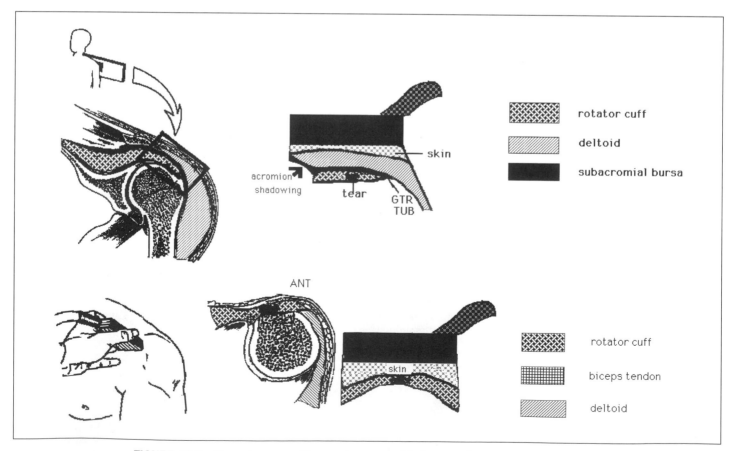

FIGURE 49-7. Transducer position and sonographic image of a rotator cuff tear.

3. Focal area or areas of echogenicity (not to be confused with calcific tendonitis)
4. Loss of the normal homogeneous echo texture of the tendon
5. A thickened tendon with irregular areas of increased or decreased echogenicity (Edema, hemorrhage, or degeneration may be present.)

Biceps Tendonitis

Thickening and irregularity of the biceps tendon are features of biceps tendonitis.

Acute Tendonitis

A thickened tendon with decreased echogenicity indicates acute tendonitis.

Chronic Tendonitis

A thickened tendon with decreased echogenicity and a nonhomogeneous appearance indicates chronic tendonitis. Calcifications are frequently present.

Subdeltoid Bursitis

In subdeltoid bursitis, an enlarged bursa usually fills with hypoechoic fluid due to inflammatory changes. The bursa will have irregular borders.

Biceps Tendon Sheath Effusion

A hypoechoic area is visualized surrounding the biceps tendon when there is a sheath effusion.

Calcific Tendonitis

When tendonitis is calcific, the tendon is usually less echogenic than normal and contains one or more echogenic foci within its substance, with or without acoustic shadowing.

Synovial Cyst

Synovial cysts are most commonly found extending along the biceps tendon and appear as well-defined hypoechoic structures with smooth borders and good through transmission.

★ PITFALLS

1. *Normal anatomy vs. pathology.* Comparison with the asymptomatic shoulder can help distinguish certain normal variants from pathology.
2. *Postoperative rotator cuff.* The surgical procedure performed as well as how it alters the anatomy of the rotator cuff should be reviewed with the surgeon before sonographic evaluation.
3. *Old fractures of the shoulder.* Any dislocation of bony anatomy may alter the appearance of the rotator cuff. Plain radiographs may be helpful in such cases.
4. *Shadowing from the acromion process.* Proper movement and positioning of the arm alleviates this problem.

SELECTED READING

Farin, P. U., and Jaroma, H. Acute traumatic tears of the rotator cuff: Value of sonography. *Radiology* 197:269–273, 1995.

Farin, P. U., and Jaroma, H. Sonographic findings of rotator cuff calcifications. *J Ultrasound Med* 14:7–14, 1995.

Hollister, M. S., Mack, L. A., Patten, R. M., Winter, T. C., III, Matsen, F. A., III, and Veith, R. R. Association of sonographically detected subacromial/subdeltoid bursal effusion and intraarticular fluid with rotator cuff tear. *AJR* 165:605–608, 1995.

Mack, L. A., Nyberg, D. A., and Matsen, F. A. III. Sonographic evaluation of the rotator cuff. *Radiol Clin North Am* 26:161–177, 1988.

Middleton, W. D., et al. Pitfalls of rotator cuff sonography. *AJR* 146:555–560, 1986.

Middleton, W. D., et al. Ultrasonography of the rotator cuff: Technique and normal anatomy. *J Ultrasound Med* 3:549–551, 1984.

Van Holsbeeck, M. T., Kolowich, P. A., Eyler, W. R., Craig, J. G., Shirazi, K. K., Habra, G. K., Vanderschueren, G. M., and Bouffard, J. A. US depiction of partial-thickness tear of the rotator cuff. *Radiology* 197:443–446, 1995.

Van Holsbeeck, M., and Strouse, P. J. Sonography of the shoulder: Evaluation of the subacromialsubdeltoid bursa. *AJR* 160:561–564, 1993.

Wiener, S. N., and Seitz, W. H. Jr. Sonography of the shoulder in patients with tears of the rotator cuff: Accuracy and value for selecting surgical options. *AJR* 160:103–107, 1993.

NEONATAL INTRACRANIAL PROBLEMS

MIMI MAGGIO

SONOGRAM ABBREVIATIONS

Ag	Cyst related to agenesis of the corpus callosum
AS	Aqueduct of Sylvius
B	Body of lateral ventricle
BS	Brain stem
Cb	Cerebrum
CC	Corpus callosum
Ce	Cerebellum
CN	Caudate nucleus
CP	Choroid plexus
CSP	Cavum septi pellucidi
F	Frontal horn
FM	Foramen of Monro
IF	Interhemispheric fissure
Me	Medulla
MI	Massa intermedia
O	Occipital horn
PF	Posterior fontanelle
Po	Pons
SP	Cavum septi pellucidi
Su	Sulci
Te	Temporal
Ten	Tentorium
Thl	Thalamus
Tr	Trigone
VC	Vermis of cerebellum
3V	Third ventricle
4V	Fourth ventricle

KEY WORDS

Aqueduct Stenosis. Congenital obstruction of the aqueduct (the duct connecting the third and fourth ventricles), causing third and lateral ventricular dilatation.

Arnold-Chiari Malformation. Congenital anomaly associated with spina bifida in which the cerebellum and brain stem are pulled toward the spinal cord and secondary hydrocephalus develops.

Asphyxia. Difficulty in breathing resulting in poor oxygenation. When asphyxia occurs in the first few minutes of life, it may be associated with intracranial hemorrhage and brain swelling (edema).

Atrium (Trigone) of the Lateral Ventricles. Site where the anterior, occipital, and temporal horns join.

Axial. Refers to a scan taken from a lateral approach through the temporal bone.

Brain Death. Damaged brain that will never again show function. Arterial pulsations are absent.

Brain Stem. Part of the brain connecting the forebrain and the spinal cord; consists of the midbrain, pons, and medulla oblongata.

Caudate Nucleus. Portion of the brain that forms the lateral borders of the frontal horns of the lateral ventricles and lies anterior to the thalamus.

Cavum Septi Pellucidi. A thin, triangular hole filled with cerebrospinal fluid that lies between the anterior horns of the lateral ventricles; it is particularly prominent in the neonate (see Fig. 50-32). It may appear to have three portions. If located posteriorly, it is termed a cavum vergae.

Cerebellum. Portion of the brain that lies posterior to the pons and medulla oblongata, below the tentorium.

Cerebrum. The largest part of the brain, consisting of two hemispheres.

Choroid Plexus. Mass of special cells located in the cerebral ventricles. The largest cluster, seen on ultrasound, is in the atrium of the lateral ventricle. These cells regulate the intraventricular pressure by secreting or absorbing cerebrospinal fluid.

Cistern. Focal enlargements of the subarachnoid space serving as a reservoir for cerebrospinal fluid.

Coronal View. Scan taken along the axis of the coronal suture (transverse in the skull).

Corpus Callosum. Large group of nerve fibers visible superior to the third ventricle that connect the left and right sides of the brain.

Cystic Encephalomalacia. An irreversibly severely damaged brain. The consequence of asphyxia, infection, and other rarer processes. The brain is more echogenic, and contains multiple cysts.

Dandy-Walker Syndrome. Congenital anomaly in which a fourth ventricular cyst splays the cerebellar hemispheres, occupying the area where the hypoplastic vermis lies, often with secondary dilatation of the third and lateral ventricles.

Dura Mater. Fibrous membrane that surrounds the brain and forms the tentorium.

Edematous Brain. A brain that is swollen, so that the ventricles appear slitlike, usually due to hypoxia (too little oxygen).

Encephalocele. Congenital anomaly in which a portion of the brain protrudes through a defect in the skull.

Encephalomalacia. An abnormal softening of the cerebrum following infarction.

Ependyma. The membrane lining the cerebral ventricles.

Falx Cerebri (Interhemispheric Fissure). A portion of the dura mater that separates the two cerebral hemispheres.

Fontanelle. Space between the bones of the skull. Ultrasound can be directed through the anterior fontanelle to examine the brain until about the age of 1 year.

Germinal Matrix. Periventricular tissue within the caudate nucleus that, prior to about 32 weeks' gestation, is fragile and bleeds easily.

Gyri. Convolutions on the surface of the brain caused by infolding of the cortex.

Hematocrit. The volume percentage of red blood cells in whole blood.

Holoprosencephaly. Grossly abnormal brain in which there is a common large central ventricle. Variations of this anomaly include alobar, semilobar, and lobar holoprosencephaly.

Horns. The recesses of the lateral ventricles; there are three horns of importance sonographically—the frontal, temporal, and occipital horns.

Hydranencephaly. Congenital anomaly in which the cortical brain structures are absent. The midbrain and brain stem tissues are present to a variable extent.

Hydrocephalus. Dilatation of the ventricles due to obstruction with accumulation of cerebrospinal fluid, usually due to blockage of cerebrospinal fluid drainage pathways. Blockage can occur at the level of the small holes (foramina) that lead from the ventricle (e.g., the aqueduct of Sylvius) or at the site of reabsorption of the cerebrospinal fluid (the brain surface). The latter form of hydrocephalus is termed communicating.

Interhemispheric Fissure. The area that separates the two cerebral hemispheres and in which the falx cerebri sits.

Leukomalacia. An abnormal softening of the white matter of the brain due to ischemia. May develop into a cyst.

Lipoma of the Corpus Callosum. An echogenic fat-filled mass within the corpus callosum.

Massa Intermedia. Portion of the brain that bulges into the third ventricle.

Meninges. The brain coverings.

Neonate. Newborn infant.

Parenchyma. General term for tissues of the cortex.

Periventricular Halo. A normal variant seen in the parasagittal view. An area of increased echogenicity along the trigone of the lateral ventricles.

Periventricular Leukomalacia. An infarct or softening of the white matter surrounding the ventricles, initially seen as echogenic. Three to six weeks later, cysts develop.

Porencephalic Cyst. Cyst arising from a ventricle that develops as a consequence of a parenchymal hemorrhage.

Sagittal View. Scan taken along the axis of the sagittal suture (longitudinal in the skull).

Seizure. A sudden episode of altered consciousness (known also as an epileptic fit).

Subependyma. The area immediately beneath the ependyma. In the caudate nucleus this area is the site of hemorrhage from the germinal matrix.

Subependymal Cyst. Cyst that occurs at the site of a previous bleed, in the germinal matrix.

Sulcus. A groove or depression on the surface of the brain, separating the gyri.

Tentorium. V-shaped echogenic structure separating the cerebrum and the cerebellum; it is an extension of the dura mater.

Thalamus. Two ovoid brain structures situated on either side of the third ventricle superior to the brain stem.

Trigone. See *Atrium of the Lateral Ventricles.*

Ventricle. A cavity within the brain containing cerebrospinal fluid.

Ventriculitis. Infection of the ventricles. The lining of the ventricles appears echogenic. The ventricles are dilated, and may contain septa and debris.

Ventriculomegaly. Enlarged ventricles, due to a variety of causes, including cerebral atrophy and congenital hydrocephalus.

 THE CLINICAL PROBLEM

Intracranial Hemorrhage

Intracranial ultrasound examination in the neonate is mainly concerned with the diagnosis and follow-up of hemorrhage, hydrocephalus, and congenital malformations. Clinical symptoms that make the pediatrician suspicious of intracranial hemorrhage include respiratory distress syndrome, a drop in hematocrit, prematurity (less than 32 weeks), and problems at delivery. It has been shown that most intracranial bleeds occur within 72 hours after birth. Diagnosis of these hemorrhages is important because although they are untreatable, once they are detected a search for alternative treatable lesions in other parts of the body can be ended. Later complications of the hemorrhage such as hydrocephalus may need treatment, so follow-up by sonography is helpful. Some hemorrhages occur without symptoms in infants born before 32 weeks' gestation.

Intracranial hemorrhages develop in premature infants in the immature subependymal germinal matrix of the caudate nucleus, in the choroid plexus, and, rarely, in the cerebellum. If the subependymal bleed is severe, it can rupture into the ventricular system or the surrounding cortical tissue. A bleed into the cortical parenchyma is a serious complication that usually results in a porencephalic cyst. Intracranial hemorrhages and their complications in the neonate are graded as follows:

Grade I. Subependymal bleed without hydrocephalus

Grade II. Subependymal and intraventricular bleed without hydrocephalus

Grade III. Subependymal and intraventricular bleed with hydrocephalus

Grade IV. Subependymal and intraventricular bleed with hydrocephalus and a parenchymal bleed

A very severe variant that is usually related to asphyxia and that has a hopeless prognosis is periventricular leukomalacia.

Ventriculomegaly (Hydrocephalus)

Ventriculomegaly can be monitored by ultrasound through the anterior fontanelle until the age of 9 months to 1 year, so that severe ventricular dilatation requiring a shunt can be recognized. Once a shunt is in place, it may become blocked, causing further ventriculomegaly. Therefore, postoperative ultrasound follow-up is important. Ventriculomegaly can be followed until the child is 6 or 7 years old, using an axial approach after the anterior fontanelle has closed.

Congenital Malformations

Congenital malformations with ventricular dilatation can be diagnosed with ultrasound—for example, hydranencephaly, Dandy-Walker syndrome, and holoprosencephaly.

Encephaloceles can be examined usefully with ultrasound because one can see how much brain tissue has prolapsed out of the skull with the meninges.

ANATOMY

The anatomy of the neonatal brain is complex. It is demonstrated in Figures 50-1 to 50-5 from three angles—the longitudinal (sagittal) views (see Figs. 50-1 and 50-2); the transverse (coronal) views using the anterior fontanelle as a window (see Figs. 50-3 to 50-5); and the axial views (from the lateral side of the head) (see Fig. 50-11).

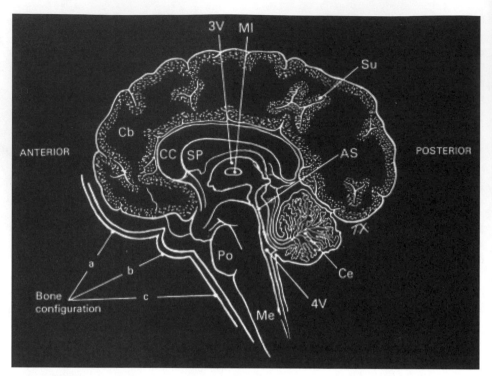

FIGURE 50-1. Normal midline sagittal view. Important structures are the cavum septi pellucidi, the third ventricle, the fourth ventricle, and the cerebellum. Note the bone configuration of a midline section: sphenoid (a), pituitary fossa (b), clivus (c).

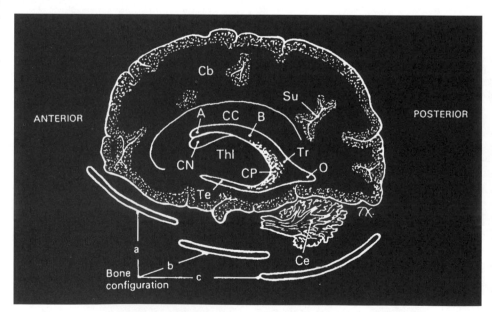

FIGURE 50-2. Normal lateral sagittal view showing the area of the caudate nucleus, the thalamus, and the occipital horn. Note the different bone configurations: anterior sphenoid (a), middle sphenoid (b), occipital fossa (c).

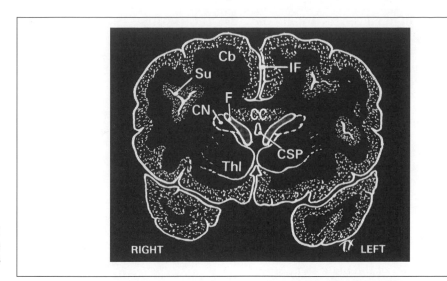

FIGURE 50-3. Normal anterior coronal view. The curvilinear frontal slits are the anterior horns; the caudate nucleus is adjacent.

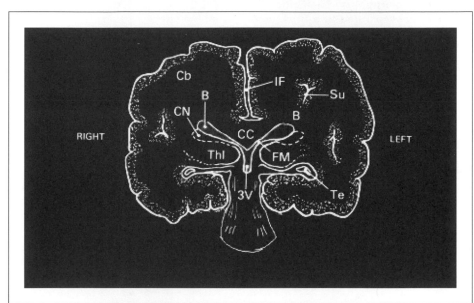

FIGURE 50-4. Normal midcoronal view, showing the body of the lateral ventricles and the third ventricular area. The thin slit of the third ventricle may not be seen unless it is slightly dilated.

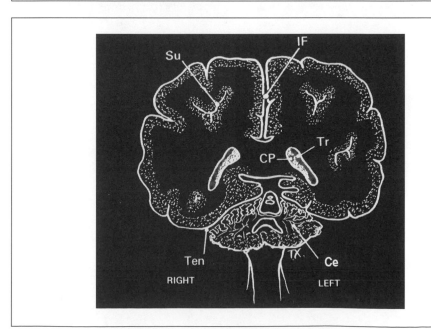

FIGURE 50-5. Normal posterior coronal view. Emphasis should be placed on seeing the choroid plexus in the trigone of the lateral ventricles.

A series of fluid spaces within the brain called ventricles, which are linked, form the framework on which the brain lies. Two lateral ventricles lie on either side of the midline and connect with the third ventricle through two small holes called the foramina of Monro. The third ventricle drains through a small tube called the aqueduct of Sylvius into a small fourth ventricle which lies in the cerebellum. The superior part of the brain, called the cerebrum (where thinking occurs), and the midbrain are separated from the cerebellum (which lies at the back of the brain) by a thick membrane called the tentorium. The brain stem connects these two regions. Above the level of the brain stem, structures are duplicated on each side. The two sides are separated by a thick membrane, called the falx, superiorly. More inferiorly, the two sides are connected by the corpus callosum, at the midbrain level, and are joined at the brain stem level. Midbrain structures are particularly sensitive to prematurity.

◢ TECHNIQUE

Most infants referred for serial scans of the neonatal brain have such a precarious hold on their health that they are in a neonatal intensive care unit (NICU). Fragile immune systems require gowns and fresh gloves for each baby. Coordinate your sterile precautions with the NICU staff; cover the transducer. If the infant has cytomegalovirus inclusion disease, it should not be examined by a pregnant sonographer.

If the infant is scanned inside an isolette, it is sometimes difficult to get access to the top of the head. After gently moving the baby and the endotracheal tube, it is helpful to build up the head—perhaps with some sterile gauze—to create more room to maneuver the transducer.

Hazards of Intracranial Scanning

1. The endotracheal tube can be displaced if the head is moved too drastically.
2. Infection can be spread from one infant to another unless the sonographer washes his or her hands between studies and covers the probe with plastic or wipes the transducer with alcohol between patients.
3. Babies have very poor temperature control and rapidly become hypothermic (too cold) if they are not warmed adequately.
4. A delicate touch is necessary for transfontanelle scanning to avoid damaging the brain.

Transducer Selection

A small footprint curved array scanner gives the best results while the anterior fontanelle is open. A linear array employed from a lateral approach (axial) can be used to follow hydrocephalus when the anterior fontanelle starts to close.

An aqueous gel should be used in both instances for good skull contact.

Sagittal Views

A 7.5- or 10-MHz transducer offers better detail for infants with a large anterior fontanelle and a small head. Use a 5-MHz transducer for infants with a small fontanelle or a medium to large head.

The time gain compensation curve should be set to identify the occipital horns properly. They cannot always be seen if the anterior fontanelle is small.

Midline

Start with sagittal scans with the baby's head in either the supine or the lateral position. Place the transducer on the anterior fontanelle along the plane of the sagittal suture (Fig. 50-6). Scan along the midline, making sure to identify the cavum septi pellucidi, the brain stem, and the area of the third and fourth ventricles (midline sagittal view).

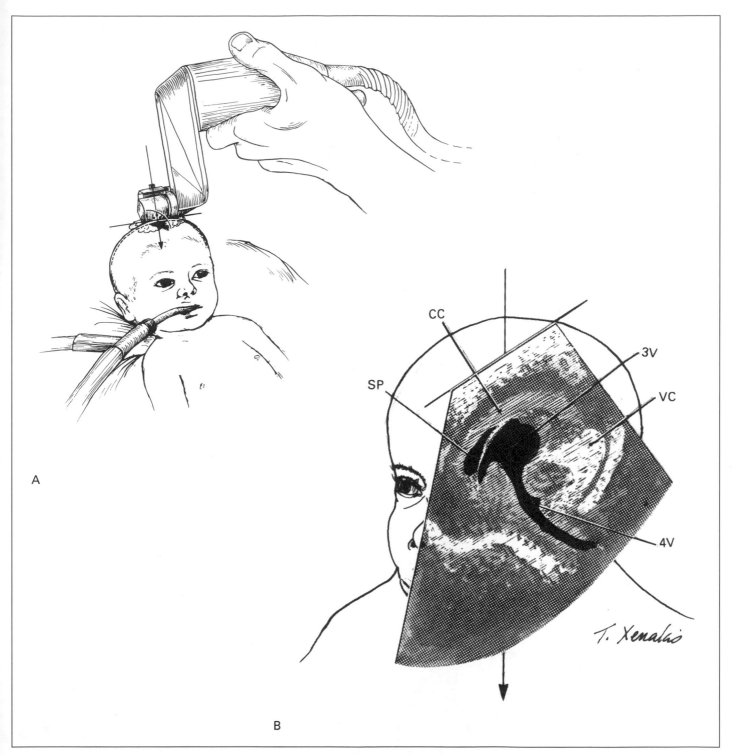

FIGURE 50-6. Midline sagittal scan. (**A**) Position for midline sagittal scan through the anterior fontanelle. (**B**) Anatomy in the midline sagittal view.

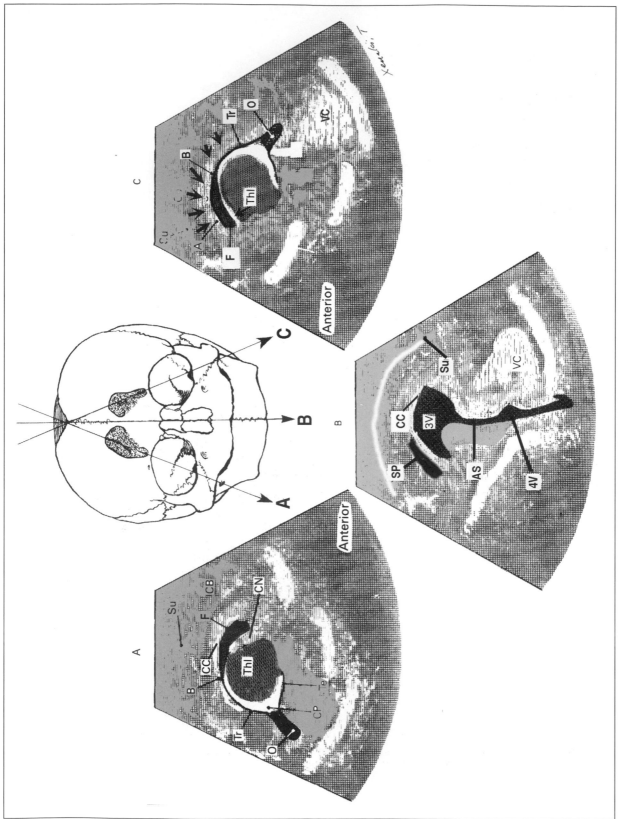

FIGURE 50-7. Parasagittal views. (**A**) Normal lateral sagittal view. Note that the anterior part of the section is facing toward the right. (**B**) Midline sagittal view. The third ventricle, the aqueduct of Sylvius, and, if possible, the fourth ventricle should be visualized. The vermis of the cerebellum should have bright-level echoes. (**C**) Normal left lateral sagittal view. Note that the anterior part is facing toward the left. The entire lateral ventricular system should be demonstrated. It normally appears as a black slit. The choroid plexus appears as bright-level echoes surrounding the thalamus. The sulci are the bright, tortuous lines in the cerebrum. The small arrows show the corpus callosum.

Parasagittal

Staying in the same position, angle out slightly to the left and right sides (Fig. 50-7). The entire lateral ventricle may not be visualized in a single view. Obtain a parasagittal view, concentrating on the anterior horn and body of the desired side. Make sure to demonstrate the interface (bright line) between the caudate nucleus and the thalamus—a common site for a bleed (Fig. 50-8).

Farther Lateral

Angle farther laterally to view the thalamus, choroid plexus, and tip of the occipital horn. This is where intraventricular blood frequently collects (see Fig. 50-8). Angle farther laterally to image the peripheral cerebral tissue.

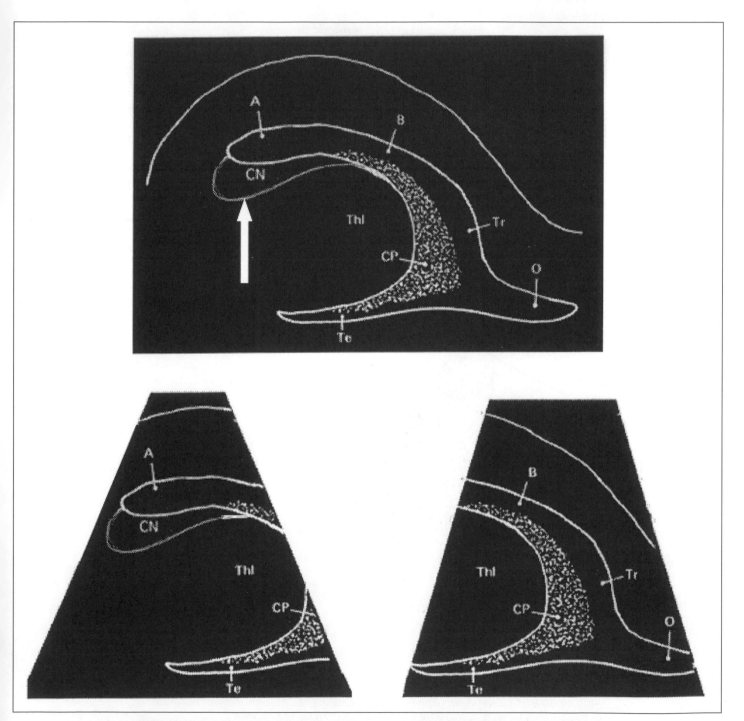

FIGURE 50-8. Lateral sagittal view demonstrating the lateral ventricle and the thalamus. Demonstrate the anterior horn (two views may be required to show the entire lateral ventricles), the body, and the thalamus. Angle slightly farther laterally to image the thalamus, choroid plexus, and tip of the occipital horn. Note the interface between the caudate nucleus and the thalamus (white arrow).

Labeling

To distinguish the left and right sagittal views, we use the following convention: left sagittal view anterior faces the sonographer's left; right sagittal view anterior faces the sonographer's right.

Coronal (Transverse) Views

The following coronal views are routine.

Posterior

Place the transducer on the anterior fontanelle along the plane of the coronal suture (Fig. 50-9). Angling posteriorly, identify the choroid plexus in the atrium of the lateral ventricles (posterior view, Fig. 50-10A).

Midcoronal

Slowly sweep anteriorly toward the body of the lateral ventricles until the foramen of Monro can be seen entering the third ventricle (see Fig. 50-10B).

Anterior Coronal

Angle more anteriorly toward the frontal horns (see Fig. 50-10C). Make sure that the orientation is correct on the coronal views. The right ventricle should be on your left as you look at the picture.

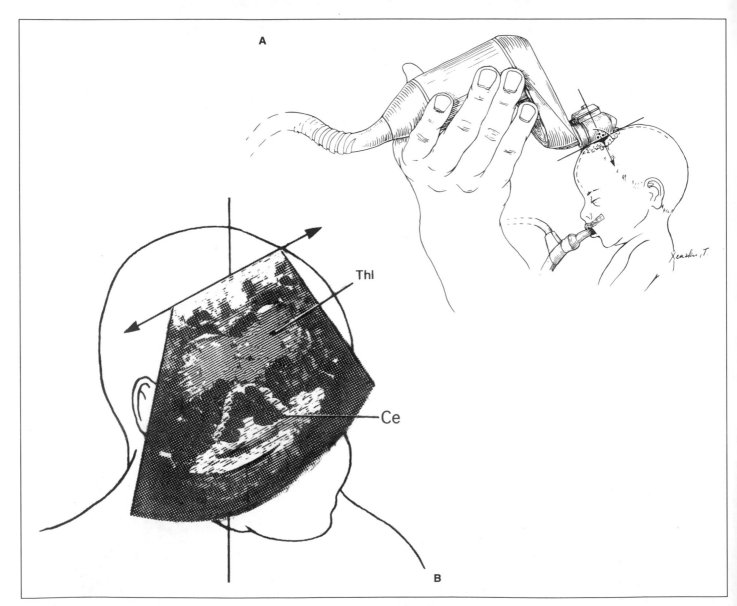

FIGURE 50-9. Coronal view. (**A**) Position for scanning the coronal views. (**B**) Anatomy of the coronal view. It is important to make the images symmetric.

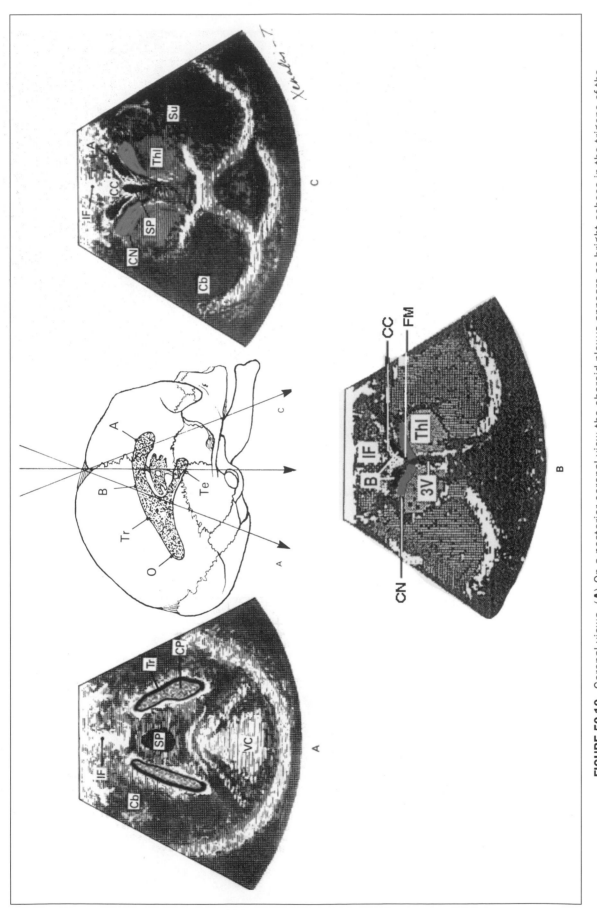

FIGURE 50-10. Coronal views. (**A**) On a posterior coronal view the choroid plexus appears as bright echoes in the trigone of the lateral ventricle. If there is dilatation of the occipital horns, a scan should be performed posterior to the choroid plexus area. Make sure that the ventricles are symmetric. (**B**) The midcoronal view demonstrates the body of the lateral ventricle. The third ventricle may be seen if it is slightly dilated, and the foramen of Monro should be demonstrated. (**C**) In the anterior coronal view, the views should be symmetric to rule out a hemorrhage in the area of the caudate nucleus and thalamus. The anterior horns will appear as narrow dark slits or may not be well seen at all if normal.

Axial Views

An axial view (Fig. 50-11) is obtained by placing the transducer on the lateral aspect of the neonatal head with either a mechanical sector scanner or a linear array. Axial views are useful for following ventricular size.

With the baby's head in the lateral position, place the probe along the temporoparietal region to demonstrate the lateral ventricular area and angle it toward the face, the area of the thalamus, and the third ventricle. The lateral ventricle on the side facing down can then be measured (Fig. 50-11A).

$$\text{Lateral ventricular ratio} = \frac{\text{Lateral ventricular width (a)}}{\text{Hemispheric width (b)}}$$

Since the near field is obscured by reverberation artifact, measurements are made from the midline to the far lateral wall and compared with the ventricle on the far side from the transducer.

The letters *a* and *b* in the equation refer to labels in Figure 50-11B.

Linear arrays using the lateral approach are less easy to use because of the difficulty in seeing small bleeds and the similarity of the choroid plexus to hemorrhage, especially when the ventricle is not dilated.

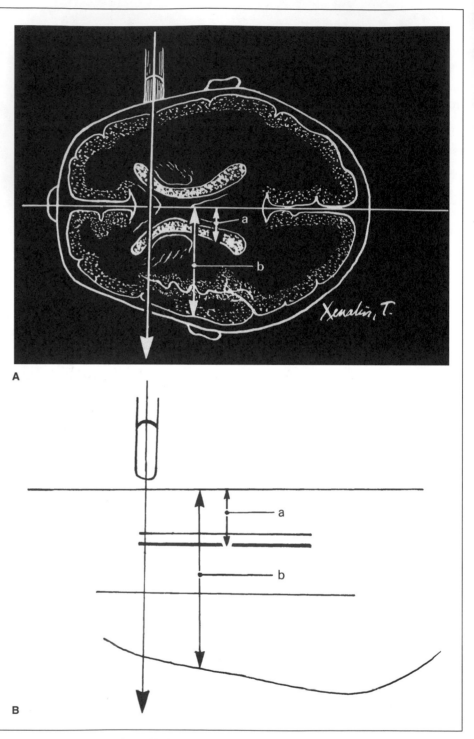

FIGURE 50-11. Axial view. (**A**) When scanning with an axial approach, the downside lateral ventricle should be measured because there is too much artifact in the near field. The progress of hydrocephalus is followed by monitoring the lateral ventricular size as it relates to hemispheric size. (**B**) Appropriate sites for measurement of the "hemisphere" (b) and ventricle (a) are shown.

Measurements

Serial sonographic measurements can be compared by measuring the occipital horn on the sagittal views (Fig. 50-12A); this is the most sensitive measurement. The normal upper limit is 16 mm. Mild dilatation can be measured in an oblique fashion in the region of the ventricular body and should not exceed 3 mm (see Fig. 50-12B). The third ventricle can be measured on coronal views (see Fig. 50-12B); it is normally 2 mm or less.

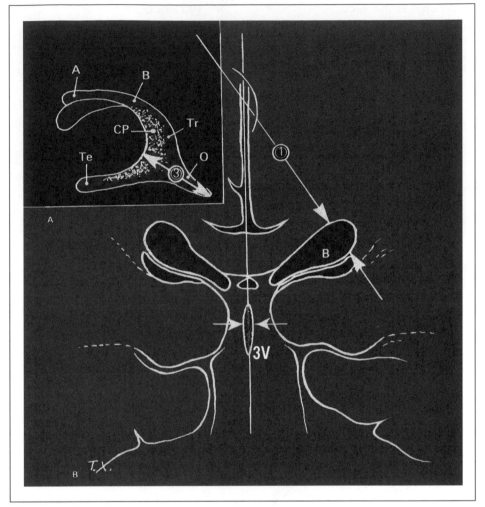

FIGURE 50-12. Measurements of lateral ventricles. (**A**) A lateral sagittal view measurement (3) taken at an oblique axis at the occipital horn can indicate ventricular enlargement at an early stage. This distance should not exceed 16 mm. (**B**) On the coronal view a measurement that should not exceed 3 mm is taken at the body of the lateral ventricle (1). The third ventricular width measurement should not exceed 2 mm.

Additional Techniques

In selected cases when the occipital horns are difficult to see, angle through the posterior fontanelle to obtain better detail of the occipital horns (Fig. 50-13). Examining the patient with the head elevated helps to visualize the occipital horns better and to demonstrate a fluid-fluid level caused by blood.

 PATHOLOGY

Hemorrhage

The appearance of intracranial hemorrhage changes with time. Early hemorrhages are echogenic. Within a couple of weeks, the increased echogenicity decreases, leaving relatively sonolucent areas.

Subependymal Hemorrhage

Increased echogenicity in the caudate nucleus can be seen on the coronal view inferior to the floor of the lateral ventricles when there is a subependymal hemorrhage (Fig. 50-14). On the sagittal view the head of the caudate nucleus is echogenic (Fig. 50-15). An affected caudate nucleus may bulge into the ventricle.

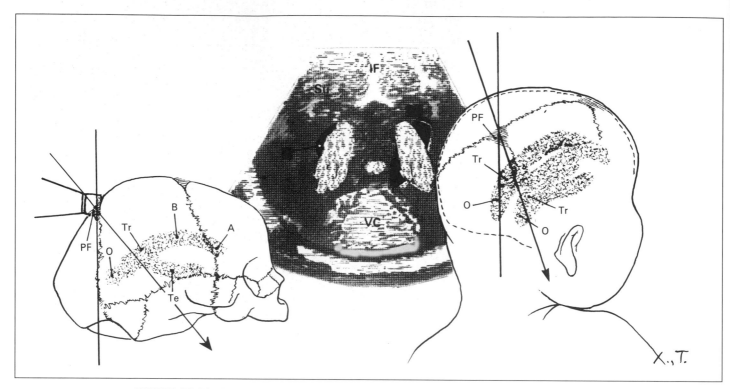

FIGURE 50-13. The posterior fontanelle approach. Sometimes it is difficult to examine the occipital horns, but by angling through the posterior fontanelle, you may be able to pick up better detail of the occipital horns.

It may be difficult to differentiate between a subependymal hemorrhage extending toward the ventricle and an intraventricular hemorrhage or clot. Such hemorrhages may not be associated with hydrocephalus initially. Occasional hemorrhages occur in the thalamus. Remember that the echogenic choroid plexus in the lateral ventricle does not extend anterior to the foramen of Monro.

Subependymal Germinal Matrix Cyst

Cysts within the germinal matrix may develop at the site of a previous bleed. These cysts have an echogenic wall and an echopenic center and bulge into the lateral ventricle. Such cysts do not normally have any long-term consequences.

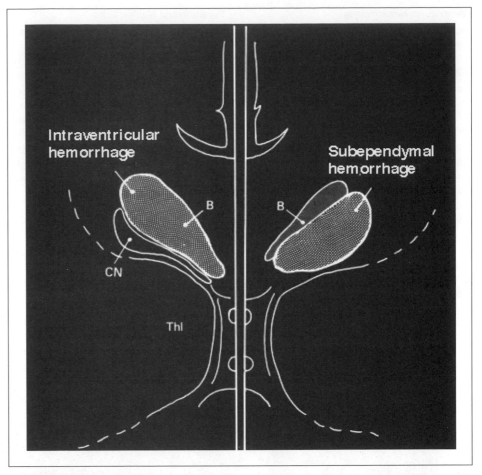

FIGURE 50-14. Sometimes it is difficult to decide whether a hemorrhage is subependymal or intraventricular. The midcoronal view is helpful for distinguishing the two lesions because the relationship to the caudate nucleus can be seen.

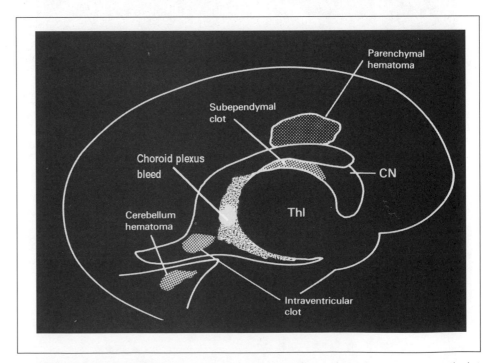

FIGURE 50-15. Lateral sagittal view. The various sites where hemorrhage and clot formation may occur are shown.

Ventricular Hemorrhage

A ventricular hemorrhage has to be distinguished from the choroid plexus. The choroid plexus rarely extends into the occipital horn (Fig. 50-16A), so detection of echoes in this area usually indicates hemorrhage. In older hemorrhages, clot is more easily discerned because hydrocephalus occurs and the clot becomes more compact (see Fig. 50-16B) and is surrounded by cerebrospinal fluid. Blood may completely fill the ventricles, forming a "cast," in which case it may be difficult to distinguish a ventricular blood clot from a large subependymal bleed and the choroid plexus (see Fig. 50-16A and B). The choroid plexus is vascular, so color flow is helpful in sorting out normal choroid plexus from intrachoroidal bleeds.

Parenchymal Hemorrhage (Bleeding Into the Brain Substance)

A dense echogenic area occurs in the brain substance at a site usually near the caudate nucleus and lateral to the ventricles (see Fig. 50-17A) when there is a parenchymal hemorrhage. This hemorrhage resolves slowly, with the formation of a porencephalic cyst (a fluid-filled cavity within the brain substance) (see Fig. 50-17B and C). Dilatation of the lateral ventricles is often associated with parenchymal hemorrhage.

Choroid and Cerebellar Bleeds

Choroid and cerebellar bleeds are very difficult to detect because they occur within echogenic structures—the choroid and cerebellum. Irregularity of the choroid outline and increased echogenicity suggest a bleed (see Fig. 50-15 and earlier discussion). If the bleed is unilateral, images which allow comparison of both choroid plexuses simultaneously, such as the posterior coronal view, are helpful (see Fig. 50-5).

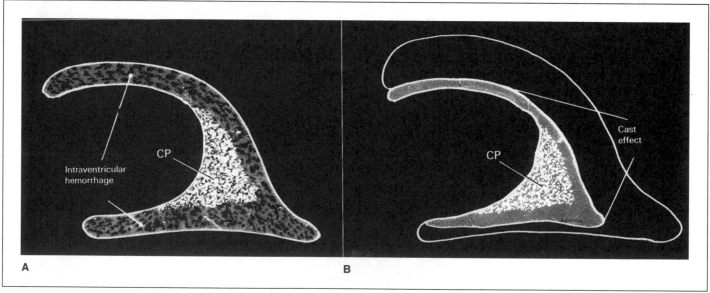

FIGURE 50-16. Intraventricular hemorrhage. (**A**) Lateral sagittal view. An intraventricular hemorrhage fills the entire lateral ventricle. The choroid plexus is difficult to distinguish from the hemorrhage without color flow. (**B**) With time, the hemorrhage takes on a cast effect and adopts the shape of the ventricle as the blood resolves. The choroid plexus is still difficult to distinguish from the clot. The ventricle is enlarged as a consequence of the intraventricular bleed.

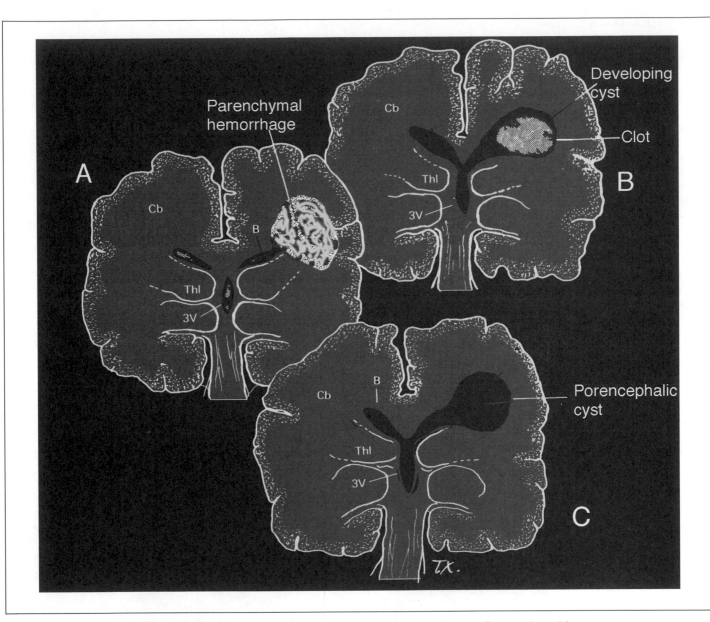

FIGURE 50-17. Parenchymal hemorrhage. (**A**) Midcoronal view of parenchymal hemorrhage. At first the parenchymal hemorrhage appears as a bright echogenic area on the brain. (**B**) The hemorrhage begins to resolve and communicate with the lateral ventricle. The parenchymal hemorrhage becomes a porencephalic cyst with a clot within. (**C**) The clot resolves completely, leaving a porencephalic cyst with lateral ventricular dilatation.

Periventricular Leukomalacia

Periventricular leukomalacia (PVL) occurs in newborn infants who have suffered asphyxia. The ultrasonic appearances are seen at two stages: stage I occurs within a day or two of birth. A dense echogenic area surrounds the ventricles, particularly in the occipital horn region (Fig. 50-18A). Stage II develops 3 to 8 weeks after birth. Cysts form around the ventricles in the areas that were previously echogenic (see Fig. 50-18B). They may be seen for only a 2- to 3-week period. Eventually, the cysts are replaced by scars, and the ventricles dilate due to cerebral atrophy.

The initial phase of PVL can sometimes be confused with the normal periventricular halo seen along the trigone of the lateral ventricles. Also, intraparenchymal hemorrhage should not be confused with the early phase of PVL. Intraparenchymal hemorrhage usually extends toward the periphery of the brain, while PVL is limited to the region surrounding the ventricles.

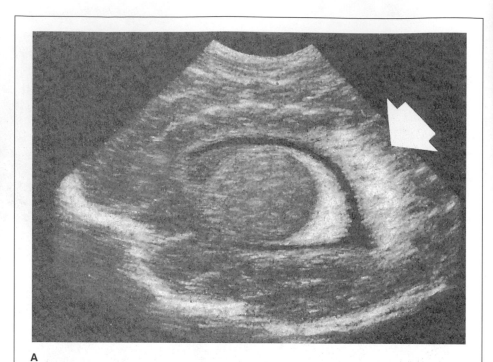

A

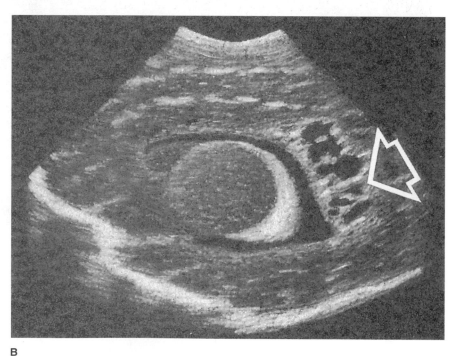

B

FIGURE 50-18. Periventricular leukomalacia. (**A**) An echogenic area surrounds the trigone of the lateral ventricle in its early stages (arrow). (**B**) Cysts develop about three to six weeks later to replace this echogenic area (arrow).

Encephalitis and Brain Edema

The overall echogenicity of the brain is increased in encephalitis and in cases of brain edema, and the ventricles become slitlike due to swelling of the brain.

Ventriculitis

Ventriculitis is usually associated with encephalitis. The brain is more echogenic, often with small cystic areas. The ventricles are dilated and contain echogenic debris (Fig. 50-19). Septa may be present within the ventricles. The ependyma (ventricular lining) is echogenic, and holes may line the borders of the ventricles.

Brain Abscess

Brain abscess presents as a cystic lesion with nonhomogeneous echogenic material within. Other signs of ventriculitis and encephalitis will be present. Abscesses can vary in size and number, and may be loculated.

Subdural Hematoma

Birth traumas can cause a tearing of the dural folds or a rupture of the medullary veins, causing blood to collect around the periphery of the brain. On the sagittal view the cerebral surfaces appear flattened; an echopenic space between the cranium and the cerebrum is seen (Fig. 50-20). On a coronal view, there is fluid within the interhemispheric fissure and a collection around the brain. The gyri become more prominent and closer together because they are compressed (see Fig. 50-20). The prominent gyri may be the clue to the presence of a hematoma not seen with a low-frequency transducer because near-field resolution is poor.

Owing to poor resolution in the near field of the ultrasound beam, subdural hematomas may be missed. A high-frequency transducer (7.5 to 10 MHz) will give a better view of the area. A stand-off pad may be of help. A small amount of fluid normally surrounds the infant brain, but it is symmetric and minimal at all sites.

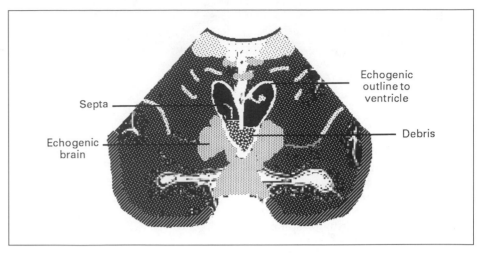

FIGURE 50-19. Ventriculitis. The ventricles are enlarged, with an echogenic border, and there is evidence of septa and debris within the ventricles.

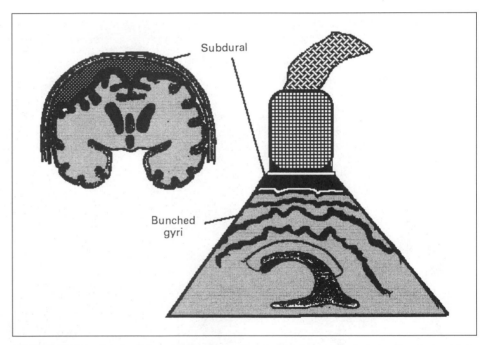

FIGURE 50-20. Subdural hematoma. Scanning in the coronal plane and using a high-frequency transducer best demonstrates the widening of the interhemispheric fissure and prominent gyri. The collection around the brain can be seen. Note that the gyri are close together.

Ventricular Dilatation

Lateral Ventricles

Normal ventricles in the neonate usually appear as tiny, barely visible slits (see Fig. 50-3). Usually the first indication of ventricular dilatation appears in the occipital horn; the body and anterior horn dilate subsequently. Ventricular dilatation of minimal, moderate, and marked degree is easy to judge on sagittal views (Fig. 50-21). The coronal views offer another plane for assessing ventricular enlargement (Fig. 50-22). Third and fourth ventricular dilatation can be seen on the sagittal midline section. Usually these structures are barely visible, so evidence of enlargement is easy to see (Fig. 50-23).

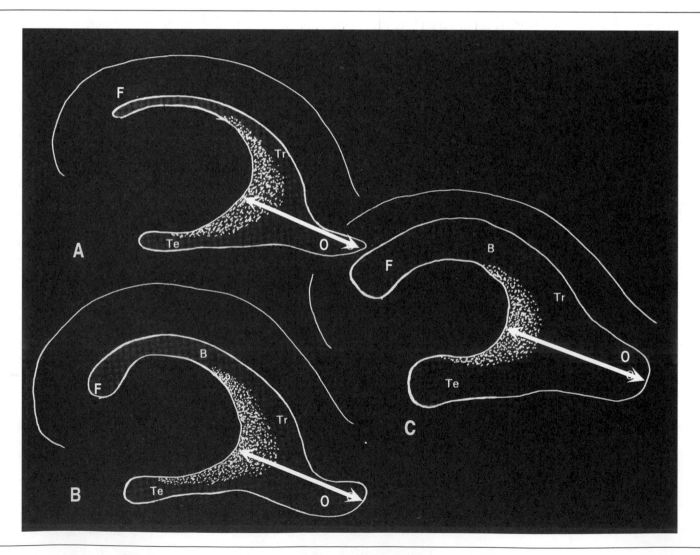

FIGURE 50-21. Lateral sagittal views with varying degrees of lateral ventricular dilatation. (**A**) Minimal ventricular dilatation. (**B**) Moderate ventricular dilatation. (**C**) Marked ventricular dilatation, with the shape of the occipital horn noticeably rounder than in (**A**). Arrows show the occipital horn site where measurements are made.

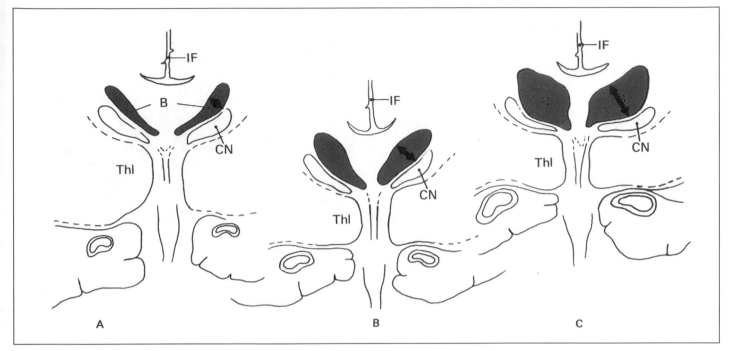

FIGURE 50-22. Varying degrees of ventricular dilatation are also measured in the midcoronal view. (**A**) Minimal ventricular dilatation. (**B**) Moderate ventricular dilatation. (**C**) Marked ventricular dilatation. Note the changes in shape of the ventricles, from slit-like, to rounded, to bulging in (**C**).

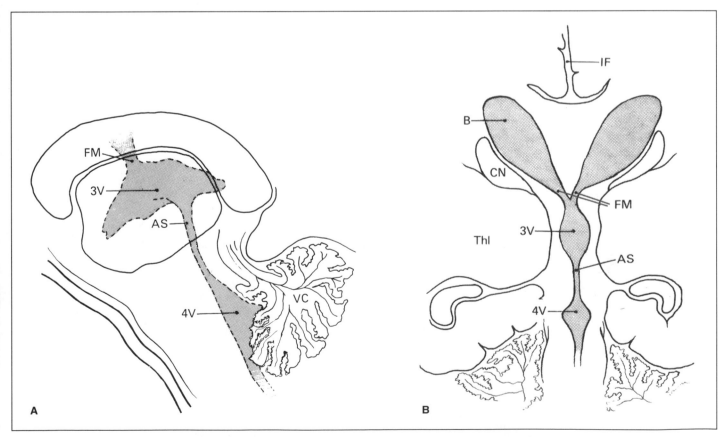

FIGURE 50-23. Midline sagittal (**A**) and coronal (**B**) view. The foramina of Monro may be seen. There may also be third and fourth ventricular dilatation.

Shunt Tube Placement

Shunts appear as dense echogenic lines. The shunt tip location should be visualized (Fig. 50-24). Sometimes a shunt tip lies in the brain parenchyma or in the choroid plexus or crosses the midline— less than ideal locations. Sometimes the fetal position affects the patency of the shunt tip; perhaps it lodges in the choroid plexus when the baby's head is on its side. This should be noted in the report.

Congenital Anomalies

There are many congenital anomalies of the brain; only the common types are described here. Some anomalies are incompatible with long-term survival. The role of the sonographer is to show the nature of the anomaly so that a decision can be made about whether resuscitation attempts are worthwhile or whether surgical intervention (usually shunting) is necessary.

Aqueductal Stenosis

Aqueductal stenosis is a moderately common condition in which both lateral ventricles and the third ventricle are dilated and the aqueduct of Sylvius is obstructed. The aqueduct can be seen leading from the third ventricle and ending abruptly before it reaches the fourth ventricle (see Fig. 50-23). The fourth ventricle is not dilated.

Communicating Hydrocephalus

The ventricles are dilated but there is a fluid space around the brain in communicating hydrocephalus. The cerebrospinal fluid is not circulating and being resorbed as is normally the case. The cisterna magna and the fourth, third, and lateral ventricles are all enlarged.

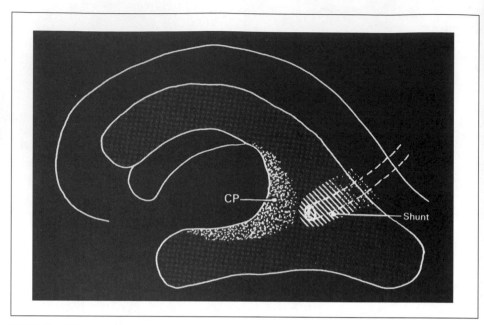

FIGURE 50-24. Lateral sagittal view. A shunt in the lateral ventricle appears as a dense group of echoes. The sonographer should demonstrate carefully where the shunt ends.

Microcephaly and Atrophy

The skull size and the brain are small in microcephaly or in atrophic brains. The ventricles are often enlarged, however, and there may be calcification within the brain or around the ventricles.

Dandy-Walker Syndrome

In Dandy-Walker syndrome a cystic cavity occupies the occipital infratentorial area, often causing symmetric dilatation of the lateral ventricles and enlargement of the third ventricle (Fig. 50-25). The cerebellum is small and malformed. The malformation is associated with an expansion of the fourth ventricle, and the cerebellar lobes are splayed on either side of the cyst. The vermis is small or absent.

Extra-axial Cyst

Extra-axial cysts are located in the posterior fossa. The fourth ventricle is normal. The cerebellum is compressed but otherwise normal, and the lobes are still joined by the vermis.

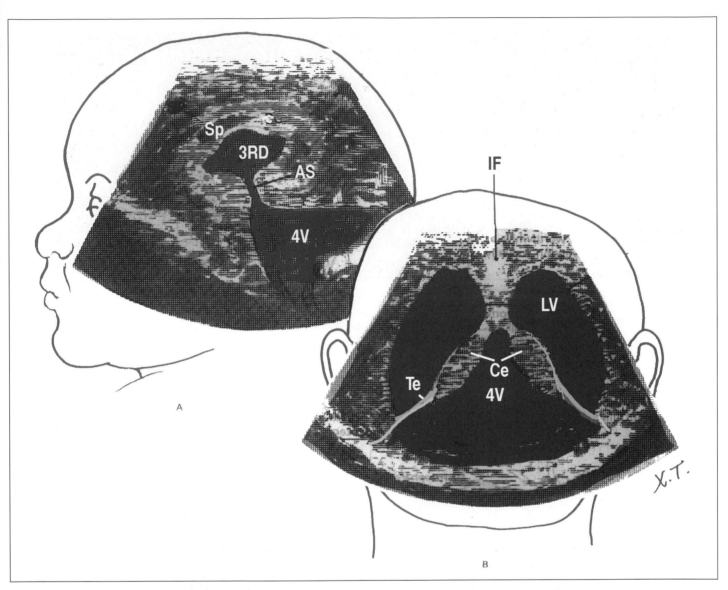

FIGURE 50-25. Dandy-Walker syndrome. (**A**) Midline sagittal view. With the Dandy-Walker syndrome there is cystic dilatation of the fourth ventricle; the third ventricle and aqueduct of Sylvius are dilated to a lesser degree. Note the abnormal cerebellar shape. (**B**) Posterior coronal view. Massive fourth ventricular enlargement and secondary lateral ventricular enlargement.

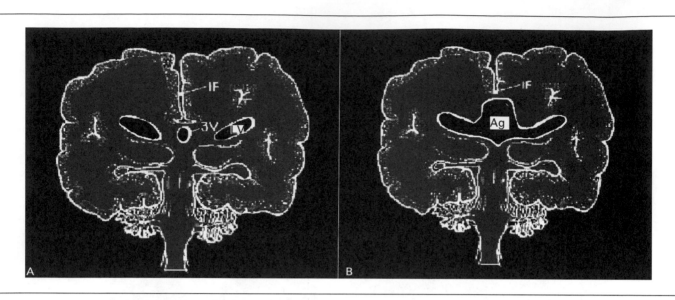

FIGURE 50-26. Agenesis of the corpus callosum. (**A**) Transverse view. The third ventricle lies high because there is no corpus callosum. The lateral ventricles are more widely separated than usual. (**B**) Agenesis of the corpus callosum with cyst. In this variant, the lateral and third ventricles are joined by a cyst (Ag) that extends superiorly from the third ventricle.

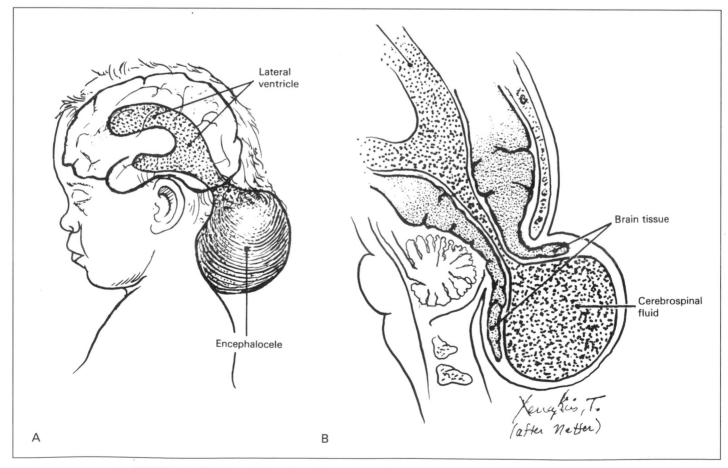

FIGURE 50-27. Encephalocele. (**A**) The lateral ventricles are usually enlarged with the presence of an encephalocele. (**B**) The lateral ventricles and brain substance extend into this encephalocele. Variable amounts of brain or ventricle may be present in an encephalocele.

Agenesis of the Corpus Callosum

Absence of the nerve tract that connects the two hemispheres (the corpus callosum) allows the third ventricle to move superiorly and separate the lateral ventricles (Fig. 50-26). The gyri are vertically rather than horizontally aligned. In association with callosal agenesis, there may be cystic extension from the roof of the third ventricle. The corpus callosum will not be visible.

Partial agenesis of the corpus callosum may be seen. Agenesis is often associated with other anomalies.

Encephalocele

In encephalocele a portion of the brain prolapses through a hole in the midline of the skull (Fig. 50-27). The hole is usually located occipitally but may be located in the nasal region. In many instances the mass is almost entirely fluid filled. The amount of brain tissue in the defect varies and affects surgical management and survival.

Holoprosencephaly

In holoprosencephaly, the brain is grossly disorganized and the lateral ventricular pattern is markedly abnormal. There is a single ventricle with a horseshoe shape (Fig. 50-28). There are three variants of holoprosencephaly:

1. In *alobar holoprosencephaly*, there is a single horseshoe-shaped ventricle with a thin cortical mantle, especially in the dorsal aspect of the brain. The thalami are fused, and the third ventricle is absent. A ridge (the hippocampal ridge) may be seen on the lateral border of the single dilated ventricle. This variant is compatible with life for only a few days or weeks.

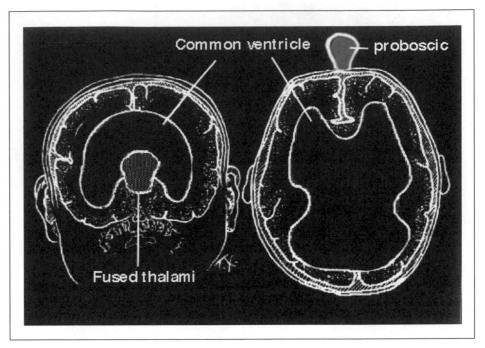

FIGURE 50-28. Alobar holoprosencephaly. Anterior coronal and axial views. A single misshaped ventricle is present. Note the proboscis which arises above the eyes. There is often no nose present in the usual location.

2. In *semilobar holoprosencephaly*, the findings are similar, with the horseshoe-shaped or partially split ventricle with fused occipital horn, but considerable cortex is present. This is a less severe variant.

3. In *lobar holoprosencephaly*, there is partial development of the occipital and temporal horns with absence of the cavum septum pellucidum and olfactory apparatus. This syndrome is also associated with mental retardation.

Midline facial anomalies are usually associated with intracranial findings of holoprosencephaly:

1. There may be a single eye or hypotelorism.

2. There may be no nose, but a proboscis (a soft tissue structure located above the eyes) may be present (see Fig. 50-28).

3. A central cleft lip and palate is often present.

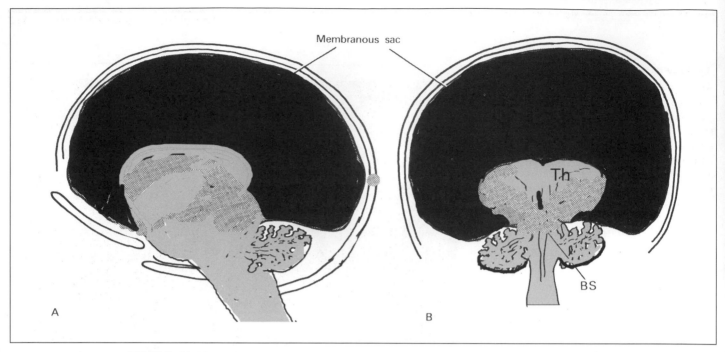

FIGURE 50-29. Hydranencephaly. Lateral sagittal (**A**) and midcoronal (**B**) views. There is no evidence of cortical tissue. A membranous fluid-filled sac replaces the brain. Only the brain stem and midbrain are present.

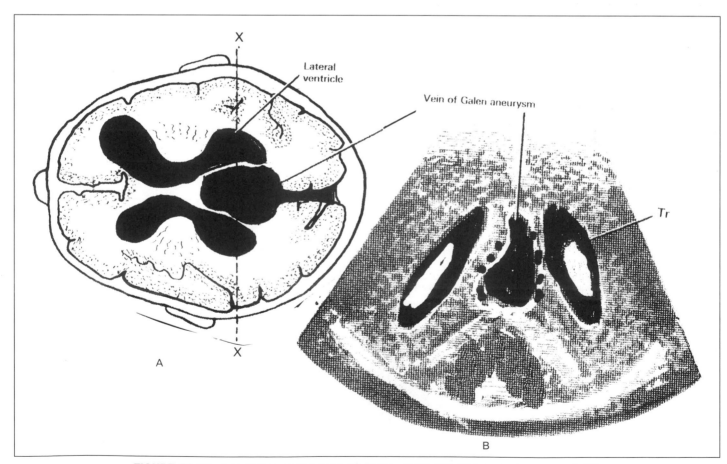

FIGURE 50-30. Aneurysm of the vein of Galen. Axial (**A**) and posterior coronal (**B**) views. An aneurysm of the vein of Galen is usually associated with lateral ventricular dilatation. Note the large draining vein. The small black dots alongside the vein of Galen aneurysm are large arterial feeders to the arterial venous fistula. The posterior coronal view was performed along line x-x.

Hydranencephaly

Absence of the cerebral hemispheres of the brain is called hydranencephaly; the condition is not compatible with survival. It is often mistaken for severe hydrocephalus. Only the midbrain and brain stem are present. The midbrain may be partially absent. No midline echo is seen (Fig. 50-29).

Vein of Galen Malformation

There is aneurysmal dilatation of the vein of Galen—a large midline vein—with secondary hydrocephalus (Fig. 50-30). Because so much blood is entering the head, there is often associated heart failure. Sonographically, one sees a large, eccentrically shaped midline cystic space with lateral ventricular dilatation. The cystic space is superior to the tentorium and posterior to the third ventricle. The dilated arteries supplying the arteriovenous malformation may be visible. A large draining vein extends posteriorly to the straight sinus.

Doppler showing flow within the cystic cavity establishes the diagnosis of vein of Galen malformation.

Arnold-Chiari Malformation

Arnold-Chiari malformation is a relatively common syndrome, usually a consequence of a spina bifida defect tethering the spinal cord so that the brain structures cannot rise into the head to their normal site. The cerebellum is pulled inferiorly. Secondary hydrocephalus develops. The sonographic findings are as follows:

1. Superior and inferior sharp angles to the lateral ventricles
2. Possible absence of the cavum septi pellucidi
3. Enlarged asymmetric ventricles
4. Inferior placement of the tentorium
5. A banana-shaped cerebellum (see Fig. 18-28)
6. An absent cisterna magna
7. Views through the upper cervical spine that may show the cerebellum within the upper spinal canal adjacent to the cord

Lipoma of Corpus Callosum

An echogenic mass is seen within the corpus callosum when there is a lipoma. Coronal views show the anterior horns to be widely separated and pointed due to the maldevelopment of the corpus callosum caused by the intervening midline lipoma.

Choroid Plexus Papilloma

Choroid plexus papilloma is a benign tumor. The choroid plexus appears enlarged and echogenic. Hydrocephalus may develop due to obstruction of ventricular foramina.

Intracranial Calcifications

Infections that may occur during pregnancy—cytomegalovirus inclusion disease or toxoplasmosis—can cause intracranial calcifications in the newborn. Echogenic areas are present in the brain that may be associated with shadowing. With cytomegalovirus inclusion disease, the echogenic areas are in a periventricular location. With toxoplasmosis, they are more diffuse and scattered throughout the brain.

✸ PITFALLS

Normal Variants

1. *Sulci.* The sulci may appear more echogenic than usual. This finding is of no pathologic significance and is seen in older infants (Fig. 50-31).

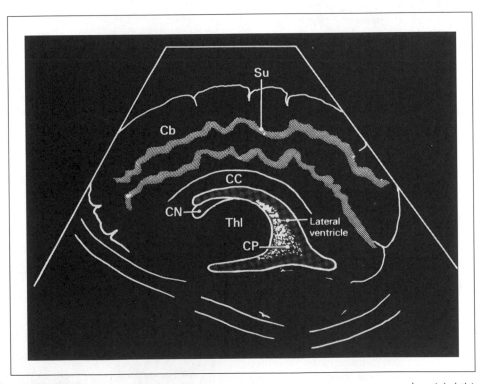

FIGURE 50-31. Lateral sagittal view. The sulci may appear as very prominent bright lines. This is a normal variant. The sulci become more prominent as the infant grows older.

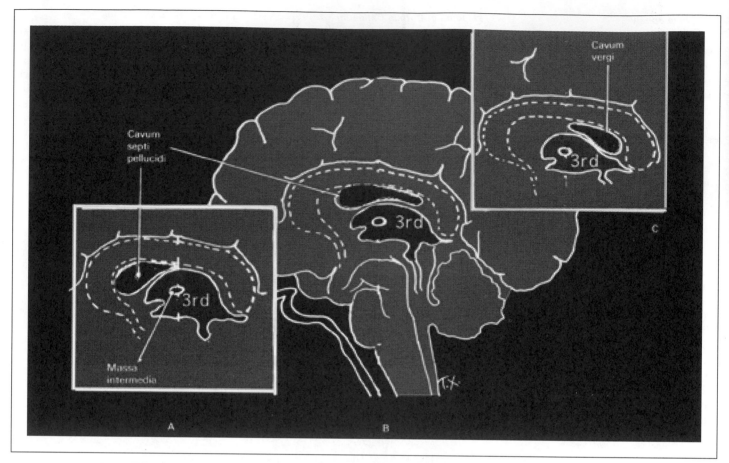

FIGURE 50-32. Cavum septi pellucidi. If the scanning angle is incorrect, this normal variant may be mistaken for a dilated ventricle. It may appear in one of three different patterns: Cavum septi pellucidi (**A**), cavum septi pellucidi and cavum vergae (**B**), and cavum vergae (**C**).

2. *Cavum septi pellucidi.* A midline sonolucent space inferior to the corpus callosum is termed the cavum septi pellucidi (Fig. 50-32A and B). In the midline sagittal view a very prominent cavum septi pellucidi may be present, and if the positioning is incorrect, it may be mistaken for a dilated ventricle. The posterior segment of this midline cavity is termed the *cavum vergae.* Only the anterior portion may be visible (see Fig. 50-32B and C). All of these cavities are normal variants.

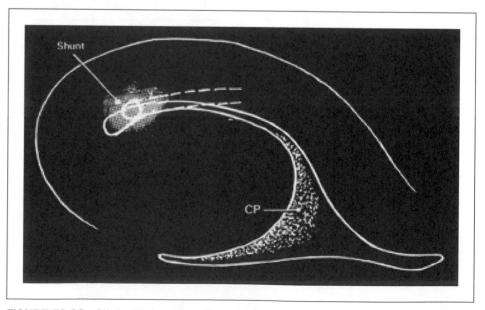

FIGURE 50-33. Clinical information is essential when scanning infants. In this lateral sagittal view, the bright echoes from a misplaced shunt could be mistaken for a hemorrhage. The wall of the ventricle collapsed around the shunt.

3. *Massa intermedia.* The massa intermedia appears as an echogenic mass in the center of the third ventricle (see Fig. 50-32).

4. *Shunts.* A shunt tube should not be mistaken for a bleed. These tubes often cause the ventricle to collapse around them (Fig. 50-33).

5. *Orientation.* Be sure that the orientation is correct to avoid confusion about which side has a bleed or is hydrocephalic. Wrong labeling will confuse follow-up studies and could have serious clinical consequences.

6. *Choroid plexus vs. bleed.* The choroid plexus may extend into the occipital horn, mimicking a bleed (Fig. 50-34). Placing the patient in the erect position may help by showing that the blood moves and forms a fluid-fluid level (Fig. 50-35), whereas the choroid plexus does not change.

7. *Choroid bleeds.* Choroid plexus bleeds may be overlooked. Compare both the choroid plexuses to see if they have the same echogenicity and outline. A lumpy outline suggests the presence of a bleed. The choroid plexus pulsates on real-time—blood clot will show no pulsation or evidence of flow on color flow or with Doppler.

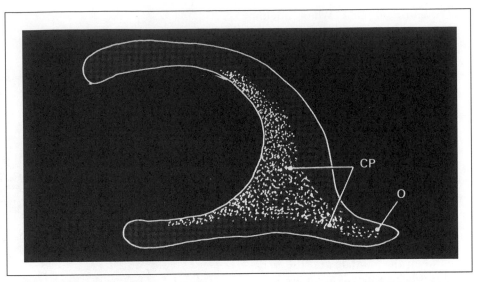

FIGURE 50-34. A variant choroid plexus may extend into the occipital horn, as seen in this lateral sagittal view.

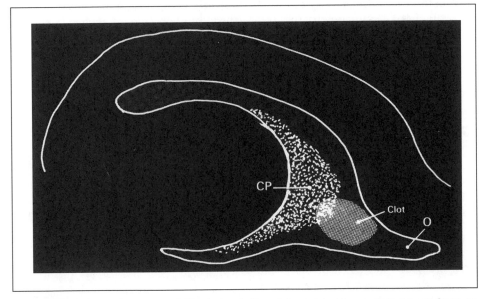

FIGURE 50-35. At times it is difficult to distinguish clot in the occipital horn from an extension of the choroid plexus, a rare variant. Positioning the patient's head erect helps to identify the clot, which will layer.

8. *Periventricular halo.* When angling in the parasagittal view posterior to the trigone of the lateral ventricles, an area of variable increased echogenicity can be seen. Do not mistake this normal echogenic area for periventricular leukomalacia (Fig. 50-36).

9. *Subependymal germinal matrix cysts.* Cysts seen within the germinal matrix develop at the site of a previous bleed. The cysts have echogenic walls and an echopenic center and bulge into the lateral ventricle.

10. *Caudothalamic notch vs. choroid plexus bleed.* The caudothalamic notch is normally a small, echogenic line between the caudate and the thalamus, whereas bleeds are more irregular in shape.

11. *Cerebellar bleeds.* Cerebellar bleeds may be overlooked because the cerebellum is normally densely echogenic. Look for asymmetry on coronal views.

12. *Missed subdurals due to low-frequency transducers.* If a low-frequency transducer is used with a poor near-field resolution, a subdural hematoma can be missed.

WHERE ELSE TO LOOK

1. *Arnold-Chiari malformation.* This condition is associated with spina bifida and myelomeningocele. In a neonate the spinal canal should be examined to make sure that no intraspinal mass is present and the cord does not extend too low.

2. *Possible hemorrhage.* If a possible, but not definite, hemorrhage is detected, follow-up studies should be performed.

3. *Vein of Galen aneurysm.* Look for increased heart size since there will be cardiac overload. Hydrops may develop (see Chapter 18).

4. *Subdural hematoma.* If fluid is noted in the interhemispheric fissure while scanning, switch to a very high frequency transducer to check the near field for subdural hematoma. An axial view may also help demonstrate this condition.

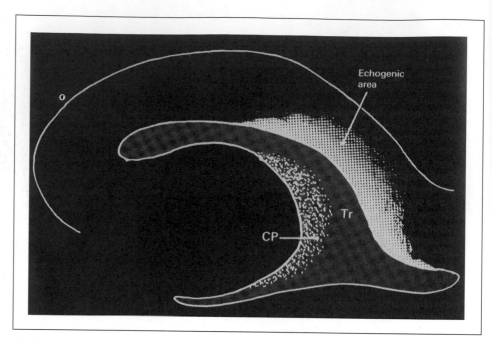

FIGURE 50-36. Sometimes there is an echogenic (bright) area behind the trigone of the lateral ventricle, as seen in this lateral sagittal view. This should not be mistaken for a bleed. Note the mild dilatation of the lateral ventricle.

SELECTED READING

Babcock, D. S. Sonography of the brain in infants: Role in evaluating neurologic abnormalities. *AJR* 165:417–423, 1995.

Naidich, T. P., et al. Hippocampal formation and related structures of the limbic lobe: Anatomic-MR correlation, Part 1. *Neuroradiology* 162:747–754, 1987.

Naidich, T. P., et al. Sonography of the internal capsule and basal ganglia in infants. *Pediatr Radiol* 161:615–621, 1986.

Naidich, T. P., Yousefzadeh, D. K., and Gusnard, D. A. Sonography of the normal neonatal head. *Neuroradiology* 28:408–427, 1986.

Siegel, M. J., and Herman, T. E. Congenital brain anomalies. *Ultrasound Quart* 13:1–24, 1995.

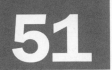

51

NEONATAL SPINE PROBLEMS

JOE ROTHGEB, ROGER C. SANDERS

KEY WORDS

Arachnoid Space. Fluid-filled space surrounding the cord and brain enclosed by a meningeal membrane called the arachnoid.

Cauda Equina. The nerve fibers arising from the terminal end of the spinal cord.

Cerebrospinal Fluid. Fluid that surrounds the spinal cord to cushion and protect it from rapid movement.

Conus Medullaris. The inferior (caudal) end of the cord that tapers to form a V shape.

Diastematomyelia. Condition in which the cord is split around an intraspinal bone fragment.

Filum Terminale. The distal tip of the spinal cord.

Lipoma. Deposit of fat that distorts the nerves in the spinal canal in the lower lumbar spine.

Myelomeningocele. Neural tube defect. A portion of the spinal cord and membranes protrude outside the spinal canal.

Pilonidal Sinus. Deep hair-containing tract in the skin that overlies the sacrum and coccyx.

Tethered Cord. Abnormal low position of the distal end of the spinal cord in the spinal canal. The cord normally ends around L2 or L3.

 THE CLINICAL PROBLEM

Since ossification of the lamina and spinous processes is incomplete at birth, a high-quality acoustic window to examine the spinal contents is available until about 1 year of age. Ultrasound is of value in the examination of a myelomeningocele to determine contents and in the detection of lipomas, cord tethering, and diastematomyelia. It is a cheaper and less threatening procedure than magnetic resonance imaging and does not require patient immobilization or sedation.

Spinal Cord

The spinal cord lies between the strong echoes of the vertebral body and the posterior elements. On sagittal views, three echogenic lines derived from the cord are seen within the normal spinal canal. Two lines represent the anterior and posterior surfaces of the cord. The middle line represents the central canal. On transverse scans, the cord is a round structure in the cervical region that is ovoid in shape as it enters the thoracic region (Fig. 51-1). Cerebrospinal fluid can be seen around the cord.

Cauda Equina

At the caudal end of the cord in the lumbar region, the cord becomes bulbous, and then tapers to the conus medullaris (see Fig. 51-1). Caudal to the conus medullaris and filling most of the arachnoid space are the nerve fibers (filaments) of the filum terminale. The nerve roots normally show movement and may pulsate.

◪ TECHNIQUE

1. A prone position with the legs flexed is preferable. A decubitus position may be useful since coronal views can be obtained.
2. A linear array of the highest frequency available (not less than 5 MHz, preferably 7 MHz or higher) should be employed.
3. If a dual function is available, obtain composite linear images. This is useful in demonstrating pathology in relation to normal structures.
4. To demonstrate superficial structures it may be helpful to place a stand-off pad between the skin and the transducer.
5. Know and label on screen the level of the spine that you are scanning. Either start at the vertebra with the lowest rib or the sacrococcygeal spine and count the ossification centers above or below.

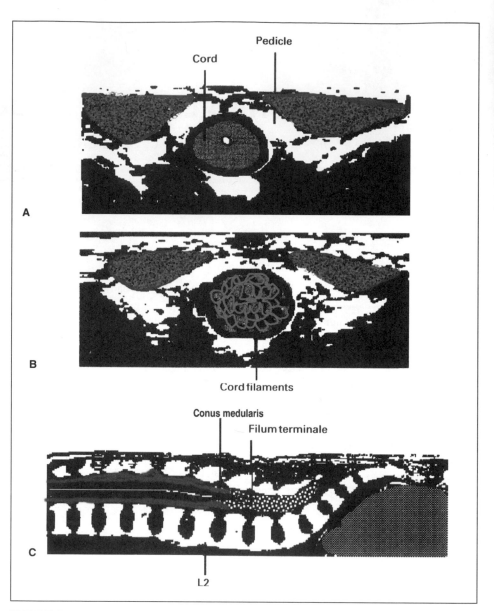

FIGURE 51-1. The spinal cord. (**A**) Transverse views of the normal cord in the thoracic region showing the spinal canal. (**B**) Transverse views of the normal cord at the level of the filum terminale. Note the small nerve fragments. (**C**) Longitudinal view of the cord showing that it ends at approximately L2.

◆ PATHOLOGY

Tethered Cord

In the normal newborn or infant, the cord ends at the level of L2. A tethered cord ends at L3 or lower (Fig. 51-2). The nerve roots in the cauda equina do not show movement or pulsations as are seen in the normal cord.

Spinal Lipoma

A deposit of fat that is connected to the pia mater or to the spinal cord is called a lipoma (see Fig. 51-2). (The pia mater is the innermost of the meninges.) Lipomas are more echogenic than the normal intraspinal tissue. Tethering of the cord or spina bifida may have associated skin findings. Spinal lipomas are suspected if a tuft of hair or a dimple is seen on the lower back, and are associated with bladder and leg dysfunction.

Diastematomyelia

Diastematomyelia is a rare condition in which the cord is split (Fig. 51-3). Two cords with spinal canals are visible on either side of a bony spur. There are abnormal vertebrae below the level of the bony spur. Transverse and coronal views show this condition best.

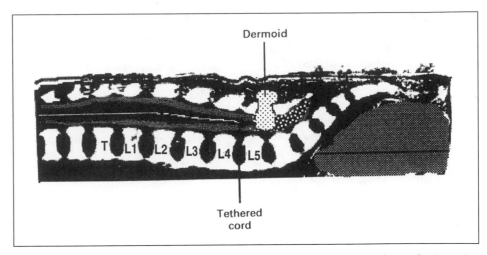

FIGURE 51-2. Sagittal view showing a lipoma. Note that the cord terminates at a much lower position than usual because it is tethered. Normal termination is at L1 to L2. In this instance, the cord terminates at L5.

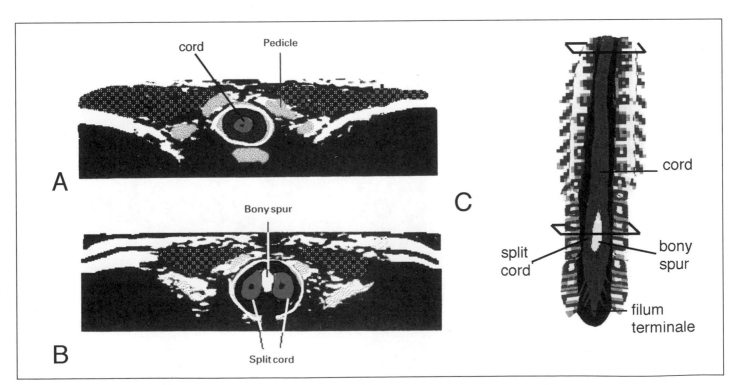

FIGURE 51-3. Transverse views of a normal cord (**A**) and of a cord with diastematomyelia (**B**). Note the bony fragment separating the two cords. Sagittal view (**C**) showing abnormalities of the vertebral bodies below the bone and splitting of the cord at the level of the bony spur.

Myelomeningocele

An ultrasound examination of spina bifida with a myelomeningocele may show neural tissue within a fluid-filled sac. The more nerves that are present the worse the prognosis.

Pilonidal Sinus

A dimple associated with a hairy area in the skin that overlies the sacrum and coccyx is known as a pilonidal sinus. The dimple and hair may indicate cord tethering.

PITFALLS

1. Lipomas may inhibit visualization of the conus medullaris. A diagnosis of tethering can then be difficult.
2. Patients with scoliosis may be difficult or even impossible to examine.
3. Do not mistake hemivertebra for diastematomyelia. Below the level of the bony spur, the vertebrae are disorganized, but there will be no splitting of the cord with hemivertebra.

SELECTED READING

Filippigh, P., Clapuyt, P., Debauche, C., and Claus, D. Sonographic evaluation of traumatic spinal cord lesions in the newborn infant. *Pediatr Radiol* 24:245–247, 1994.

Korsvik, H. E., and Keller, M. S. Sonography of occult dysraphism in neonates and infants with MR imaging correlation. *Radiographics* 12:297–306, 1992.

Naidich, T. P., et al. Sonography of the caudal spine and back: Congenital anomalies in children. *AJR* 142:1229–1242, 1984.

Raghavendra, B. N., et al. The tethered spinal cord: Diagnosis by high-resolution realtime ultrasound. *Radiology* 149:123–128, 1983.

Schumacher, R., Kroll, B., Schwarz, M., and Ermert, J. A. M-mode sonography of the caudal spinal cord in patients with meningomyelocele. *Radiology* 184:263–265, 1992.

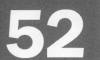

ULTRASOUND-GUIDED TECHNIQUES

NANCY SMITH MINER, DAN MINER

KEY WORDS

Coaxial Catheters. Two or more catheters nested within one another.

Cordocentesis. Puncture of the umbilical cord.

CVS. Chorionic villi sampling. Placental tissue is analyzed for the fetal karyotype. A needle is put into the region of the placenta closest to the amniotic fluid, and a portion of the placenta is sucked into a tube.

Dermatotomy. Skin incision.

French. Measure of catheter size.

Hysteroscope. A small tube with a mirror is inserted into the cervix, so the interior of the endometrial cavity can be viewed and samples can be obtained.

Indigo Carmine. A harmless dye which is inserted into the amniotic fluid when there is a possibility of twins.

Laminectomy. Surgical removal of the posterior arch of a vertebra.

Lecithin/Sphingomyelin Ratio (L/S). Surfactants present in the amniotic fluid which are used as biochemical markers to determine fetal lung maturity.

Myelotomy. Surgical incision of the spinal cord.

Needle Stop. A small clamp that screws onto any gauge needle; it prevents the needle from being inserted past the predetermined depth.

Percutaneous Umbilical Blood Sample (PUBS, Cordocentesis). A small needle is placed in the umbilical artery and fetal blood is aspirated.

Pigtail Catheter. A catheter with a circular shape at one end. It tends to remain within a cavity. The side holes are placed within the curved region that is known as the pigtail.

Syrinx. A fluid collection in the center of the spinal canal.

Tandem. A tube containing radioactive material that is put within the endometrium.

Trocar. Central insert placed within a tubular needle to give it a point. When it is withdrawn, tissue or fluid can be aspirated.

Vacutainer Tube. Tube that is used for drawing blood. Built-in suction within the tube pulls the blood out at a more rapid rate.

Ultrasound is now used to guide a variety of invasive procedures that previously relied on fluoroscopic localization or experienced guesswork. Ultrasonic localization should take place immediately before fluid aspiration or biopsy.

APPROACHES TO PUNCTURE PROCEDURES

Localization Without Guidance

If the lesion is large and close to the skin, localization is performed with ultrasound but no guidance is necessary (Fig. 52-1).

The Right-Angle Approach

If the lesion is located in the liver (Fig. 52-2) or if the needle is entering in a space that has an accessible acoustic window at a 60- to 90-degree angle, the following technique is best.

1. Choose a needle insertion site where the lesion can be seen well and where the course of the needle is safe. Try, for instance, to avoid a path where you must angle around bowel or the gallbladder.
2. Place the transducer at a nonsterile location where the lesion and needle track can be viewed and that is at approximately right angles to the needle insertion angle. The procedure is usually performed with a curved linear transducer so the angle of the transducer beam to the needle can be readily seen. The transducer should be turned so that the beam is in the same plane as the needle. It is critical to follow subtle angulation changes in the needle position with the transducer; aligning the two is essential for successful needle visualization.
3. Prior to inserting the needle, press with your finger on the skin at the approximate needle insertion site to help show where the needle is about to enter the image. The finger movement can be seen.
4. Localize the lesion in two planes.
5. Provide continuous guidance during the procedure.

Providing the needle location and axis are successfully followed by the sonographer (and this requires skill, experience, and communication between the sonologist and sonographer), even 22-gauge needles can be clearly seen.

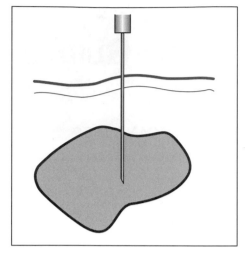

FIGURE 52-1. A large mass that is close to the skin does not require ultrasonic guidance. A site is marked on the skin over the area in front of the collection.

It is of particular importance when using a 22-gauge needle to align the bevel and the scan plane to avoid having the needle bend out of the field of view. Needles with centimeter calibrations on them can be very helpful in determining how far the needle has been inserted.

Freehand at an Oblique Axis to the Needle

The needle can be placed alongside the transducer at an oblique axis to the ultrasound beam (Fig. 52-3). The needle will generally be guided by the physician, who holds both needle and transducer. The transducer is placed within a sterile plastic bag that has some gel within it. Use a sterile rubber band or pipe cleaner to tighten the plastic bag neck around the transducer. Sterile tube gauze can be placed around the cable to keep the sterile field intact.

This technique is used when the lesion is quite large and superficial; access is limited, and some guidance is required. Recognizing the needle path requires skill, since the echoes from the needle are subtle and only the tip is easily seen. The needle cannot be seen near the skin. An up-and-down motion with the needle on insertion and removal of the trocar help with visualization.

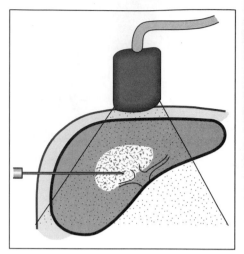

FIGURE 52-2. The right-angle technique is used predominantly in the liver and in obstetrics. The transducer is placed on the anterior or lateral aspect of the liver. The needle insertion site is found by pushing on the skin and watching the image closely. The needle is then placed at approximately right angles to the ultrasonic beam into the mass. Excellent visualization is obtained.

Using a Biopsy Attachment

Biopsy attachments are occasionally helpful when the ultrasonic access is limited and the target is small (see Fig. 52-3). Biopsy attachments are available for most transducers. The needle is inserted through a guide so the needle enters the image and the body at a preset oblique axis, shown on the monitor as a dotted line or template. The transducer axis can be changed so that the target lies in the middle of the dotted line. The needle is often not easy to see unless it is large (18 gauge or larger) because the needle is almost on the same axis as the sound beam. Needle tip visualization is improved by using a needle that has a roughened tip to make it more echogenic. A proprietary color Doppler signal passed along the needle can also enhance needle visualization.

The sonographer must be adept at recognizing subtle tissue movement as the needle enters the tissues. The needle will enter the image obliquely and may not follow the expected template route. Thin needles tend to bend out of the plane as they meet tissues of different consistency.

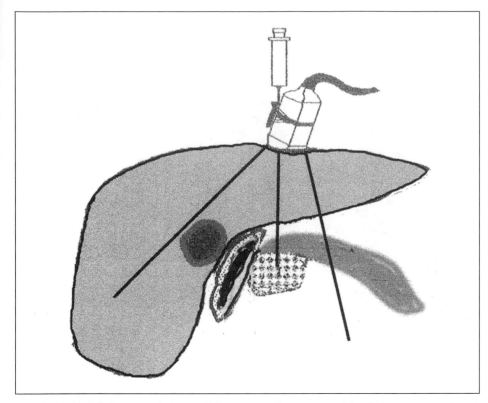

FIGURE 52-3. Oblique technique. This pancreatic mass could only be punctured with a needle alongside the transducer because the area around it was obscured by gas. It is difficult to see the needle with this oblique approach, but it can be used if the access is limited. A biopsy guide is helpful with this approach.

3. Watch the patient's respiration. Scanning and locating the site during quiet breathing is best. Respiration should be suspended when the needle is inserted. The needle may move greatly, especially in the kidney, when the patient breathes.
4. The puncture site must be marked in such a way that the mark will not be scrubbed away when the patient's skin is cleaned. A simple but effective method is to imprint the skin by pressing on it with a localizer. Among the many possible "scientific puncture site localizers" that are used are retracted ballpoint pens, plastic needle caps, and caps from a Magic Marker. Anything that is not too sharp to cause the patient discomfort will do. Press on the skin just before the skin is cleansed, and a small red circle will remain.
5. Once the lesion has been found and the puncture site has been marked, leave an image on the screen with the calipers demonstrating the depth of the lesion. This can serve as a reference during the set-up for the procedure, enabling the physician to review the depth and approximate angle.

Remove Gel

The gel that has been used in performing the scan must be thoroughly removed or the iodine-prepping solution will bead up and roll off. Alcohol is usually sufficient to remove gel.

Document the Puncture Site

Make sure that the actual puncture site has been photographed and is part of the patient's record. No matter how carefully a procedure is carried out, tissue or fluid is not always obtained, and documentation of an appropriate approach is therefore important. For example, an apparent collection may in fact be an organized hematoma, and nothing can be aspirated even though the needle is correctly placed. If a procedure using a biopsy guide allows visualization of the needle placement, this also should be documented.

PRACTICAL STEPS

Obtain Consent Forms

Punctures of any kind carry potential risks, and a full explanation of the risks and benefits of the procedure is given to the patient. The alternative diagnostic and therapeutic maneuvers that are available must be discussed. The patient must then sign a consent form prior to the puncture. Consent forms are obtained by the physician performing the procedure, but such matters can be overlooked in any busy laboratory; the sonographer should therefore double-check that the form has been signed. The sonographer usually acts as a witness to the consent.

Find the Puncture Site

Demonstrate the following:

1. Where the mass or collection is
2. How deep it is
3. What lies between the patient's skin and the mass, such as bowel or vessels

Determine the Optimum Needle Depth

1. *Make sure that the patient is comfortable.* This is important because the patient must lie still for about half an hour during the procedure. However, the position should give the physician easy access to the target, preferably in a vertical axis without the need to angle the needle. Stabilize the patient with sponges or pillows if necessary.
2. Move the patient so that as few structures as possible lie in the path of the needle. Piercing the liver or bowel is undesirable if it can be avoided by a change in the angulation of the patient or the approach.

PUNCTURE EQUIPMENT

The following sterile supplies should either be available as a basic tray or assembled before a procedure (Fig. 52-4). Prepackaged kits for specific examinations are readily available and should include the following:

Sterile drapes (one with a hole for access to the puncture site)

Two containers (for antiseptic solutions)

Glass tubes (for collecting specimens)

5-mL syringe, and 25- and 22-gauge needles (for local anesthetic)

Cleansing sponges

To be added:

Needle of choice; should have roughened tip

20-cc and 2-cc syringe for amniocentesis

Syringe of choice (depends on the size of the collection)

Extension tubing (desirable for targets that move with respiration, for example, kidney)

Sterile ruler (to measure the correct depth on the needle)

Needle stop (to screw on the needle at the correct depth)

Local anesthetic (usually lidocaine; may be 1 percent or 2 percent)

Alcohol wipes (for cleaning off the rubber stopper on any bottles, such as lidocaine, radiographic contrast media, anaerobic culture bottles)

Sterile gloves

Biopsy guide attachment for transducer if necessary

Sterile plastic bag to cover the transducer, with sterile rubber bands or sterile pipe cleaner to secure bag in place

#11 scalpel blade (to perform dermatotomy)

Syringe aspiration handle (useful for increasing suction in biopsies)

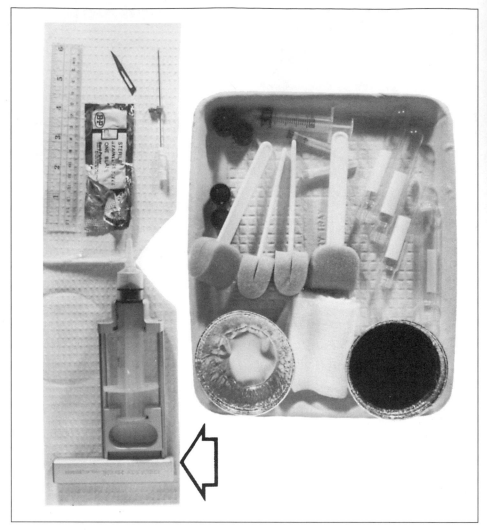

FIGURE 52-4. Supplies needed for a basic tray for a sterile procedure include containers for iodine and alcohol; prep sponges; a 5-mL syringe; 22-, and 25-gauge needles for drawing up local anesthetic; glass culture tubes; some 3 by 4 gauze pads; and sterile drapes (at least one fenestrated). A sterile ruler, a scalpel blade, and the appropriate needle and sterile needle stop must be added. The arrow points to an aspiration device that can be attached to a 20-mL syringe to help apply more negative pressure during biopsies.

OBSTETRIC PUNCTURE PROCEDURES

Prenatal Chromosomal Analysis

Needles are most commonly placed within the uterus during pregnancy to obtain material for chromosomal analysis. The technique used depends on the stage of pregnancy. In the first trimester, chorionic villi material is obtained by chorionic villi sampling. In the early second trimester, amniocentesis is the usual technique. Later in the second trimester, percutaneous umbilical blood sampling may be required because it gives the speediest result.

Amniocentesis is also performed in the third trimester to evaluate the lecithin/sphingomyelin (L/S) ratio for fetal lung maturity; this information is valuable if the obstetrician is thinking of inducing labor or considering a procedure that may precipitate labor.

Chorionic Villi Sampling (CVS)

Chromosomal material can be obtained in the first trimester by taking a sample from the placental implantation site. Most commonly, a catheter is inserted through the cervix and is guided under ultrasound to the thickest portion of the gestational sac; a portion of the chorion is aspirated. If the gestational sac is at an inaccessible site—for example, in an acutely anteverted or retroverted uterus—a needle can be placed into the uterus through the abdominal wall. This route is less likely to introduce infection than the vaginal route, but it may be more painful. Chorionic villi sampling gives material that allows chromosomal growth in 2 days at a very early stage of pregnancy, however, (1) it is statistically slightly more hazardous than amniocentesis; (2) alpha-fetoprotein amniotic fluid analysis cannot be performed; and (3) maternal cells may occasionally be confused with fetal cells. Occasionally, persistent amniotic fluid leakage may occur. CVS is a technique that requires a skilled operator, and is best performed at a site where a perinatologist is available.

In addition to the early and quick availability of chromosomal information with CVS, it is also possible to take the tissue and extract DNA to test for certain specific diagnoses, such as cystic fibrosis and sickle cell anemia.

Amniocentesis

Amniocentesis for chromosomal analysis is usually performed between 15 and 18 weeks. It is safe, with a less than 0.5 percent abortion rate; cell growth occurs within 6 to 17 days. Alpha-fetoprotein can be measured in the amniotic fluid. Second trimester amniocentesis is generally performed to rule out congenital defects at a stage early enough to give the parents the option of termination if a fetal anomaly is found. Some centers are providing that information even sooner with amniocentesis done as early as 12 weeks, but this procedure remains controversial.

In the third trimester amniocentesis is performed to obtain an L/S ratio to see whether the fetal lungs are mature. There is relative oligohydramnios in the third trimester, and the procedure can be more difficult to perform.

Percutaneous Umbilical Blood Sampling (PUBS or Cordocentesis)

Percutaneous umbilical blood sampling is performed later in pregnancy when a rapid chromosomal analysis is required. A needle is inserted into the cord at either the placental or, less often, the fetal end of the cord. Cordocentesis is done either when the pregnancy is close to the abortion limit or when the fetus may be viable, but has an anomaly that raises the question of a chromosomal abnormality. It is the most hazardous of the three techniques, although the exact abortion rate is as yet unknown. It is still surprisingly safe.

Amniocentesis Technique

When amniocentesis is performed in the second trimester, the site is easily localized. There are several important points to be remembered when choosing a site:

1. *Avoid the placenta.* This may be impossible if the placenta covers the entire anterior surface of the uterus (Fig. 52-5); then it is still possible to take a needle path through the placenta unless Rh incompatibility has been diagnosed. Penetrating the placenta will aggravate the basic condition in these cases.

2. *Avoid the fetus.* The chances of striking the fetus are slim; however, do not choose a puncture site with a fetus in the field of view. Monitor continuously during the procedure.

3. *Avoid the umbilical cord.* The cord can easily be seen floating in the fluid (see Fig. 52-5). If the puncture has to be performed through the placenta, be sure to avoid the site of the cord entrance.

4. *Avoid a site that is too lateral.* The uterine arteries run along the lateral walls of the uterus. Fortunately, these arteries are generally visible on the sonogram as large sonolucent areas (see Fig. 52-5). Color Doppler will help identify them if there is confusion.

5. *Document the site.* The site should be recorded on film using calipers to show the correct depth.

6. *Speed of needle insertion.* The needle should be inserted quickly, particularly in second trimester amniocenteses, to avoid tenting of the amniotic membrane.

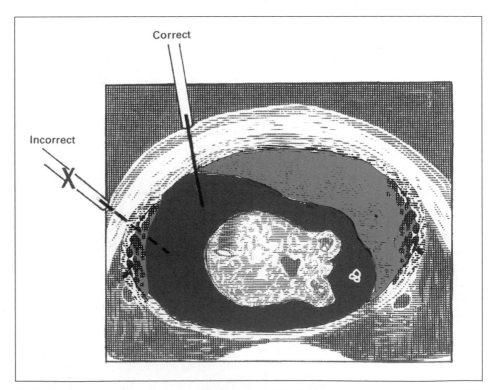

FIGURE 52-5. Transverse section through a pregnant uterus. A small area of amniotic fluid is present. The correct angle for obtaining fluid from this site is shown. Avoid the large vascular sinuses that would be punctured if a lateral approach were used.

Amniocentesis Equipment

A 3-mL syringe is used to take off the first few milliliters of fluid collected so that any maternal blood is cleared from the main sample. Either a 20- or 22-gauge needle is used for amniocentesis; those with a roughened tip can be seen in fluid with a 3.5- to 5-MHz transducer. Prepackaged amniocentesis sets are available.

Opaque tubes are necessary to keep light from reaching fluid samples and breaking down the bilirubin pigments if an Rh problem is being investigated.

Amniocentesis Guidance

Regardless of your choice of technical approach, it is important to monitor the procedure continuously on real-time during amniocentesis.

FREEHAND TECHNIQUE. With a freehand technique the operator guides the needle with one hand and holds the transducer, which has been covered with a sterile bag, with the other. Insertion at a 45-degree angle allows good needle visualization.

RIGHT-ANGLE TECHNIQUE. The right-angle technique, in which a second individual holds the transducer at a right angle to the needle, is very effective. Needle visualization is optimal with this approach. Since the transducer is used from a site outside the sterile field, a sterile bag does not have to be placed over the transducer.

USE OF A BIOPSY GUIDE. The use of a biopsy guide attached to the transducer may be helpful if the amniotic fluid volume is very limited and avoiding the fetus is tricky.

Third Trimester Problems

If it is difficult to find a big enough fluid pocket in the third trimester, turning the patient to an oblique position allows a small pool to form. If no pocket is available, the physician can push the fetal head out of the pelvis, creating a small pocket of fluid not previously seen.

Twins

When performing an amniocentesis on twins, take care to avoid tapping the same amniotic sac twice (see Fig. 17-1). Find the amniotic sac membrane and choose puncture sites on either side of the membrane. Perform the first amniocentesis and leave the needle in place, injecting a small amount of indigo carmine dye through it to color the fluid in that sac only.

Perform the second amniocentesis at a site localized on the other side of the membrane. The fluid should be a clear, yellow color. If there is any question as to whether the dye has crossed the intra-amniotic membrane, more fluid can be aspirated out of the initial needle site to compare the color of the fluid from the two different sacs.

Check Fetal Heart Motion

Before amniocentesis, check for fetal heart motion. If fetal death is found, it will not be attributed to the amniocentesis and potential legal problems can be avoided. After amniocentesis, check and document the fetal heart motion again. It is reassuring for the parents to see that the fetal heart is beating after the procedure is finished and provides legal confirmation that the fetus is viable.

Chorionic Villi Sampling Technique

Two methods of performing chorionic villi sampling are currently used. In the most popular technique, the transducer views the catheter insertion through a transvesical approach (Fig. 52-6). The catheter is followed as it is placed through the vagina and cervix. A sample of the villi is obtained from the thickest portion of the gestational sac. Ultrasound delineates the precise location of the catheter and monitors fetal heart rate. Small bleeds are not uncommon at the time of the chorionic villi sampling.

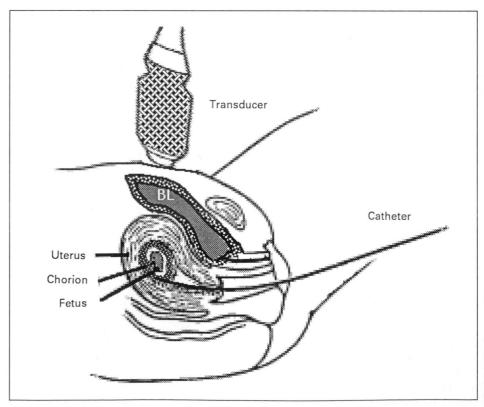

FIGURE 52-6. Chorionic villi sampling. The transducer is placed on the abdomen and views the gestational sac through the bladder. The catheter is inserted through the cervix and samples the thickest portion of the gestational sac border.

The transabdominal approach is much the same, except that the needle is placed obliquely to the transducer and enters through the abdominal wall. The transabdominal approach is similar to the technique for ovum aspiration (see Fig. 7-23). A full bladder is required, and the needle is inserted just above the bladder and placed within the gestational sac. The needle can be monitored as it proceeds through the abdominal contents by viewing it through the bladder.

Percutaneous Umbilical Blood Sampling Technique

Percutaneous umbilical blood sampling requires careful cooperation between sonographer and physician (Fig. 52-7). The cord insertion into the placenta is localized. Ideally the insertion site is anterior, but if it is posterior or lateral the procedure can still be performed. The sonographer places the transducer at right angles to the needle insertion site. The needle is carefully followed as it moves toward the umbilical artery and vein. The fetal heart is monitored at intervals to ensure that no damage has occurred.

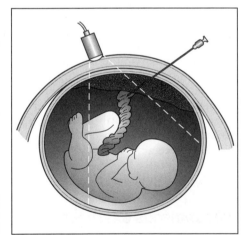

FIGURE 52-7. Percutaneous umbilical vein sampling (PUBS; cordocentesis). With the transducer in an oblique axis, the needle is inserted into the cord at the site where it leaves the placenta. The placenta in the image shown is in the optimal position. It is much more difficult to perform this procedure when the placenta is posteriorly located.

Potential Complications

Possible complications of amniocentesis, CVS, and percutaneous umbilical blood sampling include the following:

1. Premature labor
2. Vaginal fluid leakage
3. Onset of infection after a delay
4. Intrauterine bleeding
5. Cord laceration
6. Fetal damage

FLUID COLLECTION, ASPIRATION, AND DRAINAGE

Ultrasound can be used to guide cyst puncture, tapping of ascites, and fluid pocket drainage. Mark a site, preferably below the ribs, as close to the fluid pocket as possible. Then choose one of the guidance techniques described earlier to aid in obtaining fluid (see Figs. 52-1 to 52-3). Fluid is normally sent for culture and cytology. Biochemical analysis to determine whether the fluid is lymph or urine may be helpful.

If the fluid is being removed for therapeutic as opposed to diagnostic purposes, it may be desirable to leave a catheter in place. A small pigtail catheter mounted on a needle is available and is helpful when there is massive ascites or if it is desirable to drain a cyst to completion.

MASS BIOPSY

The techniques described at the beginning of this chapter are also appropriate for ultrasound guidance of mass biopsies. The freehand approach should be reserved for large or very superficial masses, such as in the thyroid.

There are two basic ways of obtaining pathologic material: thin needle aspiration and core biopsy. Both have similar set-ups. Aspiration biopsies, used for masses in the pancreas and liver, where leakage or bleeding is a concern, are done with 20- or 22-gauge needles. The length is determined by the depth of the lesion. Only a small specimen is obtained by using a syringe to suck material back into the needle. The cells are either flushed through the needle into cytology solution or immediately smeared on a slide for cytologic analysis. Ideally, a cytologist is on hand in the room to provide feedback on whether the sample contains diagnostic material.

For routine renal or liver biopsies that are performed for diffuse organ diseases, or for masses in less vascular areas, core biopsy is performed. This is most commonly done using a single-use core biopsy gun. There are a wide variety of single-use guns available, ranging in size from 14 to 22 gauge. These devices consist of a notched needle within an outer sheath which is mounted within the "gun," a spring-loaded device which allows rapid controlled passage of a needle into tissue, usually 1.8 to 2.3 cm. This minimizes bleeding and discomfort as it obtains a core of tissue. The core is sent off to the pathology lab in a formalin solution.

As with all invasive procedures, prior informed consent is necessary and premedication is helpful. Prothrombin time, partial thromboplastin time, and platelet count are generally obtained for renal and liver biopsies and when there is a history of bleeding diathesis. Although the actual biopsy takes only a few minutes, the procedure can feel quite lengthy to the patient. Make sure the patient is going to be comfortable, especially if he or she has been obliqued for the procedure. Deciding on a site, even if a small lesion has been defined by a prior computed tomography scan, can take some time. In many cases, the site can only be localized at one particular phase of respiration, so it is a good idea to practice a few times with the patient before cleansing the skin and localizing the site with ultrasound.

ABSCESS DRAINAGE

Drainage of an abscess involves the insertion of a large catheter, which is required because the infected fluid is often very thick. The procedure is painful, and premedication is given. Because the procedure can be hazardous, vital signs are obtained at appropriate intervals. The main difference from the other puncture techniques described here is that different catheters are required. Abscess drainage is best performed with an ultrasound system in the fluoroscopy suite so that guide wire and catheter placement can be visualized fluoroscopically.

One of two systems is commonly employed to access an abscess cavity. The first is a 21-gauge needle on which are mounted two coaxial catheters: a 4 French which is tapered to the needle and a 6 French mounted on the 4 French. This system can be introduced into the collection in one pass (after a small dermatotomy), or by using an 0.18-inch guide wire through the needle to allow exchange for the two coaxial catheters. Once the 6 French catheter is in the collection, the 4 French catheter and 0.18-inch wire are removed and replaced with a 0.38-inch wire, over which can then be passed a succession of dilators, enlarging the tract to the desired size. (The 0.18-inch wire is too flimsy to allow an exchange of dilators.) The second system is simpler. A thin-walled 18-gauge long needle is passed into the abscess, allowing immediate placement of a large (0.38-inch) exchange guide wire.

Systems commonly used for abscess drainage are (1) a Cope-type self-retaining pigtail catheter set; and (2) a straight or curved catheter with many side holes. The first pus aspirated is sent for culture. Platelet count and prothrombin time should be known before the procedure is done.

BILIARY DUCT DRAINAGE AND PERCUTANEOUS NEPHROSTOMY

Ultrasound plays a limited role in percutaneous nephrostomy and biliary duct drainage, but is particularly useful to guide left hepatic duct puncture as fluoroscopic guidance often results in significant dose to the operator's hands. It is mainly used to localize the site and establish the depth for the initial puncture. Because the catheter is often left in for a very long period of time, full sterile precautions including masks, gowns, and caps must be maintained.

These procedures are potentially hazardous and painful, and premedication is given. The procedure should be explained to the patient, and a consent form should be obtained in advance of the premedication. Again, one should monitor for evidence of bleeding by watching the patient's pulse and blood pressure.

BREAST INTERVENTION
Cysts

Cyst aspiration is a common procedure performed by sonologists under ultrasound guidance or, if palpable, by the clinician in the office. Small cysts can be difficult to puncture because of the extreme mobility of the breast. Often the operator will hold the transducer in one hand and the needle in the other. Sometimes assistance from the sonographer is needed to immobilize the breast for puncture.

The challenge for the sonographer is to include the needle, the mass, and the predicted needle path in the same longitudinal plane. The choice of skin site for initial needle insertion should be based on the following:

1. The nipple and the retroareola area should be avoided.
2. A superior-to-inferior approach should be used.
3. The site should be approximately 3 cm from the lesion.

The technique is similar to that used for cyst puncture, described earlier in this chapter.

The use of a vacutainer tube allows one-handed aspiration. Simple cyst aspiration is often done to alleviate symptoms and the fluid is discarded. Rarely fluid will be sent for cytology but only from complex cysts. Sterile prep is used, but local anesthesia is usually not necessary.

Core Biopsy

Unlike core biopsy of other organs, imaging-guided core biopsy of the breast usually requires at least 5 passes with a large-bore (14 gauge) biopsy needle mounted in a gun, either as a one-use device or as a reusable one. Stereotactic mammographic (radiographic) core biopsy has become extremely widespread in the last 5 years. With improved sonography and increasing interest in distinguishing benign from malignant sonographic characteristics of breast masses, there has also been a significant increase in ultrasound-guided, large-gauge core biopsy. Using large-bore needles does increase the risk of hematoma, but the risk is still small (0.5 percent). The use of local anesthesia is mandatory, however, and 2 percent lidocaine with epinephrine is used to deter bleeding.

One helpful device now used is a 13-gauge metallic sheath with cutting stylet. Prior to sterile prep, the lesion is scanned, and a skin site for puncture is picked. A site is chosen about 5 cm from the mass so a more shallow approach can be used. This facilitates visualization, is safer, and keeps the sheath stable. The skin is then prepped and infiltrated with 1 percent lidocaine. A small nick is made using the 13-gauge sheath stylet or a scalpel, and a 20-gauge spinal needle is passed along the anticipated tract to the lesion. Two percent lidocaine with epinephrine is then injected around the lesion (under ultrasound visualization) and the needle is withdrawn as the tract is infiltrated with anesthetic. The sheath is then introduced along the same tract just to the front edge of the lesion. This sheath then serves as a conduit through which passes the 14-gauge needle mounted in the biopsy gun, enabling multiple passes without traversing the entire path of breast tissue each time. Specimens are sent in formalin for analysis.

Yet another refinement in biopsy technology now available is called a mammotomy device. This consists of a 14-gauge needle with a window cut into the side. Within this a rotating blade is advanced, cutting a small specimen off and storing it inside the needle. Multiple samples can thus be obtained rapidly and very accurately by directing the window toward the lesion. This is performed under stereotactic or sonographic guidance. Although this is primarily a sampling device similar to core biopsy, there is some evidence to suggest that it may be able to remove the entire lesion in some cases, thus replacing lumpectomy.

PERCUTANEOUS GASTROSTOMY

Gastrostomy and gastrojejunostomy tubes are often placed percutaneously using fluoroscopic guidance to facilitate guide wire and catheter exchange. However, ultrasound imagery prior to the procedure is extremely useful to document the edge of the left lobe of the liver and to help choose an appropriate skin site for puncture.

VASCULAR ACCESS

Ultrasound guidance helps obtain difficult or unusual vascular access by employing duplex and color flow visualization of the vessel. The popliteal artery or vein can be accessed using this technique. Access of the popliteal artery can allow angioplasty of femoral artery stenoses that are not accessible by conventional groin puncture. Extensive deep vein thrombosis has been successfully thrombolysed using directed puncture of the popliteal vein. Central venous access (subclavian or internal jugular veins) can be expedited using ultrasound guidance. In these procedures, the sonographer finds the vessel and helps guide access by showing the best needle insertion site, the vessel depth, and appropriate angle. The needle is tracked with ultrasound as it is placed in the vessel.

INTRAOPERATIVE ULTRASOUND

Intraoperative ultrasound can help surgeons by showing masses or calculi within organs. By using high-resolution transducers directly on the surface of an organ, ultrasound can provide information not available preoperatively. Small lesions in the liver or brain can be pinpointed. This can change the surgical approach and shorten operating time.

Several dedicated OR units have been developed, but standard high-resolution equipment and probes are usable. Some transducers can be gas-sterilized (check with the manufacturer); all can be covered with sterile bags. A double-bagging routine is recommended, using sterile gel as a coupling agent between the bags. The transducer cable should also be covered, because it will inevitably lie in the sterile field. The body cavity being scanned is usually filled with saline as a further coupling aid. Generally, an initial scan is done as soon as the area of concern is exposed and before much tissue dissection has taken place. Guidance is performed as needed during surgery, then a final scan at the end of the procedure reassures the surgeon that the margin of the resection is tumor-free, the cysts are completely drained, or that all the stones have been retrieved.

Renal Surgery

In cases where renal calculi—usually staghorn—cannot be removed by means of lithotripsy or percutaneous stone extraction, intraoperative ultrasound can easily localize remaining stones, regardless of their composition. This is especially useful when the stone is surrounded by soft blood clot; the clot hinders the surgeons' ability to feel the stone but does not interfere with the ultrasound beam. A Keith needle is inserted under ultrasound guidance until it touches the stone.

More often, ultrasound is used during partial nephrectomy to localize and define the extent of renal neoplasms. If there is uncertainty from preoperative tests about whether a nephron-sparing approach is appropriate, intraoperative ultrasound can determine a tumors' relationship to the hilar structures and the capsule, and find accessory lesions. Adjacent structures can be evaluated, such as the vena cava, adrenal gland, or liver, for possible tumor extension. Ultrasound is also used for open renal biopsies and the unroofing and evaluation of renal cysts.

A transducer with multiple frequencies is optimal; a 7.5 MHz is generally used, but 10 or 5 MHz may be necessary during the procedure, and it would be time-consuming and expensive to prepare three transducers. Duplex Doppler helps to assess tumors for vascularity, differentiates renal veins and arteries from dilated collecting systems, and detects tumor spread in venous structures. If regional hypothermia is used, it is especially important to get a thorough scan before clamping the renal vessels to minimize ischemia time.

Neurosurgery

Initial intraoperative scanning of the brain takes place through a burr hole, while the dura is still intact. A multiple-frequency transducer is again preferred because the pathology may be superficial or deep-seated; a 7.5 MHz is the best compromise. A dedicated unit is not essential, but the probe should have a small foot print to enable maneuverability in the small surface available. Color Doppler is very helpful when lesions are isoechoic, particularly vascular lesions such as arteriovenous malformations or hemangioblastomas, which may show up only with color flow.

Intraoperative scanning of the spine takes place through a saline-filled cavity, after the initial laminectomy and before the dura is opened (Fig. 52-8). Well seen are the spinal cord and central canal, the dorsal surface of the dural sac, the posterior portion of the spinal subarachnoid space, and the dentate ligaments. The water path technique allows some distance between the transducer and the cord, so near-field reverberations do not interfere with the image. Usually, some air bubbles and a layer of blood are present in the saline-filled cavity. A 7.5- or 10-MHz transducer is appropriate for this technique.

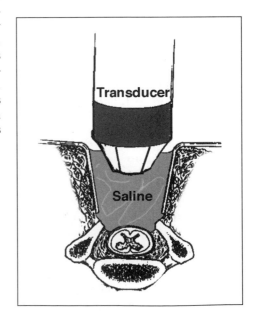

FIGURE 52-8. Intraoperative technique for examining the spine. After the spine has been exposed, saline fills the cavity and the probe is placed within the saline to view the spinal cord.

Cysts and tumors—both intramedullary and extramedullary, and intradural and extradural—and syringomyelia can be localized for resection, drainage, or biopsy. Because of the precision of the localization, the size of the myelotomy can be limited, and scans during and after the procedures verify the presence of any residual tumor or fluid collections. It is also possible to see developing intramedullary hematomas due to the surgery. Serial scans are especially important when draining fluid cavities in syringomyelia, because they may not be connected with each other and could require multiple drains.

Hepatobiliary and Pancreatic Surgery

In the abdomen, intraoperative ultrasound is used for a wide variety of procedures, from resecting tumors to localizing foreign bodies and stones. Needle and catheter placement is guided for biopsy, fluid aspiration, agent injection (e.g., alcohol into malignant tumors, chemotherapeutic drugs into arteries), and contrast media injection for radiographic studies. The biliary tree can be carefully evaluated for stones, polyps, and tumors, and decompressed under ultrasound guidance. While it is possible to use a needle-guide attachment, most needle placement is done using the freehand technique discussed earlier in this chapter.

There are flat linear-array transducers with a side-viewing capability that are optimal for obtaining good contact with the liver surface. A 7.5 MHz transducer is generally used, but ultrasound is most helpful here in demonstrating nonpalpable lesions, and a lower frequency may be needed to see them. Color Doppler is useful both for defining vascular structures and lesions, and for watching needle movement during guidance. A pencil-thin probe is preferred for biliary structures, and sometimes in the pancreas. The abdominal cavity is filled with saline, allowing the transducer to stand-off from the area of interest. Otherwise, a tiny bile duct may get lost in near-field artifact. Scan the pancreas directly on its exposed surface. If necessary, however, the pancreas can be scanned through the gastrocolic ligament, stomach, or liver.

Gynecologic Surgery

Intraoperative ultrasound decreases the risk of uterine perforation with hysteroscopic procedures such as myomectomy or endometrial adhesion resection; it is used in conjunction with the laparoscope to ensure that the resection is complete. Ultrasound has also been useful in fluid aspiration, stone and foreign body removal, and tandem radiotherapy placement. Intraoperative ultrasound may be used during uterine evacuation, both to avoid uterine perforation and to assure completion of the procedure when uterine anatomy is unusual.

Scanning is performed transabdominally, through a saline-filled bladder; a 3.5-MHz transducer is probably optimal because of the increased depth to the areas of interest. There is continuous monitoring with real-time during the procedure.

ULTRASOUND-GUIDED RADIATION TREATMENT

The outline of periaortic nodes or organs such as the prostate can be marked on the skin, prior to setting up radiotherapy ports, with ultrasound. This technique has been largely replaced with computed tomography scans which can be directly integrated into the data on the radiotherapy planning computer in a way that cannot be done with ultrasound. Since 1985, transperineal radioactive seed implantation using a template with ultrasound guidance has largely replaced open laparotomy seed placement for the treatment of early-stage prostate cancer. Specially designed 18-gauge needles are loaded with radioactive palladium 103 and iodine 125 seeds; these are placed into a custom needle holder at appropriate coordinates according to a template matched to a transrectal scan of the prostate. With the patient in lithotomy position under spinal anesthesia, an ultrasound probe is placed in the rectum and attached to a stepping unit which allows precisely controlled placement of the seeds (up to 100) throughout the entire gland.

SELECTED READING

Abati, A., Skarulis, M. C., Shawker, T., and Solomon, D. Ultrasound-guided fine-needle aspiration of parathyroid lesions: A morphological and immunocytochemical approach. *Human Pathol* 26:338–343, 1995.

Avila, N., Shawker, T., Choyke, P., and Oldfield, E. Cerebellar and spinal hemangioblastomas: Evaluation with intraoperative gray-scale and color Doppler flow US. *Radiology* 188:143–147, 1993.

Grimm, P. D., Blasko, J. C., and Ragde, H. Ultrasound-guided transperineal implantation of iodine-125 and palladium-103 for the treatment of early-stage prostate cancer. *Atlas Urolog Clin North Am* 2:113–125, 1994.

Hanbidge, A. E., Arenson, A. M., Shaw, P. A., Szalai, J. P., Hamilton, P. A., and Leonhardt, C. Needle size and sample adequacy in ultrasound-guided biopsy of thyroid nodules. *Can Assoc Radiol J* 46:199–201, 1995.

Hsu, W. H., Chiang, C. D., Hsu, J. Y., Kwan, P. C., Chen, C. L., and Chen, C. Y. Ultrasound-guided fine-needle aspiration biopsy of lung cancers. *J Clin Ultrasound* 24:225–233, 1996.

Kandarpa, K., and Aruny, J. *Handbook of Interventional Radiologic Procedures.* Boston: Little, Brown, 1996.

Letterie, G., and Kramer, D. Intraoperative ultrasound guidance for intrauterine endoscopic surgery. *Fertility and Sterility* 62:654–656, 1994.

Machi, J., Sigel, B., et al. Operative ultrasonography during hepatobiliary and pancreatic surgery. *World J Surg* 17:640–646, 1993.

McGahan, J. P. *Interventional Ultrasound.* Baltimore: Williams & Wilkins, 1990.

Parker, S., et al. Ultrasound-guided mammotomy: A new breast biopsy technique. *JDMS* 12:113–118, 1996.

Reading, C. C. Intraoperative ultrasonography. *Abdom Imaging* 21: 21–29, 1996.

53 ARTIFACTS

ROGER C. SANDERS, MIMI MAGGIO SAYLOR

SONOGRAM ABBREVIATIONS

Bl   Bladder

D   Diaphragm

GB   Gallbladder

K   Kidney

L   Liver

P   Pleural effusion

T   Tornado effect

Ut   Uterus

KEY WORDS

Analog and Digital. Analog—Echo signals that have not been computer processed have an infinite number of patterns, more than a computer can manage. This unmodified (unmodulated) signal is termed analog. Digital—To allow a computer to display the image, the picture is broken up into multiple small areas (pixels), and numerical values are given to patterns and echo levels. Glossy photographs represent an analog image, whereas the small dots that compose a newspaper photographic image were composed digitally.

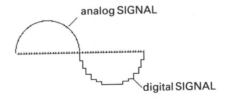

analog SIGNAL

digital SIGNAL

Azimuth. Depth axis.

Comet Tail. Artifact due to strong interface in which there is a thin line of echoes within an essentially echo-free area.

Digital. See *Analog.*

Frame Rate. Frequency of image formation; usually 30 frames per second.

Grating Artifacts. Curvilinear artifact seen with linear arrays either in front of a strong interface or behind it.

Lateral Beam Spread. Widening of the transducer focus as the beam passes through tissues at increasing depths.

Main Bang. High-level echoes at the skin's surface.

Noise. Spurious echoes throughout the image occurring in areas such as the bladder that are known to be echo-free.

Persistence. Duration of time that the image persists on the screen. If it is left on the screen it blends with the next image.

Refraction. Change in the angle of the sound beam as it passes through a substance of a different density.

Reverberation. Artifactual linear echoes parallel to a strong interface. Sound is returned to the transducer and then into the tissues again.

Ring Down. A particular type of reverberation artifact in which numerous parallel echoes are seen for a considerable distance.

Side Lobes. Secondary off-axis concentrations of energy not parallel to the beam axis; degrades lateral resolution.

Slice Thickness Artifact. Artifactual echoes seen within a cystic structure close to the distal wall due to the wide beam width.

Tornado Effect. Artifact due to gas in which there is an absence of echoes with an irregular anterior border caused by shadowing.

X-Y Axis. Horizontal axis (transverse axis).

THE CLINICAL PROBLEM

Artifacts in ultrasonic images can be classified into three categories:

1. *Artifacts related to instrument problems,* some of which relate to the type of instrumentation used (e.g., side lobes, grating lobes) and some which occur when the equipment is not functioning satisfactorily.

2. *Technique-dependent artifacts,* in which the appearance is produced by unsatisfactory operator technique.
3. *Artifacts due to the way tissues affect sound.* These artifacts cannot be avoided.

Each of these spurious sonographic appearances must be recognized so that the deceptive finding can be disregarded, eliminated, or used as a diagnostic aid.

REAL-TIME AND STATIC SCANNING ARTIFACTS

Artifacts Caused by Equipment

Artifactual Noise

Artifactual noise is caused by electrical interference from nearby equipment (e.g., in an intensive care unit; Fig. 53-1).

RECOGNITION. Such noise has a repetitive pattern unlike the overall increase in echogenicity seen with too much gain. This type of noise produces a pattern over the normal ultrasound image.

CORRECTION TECHNIQUE. Equipment can be modified to prevent such interference if it occurs in the ultrasound laboratory. You may be able to disconnect the interfering equipment during the scan. Gel warmers may be responsible.

Calibration Problems—Incorrect Distance Markers

Calibration problems may not be apparent on the image, but subsequent measurements using another ultrasonic system or phantom may show erroneous caliper measurements.

DIAGNOSTIC CONFUSION. Measurements such as the biparietal diameter may be wrong with tragic clinical consequences.

RECOGNITION. Only by comparison with other systems or by calibration check can such subtle measurement changes be detected.

CORRECTION TECHNIQUE. Calibration checks should be performed at regular intervals (see Chapter 54). Measurements should be performed in the center of the image where calibration is most correct and not at the edge of the video monitor.

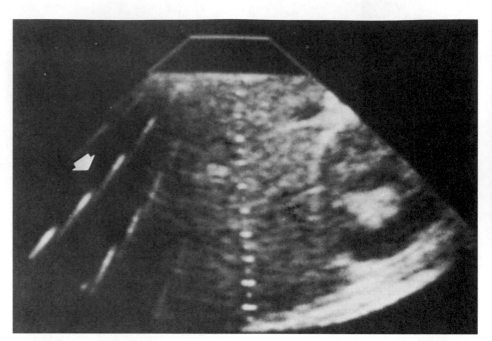

FIGURE 53-1. Interference from nearby equipment causes artifacts on the CRT (arrow).

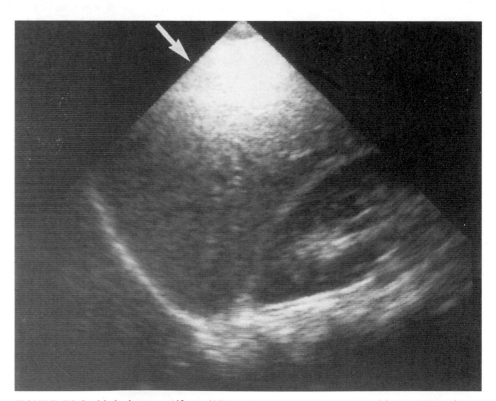

FIGURE 53-2. Main bang artifact. With older units this is caused by a strong interface between the skin and the transducer. Too much near gain (arrow) can also be a reason.

Main Bang Artifact

There can be many echoes from the skin-transducer interface in the immediate subcutaneous tissues. There is such a strong interface between the skin and the transducer that it is almost impossible to avoid the main bang artifact completely with older transducers.

The main bang is less of a problem in new transducers because the multiple matching layers give the transducer itself an impedance very close to that of the skin surface. Poor technique, such as too much near time gain compensation or rib artifact, is responsible for most superficial artifact (Fig. 53-2).

DIAGNOSTIC CONFUSION. Subcutaneous and superficial lesions will be hidden within the main bang artifact.

CORRECTION TECHNIQUE. A higher-frequency transducer diminishes the problem. Decrease the near field gain. Use of a stand-off pad will avoid a main bang artifact to some extent.

Veiling

Bands of increased echogenicity can be seen at certain depths if all focal zones are used simultaneously, producing the veiling artifact (Fig. 53-3).

DIAGNOSTIC CONFUSION. The impression of a mass may be created within the area of veiling. Masses may be overlooked at the interface of the different focal zones.

RECOGNITION. A band of increased echoes unrelated to the strong interfaces within the images is seen at a certain depth.

CORRECTION TECHNIQUE. When the veiling cannot be corrected by adjusting the time gain compensation controls, use only one focal zone.

Absence of Focusing

Electronic focusing and the use of acoustic lenses have increased the number of focal zones available with a single transducer and greatly increased the resolution of the image. If the focal zone option is not used with newer electronic systems, much blurring of echo interfaces is seen (Fig. 53-4).

DIAGNOSTIC CONFUSION. Discrete lines appear thick, and subtle masses may be overlooked.

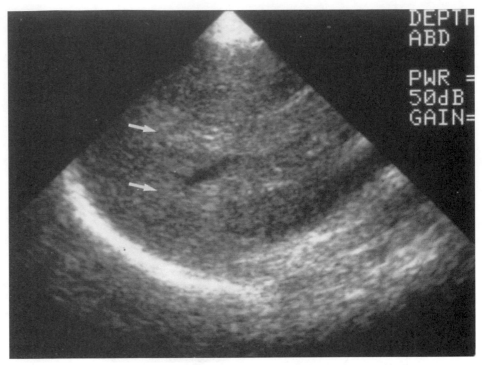

FIGURE 53-3. Veiling. Focusing zones are well delineated transverse echo areas (arrows). Utilize *only* the focusing zone in the area of interest to eliminate the focal banding.

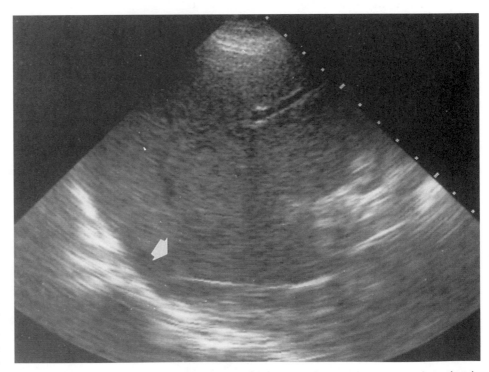

FIGURE 53-4. Absence of focusing. There is blurring of the echoes when focusing is not utilized (arrow).

RECOGNITION. The echoes in the unfocused area are large. Echoes normally seen as dots in the image are seen as a short line.

CORRECTION TECHNIQUE. Use the focal zone option, and the echoes will appear discrete. If viewing a large area, place the focusing "caret" near the bottom of the area of interest to optimize the resolution.

Focusing and Persistence Versus Fetal Heart Motion

Using multiple electronic focal zones simultaneously will increase image quality but slows the frame rate, causing a blurry or wavy appearance. If the persistence is increased, the frame rate is not reduced but the frame averaging is changed to "smooth" the image, creating the same effect.

DIAGNOSTIC CONFUSION. Structures that move rapidly such as the fetal heart may be impossible to assess and one can erroneously infer that a fetus is dead.

RECOGNITION. A wavy image motion is visible when the image is closely examined. Rapid motion of the transducer exaggerates this finding.

CORRECTION TECHNIQUE. Use only a single focal zone and a little persistence.

Pixel Mismatch (Real-Time Misregistration)

Returning sound waves are seen as analog signals. The information is converted into a digital "word" (see Key Words) when placed in location in the scan convertor. This process occurs over a period of microseconds. When the information is read into the scan converter, the image starts at the upper left-hand corner and converts the digital information back to an analog form as it is displayed on the viewing screen. Pixel mismatch occurs when the information is received as an analog signal and was misinterpreted at the time it was converted to a "word" (Fig. 53-5). This artifact occurs with a faulty scan convertor or noise in the electronic line.

DIAGNOSTIC CONFUSION. Information in the area in which the pixel mismatch is present is lowered, so subtle lesions may be overlooked.

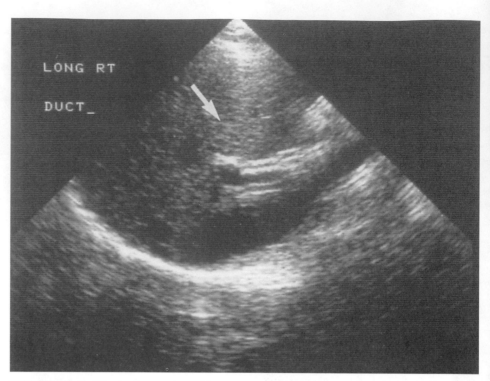

FIGURE 53-5. Pixel-mismatch artifact. Misregistration in a real-time unit occurs when the information is incorrectly placed into the scan convertor. There is a mismatch of the information between the right and the left side of the liver (arrow).

RECOGNITION. There is a band of low resolution within the image. The information on the left side of the screen does not match up with the right side.

CORRECTION TECHNIQUE. Use a different transducer. Get the transducer repaired.

Grating Lobes

A grating lobe artifact is caused by the periodic spacing of the phased array or, more commonly, linear array elements. Grating lobes travel at an angle to the main beam, and depending on whether the lobe hits the object before or after the main beam, a curvilinear echo may be seen either at a shallower or deeper depth than the structure causing the artifact (Fig. 53-6).

DIAGNOSTIC CONFUSION. An apparent septum may be present within an amniotic sac or other cystic process.

RECOGNITION. The septum, which is slightly curved, is usually related to a strong curvilinear interface in the midportion of the linear array field.

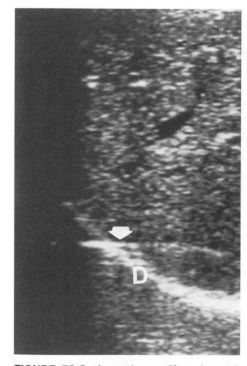

FIGURE 53-6. A grating artifact (arrow) may sometimes occur above or below a strong linear interface (e.g., the diaphragm) when using an array system, particularly a linear array.

CORRECTION TECHNIQUE. Imaging with a different transducer or using a different acoustic window or angle shows that the supposed echo is artifactual.

Side Lobes

Side lobes are secondary echoes outside the main beam that exist with all transducers.

DIAGNOSTIC CONFUSION. Noise is created within the image.

RECOGNITION. Recognition is difficult unless quality control tests are performed.

CORRECTION TECHNIQUE. Use the focusing system that comes with the transducer at the depth at which the noise is greatest.

Artifacts Caused by Technique

Noise

Noise is created by excess gain (Fig. 53-7). Gain may be turned up to a point where low-level echoes occur in unstructured fluid-filled areas such as the bladder.

DIAGNOSTIC CONFUSION. Excess gain may give the impression that the cystic lesion contains internal material or is solid.

RECOGNITION. A normally echo-free structure contains low-level echoes, which could represent pathology but may be artifact. Comparison with a known cystic structure such as the urinary bladder helps in deciding whether possible noise is a technical artifact or a real structure.

CORRECTION TECHNIQUE. Decrease gain without losing structural information in the known echogenic areas.

Transducer Selection Problems: Time Gain Compensation Problems

Artifacts created by poor time gain compensation (TGC) technique are common (see Chapter 4). Extra echoes or too few echoes may be introduced owing to wrong use of the TGC curve. Numerous echoes may be created in superficial structures and none in deep structures and vice versa (Fig. 53-8). This appearance may also be caused by the wrong choice of transducer with the result that the focal zone and frequency concentrate on superficial structures.

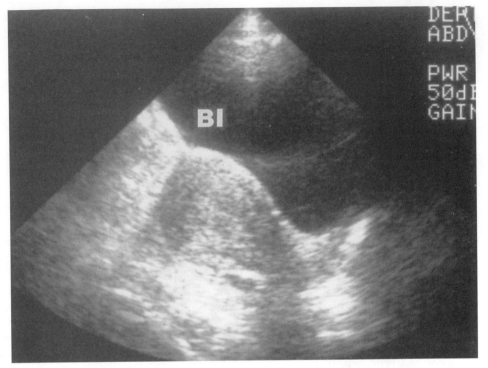

FIGURE 53-7. Low-level echoes (noise) are seen in the fluid-filled bladder.

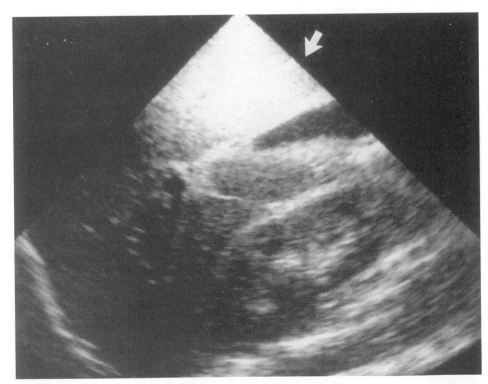

FIGURE 53-8. A longitudinal view of the right upper quadrant demonstrates the wrong use of the TGC controls. Too many echoes are displayed in the near field (arrow), with too few echoes in the far field.

DIAGNOSTIC CONFUSION. Wrong TGC settings may give rise to apparent anterior placenta previa, creation of a pseudocystic superficial lesion, or masking of a problem by too many echoes.

RECOGNITION. The relative area of increased or decreased echoes extends beyond the natural tissue boundaries. Large areas of acoustically similar tissue should have homogeneous echoes throughout.

CORRECTION TECHNIQUE. Observe the principles of TGC usage discussed in Chapter 4.

Banding

By using a finely focused transducer or excessively deep anterior TGC suppression (misuse of the slide pots), it is easy to create an area of banding across the image (Fig. 53-9). At a uniform distance from the transducer face the structures are more echogenic than structures anterior and posterior to it.

DIAGNOSTIC CONFUSION. The impression of a mass (e.g., a liver metastasis) may be created because there are more echoes in the area of banding.

CORRECTION TECHNIQUE. Use a transducer with a different frequency and alter the TGC settings.

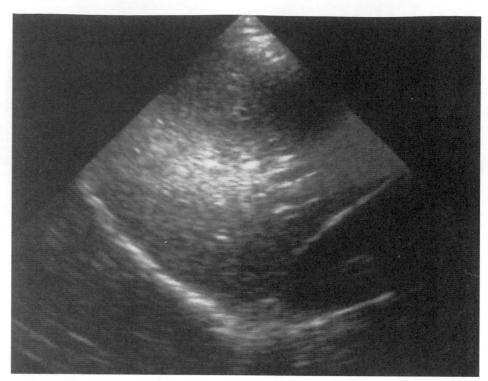

FIGURE 53-9. Banding. Misuse of the TGC slide pots can create an echogenic band at any depth in the image.

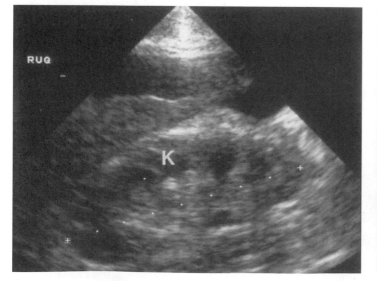

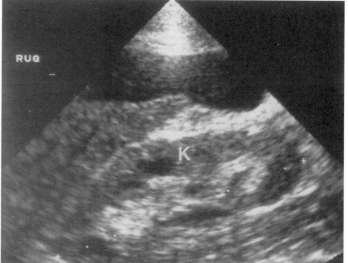

A   B

FIGURE 53-10. Breathing artifacts. (**A**) Allowing the patient to breathe shortens the kidney to 8.0 cm. (**B**) When the patient holds his breath, the kidney measures 8.7 cm.

Contact Problems

When the transducer is used in a site where contact with the skin is difficult (e.g., over ribs), portions of the image may be lost and only half of the field of view may be filled with information.

DIAGNOSTIC CONFUSION. Masses may be missed if they lie within an area obscured by poor contact.

CORRECTION TECHNIQUE. Attempt to reposition the transducer or use a transducer with a smaller face (footprint). Use a lot of gel.

Artifacts Caused by Movement

Breathing

If the patient breathes while you are scanning, the image may be distorted and blurred because part of the scan will be performed during an inspiration and part during an expiration.

DIAGNOSTIC CONFUSION. When scanning a kidney, shortening or lengthening may occur if the patient breathes during the scan (Fig. 53-10). The diaphragm and adjacent liver may be interrupted and blurred if the patient takes a breath in the middle of the scan (Fig. 53-11). Borders may be blurry or even duplicated (see. Fig. 53-9) and parenchymal echoes will appear smoothed.

CORRECTION TECHNIQUE. Ask the patient to hold his or her breath, or utilize the cine loop control to review the last frames of the scan and freeze when the most desirable image appears. If the patient is unable to suspend his or her breath, make sure the persistence is set low and that simultaneous multiple electronic focusing is not slowing the frame rate. These techniques will shorten the time it takes to stabilize the image before it can be frozen.

Operator Scanning Speed

If the sonographer scans rapidly, artifacts known as dropout lines are created (Fig. 53-12). Most digital units receive information rapidly enough to avoid this artifact. Some units appear to have gaps between the lines of the image because they have not been smoothed. Computer processing can eliminate these little gaps between beam lines in a cosmetic but uninformative fashion (i.e., the gaps are filled in with false echoes).

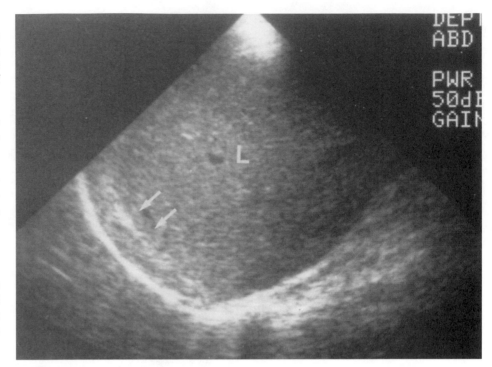

FIGURE 53-11. If the patient is breathing when you freeze an image, the diaphragm may be distorted or blurred (arrows).

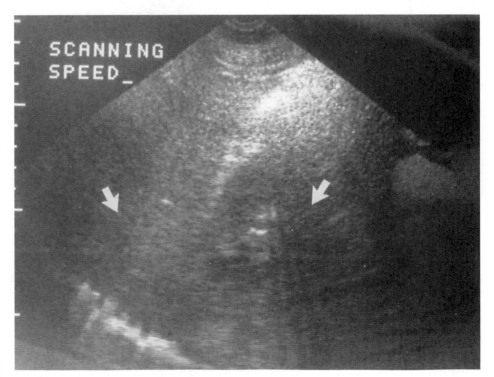

FIGURE 53-12. Dropout lines (arrows) are created when the scanning speed is too rapid.

CORRECTION TECHNIQUE. Perform the scan at a lower speed.

Operator Pressure

Applying too much or uneven pressure while scanning can distort the image.

DIAGNOSTIC CONFUSION. Scanning the fetal trunk using too much pressure with your transducer may make it appear to have a flattened ovoid shape rather than the preferred round shape (Fig. 53-13).

CORRECTION TECHNIQUE. Use only sufficient pressure to keep the transducer in contact with the skin.

Photographic Artifacts

Photographic artifacts are a major problem. If the contrast is set incorrectly, subtle metastatic lesions may be lost in the overall grayness of the image. Undue brightness may also obscure subtle textural alterations (see Chapter 55).

Dust on the Camera

If dust is allowed to settle onto a camera lens or cathode ray tube, small echogenic areas will be seen on the camera image. Similar artifacts can occur with Polaroid images.

DIAGNOSTIC CONFUSION. Echogenic foci can be mistaken for debris, hemorrhage, or gallstones within cystic structures.

RECOGNITION. A similar echogenic area occurs in the same location on every film.

CORRECTION TECHNIQUE. Make sure that the camera is dusted frequently.

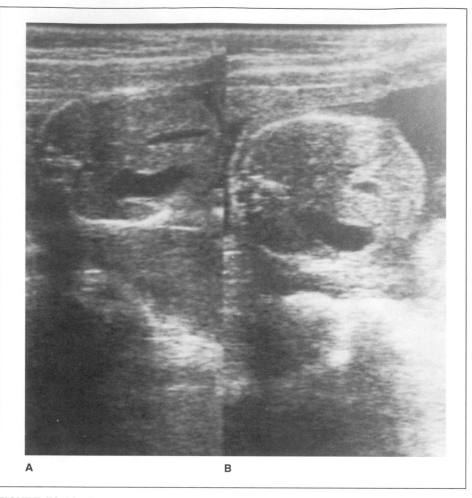

FIGURE 53-13. Pressure artifacts. (**A**) Too much pressure over the fetal trunk produces a flattened ovoid shape. (**B**) A lighter scanning pressure creates a round trunk and correct measurements.

Artifacts Caused by Sound–Tissue Interactions

Artifacts From Strongly Reflective Structures (Shadowing)

Gas, bone, and, to a much lesser extent, fatty tissues do not conduct sound well. When sound strikes a strong interface such as gas or bone, one of two responses may be produced. Either there is no sound conduction through the area (shadowing), or numerous secondary reverberations are produced, causing a series of echogenic lines extending into the tissues (*ring down*).

DIAGNOSTIC CONFUSION. Large shadowing artifacts may obscure a deep pathologic process (e.g., nodes).

RECOGNITION. The reverberation pattern seen with bone is a series of alternating lines (Fig. 53-14A), whereas that seen with gas is usually a more diffuse, vaguely outlined pattern with considerable noise—the "tornado" effect. A linear series of parallel bands may also be seen with gas—the ring down effect (see Fig. 53-14B).

CORRECTION TECHNIQUE. The sonographer should attempt to scan around gas or bone, obtaining scans of the areas below these structures from an oblique angle.

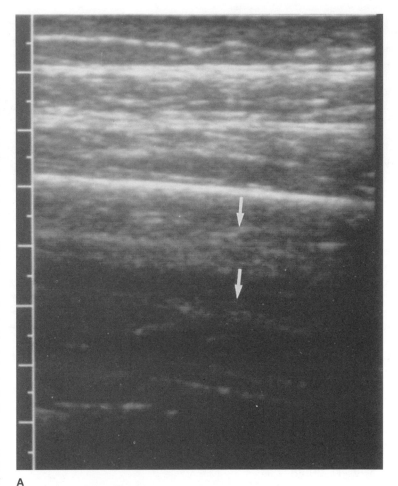

A

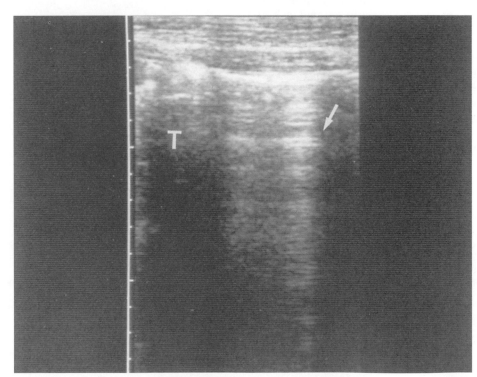

B

FIGURE 53-14. Reverberation artifacts. (**A**) A longitudinal scan of the thigh. Notice the reverberations (alternating lines) extending below the bone interface (arrows). (**B**) Gas may cause the creation of a line of reverberation echoes (arrow), the "ring down" effect, or a vague sonolucent area of acoustic shadowing, the "tornado" effect (T).

BENEFIT. Shadowing occurs when the sound beam hits a highly reflective surface such as gallstones, renal stones, or surgical clips, allowing a diagnosis of an acoustically dense structure. The shadowing can be made more obvious by increasing the frequency of the transducer (Fig. 53-15).

Reverberation Artifacts

Whenever sound passes out of a structure with an acoustic impedance that is markedly different from its neighbor, a large amount of sound is returned to the transducer. The amount of sound returning may be so great that it is sent from the transducer back into the tissues, causing a duplication of the original structure. The second wave has traveled twice as far as the first one, the third echo three times as far, and so forth. The distance between each successive echo will equal the distance between the original two interfaces. The second echo and each successive echo parallel the original interface.

DIAGNOSTIC CONFUSION. Such reverberation artifacts are most commonly seen adjacent to the bladder anterior wall (see Fig. 53-2), but also occur elsewhere in the body in soft tissue as well as fluid; they may mimic a mass. Reverberations from the anterior surface wall can make a simple cyst appear complex.

RECOGNITION. Reverberation artifacts of this type may occur at some distance from the original interface (e.g., behind the posterior wall of the bladder). A second apparent bladder resembling fluid-filled bowel appears to lie where measurement shows the sacrum should lie.

CORRECTION TECHNIQUE. Distinguish such artifacts from real structures by (1) using transducers of a different frequency; (2) bouncing the transducer on the abdominal wall and noticing that the second linear structure moves in exactly the same fashion as the strong echo nearest the transducer; and (3) scanning the same area from a different angle.

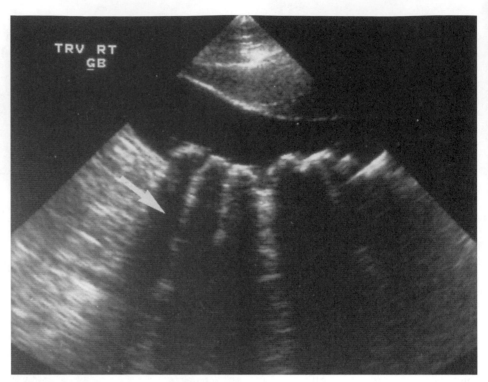

FIGURE 53-15. Large acoustic interfaces due to gallstones are associated with shadowing (arrow). Shadowing is accentuated with a higher frequency.

Mirror Artifacts

If a sonographic structure has a curved appearance, it may focus and reflect the sound like a mirror.

RECOGNITION. Mirror artifacts occur most commonly when scanning the diaphragm. Theoretically, there should be no echoes from the lungs because they are full of gas, but in fact there is a duplication of the structures within the liver above the diaphragm in all normal individuals (Fig. 53-16). This mirror image can create a false impression of a pleural effusion because the diaphragm is also duplicated. This artifact occurs when the patient is scanned in an oblique axis in the coronal position. Lesions within the liver or spleen adjacent to the diaphragm can be "duplicated" in the lung.

BENEFIT. If this mirror image is absent in the lung, it can be deduced that a pleural effusion is present (see Fig. 53-16C).

CORRECTION TECHNIQUE. Try to scan the same area from another position.

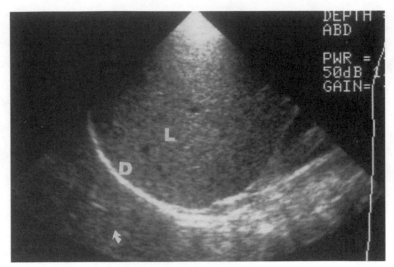

A

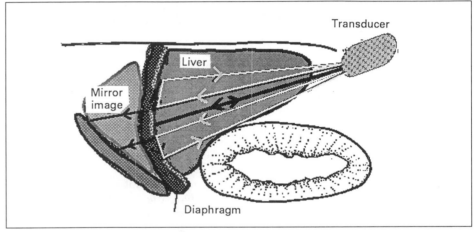

B

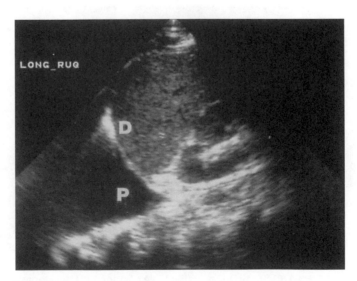

C

FIGURE 53-16. Mirror artifacts. (**A**) In the normal patient there is a mirror image of the liver tissue above the diaphragm at the site of the lung (arrow). (**B**) Diagram of how the artifact is created. (**C**) When there is a pleural effusion, an echo-free area is seen above the diaphragm.

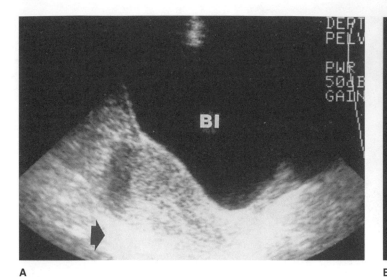

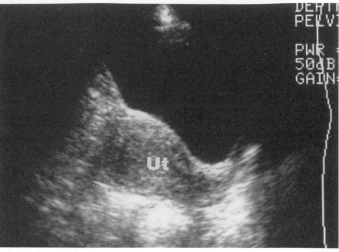

A   B

FIGURE 53-17. Enhancement effect. (**A**) Increased echoes obscure the structures behind the bladder owing to enhancement of the sound passing through the bladder (arrow). (**B**) Decreasing the gain allows the uterus to be seen clearly.

Enhancement Effect

As the sound beam passes through fluid-filled structures or structures containing many cysts, it is not attenuated and there is an increase in the amplitude (brightness) of the echoes distal to the fluid (Fig. 53-17A).

DIAGNOSTIC CONFUSION. A true pathologic condition may be obliterated by the increased gain distal to a fluid-filled structure (e.g., fibroid uterus behind the bladder).

BENEFIT. Acoustic enhancement is almost always beneficial and may be useful in differentiating between solid and cystic lesions, in addition to aiding the sonographer in seeing deep structures.

CORRECTION TECHNIQUE. The sonographer should diminish the overall gain and adjust the TGC (see Fig. 53-17B). If the condition is pathologic (e.g., renal cyst), document the increased acoustic enhancement behind the structure.

Split-Image Artifact

A duplicate image occurs when the transducer is placed in the midline in the pelvis. The curved rectus muscles cause a bending (*refraction*) of the sound beam. The beam is bent toward the midline from both sides of the muscle layer. The system is unaware that refraction has occurred. The echoes that are returned to the transducer are placed at the assumed distance and direction. The original structure is duplicated (Fig. 53-18A).

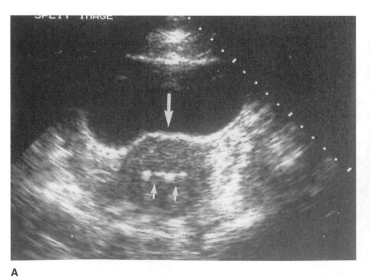

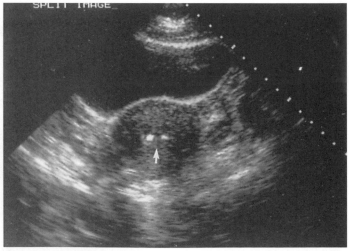

A   B

FIGURE 53-18. Split-image artifact. (**A**) Scanning transversely in the midline of the pelvis can create a duplication of the structure which is situated in the midline due to refraction. A double image of a Copper 7 IUD is seen in the uterus (arrows). Note the dimple in the contour of the uterine wall (larger arrow) at the intersection of the two images. (**B**) When scanning away from the midline in the transverse plane, a better image is displayed. The true configuration of the Cu 7 IUD is seen (arrow). The dimple has disappeared.

This artifact can occur with a phased array or a linear array probe, but is more frequent with linear array systems.

DIAGNOSTIC CONFUSION. A double image is created. A single sac can be mistaken for a twin pregnancy, or there may appear to be two IUDs.

CORRECTION TECHNIQUE. To avoid the refraction of the sound beam through the rectus muscle, scan from a site other than the midline (see Fig. 53-18B).

Slice Thickness Artifact

When the interface between a fluid-filled cyst and soft tissue is acutely angled, the beam, which is relatively wide (2–3 mm), may strike both tissue and fluid simultaneously. Low-level artifactual echoes will be displayed within the fluid (Fig. 53-19).

DIAGNOSTIC CONFUSION. Low-level echoes in the posterior aspect of a cyst may be thought to be evidence of abnormal cyst contents.

RECOGNITION. Echoes are seen at the posterior aspect of the cyst and develop as the transducer moves from the center of the cyst.

CORRECTION TECHNIQUE. Scanning from a different angle shows that there are no echoes within the area where the slice thickness artifact was seen.

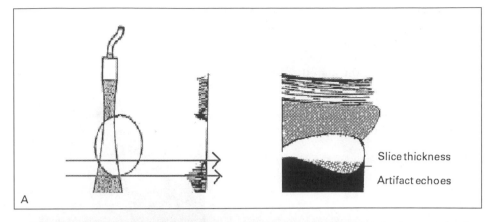

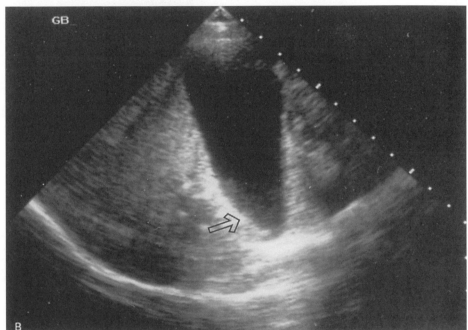

FIGURE 53-19. Slice thickness artifact. (**A**) Echoes in the posterior part of the gall-bladder relate to the slice thickness artifact. The diagram shows the beam intersecting an oblique segment of the cyst wall. (**B**) Sonogram demonstrates low-level echoes apparently in the posterior part of the gallbladder where the gallbladder angle is steep.

Comet Effect

A very strong acoustic interface, such as an air bubble or a metallic structure such as a suture, creates a dense echogenic line extending through the image known as the comet effect (Fig. 53-20).

DIAGNOSTIC CONFUSION. The echogenic line may be mistaken for a real structure.

BENEFIT. The presence of the line indicates a very strong interface and may allow recognition of metallic structures such as clips.

CORRECTION TECHNIQUE. Scan from a different angle and the line will either disappear or be projected onto a different site.

Color Misregistration Artifact

When movement occurs in nearby tissues, artifactual color signals may be generated in nearby uninvolved tissue, resulting in the transient appearance of color throughout the region. Typical situations in which this type of artifact occur are when the transducer is moved too fast; with active gut peristalsis; and adjacent to large, highly pulsatile arteries, arterial venous fistula, and pseudoaneurysm.

CORRECTION TECHNIQUE. Perform a scan at a lower speed and cut down on gain. Use of the proper color filter will eliminate most of this motion artifact.

Excessive Color Gain

If too much color gain is used, vessels will appear larger than they really are and "bleed" into surrounding tissue, and artifactual color will be seen in immobile structures (Color Plates 53-1 and 53-2).

CORRECTION TECHNIQUE. Lower gain.

Poor Angle for Color

As with pulsed Doppler, the best visualization of a vessel is with the transducer at an angle of less than 60 degrees to the vessel. If a 90-degree angle is used, flow within vessels will be poorly seen (Color Plates 53-3 and 53-4).

CORRECTION TECHNIQUE. Power Doppler is not angle sensitive and will show vessels in the same area.

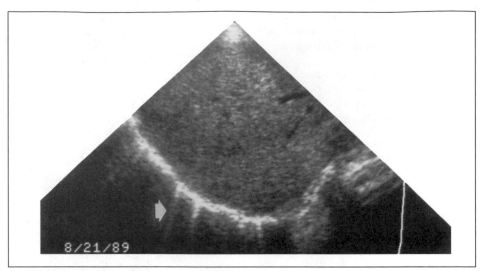

FIGURE 53-20. The comet effect is demonstrated on this longitudinal view of the liver. At the diaphragm, echogenic lines can be seen extending toward the lung (arrow).

Calcification

In areas of calcification, spurious color signals can be derived from high-level echogenic areas. The signal consists of a mixture of red and blue signals over an area of calcification. The artifact is present regardless of the velocity, wall filter setting, probe frequency, focal depth, and color Doppler system.

CORRECTION TECHNIQUE. Scan over calcification at a low speed with low gain and discount apparent color flow signals from highly echogenic structures that are calcified.

Transducer Movement

When the transducer is moved, apparent color flow signals may be derived from stronger echogenic areas such as septum. These signals disappear once the transducer is kept steady.

CORRECTION TECHNIQUE. Never attempt to obtain color flow information until the transducer has stayed motionless in a spot for at least 10 to 15 seconds.

Aliasing

As explained in Chapter 5, if the pulse repetition frequency is set at too fast a speed, signals return to the transducer after the transmission of the next signal. With color flow, this artifact induces specks of color at the opposite end of the spectrum from the rest of the color related to high-velocity areas (i.e., in areas of red, there will be a few specks of blue intermixed with the red, where aliasing is occurring) (Color Plate 53-5).

CORRECTION TECHNIQUE. Do not set the pulse repetition frequency at too rapid a rate, especially when structures are deep and at a long distance from the transducer.

SELECTED READING

Avruch, L., and Cooperberg, P. L. The ringdown artifact. *J Ultrasound Med* 4:21–28, 1985.

Goldstein, A., and Madrazo, B. L. Slice-thickness artifacts in gray-scale ultrasound. *J Clin Ultrasound* 9:365–375, 1981.

Hedrick, W. R., and Peterson, C. L. Image artifacts in real-time ultrasound. *JDMS* 11:300–308, 1995.

Hykes, D., Hedrick, W. R., and Starchman, D. (Eds.). *Ultrasound Physics and Instrumentation.* New York: Churchill Livingstone, 1993.

Laing, F. C. Commonly encountered artifacts in clinical ultrasound. *Seminars in Ultrasound, CT and MRI* 4(1):27–43, 1983.

Rahmouni, A., Bargoin, R., Herment, A., Bargoin, N., and Vasile, N. Color Doppler twinkling artifact in hyperechoic regions. *Radiology* 199:269–271, 1996.

Sanders, R. C. Normal variants that mimic tumor or fetal anomalies. *Ultrasound Quart* 7:133–189, 1989.

Sauerbrei, E. E. The split image artifact in pelvic ultrasonography: The anatomy and physics. *J Ultrasound Med* 4:29–34, 1985.

Thickman, D. I., et al. Clinical manifestations of the comet tail artifact. *J Ultrasound Med* 2:225–230, 1983.

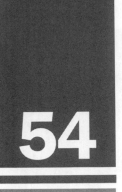

EQUIPMENT CARE AND QUALITY CONTROL

ROGER C. SANDERS, IRMA WHEELOCK TOPPER

KEY WORDS

Axial. The vertical transducer axis.

Azimuth. Depth axis.

Registration. The creation of a two-dimensional image on the monitor in the X-Y and azimuth axes.

Resolution. Ability of a system to distinguish closely spaced targets. Lateral resolution is transverse to the beam (width); axial resolution is along the beam axis (depth).

SUAR. Sensitivity, uniformity, axial resolution phantom (obtainable from RMI, Middleton, WI).

Tissue Equivalent Phantom. Phantom used to test real-time ultrasound systems, having an attenuation coefficient measured in db/cm/MHz with a consistency similar to tissue.

X-Y Axis. Transverse axis.

 THE CLINICAL PROBLEM

Ultrasound systems are like people: They don't respond well to rough treatment or lack of attention. Certain practical equipment checks decrease downtime and increase the quality of the image.

PREVENTIVE MAINTENANCE

1. Be careful if you must store gel on the equipment. Spills may cause serious equipment problems.
2. Cables and transducers should be inspected visually for worn areas or cracks. Damaged cables may be potential safety hazards or the causes of intermittent malfunctions. Gel left on the transducer and on the cable causes brittle transducer housings.
3. Careless placement of the transducer and cable on the machine can cause cable damage. Dropping a transducer on the floor may damage some of the elements. Repairs may cost thousands of dollars. Cables are often damaged on portable studies when they are run over by the system wheels. Transducers should be placed in proper holders or cables may break.
4. Air filters should be cleaned periodically (weekly). They can usually be removed, cleaned with soap and water, and replaced. Neglect may cause equipment to overheat owing to decreased airflow.

WARM-UP

When a multiformat camera or real-time system is first turned on, there is a period during which images vary in brightness. Most systems require approximately 5 minutes to become stable. Many systems do not allow imaging during the warm-up period. We suggest turning the systems off each night as well as over weekends because an unexpected breakdown in the air conditioning could give rise to major overheating problems if the equipment is left on all the time.

TRANSDUCERS

Transducers require careful handling. Dropping them sometimes damages the crystal or the backing used to damp the unwanted vibrations. Transducers should be cleaned after each patient with an alcohol sponge or transducer disinfectant, particularly if the patient has an open wound or a skin problem. Some transducers can be immersed in Cidex up to the handle for sterilization. About 10 minutes immersion is required for adequate sterilization (see Appendix 33).

CONTACT AGENTS

Use a commercial water-soluble gel couplant to ensure good acoustic contact between the transducer and patient. Thick, high-viscosity gels are desirable when scanning pleural effusions since they don't slide off a sitting patient's back. Thicker gels are also helpful for obstetric patients with large abdomens.

It is desirable to heat gel in a commercially available heating device. However, make sure that there is enough gel in the container because gel can be overheated if only a small amount is present. Do not leave older gel warmers on indefinitely because they pose a potential fire hazard. Modern gel warmers are thermostatically controlled so this is no longer a problem.

Use disposable gloves when scanning a patient to avoid the risk of infection. Spread the gel around the abdomen with the transducer rather than by hand. Do not handle the controls with gel on your hand or glove.

QUALITY ASSURANCE

Quality assurance tests are a nuisance and are tedious to perform, but are worthwhile because it is difficult or even impossible to detect major calibration and measurement distortions from examination of the image alone. Clearly, major clinical problems may occur if erroneous measurement data are produced. Component breakdown can be detected before it occurs in some instances. Quality assurance checks should be performed on a quarterly basis with most systems or more often if a problem is suspected (e.g., if a transducer has been dropped).

Quality Control Tests

The standard tests performed to ensure that the system is working satisfactorily are (1) aspect ratio and scaling tests; (2) resolution tests (both axial and lateral), including tests of focus capabilities at different depths; and (3) a comparative power output test that equates to a depth of penetration measurement. All of these tests are performed on a tissue equivalent phantom (RMI 413A or equivalent).

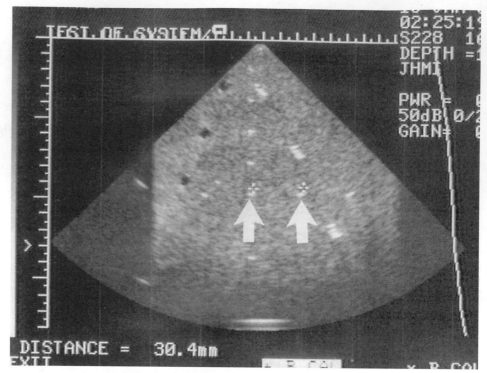

FIGURE 54-1. View of a scan of the RMI phantom showing that the horizontal measurement between pins is correct (arrows). A diagram of the arrangement of the pins within the RMI phantom is shown below.

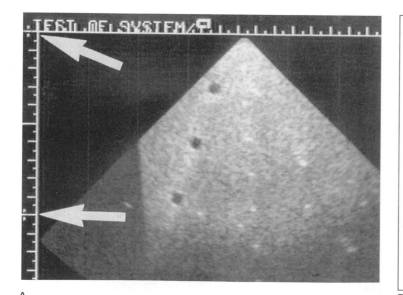

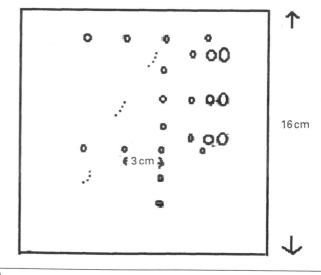

FIGURE 54-2. View of an RMI phantom showing that the vertical measurement between pins on the RMI phantom corresponds with the distance shown by the calipers on the scan (arrows).

Aspect Ratio and Scaling

The aspect ratio and scaling test measures whether distances are accurate in both directions (X [vertical], Y [horizontal]) and whether these measurements are correctly displayed on a hardcopy device (Figs. 54-1 to 54-3). When the phantom is scanned, the horizontally (spaced 3-cm apart; see Figs. 54-1 and 54-2) and vertically (spaced 2-cm apart; see Figs. 54-2 and 54-3) aligned pins should measure the correct distance apart. The distance between pins is compared with centimeter markers in both the horizontal and vertical directions (see Figs. 54-2 and 54-3) on the ultrasound monitor. This measurement should be confirmed when the vertical and horizontal scale markers are measured with a hand-held caliper. One centimeter measured vertically on an image should be equal to the same distance measured horizontally.

Resolution

Both axial (vertical) and lateral resolution are determined at each set of resolution pins. These arrays of pins appear at the 3-, 7-, and 12-cm depths on the RMI phantom. A magnified view of each group, with the focus set to that area, provides an image adequate to perform these tests (Fig. 54-4).

Axial resolution is assessed by seeing whether the spacing between the pins can be resolved. The spacings between the closest pins on the RMI phantom are 3 mm, 2 mm, 1 mm, and 0.5 mm. In Figure 54-4 the spacing can be seen between all the pins, therefore, the axial resolution is finer than the smallest distance (0.5 mm) and the lateral resolution (as measured across pin 2) is about 1.7 mm as shown by the calipers. The axial and lateral measurements are repeated for the other two sets of pins at the 7-cm and 12-cm depths and the data are recorded.

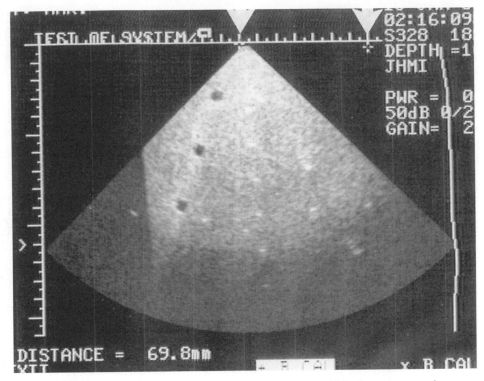

FIGURE 54-3. View of an RMI phantom confirming that width distances as shown on the calipers are correct (arrows).

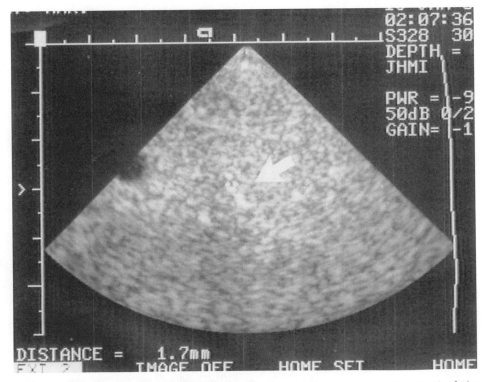

FIGURE 54-4. View of an RMI phantom with the focal zone set to the level of the pins. This is a magnified image and distinction between all five pins is possible. The smallest distance is 0.5 cm, so this resolution is resolvable.

Comparative Power Output

The test for comparative power output determines whether the sound beam emitted by the transducer can reach a depth adequate to see deep structures (Figs. 54-5 and 54-6). The test is performed at full power output (in Fig. 54-5 the highest power output is 0 db), and the time gain compensation (TGC) is set at maximum at the area of depth visualization. The measurement is taken from the top to the deepest area at which good information is still obtained. In Fig. 54-5 the deepest area satisfactorily imaged is 73.5-mm (7.35-cm) deep. This model of the RMI phantom had an attenuation factor of 0.7 db/cm/MHz, and the transducer used had a frequency of 5 MHz. These numbers are used to determine the output capabilities of the system with this transducer. The comparative power output can be calculated as follows:

Attenuation factor (0.7) $\times$ Depth (7.35) $\times$ Transducer frequency (5) = 25.725 db

This number is recorded in the quality control logbook as the output for this transducer using this phantom. Repeat tests should give the same result.

SELECTED READING

Hykes, D. L., Hendrick, W. R., Milavickas, L. R., and Starchman, D. E. Quality assurance for real-time ultrasound equipment. *JDMS* 2: 121–133, 1986.

Kremkau, F. *Diagnostic Ultrasound: Physical Principles and Exercises* (3rd ed.). New York: Grune & Stratton, 1994.

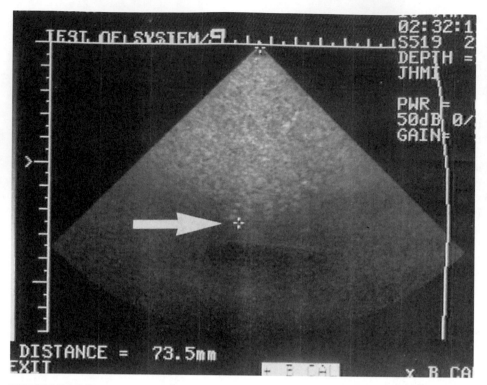

FIGURE 54-5. Image showing the depth at which structures can be viewed with a sector scan transducer (7.4 cm) (arrow).

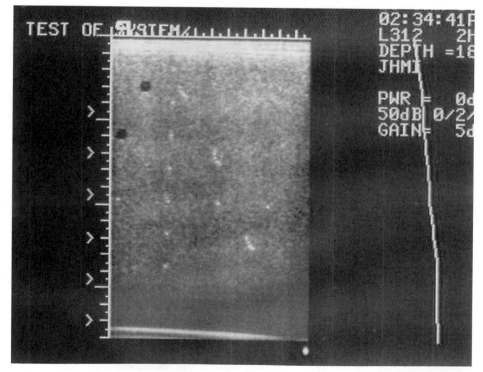

FIGURE 54-6. Linear array view showing the depth at which a satisfactory image can be obtained.

55 PHOTOGRAPHY

ROGER C. SANDERS, MIMI MAGGIO SAYLOR

KEY WORDS

Brightness. Controls the intensity of the CRT background.

Cathode Ray Tube (CRT). The sonographic image is displayed on the screen of a cathode ray tube. A second CRT displays the image for the multiformat camera.

Contrast. Controls the amount of gray-level echoes seen, that is, how many medium-level and low-level echoes are visible.

F-stop. Controls the aperture of the lens; the wider the aperture, the more light is presented to the film, but the lower the f-stop number.

Time (T). Sets the time interval of exposure (e.g., 0.5 second, 1 second).

PHOTOGRAPHIC SYSTEMS

Several different methods of recording the image are in use; each has virtues and disadvantages.

Polaroid Camera

Polaroid has the following advantages: the camera is cheap and easy to use, film development is rapid, and resolution is almost as good as that with the CRT image. However, the film is costly, fades with time, and is difficult to store. Camera settings are not easy to maintain. With approximately three patients a day and an average number of films, one can save the price of a multiformat camera during the course of a year by not using Polaroid film.

Thermal-Sensitive Paper Printer

A cheaper alternative to Polaroids is the paper printer that utilizes durable thermal paper. The camera operates much like the multiformat cameras with brightness and contrast controls. No processor is required. Image quality is good. Color images can be recorded.

At the time of writing, the cost of an image on a printer was one tenth the cost of a Polaroid image and a sheet of x-ray film cost about twice as much as a Polaroid image. Each sheet of film may contain four to nine images. Images recorded on thermal paper start to decay after about 6 months.

Multiformat Cameras

Multiformat cameras have the following advantages: they use relatively cheap film, the film is easy to store and view, and exposures are relatively easy to set. However, the initial purchase of a multiformat camera is expensive, a processor is required, and personnel are needed to handle the film, chemicals, and so on.

Multiformat cameras come with various features, some of which are well worth having. The smaller and more compact versions are as cheap as the larger systems and are preferable because they can be placed on a portable real-time system. One feature that is unimportant is whether the system is "on axis" (i.e., whether the lens lines up with the CRT image directly). A variable-format system is not of much practical importance because the sonographer almost always uses the same settings (usually six on one film). This format displays an image of satisfactory size, but putting nine images on one film provides optimum cost savings. Processing systems are now available which do not require a darkroom or additional chemicals. These "dry" systems are expensive.

There are several important features to consider in your choice of a multiformat camera:

1. Rapid exposure time
2. Compact size
3. A method of preventing double exposure
4. Convenient brightness and contrast controls (not buried inside the camera)
5. A "flat-face" screen (which means that a measurement at the periphery of the image will be reliable)

"Laser" multiformat cameras yield a consistent quality image because they compensate for poor quality image settings. They are very expensive.

35-Millimeter Camera

Cameras using 35-mm film are cheaper than multiformat cameras but less convenient. The advantages of these systems are that the film and camera are very inexpensive. More than six exposures can be made without changing the film or cassette. However, the system needs a processor. Film can be wasted when you want to photograph and view the images from a single patient because the roll of film could take many more pictures.

PACs Systems

Image acquisition to a computer is practical because new hard drives can accommodate gigabytes of data. An acquisition box connected to the ultrasound system accumulates images which are downloaded to a central computer. Image quality is excellent when the images are reviewed. Benefits of this type of system are the absence of lost films, long-term economies since no film is used, and the ability to process the image on the computer. Theoretically, comparison of ultrasound with other imaging techniques such as computed tomography and magnetic resonance imaging at the same level could be helpful.

Practical difficulties with a system of this type include frequent system failure and difficulty printing out images when they are requested by clinicians or when they are needed at another site. Comparing images from a current series with previous studies requires several display facilities. Retrieval of earlier images may be tedious unless a "juke box" is available for the optical disks on which information is stored. Since there is no standardization of computer image acquisition,

initial high expense and inability to exchange images are other drawbacks.

Videotape

Some advocate videotaping all examinations. This makes the examination difficult to view at a later date because videotape review is lengthy.

Videotapes decay with time unless they are reexamined at biannual intervals.

SETTING UP THE CAMERA

Setting the photographic controls on the ultrasound system is one of the most important and difficult parts of obtaining a satisfactory long-term record of the examination. Subtle changes in brightness and contrast greatly alter the image. Although observation of the graybars helps in setting up the image, a clinical scan showing an area such as the liver and kidney, where there are both high-level and low-level echoes, is of more value. A tissue equivalent phantom that has pseudometastatic and pseudocystic lesions within it can also be used.

Multiformat Camera Set-Up

Warm-up time adjustments may be avoided by making sure that the scanner and multiformat camera have been turned on a half hour before they are adjusted or used. Most multiformat cameras will not allow an image to be photographed until the camera is warmed up.

Practical Maneuvers

1. Lower the background and contrast all the way. Select the mode (black or white background) for display.
2. Find the optimal background display by changing the brightness level. Fine-tune settings with no image on the screen until you see an acceptable background for white or black imaging. Note the setting.
3. Put graybars on the screen. Move the contrast to a level at which all graybars can be seen at the same time, keeping the background brightness at an optimal level, perhaps by reducing the brightness slightly.
4. Obtain a good-quality image of the liver and right kidney on a longitudinal view; include a gallbladder with some artifactual echoes, and see if you can reproduce those low-level echoes.

5. Now vary the contrast and compensate with the brightness until you achieve an optimal setting. Photograph each setting, and record the different levels. Unfortunately, both controls usually need to be varied at the same time.
6. Once the ideal photographic settings have been obtained, lock and record them (Fig. 55-1). It takes time to set up a camera correctly; a casual knob-fiddler can destroy an hour's work.
7. Multiformat cameras are not very sturdy and can easily malfunction if mistreated. An important part of practical maintenance is keeping the air filters clean (check daily for dust accumulation). Do not put the multiformat camera in too confined a space because it tends to overheat. The internal monitor must be adjusted periodically to maintain optimum photographic capability.

Polaroid Camera

Technique is different on Polaroid cameras; the f-stop and time (shutter speed) must be adjusted. The f-stop on Polaroid cameras has an opposite effect on exposure from that in a multiformat camera because the Polaroid image is a positive image. A decrease in the f-stop number brightens the picture. Polaroid camera set-up includes adjusting the camera CRT to display an acceptable image and then varying the f-stop and time to capture the image properly on film.

Ideally, only one variable should be changed at a time (i.e., the background is adjusted for optimum brightness and the contrast is then varied for proper echo levels superimposed on this brightness level), but this is not entirely practical. The adjustment of either brightness or contrast could change the background.

Maintenance of Polaroid cameras requires cleaning the rollers with an alcohol swab on a daily basis. The rollers are easily detachable from most Polaroid cameras. Do not unwrap Polaroid film before it is to be used because humidity and heat decrease the sensitivity of the film. Develop the film within a few minutes. If the film is left undeveloped for longer than this, it adheres to the film back. Pull the Polaroid tab straight through the rollers or streaks may appear on the image and paper segments may break off in the rollers.

Thermal-Sensitive Paper

Thermal-sensitive paper printers require special maintenance procedures. Dust and dirt can collect on the thermal printing head. A head cleaning sheet is usually provided. If the thermal head overheats, prints may come out totally black. Allow the temperature of the printing head to drop by not printing, then continue. When the printer is suddenly exposed to a temperature change, moisture may condense inside the unit and the paper can adhere to the roller, causing a jam. Let the printer dry out for a couple of hours and then pull the paper out gently.

FILM CHOICE AND STORAGE

Film

There is a choice of film that can be used with multiformat cameras. All manufacturers make both a film with a clear base and one with a blue-green base. We prefer the clear base because we think there is a chance that low-level echoes may be overlooked against a blue-green background, but many feel that the blue-green format is more attractive.

Silver-Coated Paper

Some systems use standard multiformat cameras but use silver-coated paper instead of film. Because paper cannot be viewed through a viewbox, this system is cumbersome for teaching large groups. However, this method is acceptable if showing the image to an audience is not part of your practice, because paper is inexpensive and is easily stored.

Thermal-Sensitive Paper

Store paper rolls in a cool, dry area away from heat and sunlight. Printed images are said to last approximately 5 years if kept in a clear plastic case. The print could be damaged if brought into contact with solvent such as alcohol.

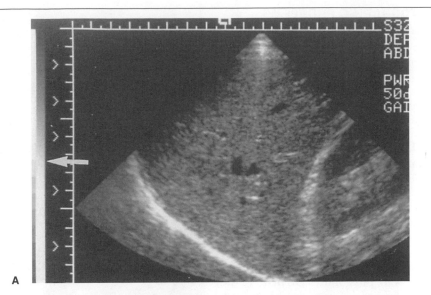
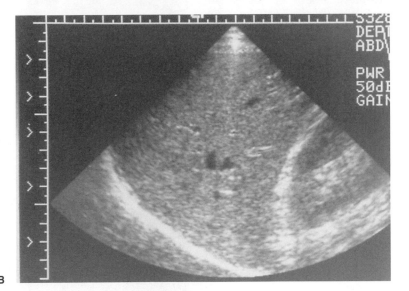
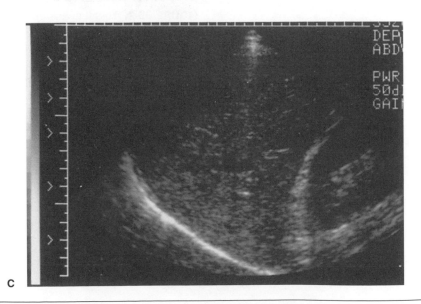

FIGURE 55-1. Obtaining correct photographic settings. (**A**) A satisfactory photographic image. Note the gray scale bars (arrow). (**B**) Excessive brightness. Compare the gray scale bars with those in A. (**C**) Incorrect contrast settings with suboptimal gray scale bar display.

PHOTOGRAPHIC PROBLEMS

1. *Fogging* along the edge of the film may occur (Fig. 55-2). Either the cassette has not been pushed completely into the multiformat camera or there is a light leak along one edge of the cassette. Cassettes are fragile and develop light leaks with rough usage.

2. There may be *white marks* on the film (when using white-on-black mode) that appear in the same place on sequential films (Fig. 55-3). Dust is present on the camera lens or on the CRT face. Clean the camera.

3. The *film won't expose,* although it seems to be in a good position. Push the cassette properly into its housing.

4. The film may be *unexpectedly dark or light.* The possibilities are that (1) the multiformat camera or ultrasound system has not warmed up; (2) the wrong type of film is in the cassette; (3) the processor has not been warmed up (is the film damp?); (4) the developing mixture is wrong; or (5) someone has altered the camera settings.

5. If the processed image is crisscrossed with *diagonal lines* (Fig. 55-4), the horizontal hold of the CRT is out of adjustment. You won't be aware of this unless you look at the camera monitor.

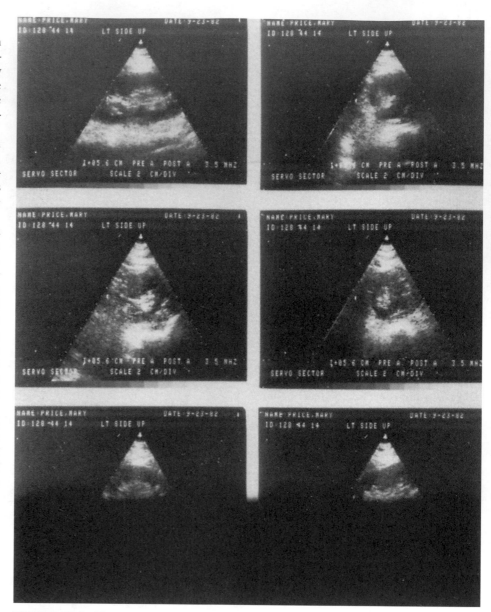

FIGURE 55-2. This film has been partially exposed to light at the bottom. Check the cassette for cracks and light leaks.

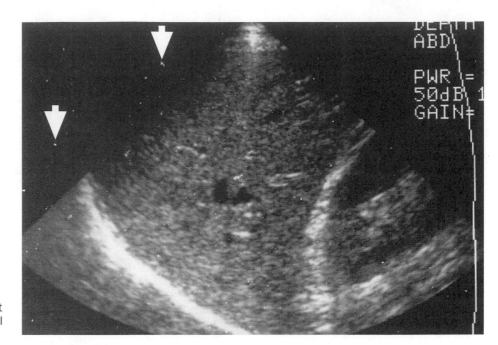

FIGURE 55-3. White marks due to dust on the CRT will appear on sequential films in the same area.

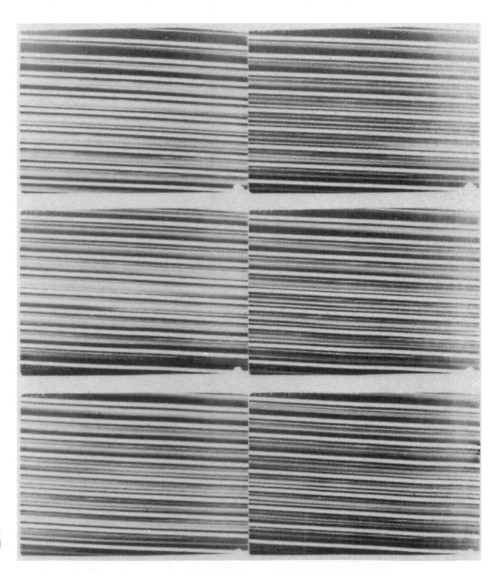

FIGURE 55-4. Diagonal linear artifact usually due to defective horizontal hold on the CRT.

56 NURSING PROCEDURES

DEROSHIA B. STANLEY

KEY WORDS

Ambu Bag. A bag used for emergency inflation of the lungs through a face mask.

Body Mechanics. The use of the human body as a machine. Performed properly, body mechanics aid in the safe movement of people and objects.

CPR Barrier Device. Various devices such as an ambu bag and a mask with a one-way valve which allow performance of rescue breathing without direct mouth-to-mouth contact.

Effective Communication. The use of spoken words, body language, and the environment to reduce patient anxiety and obtain patient cooperation and satisfaction.

Fowler's Position. A sitting position.

Handwashing. The reduction of microorganisms on the hands through the use of water, soap, and friction. It is the single most important aspect of infection control.

High Filtration Mask. A nose/mouth mask worn when providing direct care to a patient with active tuberculosis.

Infiltration. If an intravenous needle becomes dislocated from the vein, fluid continues to infuse into the soft tissues. This mishap is termed infiltration.

Mask with a One-Way Valve. Device that allows performance of mouth-to-mouth resuscitation without the risk that the stomach contents of the dying patient may return into your mouth.

NPO. Abbreviation for nothing by mouth.

Orthostatic (Postural) Hypotension. Low blood pressure occurring as a result of the patient sitting or standing too quickly. It is commonly experienced in the elderly and patients with significant blood loss. It can cause dizziness and syncope and lead to a fall.

Sims' Position. Semiprone position with one leg flexed.

Stat. A term used when a task has to be done immediately.

Sterile (Aseptic) Technique. A procedure which prevents the contamination or introduction of microorganisms and spores into/onto a person, object, or solution. Sterile technique is required when penetrating the skin and accessing the urinary system.

Universal Precautions. Practices mandated by the Centers for Disease Control and Prevention which reduce the transmission of blood-borne pathogens such as hepatitis B virus and human immunodeficiency virus.

Water Seal. When catheters are placed into the pleural space, there is a risk that if the catheter becomes detached, air may be introduced, causing a tension pneumothorax. To prevent this mishap, catheters are attached to a water-filled bottle.

PATIENT RELATIONS

Nursing care is an important aspect of patient service. A patient has physical, emotional, and cultural needs. The sonographer, therefore, must not only obtain the best scans possible, but also provide a level of nursing care that promotes patient cooperation and satisfaction.

Effective Communication

Patient cooperation and satisfaction depend on how the patient feels about you. To cultivate a positive feeling, you must demonstrate an understanding and acceptance of the anxiety and possible limitations that a real or potential medical problem can impose on a patient.

The following help demonstrate understanding and acceptance:

1. Address the patient by his or her last name unless the patient is a child.
2. Introduce yourself.
3. Maintain eye contact when speaking.
4. Speak in a positive tone.
5. Avoid distracting or annoying habits, such as chewing gum.
6. Eliminate irrelevant noise.
7. Explain delays as well as procedures.
8. Provide privacy: close the exam room door and drape the patient.
9. Maintain patient confidentiality.
10. Apologize when necessary.
11. If necessary, assist the patient with hygienic needs.

Patient Hygiene

Dressing and Undressing the Patient

The patient who has limited mobility in an extremity may require your help to change into the gown. To remove clothes easily, start with the patient's unaffected extremity and proceed to the affected one; reverse the order to redress.

Bedpan Assistance

Direct (or assist) the patient who needs to evacuate to the nearest toilet or provide the patient with a bedpan (Fig. 56-1) or urinal. Wear gloves (and gown if necessary) when assisting the patient. When applicable, measure and record intake and output (I&O). To position a regular bedpan (see Fig. 56-1), tell the patient to raise his or her buttocks. Slide the bedpan (the broad flat end toward the sacrum) under the buttocks. Tell the patient to lower buttocks onto the bedpan (the high narrow end should be visible under the upper thighs). If the patient is unable to raise the buttocks, turn the patient onto his or her side, place the bedpan, and adjust if necessary. To simulate the normal position of evacuation, elevate the head of the stretcher unless it is contraindicated.

The elderly patient, debilitated patient, or patient in traction may need a fracture bedpan (see Fig. 56-1); the use of this bedpan requires very minimal patient movement. To position a fracture bedpan, use the same technique as for a regular bedpan, except place the flat narrow end under the patient's sacrum and the handle end under the patient's upper thighs for easy removal.

After placing a female patient on a bedpan, tell her to part her thighs slightly to prevent the deflection of any urine. Stabilize the bedpan when removing it from under the patient. Once it is removed, cover and dispose of contents as soon as possible. If necessary, clean the patient's perineal area from urethral meatus to anus. Remove gloves (and gown) and wash hands.

Urinal Assistance

When assisting a male patient with a urinal, wear gloves. Hold the urinal by the handle and use the rim to lift and place the penis within. Advance the urinal along the shaft of the penis, then rest it between the patient's thighs. After use, remove the urinal, cover, and empty as soon as possible. Remove gloves and wash hands.

Patient Preparation

Drinking Liquids

Consider where your patient is going after the sonogram: if to surgery (r/o ectopic pregnancy) or another test that requires them to be NPO (r/o gallstones, epigastric pain, etc.), then drinking to fill the bladder may be inappropriate. Catheterizing an emergency patient is an option if questions cannot be answered by endovaginal scanning. Rescheduling the exam may be necessary for others.

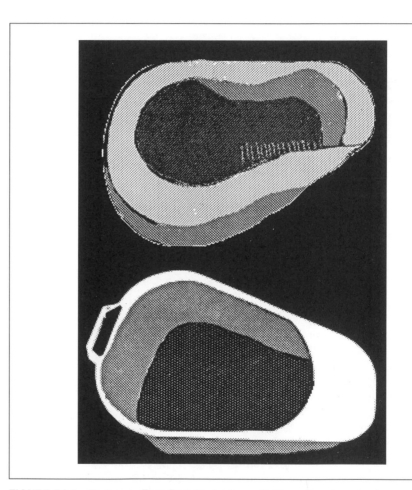

FIGURE 56-1. Bedpans. Top: Regular bedpan. Bottom: Fracture bedpan.

CLAMP THE PATIENT'S INDWELLING URINARY RETENTION CATHETER. Before clamping the catheter, check the patient's diagnosis and medical history. If he or she has a urinary tract infection (UTI), recent renal transplant, paraplegia, or bladder spasms, do not clamp the catheter. Providing there are no contraindications, clamp the catheter using a Hoffman clamp or a padded straight forceps (Fig. 56-2) (these clamps will not puncture the catheter). Check the patient for bladder distention or discomfort every 20 to 30 minutes. Unclamp the catheter once the scan is completed.

INCREASE THE RATE OF THE PATIENT'S INTRAVENOUS (IV) INFUSION. Prior to increasing the flow rate of an IV solution, obtain permission from the patient's physician. Diseases affecting fluid and electrolyte balance and solutions containing medications may contraindicate this method. After increasing the rate, tell the patient to notify you when he or she feels the urge to void. Once a full bladder is present, reduce the rate. While the IV solution is infusing rapidly, monitor the patient for fluid overload. If he or she experiences headache, difficulty breathing, or lightheadedness, reduce the rate. If symptoms persist or worsen, notify the physician or nurse.

FILL THE PATIENT'S BLADDER THROUGH A CATHETER. If the patient does not have a catheter, the bladder may be catheterized by the physician or nurse. Retrograde filling of the bladder carries the risk of contamination and urinary tract infection, therefore, adhere to sterile technique when preparing the set-up.

1. Connect irrigation tubing to a bag of irrigation saline (0.9 percent sodium chloride).
2. Position the roller clamp under the drip chamber and close it.
3. Suspend the solution bag and squeeze the drip chamber several times to fill it.
4. Open the clamp and purge the tubing of air by allowing some of the saline to flow through; close the clamp.
5. Clamp the catheter (see Fig. 56-2) and disconnect the urinary drainage bag. Wrap the exposed end of the drainage bag tubing inside an alcohol wipe or sterile 4 × 3 gauze and lay it aside.

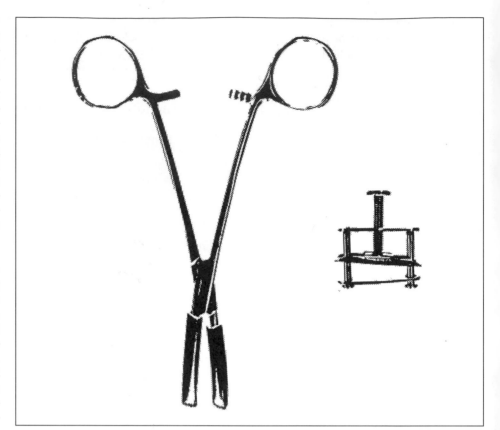

FIGURE 56-2. Clamps. Left: Hoffman. Right: Padded Halsted (gauze can also be used for padding).

6. Connect the irrigation set to the catheter and unclamp both. Allow the saline to flow into the bladder gradually.
7. Once the bladder is full, close the tubing clamp and perform scan.
8. After scanning, decompress the bladder by lowering the bag below the level of the bladder. Open the tubing clamp thus allowing drainage. To prevent the possibility of an inaccuracy in a patient's I&O measurement, drain the same amount of fluid that was instilled.

Water Enema

When the distinction between a pelvic mass and colon is unclear, a water enema may be needed.

1. Close the clamp on an enema bag and fill the bag with 500 to 700 cc warm water. Purge the tubing of air by allowing some of the water to flow through and reclamp.
2. Place the patient in the Sims' position (on left side with right knee bent and left leg straight).

3. Liberally lubricate the tip of the enema tubing. Unless contraindicated, lidocaine jelly may be used as a lubricant to ease discomfort.
4. Separate the patient's buttocks to see the anus.
5. Angle the enema tip toward the patient's umbilicus and gently insert and advance it 3 to 4 inches into the rectum. To help the patient relax the abdominal muscles, instruct him or her to breath deeply and slowly through the mouth. If you feel resistance while inserting the tip, reangle or allow a little of the water to flow through. If resistance is still felt, stop and notify the sonologist or nurse.
6. Once the tip is inserted, tape it in place. Tell the patient to tighten the anal sphincter to help retain the water.
7. Position the patient supine and unclamp the tubing. Allow the water to flow in gradually.
8. After scanning, direct (or assist) the patient to a toilet or provide a bedpan.

Fatty Meal

To properly examine the gallbladder and common bile duct, the patient should not eat anything 5 to 6 hours before the scan. This helps to ensure that the gallbladder will be distended. Clear liquids such as water and jello are permitted.

If the initial scan shows a greatly dilated gallbladder or a mildly dilated common bile duct, Neo Cholex or another liquid fatty agent may be given to the patient by mouth to stimulate gallbladder contraction or bowel excretion. If the patient is not permitted anything by mouth, cholecystokinin (CCK) may be administered IV. Nausea and vomiting are common transient adverse effects of Neo Cholex and CCK. After administering the agent, rescan the gallbladder in 15 to 20 minutes.

Drug Administration

With the exception of a "fatty meal," very few diagnostic or contrast agents are administered as a part of ultrasonography. If you are required to administer any drugs to a patient, follow these guidelines:

1. Obtain a doctor's order.
2. Prepare the correct drug by reading the label on the container three times: when taking the container off the shelf, while preparing the dose, and when discarding or returning the container.
3. Prepare the correct dose by having a conversion chart or table of equivalents available.
4. Identify the patient by checking the ID bracelet or asking his or her name (as opposed to saying "Are you Mrs. X?").
5. Check the patient's allergy history.
6. Administer the drug at the correct time and by the correct route.
7. Document the administration in the patient's medical record.

BODY MECHANICS

Many scans can be performed with the patient on the transport stretcher but regardless of how a patient arrives, proper transport, transfer, and positioning techniques help to ensure patient safety and handling. Proper body mechanics decrease the risk of injury, increase comfort, and conserve energy for yourself as well as the patient.

Transport

When transporting a patient, reduce personal back strain and protect the patient's head from possible injury. Push a wheelchair from the handles and a stretcher from the two adjacent corners nearest to the patient's head. Walk beside an ambulatory patient and, if needed, hold his or her arm to provide support and guidance.

Transfer

Prior to transferring a patient onto the exam table, assess his or her ability to assist with the move, then decide on the best method of transfer. Guidelines to follow are as follows:

1. Transfer across the shortest distance; place a wheelchair as close to the exam table as possible, and place a stretcher level with the table and against it.
2. Stabilize the transport vehicle and exam table; lock the brakes; raise the footrests on a wheelchair.

3. Do not permit a patient to climb onto the exam table; place a stepstool beside the table, turn the patient's back toward the table, and tell the patient to step onto the stepstool from the side.
4. Support, if necessary, the patient's head or neck, spine, and/or legs during a transfer; do not permit the patient to support himself or herself by holding the back of your neck.
5. When returning a patient from an exam table to a wheelchair, tell the patient to sit momentarily on the side of the table to avoid orthostatic hypotension. If the patient stands suddenly, his or her blood pressure may drop, causing dizziness and loss of balance, which could lead to a fall.
6. Use the two-carrier lift (Fig. 56-3) to transfer the patient who cannot stand.
7. Before leaving a patient alone, secure the safety straps and railings. Place a call bell within reach.

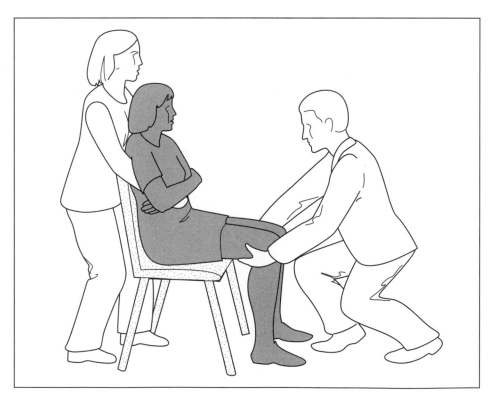

FIGURE 56-3. The two-carrier lift. Place patient's arms across his or her chest; bend your knees slightly and place your arms around the patient's chest and knees. On signal, lift the patient and place on stretcher.

Positioning

Occasionally, limb restraints are necessary to aid positioning or protect the patient and others from harm. Before applying restraints, obtain a doctor's order and explain the need to the patient. Pad the skin to protect it from possible abrasions. Secure the restraint to the stretcher or exam table frame out of the patient's grasp and in a way that allows for quick release and removal in case of an emergency. Restraints should be loose enough to allow adequate circulation to the extremity. Signs and symptoms of impaired circulation include an absent or weak pulse, coldness, numbness, burning, tingling, cyanosis (or pallor), and edema in the affected extremity.

INFECTION CONTROL

Many different patients with various illnesses are scanned daily on the same system so there is a hazard of cross infections. Hospital acquired (nosocomial) infections are especially dangerous because they prolong hospitalization and may increase morbidity.

Handwashing

Touch is the predominant mode of microbial transmission; therefore, effective handwashing is crucial to infection control. Wearing exam gloves does not replace the need for handwashing.

Hands should be washed frequently: between patients, after toileting or blowing your nose, before setting up sterile procedures, before preparing drugs, and whenever else you deem necessary. Lather and wash hands for at least 10 to 15 seconds. After washing your hands, turn off the faucet using a paper towel.

Transducer Care

The probe and stand-off pad should be disinfected after each use. Use isopropyl alcohol, 70 percent, or follow manufacturer's or institution's recommendations. Wipe the probe several times to thoroughly clean it. Prior to using an endoprobe, cover it with a disposable sheath, such as a condom. After use, discard the sheath, wipe off the couplant, and disinfect the endoprobe by immersing it in an activated glutaraldehyde solution such as Cidex for a minimum of 10 minutes. (Do not immerse the cable connection.) Use a longer period if gross contamination occurs, but do not exceed 10 hours. Do not sterilize transducers using gas sterilization, ultraviolet sterilization, dry heat sterilization, autoclaving, or soaking in chlorine bleach. After immersion, rinse the endoprobe thoroughly with tap water and dry it (see Appendix 33).

Sanitation

Use an acceptable disinfectant for routine cleaning of counters, tables, technical units, and probe cables. To prevent dust and dirt accumulation (which may harbor spores), cover bedpans and urinals until they are emptied, then rinse and dispose of them properly. Handle soiled linen gently to avoid spreading microorganisms.

Isolation Precautions

Because you cannot be certain whether a patient is infected with the human immunodeficiency virus (HIV), which is responsible for acquired immunodeficiency syndrome (AIDS), or hepatitis B virus (HBV), blood and body fluid precautions or Universal Precautions are recommended for use with everyone. Always wear gloves when there is a possibility of coming in contact with any blood or body fluid. When splattering may occur, wear a gown, mask, and goggles. Do not recap, clip, or bend needles or blades; place them directly into a designated and impervious container from which they cannot be removed. Precautions instituted for other means of transmission as well as Universal Precautions are outlined in Table 56-1.

When requested to do a portable scan on a patient in isolation, consult with the patient's nurse before entering the room.

TABLE 56-1. REQUIRED ELEMENTS FOR PRECAUTION CATEGORIES

	Universal	AFB	Strict	Contact	Contact w/ Mask	RSV
Mask	fluid splatter	yes*	yes	no	close to patient	
Goggles	fluid splatter	no	no	no	no	no
Gown	fluid splatter	no	yes	contact with patient	contact with patient	contact with patient
Gloves	contact with blood or body fluid	no	yes	contact with infected material	contact with infected material	yes
Probe cover	contact with blood or body fluid	no	yes	yes	yes	yes
Disposable Items: Biohazard bag	soiled with blood or body fluid	sputum	yes	soiled with infected material	soiled with infected material	sputum
Linen	Place in moisture resistant laundry bag in room					
Disinfect Equipment Supplies	yes — Use Wescodyne (povidone–iodine) or Sodium Hypochlorite .05% (bleach solution) →					
Specimens	← Place in special transport bags →					
Handwashing	yes ← Use Chlorhexidine gluconate →					

*Requires a high filtration mask

Sterile Techniques

Procedures that pierce the skin or mucosa and those that invade the urinary tract or vascular system demand the use of sterile techniques (Table 56-2) to prevent contamination and possible infection.

Skin Prep

The skin is the body's first line of defense against microbes. A percutaneous invasive procedure such as a biopsy, drainage, or aspiration requires the skin to be cleaned with a povidone-iodine solution and isopropyl alcohol, 70 percent (do not use alcohol on mucous membranes). A sterile drape is then placed around the site to create a sterile field. After the procedure, cover the puncture site with a Band-Aid or sterile gauze dressing.

Scanning for guidance during a sterile procedure is often required. To scan within a sterile field, (1) wear sterile gloves; (2) use a sterile acoustic couplant that is hypoallergenic and easily removed; and (3) use a probe that has been rendered sterile.

Probe Sterilization Techniques

GAS STERILIZATION. Equipment other than transducers may be sterilized by ethylene oxide gas. The equipment remains sterile until the integrity of the package is compromised or the date expires. Gas sterilization takes at least 24 to 48 hours.

TABLE 56-2. PRINCIPLES OF SURGICAL ASEPSIS

Field	Dry Items	Solutions	Non-Scrubbed Person	Scrubbed Person
Prepare as close as possible to time of use. Do not leave it unattended. Open and place sterile drape over table to create a sterile field (handle edges only). Consider edges unsterile. Any item extending off the field is contaminated and removed. Cover contaminated area with sterile folded drape.	Open wrapped item distal, lateral, lateral, proximal. Open pouched items by "peeling down" from the top. Consider edge of pouch contaminated; do not allow item to touch edge. Consider a sterile item that has been touched by an unsterile item/person contaminated. Keep handling of pouch to a minimum (pressure forces sterile air out and replaces it with room air).	Do not discard antiseptics/disinfectants unless expired, contaminated, or left open. Before pouring into a sterile container, pour off some; pour with label facing you. Lay caps/lids/tops down with the insides facing up. Date multiple dose vials on initial use; discard within 30 days unless an earlier expiration is indicated. Prep the entry site of vial with alcohol wipe before inserting the needle. Discard hydrogen peroxide 7 days after opening. Discard solutions without preservatives (irrigation saline/water) 24 hours after initial use.	Open sterile packages and flip items onto field. Pour solution into sterile containers and avoid splashing. Refrain from reaching over field. Do not turn back to field. Face field when passing and allow one foot of margin safety. Keep exam room door/curtain closed.	Must wear sterile gloves (gown is optional). Put gown on first then gloves. Don gown —Open wrap. —Lift gown by neck, gently shake loose. —Slide arms into sleeves. —Have non-scrubbed person secure ties. Face field when passing. Avoid leaning over an unsterile area. Don gloves —Peel down pouch. —Remove inner wrap. —Expose gloves by pulling back flaps. —Pick up first glove at the fold of cuff. —Hold the opposite hand palm up and slide into glove. —Using the gloved hand, pick up the second glove by slipping fingers under the edge of cuff. —Palm up, slide hand inside glove. —Adjust for proper fit. —Cuffs must extend over cuffs of gown. Keep hands above waist and in front of chest.

PROBE IMMERSION. Immerse the probe for a minimum of 10 hours in an activated glutaraldehyde solution (do not immerse the cable connection). Don sterile gloves; remove and rinse the probe using sterile water. Wrap and seal the probe in a double-folded sterile towel. The probe remains sterile only a few hours.

STERILE PLASTIC COVERS. With the exception of some needle guide transducers, most probes can be rendered sterile by using sterile covers. After placing a sterile cover onto a sterile field, don sterile gloves. Open the sterile probe cover and allow an unscrubbed person to put couplant inside the cover (or the couplant may be put directly on the probe). The unscrubbed person then places the probe within the cover. Unfold the sterile cover over the probe and secure it with a rubber band or tie (Fig. 56-4). An unscrubbed person can place sterile gel inside the bag or on the probe before covering; keep a supply of sterilized rubber bands on hand to keep the bag tight around the transducer face so air won't interfere with the image (see Fig. 56-4). Remember that the cable will drag across the sterile field, so decide whether it is necessary to put a sterile "sleeve" or stockinette over it.

STERILE BARRIER. To scan over a fresh or recent postoperative site, such as a renal transplant wound, a sterile gel-film skin barrier (Fig. 56-5) may be used. The skin barrier eliminates the need for a sterile probe and sterile acoustic couplant. Handle the skin barrier by the edges and extend it at least 1 inch beyond the periphery of the wound.

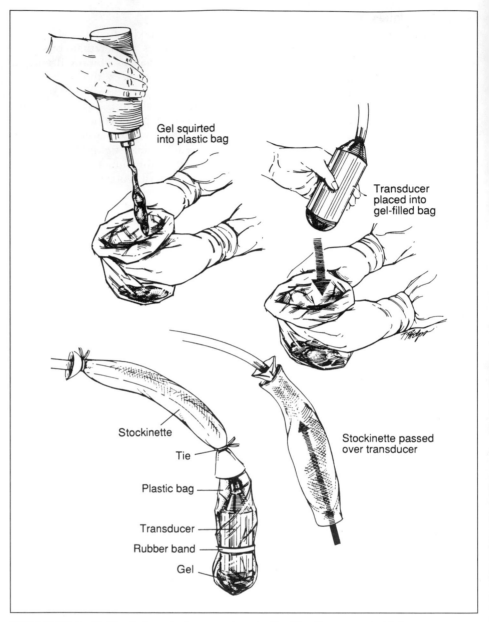

Gel squirted into plastic bag

Transducer placed into gel-filled bag

Stockinette passed over transducer

Stockinette

Tie

Plastic bag

Transducer

Rubber band

Gel

FIGURE 56-4. Method of rendering a probe sterile. Sterile covers (which are commercially available in various sizes) can be fabricated from 6 × 3 × 15-inch plastic bags as shown. Application of sterile covers: The sterile bag is folded open; fingers are placed under the fold. Gel (sufficient to cover probe face) is squirted into the bag away from the seam. The probe is placed onto the gel inside the bag. The bag is rolled over the probe and secured. Sterile stockinette, if needed, is slipped over bag to cable and secured. (Reprinted with permission of Raven Press, from The nurse's role in ultrasound, *Ultrasound Quarterly* 7(1) : 73–104, 1989.)

If a sterile dressing impedes your ability to scan around an area, remove the dressing (unless contraindicated) and apply another one afterwards. Remove suture strips only after consulting with the patient's physician or nurse; this is usually unnecessary.

INTRAVENOUS THERAPY

The care of an IV line (Fig. 56-6) is the responsibility of the sonographer while the patient is in the ultrasound division. The constant flow of solution into a vein carries the risk of contaminants being flushed directly into the patient's body; and the insertion site acts as an entry site for microbes. Problems that may occur with an IV line are as follows:

1. The line may inadvertently become disconnected.
2. The line may "run dry."
3. The IV device may clot.

Check the patient's IV line before, during, and after scanning.

Infusion Rate

The flow of a solution is checked by observing the drip rate in the chamber (on the administration set). Confirm a "wide open" or very rapid rate with the patient's nurse. If the solution is not dripping, check the clamp and stopcock. If they are open, eliminate any kinks or sharp bends in the tubing that could be impeding the flow, and/or raise the height of the container. If the clamp or stopcock is closed, another solution may be infusing into the same IV device. If there is none, notify the nurse.

An infusion pump is used for an IV solution that requires strict monitoring. The pump regulates the flow. When various problems occur, they are displayed and an alarm sounds. To avoid the low battery alarm, keep the pump plugged in when possible.

Check the fluid level in the container. If the level is under 100 cc, notify the patient's nurse. If the container is empty, close the roller clamp and notify the nurse unless instructed otherwise. If a container breaks, immediately close the clamp at a point closest to the insertion site, then notify the nurse.

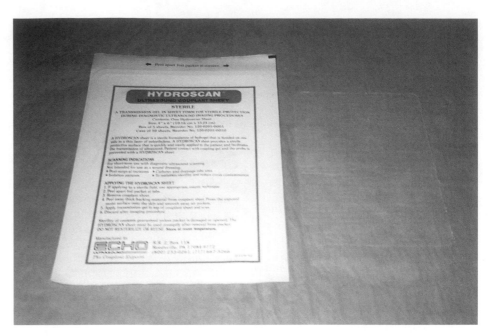

FIGURE 56-5. "Hydroscan Ultrasound Couplant Sheet, 4 × 6 inches, are distributed by Echo Ultrasound; Reedsville, PA."

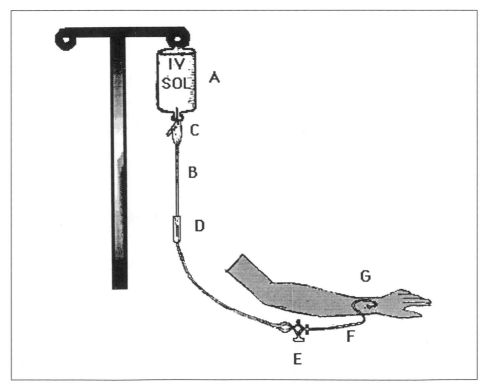

FIGURE 56-6. An IV line. (**A**) Solution. (**B**) Administration set. (**C**) Drip chamber. (**D**) Clamp. (**E**) Fourway stopcock. (**F**) Extension tubing. (**G**) Insertion site.

IV Disconnection

When handling the IV line, avoid putting tension on it. Tension may cause the line to disconnect or the device to dislodge. The following guidelines should be observed:

1. Do not allow IV tubing to dangle near the wheels of a transport vehicle; it could become entangled with the wheels.
2. Avoid having the patient sit or lie on the IV. When transferring the patient, keep the tubing in front of or beside the patient.
3. Keep the IV pole close to the insertion site.
4. The primary responsibility, should a line disconnect, is to prevent solution and blood loss. When an administration set disconnects from an extension tubing, clamp both. If the exposed ends did not touch the floor or other soiled surface, and air did not enter the extension tubing, wipe both ends with an alcohol wipe or povidone-iodine solution and reconnect. If tubing disconnects from the hub of an IV device, clamp the tubing and apply pressure over the vein one-half to one inch above the insertion site or insert the tip of a 1 cc syringe into the hub. Notify the nurse.
5. When an IV device is pulled out inadvertently, check it immediately for breakage. If the tip is missing, apply a light tourniquet high on the affected extremity and immobilize the patient. Promptly notify the patient's physician. Apply a sterile dressing over the insertion site; it is usually necessary to apply pressure.

IV Site Care

If a patient complains of pain at the insertion site, inspect it for infiltration and phlebitis. Infiltration occurs when the IV device dislodges from the vein into the tissue. Signs and symptoms include edema (compare muscle mass to the opposite extremity), pain, cool skin over the site, and a wet dressing due to solution leaking out of the site. Clamp off the infusion and notify the nurse.

Phlebitis is inflammation of a vein due to overuse of the vein, rubbing of the device against the vein wall, or irritating drugs (e.g., potassium and antibiotics). Signs and symptoms include redness, warmth, and pain and induration along the course of a vein. Notify the nurse.

CATHETERS AND DRAINAGE TUBINGS

As with an IV line, avoid putting tension on any catheter or tubing that may be attached to the patient. Subsequent disconnections and dislodgements may require the patient to undergo a painful reinsertion or place the patient at risk for a serious complication. Guidelines to follow are similar to those listed under IV Disconnection.

To prevent drainage from backflowing into the patient, do not drape tubings over a side rail, and keep receptacles upright and below or at the level of the site being drained.

If a catheter or tube does fall out, cover the skin site (if applicable) with a sterile gauze dressing and notify the physician or nurse.

Nasogastric/Nasoenteric Tubes

The patient with an NG or NE tube should always be placed in a Fowler's position (head/chest elevated 35 to 90 degrees). When decompression tubes remain off suction or straight drainage for any length of time, the patient may vomit around the tube. If the patient complains of nausea, position him or her in an upright sitting position. If unable to sit, place the patient on the right side with the head elevated 45 degrees. This may relieve pressure on the cardiac sphincter and in case of vomiting prevent aspiration of secretions. Notify the nurse.

Chest and Abdominal Catheter

A disruption in a water seal chest catheter requires immediate correction to prevent the possibility of the patient experiencing a tension pneumothorax. If the receptacle breaks or the tubing disconnects from the catheter, clamp the catheter at a point close to the chest wall. If the catheter falls out, place an occlusive dressing, such as petrolatum gauze, over the site. Elevate the patient's head 45 degrees and notify the physician or nurse.

If a biliary abdominal catheter, surgical drain, or nephrostomy tube falls out, discard it and cover the site with a sterile dressing. Notify the patient's physician or nurse.

OXYGEN THERAPY

When a patient receiving oxygen arrives in the ultrasound division, check the two gauges on the cylinder's regulator. One gauge registers the oxygen pressure; the other, the liter flow per minute. Make a mental note of the liter flow rate, then turn off the oxygen. Disconnect the oxygen tubing from the cylinder and connect it to a regulator that has been inserted into a wall oxygen outlet. Wall regulators have only one gauge which is used for setting the flow rate. Set the gauge to the same rate that was registered on the cylinder regulator.

To eliminate the need to check and possibly replace a cylinder, use wall oxygen whenever it is available. When a cylinder's regulator pressure gauge registers 500 or less, the cylinder will soon need replacing. When both gauges register 0, the cylinder is empty. Call the oxygen therapy division for replacement or notify the nurse.

Humidity may be added to the oxygen delivery system to prevent excessive drying of the mucous membranes. If a distilled water container is attached, keep it upright to prevent spillage. When condensation builds in the aerosol hose, it can prevent the flow of oxygen. Disconnect the hose from the container and the patient's mask. Dump the water and reconnect the hose.

Do not permit anyone to smoke within the vicinity of a patient receiving oxygen; there is a danger of explosion.

INFANT WARMERS

To maintain a premature baby's temperature, he or she is placed in an isolette or a warmer. You may be asked to plug in the warmer or isolette. Refrain from unduly opening the isolette or removing the baby from the warmer. If the scan cannot be performed with the baby in an isolette, maintain the baby's temperature outside the isolette by using a heating lamp. Position the lamp 2½ to 4½ feet from the baby.

EMERGENCIES

Medical emergencies rarely occur during ultrasonic scanning, but when one occurs, you need to be prepared.

General Guidelines

1. Plan ahead; have equipment available or know where to obtain it.
2. Do not leave the patient alone; call out for help.
3. If the patient stops breathing, note the time.
4. Notify the physician; stat page if necessary; tell the operator the type of emergency and your exact location; hang up last.
5. Keep the area clear of spectators; move ultrasound equipment out of the way when a cardiopulmonary resuscitation (CPR) team is coming.
6. Document the emergency in the medical record and, if required, fill out an incident report.
7. Clean and replace the equipment and supplies afterwards.

Syncope (Fainting)

Position the patient supine and loosen tight clothing. Place inhalant ammonia, a respiratory stimulant, under the patient's nose to attempt to arouse him or her.

Insulin Reaction

A diabetic patient required not to eat in preparation for a scan may experience low blood sugar (hypoglycemia). Signs and symptoms occur suddenly and include headache, nervousness, shaking, dizziness, sweating, cold-clammy skin, blurred vision, numbness of lips or tongue, and hunger. Give the patient sugar, such as hard candy or orange juice. If the patient must remain NPO, the physician may request you to prepare dextrose, 50 percent, for IV bolus or glucagon, 1 mg, for subcutaneous or intramuscular injection. Diabetic patients should have early morning appointments when required to be NPO.

Vasvagal Reaction

Patients undergoing transrectal exams, carotid studies, and invasive procedures such as biopsies may experience a decrease in blood pressure and pulse brought on by stimulation of the vagus nerve. Pain or anxiety usually triggers this reaction. Signs and symptoms include pallor, warmth, nausea/vomiting, dizziness, and cold-clammy skin. Immediately stop the procedure and remove the offending device such as the needle or rectal probe. Place a cool damp cloth to the patient's forehead and position him or her supine. Notify the physician or nurse. If the patient does not improve, IV fluids and atropine, 1 mg, may need to be administered.

Seizure

Protect the patient from injury by placing padding under his or her head and removing sharp or hard objects out of the way. Do not restrain the patient. Loosen tight clothing. Observe and time the seizure closely. After the seizure, turn the patient onto the side nearest you and check for breathing. If respirations are absent, open the airway by tilting the head and lifting the chin. If breathing does not resume, initiate CPR.

Cardiac/Respiratory Arrest

Whenever a patient becomes unresponsive, with chest movement barely visible or pulse extremely weak, stat page and initiate cardiopulmonary resuscitation. To eliminate mouth-to-mouth contact when administering breaths, use an ambu bag, resuscitative airway, or mask with a one-way valve. Attend annual CPR training classes to remain current.

SELECTED READING

Aehlert, B. Providing life support: Would you pass the test? Part I. *Nursing 95* 25:50–52, 1995.

Antai-Ontong, D. When your patient is angry. *Nursing 88* 18:44–45, 1988.

Boutotte, J. Protecting yourself against hepatitis B. *Nursing 93* 23:64–65, 1993.

Brider, P. OSHA stiffens bloodborne rules, decrees free hepatitis B vaccine. *AJN* 92:82–84, 1992.

Brider, P. Regs put new legal force behind Universal Precautions. *AJN* 92:82, 84, 1992.

Cahill, M., et al. (Eds.). *Signs and Symptoms. Nurse's Reference Library.* Springhouse, PA: Springhouse Publishing, 1986.

Calianno, C., et al. Oxygen therapy: Giving your patient breathing room. *Nursing 95* 25:33–38, 1995.

Ceron, G., and Rakowski-Reinhardt, A. Action stat! Autonomic dysreflexia. *Nursing 91* 21:33, 1991.

Colizza, D. F. Action stat! Dislodged chest tube. *Nursing 95* 25:33, 1995.

Ehrlich, R. A., and McCloskey, E. D. *Patient Care in Radiology* (4th ed.). St. Louis: Mosby, 1993.

Harrison, A. Easing a patient's anxiety. *Nursing 92* 22:32c–32f, 1992.

Huston, C. J., and Boelman, R. Emergency! Autonomic dysreflexia. *AJN* 95:55, 1995.

Lampmann, L. E. H., and Versteylen, R. J. Hydrogel wound dressing: A versatile aid in troublesome sonography. *Am J Roentgenol* 148:1274, 1987.

Laskowski-Jones, L. First-line emergency care. *Nursing 95* 25:34–43, 1995.

Loeb, S., et al. (Eds.). *Nursing Procedures.* Springhouse, PA: Springhouse Corp., 1992.

Peterson, A., and Drass, J. Managing acute complications of diabetes. *Nursing 91* 21:34–38, 1991.

Reising, D. Acute hypoglycemia. *Nursing 95* 25: 41–48, 1995.

Saver, C. Decoding the ACLS algorithms. *AJN* 24:27–35, 1994.

Seago, K. Scoring a radiology department's niceness factor. *Applied Radiol* 15:49–57, 1986.

Stanley, D. B. The nurse's role in ultrasound. *Ultrasound Quart* 7:73–104, 1989.

Stolley, J. Freeing your patients from restraints. *AJN* 25:26–30, 1995.

Ziemba, S. K. Seizures. *AJN* 25:32, 33, 1995.

57 PRELIMINARY REPORTS

SANDRA L. HUNDLEY, ROGER C. SANDERS

KEY WORDS

Anechoic. Echo free.

Attenuating Lesion. A sound-absorbing lesion.

Contour. The shape and borders of a lesion or organ.

Echogenicity. The number of echoes within a structure.

Echotexture. The arrangement of echoes within tissue.

Posterior Enhancement. Increased echogenicity directly behind a structure.

Preliminary Report. The unofficial report that precedes the final, detailed report.

PRELIMINARY REPORTS

Preliminary reports should give the key sonographic findings so that the clinician does not have to wait for the official dictation to be typed (which may take several days). Immediate action may be indicated by the sonogram findings. Preliminary reports by the sonographer are required when the sonologist is not present at the exam.

Who Writes Them?

Some ultrasound departments are well staffed with physicians who write preliminary reports; others depend on the sonographer. Sonographers entrusted with this task should confine themselves to describing the sonographic findings without offering a conclusion about pathology unless prior physician approval has been obtained.

Typical Reports

Normal Study

LIVER No lesion seen; normal size.

CBD 4 mm (normal for age).

GB No evidence of sludge or calculi. Normal wall thickness.

PANCREAS No abnormality seen. No evidence of dilated ducts or focal lesions.

SPLEEN No focal lesions seen; normal size.

KIDNEYS Right 10 cm. Left 10 cm. No evidence of hydronephrosis, calculi, or mass.

No fluid seen in the abdomen.

Abnormal Study

(The pathologic lesion described is noted here in parentheses.)

LIVER Echopenic region in the right posterior lobe 4 × 5 × 3 cm. (Primary or metastatic lesion in the liver.)

GB Gallstones. Gallbladder wall 5-mm thick. Local tenderness over the gallbladder. (Acute cholecystitis.)

PANCREAS Highly echogenic pancreas with irregular border and calcification. (Chronic pancreatitis.)

KIDNEY Cystic structure at the right lower pole with septation and irregular superior border. (Complex cyst suggesting a neoplasm.)

OB

1. The lateral ventricles are 16 mm at the level of the atrium (top normal 10 mm) with an abnormal shape to the cerebellum and skull. The distance between the posterior elements of the spine is increased, and there is an adjacent cystic area at L3–S1. (Spina bifida with hydrocephalus.)
2. There is a fluid pocket of greater than 8 cm noted. (Polyhydramnios.)
3. There is an anterior placenta that completely/partially covers the internal os. (Placenta previa before or after 20 weeks.)

Pathologic descriptions can be used if there is well-accepted standard terminology and there is not a subjective element involved.

For the clinician, the report gives an indication of relevant sonographic findings without a conclusion about the pathologic diagnosis. (This is considered the physician's privilege/liability/burden.)

The sonologist conveys a clinical opinion in addition to the factual data.

INTERPRETATION AND DOCUMENTATION

Measurements

If the exam includes a description of organs that are measurable, it is good practice to include these measurements in the report. Consistent measurement (e.g., inner to outer, inner to inner, or outer to outer) should be used. The same charts and tables should be used all the time, and the measurements described by the author when the chart was developed must be followed (see Appendixes 2–24).

Established normal measurements may be mentioned in the report. Organs that need measuring on a routine basis include the following:

1. *Kidney*
   a. Length (longest possible length, with even cortex surrounding the sinus).
   b. A-P (perpendicular to the length measurement on the same image).
   c. Width (90 degrees from the length view at the level of renal vein) may be helpful.
2. *Common Bile Duct*
   In the sagittal plane, measured at the point where it crosses anterior to the main portal vein and the hepatic artery. Measure from inner wall to inner wall. Magnify an image before measuring to increase the accuracy.
3. *Uterus*
   a. Length (showing the linear endometrial canal).
   b. A-P (perpendicular to the length measurement on the same image).
   c. Width (obtained at the widest diameter of the uterus, 90 degrees from the length view).
4. *Ovary*
   a. Length (sagittal plane).
   b. A-P (perpendicular to the length measurement on the same image).
   c. Width (90 degrees to the length view, in the transverse plane).
5. *Prostate*
   a. Length (obtained in the sagittal plane).
   b. A-P (perpendicular to the length measurement on the same image).
   c. Width (transverse plane, widest diameter of gland).
6. *Urinary bladder*
   a. Length (greatest length measured postvoid, sagittal plane).
   b. A-P (perpendicular to the length measurement on the same image).
   c. Width (90 degrees to the length view at the widest diameter of the bladder in the transverse plane). Prevoid measurements are given only if your sonologist requests it. Postvoid measurements are required if the patient has prostate problems, urinary tract infections, or neurologic problems.
7. All masses should be measured.

Sonographic Appearances

Organs that need to be evaluated for texture and mentioned in the preliminary report are the liver, kidneys, pancreas, and spleen. Statements of relative echogenicity are acceptable in the preliminary report.

Echogenicity

The echogenicity of an organ can indicate the functional state of that organ. The normal range of echogenicity of abdominal viscera from greatest to least is as follows:

renal sinus → pancreas → spleen → liver → renal cortex → renal medullary (pyramids)

A kidney with echogenicity greater than the adjacent liver or spleen suggests renal pathology, except in the neonate. A pancreas that is less echogenic than the adjacent liver makes one suspicious of acute pancreatitis, except in the small child.

Through Transmission

The echogenicity posterior to a structure or lesion should be mentally quantitated because it relates to the internal composition of that structure. Enhanced echogenicity behind an area of interest usually indicates a fluid-filled structure. Decreased echogenicity posterior to a structure indicates a solid, sound-absorbing lesion.

Contour

DEMARCATION. A structure that is well circumscribed should be described as such; this indicates a confined process with no surrounding tissue invasion. Irregular borders raise the question of tissue intrusion as by inflammation or neoplasm.

SHAPE CHANGES. Note whether a structure appears enlarged or smaller than usual. Changes in shape with time may occur on a physiological basis—for example, the kidney enlarges when fluid is administered. The uterine size changes with puberty, the menstrual cycle, and menopause. Most often, however, shape changes indicate pathology.

WHEN TO TELEPHONE

Findings that require urgent management change should be conveyed to the patient's physician immediately.

1. Strong suspicion of ectopic pregnancy
2. Fetal death
3. Major fetal anomalies
4. Abruptio placentae
5. Markedly abnormal fetal heart rate
6. Leaking aneurysm
7. Unexpected neoplastic mass
8. Unexpected periorgan hematoma
9. Renal artery occlusion in a transplant
10. Obstructed bile ducts
11. Placenta previa if there is vaginal bleeding
12. Unexpected renal obstruction
13. Tendon or muscle tear
14. Undiagnosed deep vein thrombosis
15. Markedly narrowed carotid or limb vessels
16. Incompetent cervix
17. Absent fetal movement and low fluid, especially with marked intrauterine growth restriction
18. Testicular fragmentation by trauma
19. Testicular torsion

Information that is too sensitive for the patient to carry should also prompt a telephone call.

1. Fetal death
2. Fetal anomalies if not discussed with the patient previously
3. Findings indicative of AIDS
4. Neoplastic mass if not discussed with the patient previously

Findings that are subjective in nature may be better conveyed by a phone call.

1. Unexpected absence of fetal movement in the presence of normal measurements
2. Reporting on structures inadequately visualized that are strongly suspicious for pathology, such as the fetal head being deep in the pelvis, but appearing to contain an intracranial abnormality

PITFALLS

Legal Hazards

A preliminary report is not considered legally hazardous as long as the sonographer does not attempt to make a diagnosis. If a sonographer is working for a sonologist, the sonographer is not responsible for errors in the study, providing that the study is performed according to standards set by the sonologist, even if the study is of poor quality. The sonographer is not liable in cases of falsely created pathology. Some examples of misleading findings or wrong technique that are not the sonographer's legal responsibility if uncorrected by the sonologist are the following:

1. Pseudohydronephrosis due to a full urinary bladder
2. Sludge-filled gallbladder due to an overgained image

3. Not following up on a pathologic finding, such as missing hydronephrosis with a pelvic mass
4. Missing a pancreatic mass by not trying different scanning techniques such as erect scanning or having the patient drink to fill the stomach to create an acoustic window
5. Missing stones in the gallbladder or kidneys due to a failure to use a high-frequency transducer

Although the sonographer is not legally responsible for these errors, the sonographer is morally and ethically responsible for the consequences of these types of misdiagnoses.

The sonologist is not legally responsible for a sonographer who deviates from the standards of practice. Breaches of standards of practice include the following:

1. Working under the influence of alcohol or drugs
2. Molesting a patient (e.g., endovaginally or transrectally)
3. Unnecessarily depriving a patient of modesty
4. Giving a patient an inaccurate diagnosis
5. Not securing a patient's safety (falling from a table or chair)

The sonographer should not tell the patient the diagnosis, unless the sonographer will be issuing the final report. Giving the final report to the patient means that the sonographer undertakes the malpractice risks.

Inadequate quality of films, loss of films due to a poor filing system, or misplacement of reports can result in liability, but the risk will not be borne by the sonographer if he or she is under the supervision of a sonologist.

MALPRACTICE INSURANCE: WHO NEEDS IT?

Any sonographer doing freelance work (i.e., moonlighting or on a mobile service) should invest in malpractice insurance. Sonographers employed by a hospital or other institution do not generally need to purchase insurance because they are covered by the hospital policy.

APPENDIXES

AAA	Abdominal aortic aneurysm	D ≠ E	Dates do not equal exam	IBD	Inflammatory bowel disease
Ab	Abortion	DM	Diabetes mellitus	IC	Iliac crest
A and B	Apnea and bradycardia	D<E	Small for dates	IDDM	Insulin-dependent diabetes mellitus
AFM	After fatty meal	D>E	Large for dates		
AFP	Alpha fetoprotein	DFHT	Documentated fetal heart tone	ITTP	Idiopathic thrombotic thrombocytopenic purpura
ALL	Acute leukocytic leukemia	D.T.'s	Delirium tremens		
AM	Adnexal mass	DTR	Deep tendon reflex	IUCD (IUD)	Intrauterine contraceptive device
AML	Acute monocytic leukemia	DUB	Dysfunctional uterine bleeding		
A-Mode	Amplitude modulation	Dx	Diagnosis	IUGR	Intrauterine growth restriction (intrauterine growth retardation)
AODM	Adult onset of diabetes mellitus				
ARC	Aids related complex			IUP	Intrauterine pregnancy
ARDS	Adult respiratory distress syndrome	EDC	Estimated date of confinement	IVC	Inferior vena cava
AROM	Artificial rupture of membranes	EFW	Estimated fetal weight	IVDA	Intravenous drug abuser
ATB	Antibiotic	ESWL	Extracorporeal shock wave lithotripsy	IVP	Intravenous pyelogram
ATN	Acute tubular necrosis	ETOH'er	Ethanol (alcohol) abuser		
		EUA	Examination under anesthesia	JODM	Juvenile onset diabetes mellitus
BE	Barium enema				
B-H	Braxton-Hicks' contraction				
BIP (BPD)	Biparietal diameter	F	Fahrenheit	K+	Potassium
B-Mode	Brightness modulation	FCD	Fibrocystic disease		
BMT	Bone marrow transplant	FDIU	Fetal death in utero		
BOE	Best obstetrical estimate	FH	Fundal height, fetal heart, or family history	LAP	Lower abdominal pain
BP	Blood pressure			LE	Lower extremity
BPD (BIP)	Biparietal diameter	FSH	Follicle-stimulating hormone	LFT	Liver function test (e.g., SGPT, SGOT, alk phos)
BPH	Benign prostatic hypertrophy	FUO	Fever of unknown origin		
BSO	Bilateral salpingo-oophorectomy	FTT	Failure to thrive	LH	Luteinizing hormone
BTD	Biliary tract disease			LK	Left kidney
BUN	Blood urea nitrogen			LLQ	Left lower quadrant
BX	Biopsy	G	Gravida	LMP	Last menstrual period
		GB	Gallbladder	LNMP	Last normal menstrual period
		GBM	Glioblastoma multiforme	LOLINAD	Little old lady in apparent distress
C	Celsius (centigrade)	GI	Gastrointestinal		
c̄	With	GNR	Gram negative rods	LPO	Left posterior oblique
CBD	Common bile duct	GTD	Gestational trophoblastic disease	LSO	Left salpingo-oophorectomy
CEC	Central echo complex			LSU	Left side up
CHD	Common hepatic duct	GU	Genitourinary	LT	Ligamentum teres
cm	Centimeter	GVHD	Graft-versus-host disease	LUQ	Left upper quadrant
CML	Chronic myeloid leukemia	Gyn	Gynecology		
CMT	Cervical motion tenderness				
CNS	Central nervous system			MAB	Missed abortion
CP	Cerebral palsy	HAPA HAPA	"Here a pain, there a pain, etc." syndrome	MCA	Multiple congenital anomaly
Cr	Creatinine			MHz	Megahertz
CRT	Cadaveric renal transplant	HBP	High blood pressure	MIF	Medium internal focus (transducer)
CRT	Cathode ray tube	HC	Hepatocellular, or head circumference		
C/S	Cesarean section			ML	Midline
CST	Contraction stress test	HCG	Human chorionic gonadotropin	mm	Millimeter
Cx	Cervix			M-Mode	Time motion modulation
		HCT	Hematocrit	MRCP	Mental retardation and cerebral palsy
dB	Decibel	HIV	Human immune virus		
D & C	Dilatation and curettage	HSM	Hepatosplenomegaly	ΔMS	Altered mental status
D = E	Dates equal exam	Hydro	Hydrocephalus, or Hydronephrosis		
D = E = S	Dates equal exam equal sonogram				

N	Notch (sternal)	PTA	Prior to admission	TCC	Transitional cell cancer
NEFG	Normal external female genitalia	PTT	Prothrombin time	TCG	Time compensation gain
		PUD	Peptic ulcer disease	TGC	Time gain compensation
NGT	Nasogastric tube	PV	Portal vein	TIUV	Total intrauterine volume
NPO	Nothing by mouth			TMO	"Take me out" (refers to a pelvic mass, e.g., huge fibroid uterus)
NSS	Normal size and shape				
NST	Nonstress test	RBC	Red blood cell		
NSVD	Normal spontaneous vaginal delivery	RCM	Right costal margin	TOA	Tubo-ovarian abscess
		RK	Right kidney	TTP	Thrombotic thrombocytopenic purpura
		RLL	Right lower lobe		
Ob	Obstetrics	RLQ	Right lower quadrant	TURP	Transurethral resection of prostate
OCT	Oxytocin challenge test	R/O	Rule out	TVH	Total vaginal hysterectomy
OCG	Oral cholecystogram	ROM	Rupture of membranes	Tx	Transplant
OR	Operating room	RPO	Right posterior oblique		
OCP	Oral contraceptives	RSO	Right salpingo-oophorectomy		
		RT	Real-time (dynamic imaging)	U	Umbilicus
		RUQ	Right upper quadrant	UE	Upper extremity
p	After	Rx	Treatment	UGI	Upper gastrointestinal series
PA	Popliteal artery, or popliteal aneurysm			UPJ	Ureteropelvic junction
				US	Ultrasound
Para 1234	(1) Number of pregnancies, (2) number of premature births, (3) number of abortions, (4) number of living children	S/P	Surgical procedure	UTI	Urinary tract infection
		SAB	Spontaneous abortion	UVJ	Ureterovesical junction
		S	Symphisis pubis (SP or P)		
		SBE	Subacute bacterial endocarditis		
		SBO	Small bowel obstruction	VBAC	Vaginal birth after Caesarean section
PE	Pleural effusion, or pulmonary embolus	SBP	Spontaneous bacterial peritonitis	VTX	Vertex presentation
		SIF	Short internal focus (transducer)		
PID	Pelvic inflammatory disease	SMA	Superior mesenteric artery		
PIH	Pregnancy induced hypertension	SMV	Superior mesenteric vein	WBC	White blood cell
PMB	Postmenopausal bleeding	SSCP	Substernal chest pain	WFGOF	"We found grandmother on the floor"
POD#	Post-op day (#??)	SVD	Spontaneous vaginal delivery		
PP	Postpartum				
PPD	Test for tuberculosis				
PROM	Preterm rupture of membranes	TAB	Therapeutic abortion	X	Xyphoid
PSI	Postsaline injection	TAH	Total abdominal hysterectomy		
PT	Pregnancy test	TC	Trunk circumference		

Appendix 2.
Length of Fetal Long Bones (mm)

Week No.	Humerus Percentile			Ulna Percentile			Radius Percentile			Femur Percentile			Tibia Percentile			Fibula Percentile		
	5	50	95	5	50	95	5	50	95	5	50	95	5	50	95	5	50	95
11	—	6	—	—	5	—	—	5	—	—	6	—	—	4	—	—	2	—
12	3	9	10	—	8	—	—	7	—	—	9	—	—	7	—	—	5	—
13	5	13	20	3	11	18	—	10	—	6	12	19	4	10	17	—	8	—
14	5	16	20	4	13	17	8	13	15	5	15	19	2	13	19	6	11	10
15	11	18	26	10	16	22	12	15	19	11	19	26	5	16	27	10	14	18
16	12	21	25	8	19	24	9	18	21	13	22	24	7	19	25	6	17	22
17	19	24	29	11	21	32	11	20	29	20	25	29	15	22	29	7	19	31
18	18	27	30	13	24	30	14	22	26	19	28	31	14	24	29	10	22	28
19	22	29	36	20	26	32	20	24	29	23	31	38	19	27	35	18	24	30
20	23	32	36	21	29	32	21	27	28	22	33	39	19	29	35	18	27	30
21	28	34	40	25	31	36	25	29	32	27	36	45	24	32	39	24	29	34
22	28	36	40	24	33	37	24	31	34	29	39	44	25	34	39	21	31	37
23	32	38	45	27	35	43	26	32	39	35	41	48	30	36	43	23	33	44
24	31	41	46	29	37	41	27	34	38	34	44	49	28	39	45	26	35	41
25	35	43	51	34	39	44	31	36	40	38	46	54	31	41	50	33	37	42
26	36	45	49	34	41	44	30	37	41	39	49	53	33	43	49	32	39	43
27	42	46	51	37	43	48	33	39	45	45	51	57	39	45	51	35	41	47
28	41	48	52	37	44	48	33	40	45	45	53	57	38	47	52	36	43	47
29	44	50	56	40	46	51	36	42	47	49	56	62	40	49	57	40	45	50
30	44	52	56	38	47	54	34	43	49	49	58	62	41	51	56	38	47	52
31	47	53	59	39	49	59	34	44	53	53	60	67	46	52	58	40	48	57
32	47	55	59	40	50	58	37	45	51	53	62	67	46	54	59	40	50	56
33	50	56	62	43	52	60	41	46	51	56	64	71	49	56	62	43	51	59
34	50	57	62	44	53	59	39	47	53	57	65	70	47	57	64	46	52	56
35	52	58	65	47	54	61	38	48	57	61	67	73	48	59	69	51	54	57
36	53	60	63	47	55	61	41	48	54	61	69	74	49	60	68	51	55	56
37	57	61	64	49	56	62	45	49	53	64	71	77	52	61	71	55	56	58
38	55	61	66	48	57	63	45	49	53	62	72	79	54	62	69	54	57	59
39	56	62	69	49	57	66	46	50	54	64	74	83	58	64	69	55	58	62
40	56	63	69	50	58	65	46	50	54	66	75	81	58	65	69	54	59	62

Source: Jeanty, P. Re: Fetal limb biometry. *Radiology* 147:602, 1983.

Appendix 3.
Gestational Sac Measurement Table

MEAN DIAMETER OF GESTATIONAL SAC AND CORRESPONDING ESTIMATES OF GESTATIONAL AGE*

Mean sac diameter, mm	Mean gestational age, wk	Gestational age, d		
		Mean	95% confidence interval	95% prediction interval
2	5.0	34.9	34.3–35.5	31.6–38.2
3	5.1	35.8	35.2–36.3	32.5–39.1
4	5.2	36.6	36.1–37.2	33.3–39.9
5	5.4	37.5	37.0–38.0	34.2–40.8
6	5.5	38.4	37.9–38.9	35.1–41.7
7	5.6	39.3	38.9–39.7	36.0–42.6
8	5.7	40.2	39.8–40.6	36.9–43.5
9	5.9	41.1	40.7–41.4	37.8–44.3
10	6.0	41.9	41.6–42.3	38.7–45.2
11	6.1	42.8	42.5–43.2	39.5–46.1
12	6.2	43.7	43.4–44.0	40.4–47.0
13	6.4	44.6	44.3–44.9	41.3–47.9
14	6.5	45.5	45.2–45.8	42.2–48.7
15	6.6	46.3	46.0–46.6	43.1–49.6
16	6.7	47.2	46.9–47.5	44.0–50.5
17	6.9	48.1	47.8–48.4	44.8–51.4
18	7.0	49.0	48.6–49.4	45.7–52.3
19	7.1	49.9	49.5–50.3	46.6–53.2
20	7.3	50.8	50.3–51.2	47.5–54.0
21	7.4	51.6	51.2–52.1	48.3–54.9
22	7.5	52.5	52.0–53.0	49.2–55.8
23	7.6	53.4	52.9–53.9	50.1–56.7
24	7.8	54.3	53.7–54.8	51.0–57.6
25	7.9	55.2	54.6–55.7	51.9–58.5
26	8.0	56.0	55.4–56.7	52.7–59.4
27	8.1	56.9	56.3–57.6	53.6–60.3
28	8.3	57.8	57.1–58.5	54.5–61.1
29	8.4	58.7	58.0–59.4	55.4–62.0
30	8.5	59.6	58.8–60.4	56.2–62.9

*The mean gestational age was calculated with the regression equation shown in the legend to Fig. 1.

Source: Early pregnancy assessment with transvaginal ultrasound scanning. Reprinted with permission of the publisher from *CMAJ* 144(4):441–446, 1991.

Appendix 4.
Predicted Menstrual Age (Weeks) From CRL Measurements (cm)

CRL (cm)	MA (wk)	CRL (cm)	MA (wk)	CRL (cm)	MA (wk)	CRL (cm)	MA (wk)	CRL (cm)	MA (wk)	CRL (cm)	MA (wk)
0.2	5.7	2.2	8.9	4.2	11.1	6.2	12.6	8.2	14.2	10.2	16.1
0.3	5.9	2.3	9.0	4.3	11.2	6.3	12.7	8.3	14.2	10.3	16.2
0.4	6.1	2.4	9.1	4.4	11.2	6.4	12.8	8.4	14.3	10.4	16.3
0.5	6.2	2.5	9.2	4.5	11.3	6.5	12.8	8.5	14.4	10.5	16.4
0.6	6.4	2.6	9.4	4.6	11.4	6.6	12.9	8.6	14.5	10.6	16.5
0.7	6.6	2.7	9.5	4.7	11.5	6.7	13.0	8.7	14.6	10.7	16.6
0.8	6.7	2.8	9.6	4.8	11.6	6.8	13.1	8.8	14.7	10.8	16.7
0.9	6.9	2.9	9.7	4.9	11.7	6.9	13.1	8.9	14.8	10.9	16.8
1.0	7.1	3.0	9.9	5.0	11.7	7.0	13.2	9.0	14.9	11.0	16.9
1.1	7.2	3.1	10.0	5.1	11.8	7.1	13.3	9.1	15.0	11.1	17.0
1.2	7.4	3.2	10.1	5.2	11.9	7.2	13.4	9.2	15.1	11.2	17.1
1.3	7.5	3.3	10.2	5.3	12.0	7.3	13.4	9.3	15.2	11.3	17.2
1.4	7.7	3.4	10.3	5.4	12.0	7.4	13.5	9.4	15.3	11.4	17.3
1.5	7.9	3.5	10.4	5.5	12.1	7.5	13.6	9.5	15.3	11.5	17.4
1.6	8.0	3.6	10.5	5.6	12.2	7.6	13.7	9.6	15.4	11.6	17.5
1.7	8.1	3.7	10.6	5.7	12.3	7.7	13.8	9.7	15.5	11.7	17.6
1.8	8.3	3.8	10.7	5.8	12.3	7.8	13.8	9.8	15.6	11.8	17.7
1.9	8.4	3.9	10.8	5.9	12.4	7.9	13.9	9.9	15.7	11.9	17.8
2.0	8.6	4.0	10.9	6.0	12.5	8.0	14.0	10.0	15.9	12.0	17.9
2.1	8.7	4.1	11.0	6.1	12.6	8.1	14.1	10.1	16.0	12.1	18.0

Note: MA = menstrual age. The 95% confidence interval is ±8% of the predicted age.

Source: Reprinted with permission of the publisher (*Radiology* 182: 504).

Appendix 5.

Crown-Rump Length Studies Based on Last Menstrual Period

Data	Robinson et al (1,2)	Drumm et al (3,4)	Bovicelli et al (8)	Nelson (9)	Selbing (5)	Pedersen (6)	Current Series
Year	1973–1975	1976–1977	1981	1981	1982	1982	1991
Site	Scotland	Ireland	Italy	United States	Sweden	Denmark	United States
Scanner	Static	Static	Real-Time	Real-Time	Static	Static	Real-Time
Technique	TA	TA	TA	TA	TA	TA	TA, TV
Number	80	253	237	83	13	101	452
Analysis	Mixed	Mixed	CS	CS	Mixed	Mixed	CS
Weeks	6–14	6.7–14.4	7–13	7.7–17	5.7–14.3	6.7–14	5–18
Dates	LMP	LMP	LMP	LMP	LMP	LMP	LMP
95% confidence interval	±4.7 d	±3 d	±4.6 d	NG	±6.6 d	±4–6 d	±8.3 d
			PREDICTED MENSTRUAL AGE FROM CROWN-RUMP LENGTH TABLES OR REGRESSION EQUATIONS				
2 mm	ND	ND	ND	ND	ND	ND	5.7
10 mm	7.0	6.9	ND	ND	7.2	7.0	7.1
20 mm	8.6	8.5	8.4	9.0	8.6	8.6	8.6
30 mm	9.8	9.7	9.8	9.9	9.9	9.8	9.9
40 mm	10.8	10.8	10.8	10.7	11.0	10.9	10.9
50 mm	11.5	11.6	11.7	11.6	12.0	11.6	11.7
60 mm	12.6	12.4	12.4	12.4	12.8	12.6	12.5
70 mm	13.4	13.2	13.3	13.3	13.6	13.3	13.2
80 mm	14.1	13.8	ND	14.1	14.2	13.9	14.0
90 mm	ND	ND	ND	15.0	ND	ND	14.9
100 mm	ND	ND	ND	15.9	ND	ND	15.9
110 mm	ND	ND	ND	16.7	ND	ND	16.9
120 mm	ND	ND	ND	17.6	ND	ND	17.9

Note: CS = cross-sectional analysis, LMP = last menstrual period, Mixed = cross-sectional data analyzed in a longitudinal manner, ND = no data, TA = transabdominal, TV = transvaginal.

Source: Reprinted with permission of the publisher (*Radiology* 182: 504

Appendix 6.
Abdominal Circumference: Normal Values

Menstrual Age (weeks)	Lower Limit* (cm)	Predicted Value† (cm)	Upper Limit‡ (cm)	−2 S.D.// (cm)	Predicted Value§ (cm)	+2 S.D.// (cm)
12	5.4	6.3	7.1	3.1	5.6	8.1
13	6.4	7.4	8.3	4.4	6.9	9.4
14	7.4	8.4	9.5	5.6	8.1	10.6
15	8.3	9.5	10.8	6.8	9.3	11.8
16	9.3	10.6	12.0	8.0	10.5	13.0
17	10.2	11.7	13.3	9.2	11.7	14.2
18	11.2	12.8	14.5	10.4	12.9	15.4
19	12.1	13.9	15.7	11.6	14.1	16.6
20	13.1	15.0	17.0	12.7	15.2	17.7
21	14.0	16.1	18.2	13.9	16.4	18.9
22	15.0	17.2	19.5	15.0	17.5	20.0
23	16.0	18.3	20.7	16.1	18.6	21.1
24	16.9	19.4	22.0	17.2	19.7	22.2
25	17.9	20.5	23.2	18.3	20.8	23.3
26	18.8	21.6	24.4	19.4	21.9	24.4
27	19.8	22.7	25.7	20.4	22.9	25.4
28	20.7	23.8	26.9	21.5	24.0	26.5
29	21.7	24.9	28.2	22.5	25.0	27.5
30	22.6	26.0	29.4	23.5	26.0	28.5
31	23.6	27.1	30.6	24.5	27.0	29.5
32	24.6	28.2	31.9	25.5	28.0	30.5
33	25.5	29.3	33.1	26.5	29.0	31.5
34	26.5	30.4	34.4	27.5	30.0	32.5
35	27.4	31.5	35.6	28.4	30.9	33.4
36	28.4	32.6	36.9	29.3	31.8	34.3
37	29.3	33.7	38.1	30.2	32.7	35.2
38	30.3	34.8	39.3	31.1	33.6	36.1
39	31.2	35.9	40.6	32.0	34.5	37.0
40	32.2	37.0	41.8	32.9	35.4	37.9

*Predicted value −.13 (predicted value).

†AC = −6.9300 + 1.0985 (MA)[R^2 = 95.5%].

‡Predicted value + .13 (predicted value).
§AC = −10.4997 + 1.4256 (MA) −.00697 (MA)^2 [R^2 = 97.9%].

//2 S.D. = 2.5 cm.

Source: Adapted from Callen, P. W. *Ultrasonography in Obstetrics and Gynecology.* Boston: Saunders, 1983. With permission.

Appendix 7.

Head Circumference: Normal Growth Rates

Menstrual Age Interval (weeks)	−2 S.D. (cm/wk)	Predicted Value (cm/wk)	+2 S.D. (cm/wk)
12–13	1.4	1.6	1.8
13–14	1.3	1.5	1.7
14–15	1.3	1.5	1.7
15–16	1.3	1.5	1.7
16–17	1.3	1.5	1.7
17–18	1.2	1.4	1.6
18–19	1.2	1.4	1.6
19–20	1.2	1.4	1.6
20–21	1.1	1.3	1.5
21–22	1.1	1.3	1.5
22–23	1.2	1.3	1.4
23–24	1.1	1.2	1.3
24–25	1.1	1.2	1.3
25–26	1.1	1.2	1.3
26–27	1.0	1.1	1.2
27–28	1.0	1.1	1.2
28–29	0.9	1.0	1.1
29–30	0.9	1.0	1.1
30–31	0.8	0.9	1.0
31–32	0.8	0.9	1.0
32–33	0.7	0.8	0.9
33–34	0.6	0.8	1.0
34–35	0.5	0.7	0.9
35–36	0.5	0.7	0.9
36–37	0.4	0.6	0.8
37–38	0.4	0.6	0.8
38–39	0.3	0.5	0.7
39–40	0.1	0.4	0.7

Source: Callen, P. W. *Ultrasonography in Obstetrics and Gynecology.* Boston: Saunders, 1983. With permission.

Appendix 8.
Head Circumference: Normal Values

Menstrual Age (weeks)	Lower Limit (cm)	Predicted Value (cm)	Upper Limit (cm)	−2 S.D. (cm)	Predicted Value (cm)	+2 S.D. (cm)
12	5.8	7.3	8.8	5.1	7.0	8.9
13	7.2	8.7	10.2	6.5	8.9	10.3
14	8.6	10.1	11.6	7.9	9.8	11.7
15	9.9	11.4	12.9	9.2	11.1	13.0
16	11.3	12.8	14.3	10.5	12.4	14.3
17	12.6	14.1	15.6	11.8	13.7	15.6
18	13.9	15.4	16.9	13.1	15.0	16.9
19	15.2	16.7	18.2	14.4	16.3	18.2
20	16.4	17.9	19.4	15.6	17.5	19.4
21	17.7	19.2	20.7	16.8	18.7	20.6
22	18.9	20.4	21.9	18.0	19.9	21.8
23	20.0	21.5	23.0	19.1	21.0	22.9
24	21.2	22.7	24.2	20.2	22.1	24.0
25	22.3	23.8	25.3	21.3	23.2	25.1
26	23.4	24.9	26.4	22.3	24.2	26.1
27	24.4	25.9	27.4	23.3	25.2	27.1
28	24.4	26.9	29.4	24.3	26.2	28.1
29	25.4	27.9	30.4	25.2	27.1	29.0
30	26.3	28.8	31.3	26.1	28.0	29.9
31	27.2	29.7	32.2	27.0	28.9	30.8
32	28.1	30.6	33.1	27.8	29.7	31.6
33	28.9	31.4	33.9	28.5	30.4	32.3
34	29.7	32.2	34.7	29.3	31.2	33.1
35	30.4	32.9	35.4	29.9	31.8	33.7
36	31.1	33.6	36.1	30.6	32.5	34.4
37	31.7	34.2	36.7	31.1	33.0	34.9
38	32.3	34.8	37.3	31.9	33.6	35.5
39	32.9	35.4	37.9	32.2	34.1	36.0
40	33.4	35.9	38.4	32.6	34.5	36.4

Source: Adapted from Callen, P. W., *Ultrasonography in Obstetrics and Gynecology*. Boston: Saunders, 1983. With permission.

Appendix 9.

Correlation of Predicted Menstrual Age Based Upon Biparietal Diameters

Menstrual Age (weeks)	Bpd mean values (mm)					
	Composite Sabbagha and Hughey[1]	Composite Kurtz et al.[2]	Kurtz et al.[2] < 1974	Kurtz et al.[2] > 1974	Hadlock et al.[3] 1982	Shepard and Filly[4] 1982
14	28	27	28	26	27	28
15	32	31	31	29	30	31
16	36	34	35	33	33	34
17	39	38	39	36	37	37
18	42	41	42	40	40	40
19	45	45	46	43	43	43
20	48	48	49	46	46	46
21	51	51	52	50	50	49
22	54	54	55	53	53	52
23	58	57	58	56	56	55
24	61	60	61	59	58	57
25	64	63	64	61	61	60
26	67	66	67	64	64	63
27	70	69	69	67	67	65
28	72	71	72	70	70	68
29	75	74	75	72	72	71
30	78	76	77	75	75	73
31	80	79	79	77	77	76
32	82	81	81	79	79	78
33	85	83	83	82	82	80
34	87	85	85	84	84	83
35	88	87	87	86	86	85
36	90	89	89	88	88	88
37	92	91	91	90	90	90
38	93	92	92	92	91	92
39	94	94	94	94	93	95
40	95	95	95	95	95	97

[1]Sabbagha, R. E., and Hughey, M. Standardization of sonar cephalometry and gestational age. *Obstet Gynecol* 52:402, 1978.

[2]Kurtz, A. B., Wapner, R. J., Kurtz, R. J., et al. Analysis of biparietal diameter as an accurate indicator of gestational age. *J Clin Ultrasound,* 8:319, 1980.

[3]Hadlock, F. P., Deter, R. L., Harrist, R. B., et al. Fetal biparietal diameter: A critical re-evaluation of the relation to menstrual age by means of real-time ultrasound. *J Ultrasound Med,* 1:97–104, 1982.

[4]Shepard, M., and Filly, R. A. A standardized plane for biparietal diameter measurement. *J Ultrasound Med,* 1:145–150, 1982.

Source: Callen, P. W. *Ultrasonography in Obstetrics and Gynecology.* Boston: Saunders, 1983. With permission.

Appendix 10.

Cephalic Index Formula

$$\text{Cephalic Index}* = \frac{\text{Short Axis (Biparietal Diameter) (mm)}}{\text{Long Axis (Frontal Occipital Diameter) (mm)}} \times 100 = 78.3$$

Normal range of index:
At 1 Standard Deviation = 74 to 83
At 2 Standard Deviation = 70 to 86

*Measurements of short and long axis taken from outer to outer margins of head.

Source: Hadlock, F. P., Deter, R. L., Carpenter, R. J., Park, S. K. Estimating fetal age: Effect of head shape on BPD. *AJR* 137:83–85, 1981.

© by American Roentgen Ray Society. Reprinted by permission.

Appendix 11.
Comparison of Predicted Femur Lengths at Points in Gestation

Menstrual Age (weeks)	Femur length (mm)			
	Filly et al.[1] *1981*	*Jeanty et al.*[2] *1981†*	*Hadlock et al.*[3] *1982**	*Hadlock et al.*[3] *1982†*
12		09	14	08
13		12	16	11
14	16	16	19	15
15	19	19	21	18
16	22	23	23	21
17	25	26	26	24
18	28	30	28	27
19	32	33	30	30
20	35	36	33	33
21	38	39	35	36
22	41	42	38	39
23	44	45	40	42
24	47	48	42	44
25	50	51	45	47
26	53	54	47	49
27	55	57	49	52
28	57	59	52	54
29	61	62	54	56
30	63	65	57	58
31		67	59	61
32		70	61	63
33		72	64	65
34		74	66	66
35		77	69	68
36		79	71	70
37		81	73	72
38		83	76	73
39		85	78	75
40		87	80	76

*Linear function
†Linear quadratic function

[1]Filly, R. A., Golbus, M. S., Carey, J. C., et al. Short-limbed dwarfism: Ultrasonographic diagnosis by mensuration of fetal femoral length. *Radiology,* 138:653–656, 1981.

[2]Jeanty, P., Kirkpatrick, C., Dramaix-Wilmet, M., et al. Ultrasonic evaluation of fetal limb growth. *Radiology* 140:165–168, 1981.

[3]Hadlock, F. P. et al. Fetal femur length as a predictor of menstrual age: Sonographically measured. *AJR,* 138:875–878, 1982.

Source: Callen, P. W. *Ultrasonography in Obstetrics and Gynecology.* Boston: Saunders, 1983. With permission.

Appendix 12.
Abdominal Diameter Measurement Table

Gestational Age (Weeks)	Transverse Diameter (mm)		Anterior-Posterior Diameter (mm)	
	Mean	Range from 5th to 95%	Mean	Range from 5th to 95th%
15	29	25 to 33	29	23 to 32
16	32	27 to 36	33	27 to 36
17	35	30 to 39	37	31 to 40
18	39	34 to 43	40	35 to 43
19	42	37 to 47	43	39 to 46
20	45	40 to 50	47	43 to 49
21	48	43 to 54	50	46 to 53
22	51	45 to 57	54	50 to 57
23	54	48 to 60	57	53 to 61
24	57	51 to 64	60	56 to 65
25	61	54 to 67	64	59 to 69
26	64	57 to 70	68	62 to 74
27	68	59 to 74	72	66 to 80
28	71	62 to 77	76	69 to 87
29	74	65 to 81	80	73 to 92
30	77	68 to 84	84	76 to 95
31	80	71 to 88	87	79 to 98
32	83	73 to 91	91	82 to 103
33	86	76 to 95	94	86 to 108
34	88	78 to 99	98	89 to 112
35	91	80 to 103	101	92 to 117
36	94	82 to 107	104	95 to 118
37	96	84 to 110	107	99 to 120
38	98	86 to 113	110	101 to 121
39	100	87 to 115	112	102 to 124
40	101	88 to 116	113	102 to 125

Source: Fescina, R. H., Ucieda, F. J., Cordano, M. C., Nieto, F., Tenzer, S. M., Lopez, R. Ultrasonic patterns of intrauterine fetal growth in a latin american country. *Early Human Development* 6:239–248, 1982. With permission.

Abdominal Circumference Measurement Table

Abdominal Circumference (mm)	Gestational Age (Weeks)		Abdominal Circumference (mm)	Gestational Age (Weeks)	
	Predicted Mean Values	95% Confidence Limits		Predicted Mean Values	95% Confidence Limits
100	15.6	13.7 to 17.5	235	27.7	25.5 to 29.9
105	16.1	14.2 to 18.0	240	28.2	26.0 to 30.4
110	16.5	14.6 to 18.4	245	28.7	26.5 to 30.9
115	16.9	15.0 to 18.8	250	29.2	27.0 to 31.4
120	17.3	15.4 to 19.2	255	29.7	27.5 to 31.9
125	17.8	15.9 to 19.7	260	30.1	27.1 to 33.1
130	18.2	16.2 to 20.2	265	30.6	27.6 to 33.6
135	18.6	16.6 to 20.6	270	31.1	28.1 to 34.1
140	19.1	17.1 to 21.1	275	31.6	28.6 to 34.6
145	19.5	17.5 to 21.5	280	32.1	29.1 to 35.1
150	20.0	18.9 to 22.0	285	32.6	29.6 to 35.6
155	20.4	18.4 to 22.4	290	33.1	30.1 to 36.1
160	20.8	18.8 to 22.8	295	33.6	30.6 to 36.6
165	21.3	19.3 to 23.3	300	34.1	31.1 to 37.1
170	21.7	19.7 to 23.7	305	34.6	31.6 to 37.6
175	22.2	20.2 to 24.2	310	35.1	32.1 to 38.1
180	22.6	20.6 to 24.6	315	35.6	32.6 to 38.6
185	23.1	21.1 to 25.1	320	36.1	33.6 to 38.6
190	23.6	21.6 to 25.6	325	36.6	34.1 to 39.1
195	24.0	21.8 to 26.2	330	37.1	34.6 to 39.6
200	24.5	22.3 to 26.7	335	37.6	35.1 to 40.1
205	24.9	22.7 to 27.1	340	38.1	35.6 to 40.6
210	25.4	23.2 to 27.6	345	38.7	36.2 to 41.2
215	25.9	23.7 to 28.1	350	39.2	36.7 to 41.7
220	26.3	24.1 to 28.5	355	39.7	37.2 to 42.2
225	26.8	24.6 to 29.0	360	40.2	37.7 to 42.7
230	27.3	25.1 to 29.5	365	40.8	38.3 to 43.3

Source: Hadlock, F. P., Deter, R. L., Harrist, R. B., Park S. K. Fetal abdominal circumference as a predictor of menstrual age. *AJR* 139:367–370, 1982. With permission.

Appendix 13.
Predicting Fetal Weight by Ultrasound

Biparietal diameters	Abdominal circumferences											
	15.5	16.0	16.5	17.0	17.5	18.0	18.5	19.0	19.5	20.0	20.5	21.0
3.1	224	234	244	255	267	279	291	304	318	332	346	362
3.2	231	241	251	263	274	286	299	312	326	340	355	371
3.3	237	248	259	270	282	294	307	321	335	349	365	381
3.4	244	255	266	278	290	302	316	329	344	359	374	391
3.5	251	262	274	285	298	311	324	338	353	368	384	401
3.6	259	270	281	294	306	319	333	347	362	378	394	411
3.7	266	278	290	302	315	328	342	357	372	388	404	422
3.8	274	286	298	310	324	337	352	366	382	398	415	432
3.9	282	294	306	319	333	347	361	376	392	409	426	444
4.0	290	303	315	328	342	356	371	386	403	419	437	455
4.1	299	311	324	338	352	366	381	397	413	430	448	467
4.2	308	320	333	347	361	376	392	408	424	442	460	479
4.3	317	330	343	357	371	387	402	419	436	453	472	491
4.4	326	339	353	367	382	397	413	430	447	465	484	504
4.5	335	349	363	377	393	408	425	442	459	478	497	517
4.6	345	359	373	388	404	420	436	454	472	490	510	530
4.7	355	369	384	399	415	431	448	466	484	503	523	544
4.8	366	380	395	410	426	443	460	478	497	517	537	558
4.9	376	391	406	422	438	455	473	491	510	530	551	572
5.0	387	402	418	434	451	468	486	505	524	544	565	587
5.1	399	414	430	446	463	481	499	518	538	559	580	602
5.2	410	426	442	459	476	494	513	532	552	573	595	618
5.3	422	438	455	472	489	508	527	547	567	589	611	634
5.4	435	451	468	485	503	522	541	561	582	604	627	650
5.5	447	464	481	499	517	536	556	577	598	620	643	667
5.6	461	477	495	513	532	551	571	592	614	636	660	684
5.7	474	491	509	527	547	566	587	608	630	653	677	701
5.8	488	505	524	542	562	582	603	625	647	670	695	719
5.9	502	520	539	558	578	598	619	642	664	688	713	738
6.0	517	535	554	573	594	615	636	659	682	706	731	757
6.1	532	550	570	590	610	632	654	677	700	725	750	777
6.2	547	566	586	606	627	649	672	695	719	744	770	797
6.3	563	583	603	624	645	667	690	714	738	764	790	817
6.4	580	600	620	641	663	686	709	733	758	784	811	838
6.5	597	617	638	659	682	705	728	753	778	805	832	860
6.6	614	635	656	678	701	724	748	773	799	826	853	882
6.7	632	653	675	697	720	744	769	794	820	848	876	905
6.8	651	672	694	717	740	765	790	816	842	870	898	928
6.9	670	691	714	737	761	786	811	838	865	893	922	952

Source: Shepard, M. J., Richards, V. A., Berkowitz, R. L., Warsof, S. L., Hobbins, J. C. An evaluation of two equations for predicting fetal weight by ultrasound. *Am J Obstet Gynecol* 156:80–85, January 1987. ©1982 The C. V. Mosby Co.

Abdominal circumferences

21.5	22.0	22.5	23.0	23.5	24.0	24.5	25.0	25.5	26.0	26.5	27.0	27.5
378	395	412	431	450	470	491	513	536	559	584	610	638
388	405	423	441	461	481	502	525	548	572	597	624	651
397	415	433	452	472	493	514	537	560	585	611	638	666
408	425	444	463	483	504	526	549	573	598	624	652	680
418	436	455	475	495	517	539	562	587	612	638	666	695
429	447	466	486	507	529	552	575	600	626	653	681	710
440	458	478	498	519	542	565	589	614	640	667	696	725
451	470	490	510	532	554	578	602	628	654	682	711	741
462	482	502	523	545	568	592	616	642	669	697	727	757
474	494	514	536	558	581	606	631	657	684	713	743	773
486	506	527	549	572	595	620	645	672	700	729	759	790
498	519	540	562	585	609	634	660	688	716	745	776	807
511	532	554	576	600	624	649	676	703	732	762	793	825
524	545	567	590	614	639	665	692	719	749	779	810	843
538	559	581	605	629	654	680	708	736	765	796	828	861
551	573	596	620	644	670	696	724	753	783	814	846	880
565	588	611	635	660	686	713	741	770	801	832	865	899
580	602	626	650	676	702	730	758	788	819	851	884	919
594	617	641	666	692	719	747	776	806	837	870	903	938
610	633	657	683	709	736	765	794	824	856	889	923	959
625	649	674	699	726	754	783	812	843	876	909	944	980
641	665	690	717	744	772	801	831	863	895	929	964	1,001
657	682	708	734	762	790	820	851	883	916	950	986	1,023
674	699	725	752	780	809	839	870	903	936	971	1,007	1,045
691	717	743	771	799	828	859	891	924	958	993	1,030	1,068
709	735	762	789	818	848	879	911	945	979	1,015	1,052	1,091
727	753	780	809	838	869	900	933	966	1,001	1,038	1,075	1,114
745	772	800	829	858	889	921	954	989	1,024	1,061	1,099	1,139
764	792	820	849	879	911	943	977	1,011	1,047	1,085	1,123	1,163
784	811	840	870	900	932	965	999	1,035	1,071	1,109	1,148	1,189
804	832	861	891	922	955	988	1,023	1,058	1,095	1,134	1,173	1,214
824	853	882	913	945	977	1,011	1,046	1,083	1,120	1,159	1,199	1,241
845	874	904	935	967	1,001	1,035	1,071	1,107	1,145	1,185	1,226	1,268
867	896	927	958	991	1,025	1,059	1,096	1,133	1,171	1,211	1,253	1,295
889	919	950	982	1,015	1,049	1,084	1,121	1,159	1,198	1,238	1,280	1,323
911	942	973	1,006	1,039	1,074	1,110	1,147	1,185	1,225	1,266	1,308	1,352
935	965	997	1,030	1,065	1,100	1,136	1,174	1,213	1,253	1,294	1,337	1,381
958	990	1,022	1,056	1,090	1,126	1,163	1,201	1,241	1,281	1,323	1,367	1,411
983	1,015	1,048	1,082	1,117	1,153	1,190	1,229	1,269	1,310	1,353	1,397	1,442

(continued)

Appendix 13.
Predicting Fetal Weight by Ultrasound (*continued*)

Biparietal diameters	Abdominal circumferences											
	15.5	16.0	16.5	17.0	17.5	18.0	18.5	19.0	19.5	20.0	20.5	21.0
7.0	689	711	734	758	782	807	833	860	888	916	946	976
7.1	709	732	755	779	804	830	856	883	912	941	971	1,002
7.2	730	763	777	801	827	853	880	907	936	965	996	1,027
7.3	751	775	799	824	850	876	904	932	961	991	1,022	1,054
7.4	773	797	822	847	874	901	928	957	987	1,017	1,049	1,081
7.5	796	820	845	871	898	925	954	983	1,013	1,044	1,076	1,109
7.6	819	844	870	896	923	951	980	1,009	1,040	1,072	1,104	1,137
7.7	843	868	894	921	949	977	1,007	1,037	1,068	1,100	1,133	1,167
7.8	868	894	920	947	975	1,004	1,034	1,065	1,096	1,129	1,162	1,197
7.9	893	919	946	974	1,003	1,032	1,062	1,094	1,126	1,159	1,193	1,228
8.0	919	946	973	1,002	1,031	1,061	1,091	1,123	1,156	1,189	1,224	1,259
8.1	946	973	1,001	1,030	1,060	1,090	1,121	1,153	1,187	1,221	1,256	1,292
8.2	974	1,001	1,030	1,059	1,089	1,120	1,152	1,185	1,218	1,253	1,288	1,325
8.3	1,002	1,030	1,059	1,089	1,120	1,151	1,183	1,217	1,251	1,286	1,322	1,359
8.4	1,032	1,060	1,090	1,120	1,151	1,183	1,216	1,249	1,284	1,320	1,356	1,394
8.5	1,062	1,091	1,121	1,151	1,183	1,216	1,249	1,283	1,318	1,355	1,392	1,430
8.6	1,093	1,122	1,153	1,184	1,216	1,249	1,283	1,318	1,354	1,390	1,428	1,467
8.7	1,125	1,155	1,186	1,218	1,250	1,284	1,318	1,353	1,390	1,427	1,465	1,505
8.8	1,157	1,188	1,220	1,252	1,285	1,319	1,354	1,390	1,427	1,465	1,504	1,543
8.9	1,191	1,222	1,254	1,287	1,321	1,356	1,391	1,428	1,465	1,503	1,543	1,583
9.0	1,226	1,258	1,290	1,324	1,358	1,393	1,429	1,456	1,504	1,543	1,583	1,624
9.1	1,262	1,294	1,327	1,361	1,396	1,432	1,468	1,506	1,544	1,584	1,624	1,666
9.2	1,299	1,332	1,365	1,400	1,435	1,471	1,508	1,546	1,586	1,626	1,667	1,709
9.3	1,337	1,370	1,404	1,439	1,475	1,512	1,550	1,588	1,628	1,668	1,710	1,753
9.4	1,376	1,410	1,444	1,480	1,516	1,554	1,592	1,631	1,671	1,712	1,755	1,798
9.5	1,416	1,450	1,486	1,522	1,559	1,597	1,635	1,675	1,716	1,758	1,800	1,844
9.6	1,457	1,492	1,528	1,565	1,602	1,641	1,680	1,720	1,762	1,804	1,847	1,892
9.7	1,500	1,535	1,572	1,609	1,547	1,686	1,726	1,767	1,809	1,852	1,895	1,940
9.8	1,544	1,580	1,617	1,654	1,693	1,733	1,773	1,815	1,857	1,900	1,945	1,990
9.9	1,589	1,625	1,663	1,701	1,740	1,781	1,822	1,864	1,907	1,951	1,996	2,042
10.0	1,635	1,672	1,710	1,749	1,789	1,830	1,871	1,914	1,958	2,002	2,048	2,094

SD = ±106.0 gm/kg of birth weight.

Abdominal circumferences

21.5	22.0	22.5	23.0	23.5	24.0	24.5	25.0	25.5	26.0	26.5	27.0	27.5
1,008	1,040	1,074	1,108	1,144	1,181	1,219	1,258	1,298	1,340	1,383	1,427	1,473
1,033	1,066	1,100	1,135	1,171	1,209	1,247	1,287	1,328	1,370	1,414	1,459	1,505
1,060	1,093	1,128	1,163	1,200	1,238	1,277	1,317	1,358	1,401	1,445	1,491	1,538
1,087	1,121	1,156	1,192	1,229	1,267	1,307	1,348	1,390	1,433	1,478	1,524	1,571
1,114	1,149	1,184	1,221	1,259	1,297	1,338	1,379	1,421	1,465	1,511	1,557	1,605
1,143	1,178	1,214	1,251	1,289	1,328	1,369	1,411	1,454	1,499	1,544	1,592	1,640
1,172	1,207	1,244	1,281	1,320	1,360	1,401	1,444	1,487	1,533	1,579	1,627	1,676
1,202	1,238	1,275	1,313	1,352	1,393	1,434	1,477	1,522	1,567	1,614	1,663	1,712
1,232	1,269	1,306	1,345	1,385	1,426	1,468	1,512	1,557	1,603	1,650	1,699	1,749
1,264	1,301	1,339	1,378	1,418	1,460	1,503	1,547	1,592	1,639	1,687	1,737	1,787
1,296	1,333	1,372	1,412	1,453	1,495	1,538	1,583	1,629	1,676	1,725	1,775	1,826
1,329	1,367	1,406	1,446	1,488	1,531	1,575	1,620	1,666	1,714	1,763	1,814	1,866
1,363	1,401	1,441	1,482	1,524	1,567	1,612	1,657	1,704	1,753	1,803	1,854	1,906
1,397	1,436	1,477	1,518	1,561	1,605	1,650	1,696	1,744	1,793	1,843	1,895	1,948
1,433	1,473	1,513	1,555	1,599	1,643	1,689	1,735	1,784	1,833	1,884	1,936	1,990
1,469	1,510	1,551	1,594	1,637	1,682	1,728	1,776	1,825	1,875	1,926	1,979	2,033
1,507	1,548	1,589	1,633	1,677	1,722	1,769	1,817	1,866	1,917	1,969	2,022	2,077
1,545	1,586	1,629	1,673	1,717	1,764	1,811	1,859	1,909	1,960	2,013	2,067	2,122
1,584	1,626	1,669	1,714	1,759	1,806	1,854	1,903	1,953	2,005	2,058	2,113	2,169
1,625	1,667	1,711	1,756	1,802	1,849	1,897	1,947	1,998	2,050	2,104	2,159	2,216
1,666	1,709	1,753	1,799	1,845	1,893	1,942	1,992	2,044	2,097	2,151	2,207	2,264
1,708	1,752	1,797	1,843	1,890	1,938	1,988	2,039	2,091	2,144	2,199	2,255	2,313
1,752	1,796	1,841	1,888	1,936	1,984	2,035	2,086	2,139	2,193	2,248	2,305	2,363
1,796	1,841	1,887	1,934	1,982	2,032	2,083	2,135	2,188	2,242	2,298	2,356	2,414
1,842	1,887	1,934	1,982	2,030	2,080	2,132	2,184	2,238	2,293	2,350	2,407	2,467
1,889	1,935	1,982	2,030	2,080	2,130	2,182	2,235	2,289	2,345	2,402	2,460	2,520
1,937	1,984	2,031	2,080	2,130	2,181	2,233	2,287	2,342	2,398	2,456	2,515	2,575
1,986	2,033	2,082	2,131	2,181	2,233	2,286	2,340	2,396	2,452	2,510	2,570	2,631
2,037	2,085	2,133	2,183	2,234	2,286	2,340	2,395	2,451	2,508	2,567	2,627	2,688
2,089	2,137	2,186	2,237	2,288	2,341	2,395	2,450	2,507	2,565	2,624	2,684	2,746
2,142	2,191	2,241	2,292	2,344	2,397	2,452	2,507	2,564	2,623	2,682	2,743	2,806

(continued)

Appendix 13.

Predicting Fetal Weight by Ultrasound (*continued*)

Biparietal diameters	Abdominal circumferences											
	28.0	*28.5*	*29.0*	*29.5*	*30.0*	*30.5*	*31.0*	*31.5*	*32.0*	*32.5*	*33.0*	*33.5*
3.1	666	696	726	759	793	828	865	903	943	985	1,029	1,075
3.2	680	710	742	774	809	844	882	921	961	1,004	1,048	1,094
3.3	695	725	757	790	825	861	899	938	979	1,022	1,067	1,114
3.4	710	740	773	806	841	878	916	956	998	1,041	1,087	1,134
3.5	725	756	789	823	858	896	934	975	1,017	1,061	1,107	1,154
3.6	740	772	805	840	876	913	953	993	1,036	1,080	1,127	1,175
3.7	756	788	822	857	893	931	971	1,012	1,056	1,101	1,147	1,196
3.8	772	805	839	874	911	950	990	1,032	1,076	1,121	1,168	1,218
3.9	789	822	856	892	930	969	1,009	1,052	1,096	1,142	1,190	1,240
4.0	806	839	874	911	949	988	1,029	1,072	1,117	1,163	1,212	1,262
4.1	828	857	892	929	968	1,008	1,049	1,093	1,138	1,185	1,234	1,285
4.2	841	875	911	948	987	1,028	1,070	1,114	1,159	1,207	1,256	1,308
4.3	859	893	930	968	1,007	1,048	1,091	1,135	1,181	1,229	1,279	1,331
4.4	877	912	949	987	1,027	1,069	1,112	1,157	1,204	1,252	1,303	1,355
4.5	896	932	969	1,008	1,048	1,090	1,134	1,179	1,226	1,275	1,326	1,380
4.6	915	951	989	1,028	1,069	1,112	1,156	1,202	1,249	1,299	1,351	1,404
4.7	934	971	1,010	1,049	1,091	1,134	1,178	1,225	1,273	1,323	1,375	1,430
4.8	954	992	1,031	1,071	1,113	1,156	1,201	1,248	1,297	1,348	1,401	1,455
4.9	975	1,013	1,052	1,093	1,135	1,179	1,225	1,272	1,322	1,373	1,426	1,482
5.0	996	1,034	1,074	1,115	1,158	1,203	1,249	1,297	1,347	1,399	1,452	1,508
5.1	1,017	1,056	1,096	1,138	1,181	1,226	1,273	1,322	1,372	1,425	1,479	1,535
5.2	1,039	1,078	1,119	1,161	1,205	1,251	1,298	1,347	1,398	1,451	1,506	1,563
5.3	1,061	1,101	1,142	1,185	1,229	1,276	1,323	1,373	1,425	1,478	1,533	1,591
5.4	1,084	1,124	1,166	1,209	1,254	1,301	1,349	1,399	1,452	1,506	1,562	1,620
5.5	1,107	1,148	1,190	1,234	1,279	1,327	1,376	1,426	1,479	1,534	1,590	1,649
5.6	1,131	1,172	1,215	1,259	1,305	1,353	1,402	1,454	1,507	1,562	1,619	1,678
5.7	1,155	1,197	1,240	1,285	1,332	1,380	1,430	1,482	1,535	1,591	1,649	1,709
5.8	1,180	1,222	1,266	1,311	1,358	1,407	1,458	1,510	1,564	1,621	1,679	1,739
5.9	1,205	1,248	1,292	1,338	1,386	1,435	1,486	1,539	1,594	1,651	1,710	1,770
6.0	1,231	1,274	1,319	1,366	1,414	1,464	1,515	1,569	1,624	1,682	1,741	1,802
6.1	1,257	1,301	1,346	1,393	1,442	1,493	1,545	1,599	1,655	1,713	1,773	1,835
6.2	1,284	1,328	1,374	1,422	1,471	1,522	1,575	1,630	1,686	1,745	1,805	1,868
6.3	1,311	1,356	1,403	1,451	1,501	1,552	1,606	1,661	1,718	1,777	1,838	1,901
6.4	1,339	1,385	1,432	1,481	1,531	1,583	1,637	1,693	1,751	1,810	1,872	1,935
6.5	1,368	1,414	1,462	1,511	1,562	1,615	1,669	1,725	1,784	1,844	1,906	1,970
6.6	1,397	1,444	1,492	1,542	1,594	1,647	1,702	1,759	1,817	1,878	1,941	2,006
6.7	1,427	1,474	1,523	1,574	1,626	1,679	1,735	1,792	1,852	1,913	1,976	2,042
6.8	1,458	1,505	1,555	1,606	1,658	1,713	1,769	1,827	1,887	1,949	2,012	2,078
6.9	1,489	1,537	1,587	1,639	1,692	1,747	1,803	1,862	1,922	1,985	2,049	2,116
7.0	1,521	1,570	1,620	1,672	1,726	1,781	1,839	1,898	1,959	2,022	2,087	2,154

Abdominal circumferences

34.0	34.5	35.0	35.5	36.0	36.5	37.0	37.5	38.0	38.5	39.0	39.5	40.0
1,123	1,173	1,225	1,279	1,336	1,396	1,458	1,523	1,591	1,661	1,735	1,812	1,893
1,143	1,193	1,246	1,301	1,358	1,418	1,481	1,546	1,615	1,686	1,761	1,838	1,920
1,163	1,214	1,267	1,323	1,381	1,441	1,504	1,570	1,639	1,711	1,786	1,865	1,946
1,183	1,235	1,289	1,345	1,403	1,464	1,528	1,595	1,664	1,737	1,812	1,891	1,973
1,204	1,256	1,311	1,367	1,426	1,488	1,552	1,619	1,689	1,762	1,839	1,918	2,001
1,226	1,278	1,333	1,390	1,450	1,512	1,577	1,645	1,715	1,789	1,865	1,945	2,029
1,247	1,300	1,356	1,413	1,474	1,536	1,602	1,670	1,741	1,815	1,893	1,973	2,057
1,269	1,323	1,379	1,437	1,498	1,561	1,627	1,696	1,768	1,842	1,920	2,001	2,086
1,292	1,346	1,402	1,461	1,523	1,586	1,653	1,722	1,794	1,870	1,948	2,030	2,115
1,315	1,369	1,426	1,486	1,548	1,612	1,679	1,749	1,822	1,898	1,977	2,059	2,145
1,338	1,393	1,451	1,511	1,573	1,638	1,706	1,776	1,849	1,926	2,005	2,088	2,174
1,361	1,417	1,475	1,536	1,599	1,664	1,733	1,804	1,878	1,954	2,035	2,118	2,205
1,385	1,442	1,500	1,562	1,625	1,691	1,760	1,832	1,906	1,984	2,064	2,148	2,236
1,410	1,467	1,526	1,588	1,652	1,718	1,788	1,860	1,935	2,013	2,094	2,179	2,267
1,435	1,492	1,552	1,614	1,679	1,746	1,816	1,889	1,964	2,043	2,125	2,210	2,298
1,460	1,518	1,579	1,641	1,706	1,774	1,845	1,918	1,994	2,073	2,156	2,241	2,330
1,486	1,545	1,605	1,669	1,734	1,803	1,874	1,948	2,024	2,104	2,187	2,273	2,363
1,512	1,571	1,633	1,697	1,763	1,832	1,904	1,978	2,055	2,136	2,219	2,306	2,396
1,539	1,599	1,661	1,725	1,792	1,861	1,934	2,009	2,086	2,167	2,251	2,339	2,429
1,566	1,626	1,689	1,754	1,821	1,891	1,964	2,040	2,118	2,200	2,284	2,372	2,463
1,594	1,655	1,718	1,783	1,851	1,922	1,995	2,071	2,150	2,232	2,317	2,406	2,498
1,622	1,683	1,747	1,813	1,882	1,953	2,027	2,103	2,183	2,266	2,351	2,440	2,532
1,651	1,713	1,777	1,843	1,913	1,984	2,059	2,136	2,216	2,299	2,386	2,475	2,568
1,680	1,742	1,807	1,874	1,944	2,016	2,091	2,169	2,250	2,333	2,420	2,510	2,604
1,710	1,773	1,838	1,906	1,976	2,049	2,124	2,203	2,284	2,368	2,456	2,546	2,640
1,740	1,803	1,869	1,938	2,008	2,082	2,158	2,237	2,319	2,403	2,491	2,582	2,677
1,770	1,835	1,901	1,970	2,041	2,115	2,192	2,272	2,354	2,439	2,528	2,619	2,714
1,802	1,866	1,934	2,003	2,075	2,150	2,227	2,307	2,390	2,475	2,564	2,657	2,752
1,834	1,899	1,966	2,037	2,109	2,184	2,262	2,342	2,426	2,512	2,602	2,694	2,790
1,866	1,932	2,000	2,071	2,144	2,219	2,298	2,379	2,463	2,550	2,640	2,733	2,829
1,899	1,965	2,034	2,105	2,179	2,255	2,334	2,416	2,500	2,588	2,678	2,772	2,869
1,932	1,999	2,069	2,140	2,215	2,291	2,371	2,453	2,538	2,626	2,717	2,811	2,909
1,967	2,034	2,104	2,176	2,251	2,328	2,408	2,491	2,577	2,665	2,757	2,851	2,949
2,001	2,069	2,140	2,213	2,288	2,366	2,446	2,530	2,616	2,705	2,797	2,892	2,991
2,037	2,105	2,176	2,250	2,326	2,404	2,485	2,569	2,656	2,745	2,838	2,933	3,032
2,073	2,142	2,213	2,287	2,364	2,443	2,524	2,609	2,696	2,786	2,879	2,975	3,075
2,109	2,179	2,251	2,326	2,403	2,482	2,564	2,649	2,737	2,827	2,921	3,018	3,117
2,147	2,217	2,290	2,365	2,442	2,522	2,605	2,690	2,778	2,869	2,964	3,061	3,161
2,184	2,255	2,329	2,404	2,482	2,563	2,646	2,732	2,821	2,912	3,007	3,104	3,205
2,223	2,295	2,368	2,444	2,523	2,604	2,688	2,774	2,863	2,955	3,050	3,149	3,250

(*continued*)

Appendix 13.
Predicting Fetal Weight by Ultrasound (*continued*)

Biparietal diameters	Abdominal circumferences											
	28.0	28.5	29.0	29.5	30.0	30.5	31.0	31.5	32.0	32.5	33.0	33.5
7.1	1,553	1,603	1,654	1,706	1,761	1,817	1,875	1,934	1,996	2,059	2,125	2,193
7.2	1,586	1,636	1,688	1,741	1,796	1,853	1,911	1,971	2,044	2,098	2,164	2,232
7.3	1,620	1,671	1,723	1,777	1,832	1,890	1,948	2,009	2,072	2,137	2,203	2,272
7.4	1,655	1,706	1,759	1,813	1,869	1,927	1,987	2,048	2,111	2,176	2,244	2,313
7.5	1,690	1,742	1,795	1,850	1,907	1,965	2,025	2,087	2,151	2,217	2,265	2,354
7.6	1,727	1,779	1,833	1,888	1,945	2,004	2,065	2,127	2,192	2,258	2,326	2,397
7.7	1,764	1,816	1,871	1,927	1,985	2,044	2,105	2,168	2,233	2,300	2,369	2,440
7.8	1,801	1,855	1,910	1,966	2,025	2,085	2,146	2,210	2,275	2,343	2,412	2,484
7.9	1,840	1,894	1,949	2,006	2,065	2,126	2,188	2,252	2,318	2,386	2,456	2,528
8.0	1,879	1,934	1,990	2,048	2,107	2,168	2,231	2,296	2,362	2,431	2,501	2,574
8.1	1,919	1,975	2,031	2,089	2,149	2,211	2,275	2,340	2,407	2,476	2,547	2,620
8.2	1,960	2,016	2,073	2,132	2,193	2,255	2,319	2,385	2,462	2,522	2,594	2,667
8.3	2,002	2,059	2,116	2,176	2,237	2,300	2,364	2,431	2,499	2,569	2,641	2,715
8.4	2,045	2,102	2,160	2,220	2,282	2,345	2,410	2,477	2,546	2,617	2,689	2,764
8.5	2,089	2,146	2,205	2,266	2,328	2,392	2,457	2,525	2,594	2,665	2,739	2,814
8.6	2,134	2,192	2,251	2,312	2,375	2,439	2,505	2,573	2,643	2,715	2,789	2,864
8.7	2,179	2,238	2,298	2,359	2,423	2,488	2,554	2,623	2,693	2,765	2,840	2,916
8.8	2,226	2,285	2,346	2,408	2,472	2,537	2,604	2,673	2,744	2,817	2,892	2,968
8.9	2,274	2,333	2,394	2,457	2,521	2,587	2,655	2,725	2,796	2,869	2,944	3,021
9.0	2,322	2,382	2,444	2,507	2,572	2,639	2,707	2,777	2,849	2,923	2,998	3,076
9.1	2,372	2,433	2,495	2,559	2,624	2,691	2,760	2,830	2,903	2,977	3,053	3,131
9.2	2,423	2,484	2,547	2,611	2,677	2,744	2,814	2,885	2,958	3,032	3,109	3,187
9.3	2,475	2,536	2,599	2,664	2,731	2,799	2,869	2,940	3,014	3,089	3,166	3,245
9.4	2,527	2,590	2,653	2,719	2,786	2,854	2,925	2,997	3,070	3,146	3,224	3,303
9.5	2,582	2,644	2,709	2,774	2,842	2,911	2,982	3,054	3,129	3,205	3,283	3,362
9.6	2,637	2,700	2,765	2,831	2,899	2,969	3,040	3,113	3,188	3,264	3,343	3,423
9.7	2,693	2,757	2,822	2,889	2,958	3,028	3,099	3,173	3,248	3,325	3,404	3,484
9.8	2,751	2,815	2,881	2,948	3,017	3,088	3,160	3,234	3,309	3,387	3,466	3,547
9.9	2,810	2,874	2,941	3,009	3,078	3,149	3,222	3,296	3,372	3,450	3,529	3,611
10.0	2,870	2,935	3,002	3,070	3,140	3,211	3,285	3,359	3,436	3,514	3,594	3,676

Abdominal circumferences

34.0	34.5	35.0	35.5	36.0	36.5	37.0	37.5	38.0	38.5	39.0	39.5	40.0
2,262	2,334	2,409	2,485	2,564	2,646	2,730	2,817	2,907	2,999	3,095	3,193	3,295
2,302	2,375	2,450	2,527	2,607	2,689	2,773	2,861	2,951	3,044	3,140	3,239	3,341
2,343	2,416	2,491	2,569	2,649	2,732	2,817	2,905	2,996	3,089	3,186	3,285	3,388
2,384	2,458	2,534	2,612	2,693	2,776	2,862	2,950	3,041	3,135	3,232	3,332	3,435
2,426	2,501	2,577	2,656	2,737	2,821	2,907	2,996	3,088	3,182	3,279	3,380	3,483
2,469	2,544	2,621	2,700	2,782	2,866	2,953	3,042	3,134	3,229	3,327	3,428	3,531
2,513	2,588	2,666	2,746	2,828	2,912	3,000	2,090	3,182	3,277	3,376	3,477	3,581
2,557	2,633	2,711	2,792	2,874	2,959	3,047	3,137	3,230	3,326	3,425	3,526	3,631
2,603	2,679	2,757	2,838	2,921	3,007	3,095	3,186	3,279	3,376	3,475	3,576	3,681
2,649	2,725	2,804	2,886	2,969	3,056	3,144	3,235	3,329	3,426	3,525	3,627	3,733
2,695	2,773	2,852	2,934	3,018	3,105	3,194	3,286	3,380	3,477	3,577	3,679	3,785
2,743	2,821	2,901	2,983	3,068	3,155	3,244	3,336	3,431	3,529	3,629	3,732	3,838
2,791	2,870	2,950	3,033	3,118	3,206	3,296	3,388	3,483	3,581	3,682	3,785	3,891
2,841	2,920	3,001	3,084	3,169	3,257	3,348	3,441	3,536	3,634	3,735	3,839	3,945
2,891	2,970	3,052	3,135	3,221	3,310	3,401	3,494	3,590	3,688	3,790	3,894	4,000
2,942	3,022	3,104	3,188	3,274	3,363	3,454	3,548	3,644	3,743	3,845	3,949	4,056
2,994	3,074	3,157	3,241	3,328	3,417	3,509	3,603	3,700	3,799	3,901	4,005	4,113
3,047	3,128	3,210	3,295	3,383	3,472	3,565	3,659	3,756	3,855	3,958	4,063	4,170
3,101	3,182	3,265	3,351	3,438	3,528	3,621	3,716	3,813	3,913	4,015	4,120	4,228
3,155	3,237	3,321	3,407	3,495	3,585	3,678	3,773	3,871	3,971	4,074	4,179	4,287
3,211	3,293	3,377	3,464	3,552	3,643	3,736	3,832	3,930	4,030	4,133	4,239	4,347
3,268	3,350	3,435	3,522	3,611	3,702	3,795	3,891	3,989	4,090	4,193	4,299	4,408
3,326	3,409	3,494	3,581	3,670	3,761	3,855	3,951	4,050	4,151	4,254	4,361	4,469
3,384	3,468	3,553	3,641	3,738	3,822	3,916	4,013	4,111	4,213	4,316	4,423	4,532
3,444	3,528	3,614	3,701	3,791	3,884	3,978	4,075	4,174	4,275	4,379	4,486	4,595
3,505	3,589	3,675	3,763	3,854	3,946	4,041	4,138	4,237	4,339	4,443	4,550	4,659
3,567	3,651	3,738	3,826	3,917	4,010	4,105	4,202	4,302	4,404	4,508	4,615	4,724
3,630	3,715	3,802	3,890	3,981	4,074	4,170	4,267	4,367	4,469	4,573	4,680	4,790
3,694	3,779	3,866	3,956	4,047	4,140	4,236	4,333	4,433	4,536	4,640	4,747	4,857
3,759	3,845	3,932	4,022	4,113	4,207	4,303	4,400	4,501	4,603	4,708	4,815	4,924

Appendix 14.

Tenth Percentile of Birth Weight (g) for Gestational Age by Gender:
U.S. 1991 Single Live Births to Resident Mothers

Gestational age (wk)	Male	Female	
20	270	256	
21	328	310	
22	388	368	
23	446	426	
24	504	480	
25	570	535	
26	644	592	
27	728	662	
28	828	760	
29	956	889	
30	1117	1047	
31	1308	1234	
32	1521	1447	
33	1751	1675	
34	1985	1901	
35	2205	2109	
36	2407	2300	
37	2596	2484	
38	2769	2657	
39	2908	2796	
40	2986	2872	
41	3007	2891	
42	2998	2884	
43	2977	2868	
44	2963	2853	

Source: Alexander, G. R., Himes, J. H., Kaufman, R. B., Mor, J., Kogan, M. A United States national reference for fetal growth. *Obstet Gynecol* 87(2):167, 1996. Reprinted with permission from The American College of Obstetrics and Gynecologists.

Appendix 15.

Ratio of Head Circumference to Abdominal Circumference: Normal Values

Menstrual Age (weeks)	−2 S.D.† (cm)	Predicted Value* (cm)	+2 S.D.† (cm)	−2 S.D.§ (cm)	Predicted Value‡ (cm)	−2 S.D.§ (cm)
12	1.16	1.29	1.41	1.12	1.22	1.31
13	1.15	1.28	1.40	1.11	1.21	1.30
14	1.14	1.27	1.39	1.11	1.20	1.30
15	1.13	1.26	1.38	1.10	1.19	1.29
16	1.12	1.25	1.37	1.09	1.18	1.28
17	1.11	1.24	1.36	1.08	1.18	1.27
18	1.10	1.22	1.35	1.07	1.17	1.26
19	1.09	1.21	1.34	1.06	1.16	1.25
20	1.08	1.20	1.33	1.06	1.15	1.24
21	1.07	1.19	1.32	1.05	1.14	1.24
22	1.06	1.18	1.30	1.04	1.13	1.23
23	1.05	1.17	1.29	1.03	1.12	1.22
24	1.04	1.16	1.28	1.02	1.12	1.21
25	1.03	1.15	1.27	1.01	1.11	1.20
26	1.02	1.14	1.26	1.00	1.10	1.19
27	1.01	1.13	1.25	1.00	1.09	1.18
28	1.00	1.12	1.24	.99	1.08	1.18
29	.99	1.11	1.23	.98	1.07	1.17
30	.97	1.10	1.22	.97	1.07	1.16
31	.96	1.09	1.21	.96	1.06	1.15
32	.95	1.08	1.20	.95	1.05	1.14
33	.94	1.07	1.19	.95	1.04	1.13
34	.93	1.05	1.18	.94	1.03	1.13
35	.92	1.04	1.17	.93	1.02	1.12
36	.91	1.03	1.16	.92	1.01	1.11
37	.90	1.02	1.15	.91	1.01	1.10
38	.89	1.01	1.13	.90	1.00	1.09
39	.88	1.00	1.12	.89	.99	1.08
40	.87	.99	1.11	.89	.98	1.08

*HC/AC = 1.42104 − .0106229(MA)[R^2 = 58.9%].

†2 S.D. = 0.12.

‡HC/AC = 1.32293 − .0084471(MA)[R^2 = 67.2%].

§2 S.C. = 0.10

Source: Adapted from Callen, P. W. *Ultrasonography in Obstetrics and Gynecology.* Boston: Saunders, 1983. With permission.

Appendix 16.

Renal to Abdominal Ratio in the Fetus

Range Throughout Second and Third Trimester	Ratio
Renal to Abdominal Circumferences	0.27 to 0.30
Renal to Abdominal Anterior-Posterior Diameters	0.25 to 0.31
Renal to Abdominal Transverse Diameters	0.27 to 0.31

Source: Grannum, P., Bracken, M., Silverman, R., Hobbins, J. C. Assessment of fetal kidney size in normal gestation by comparison of ratio of kidney circumference to abdominal circumference. *Am J Obstet Gynecol* 136:249–254, 1980. With permission.

Appendix 17.

Mean Renal Lengths for Various Gestational Ages

Gestational Age (weeks)	Mean Length (cm)	SD	95% CI	n
18	2.2	0.3	1.6–2.8	14
19	2.3	0.4	1.5–3.1	23
20	2.6	0.4	1.8–3.4	22
21	2.7	0.3	2.1–3.2	20
22	2.7	0.3	2.0–3.4	18
23	3.0	0.4	2.2–3.7	13
24	3.1	0.6	1.9–4.4	13
25	3.3	0.4	2.5–4.2	9
26	3.4	0.4	2.4–4.4	9
27	3.5	0.4	2.7–4.4	15
28	3.4	0.4	2.6–4.2	19
29	3.6	0.7	2.3–4.8	12
30	3.8	0.4	2.9–4.6	24
31	3.7	0.5	2.8–4.6	23
32	4.1	0.5	3.1–5.1	23
33	4.0	0.3	3.3–4.7	28
34	4.2	0.4	3.3–5.0	36
35	4.2	0.5	3.2–5.2	17
36	4.2	0.4	3.3–5.0	36
37	4.2	0.4	3.3–5.1	40
38	4.4	0.6	3.2–5.6	32
39	4.2	0.3	3.5–4.8	17
40	4.3	0.5	3.2–5.3	10
41	4.5	0.3	3.9–5.1	4

Source: Cohen, HL et al, Normal length of fetal kidneys: Sonographic study in 397 obstetric patients. *AJR* 157:545–548, 1991. Reprinted with permission from the American Roentgen Ray Society.

Appendix 18.
Ocular, Binocular, and Interocular Distance

Predicted BPD and Weeks Gestation from the Inner and Outer Orbital Distances
Measure "Outer to Outer Margins of Eyes"

BPD (cm)	Gestation (wk)	IOD (cm)	OOD (cm)	BPD (cm)	Gestation (wk)	IOD (cm)	OOD (cm)
1.9	11.6	0.5	1.3	5.8	24.3	1.6	4.1
2.0	11.6	0.5	1.4	5.9	24.3	1.6	4.2
2.1	12.1	0.6	1.5	6.0	24.7	1.6	4.3
2.2	12.6	0.6	1.6	6.1	25.2	1.6	4.3
2.3	12.6	0.6	1.7	6.2	25.2	1.6	4.4
2.4	13.1	0.7	1.7	6.3	25.7	1.7	4.4
2.5	13.6	0.7	1.8	6.4	26.2	1.7	4.5
2.6	13.6	0.7	1.9	6.5	26.2	1.7	4.5
2.7	14.1	0.8	2.0	6.6	26.7	1.7	4.6
2.8	14.6	0.8	2.1	6.7	27.2	1.7	4.6
2.9	14.6	0.8	2.1	6.8	27.6	1.7	4.7
3.0	15.0	0.9	2.2	6.9	28.1	1.7	4.7
3.1	15.5	0.9	2.3	7.0	28.6	1.8	4.8
3.2	15.5	0.9	2.4	7.1	29.1	1.8	4.8
3.3	16.0	1.0	2.5	7.3	29.6	1.8	4.9
3.4	16.5	1.0	2.5	7.4	30.0	1.8	5.0
3.5	16.5	1.0	2.6	7.5	30.6	1.8	5.0
3.6	17.0	1.0	2.7	7.6	31.0	1.8	5.1
3.7	17.5	1.1	2.7	7.7	31.5	1.8	5.1
3.8	17.9	1.1	2.8	7.8	32.0	1.8	5.2
4.0	18.4	1.2	3.0	7.9	32.5	1.9	5.2
4.2	18.9	1.2	3.1	8.0	33.0	1.9	5.3
4.3	19.4	1.2	3.2	8.2	33.5	1.9	5.4
4.4	19.4	1.3	3.2	8.3	34.0	1.9	5.4
4.5	19.9	1.3	3.3	8.4	34.4	1.9	5.4
4.6	20.4	1.3	3.4	8.5	35.0	1.9	5.5
4.7	20.4	1.3	3.4	8.6	35.4	1.9	5.5
4.8	20.9	1.4	3.5	8.8	35.9	1.9	5.6
4.9	21.3	1.4	3.6	8.9	36.4	1.9	5.6
5.0	21.3	1.4	3.6	9.0	36.9	1.9	5.7
5.1	21.8	1.4	3.7	9.1	37.3	1.9	5.7
5.2	22.3	1.4	3.8	9.2	37.8	1.9	5.8
5.3	22.3	1.5	3.8	9.3	38.3	1.9	5.8
5.4	22.8	1.5	3.9	9.4	38.8	1.9	5.8
5.5	23.3	1.5	4.0	9.6	39.3	1.9	5.9
5.6	23.3	1.5	4.0	9.7	39.8	1.9	5.9
5.7	23.8	1.5	4.1				

Source: Mayden, K. L., Tortora, M., Berkowitz, R. L. Orbital diameters: A new parameter for prenatal diagnosis and dating. *Am J Obstet Gynecol* 144:289–297, 1982. With permission.

Appendix 19.
Normal Ocular Values

Week	Ocular Diameter			Binocular Distance			Interocular Distance		
	Percentile			*Percentile*			*Percentile*		
	5th	*50th*	*95th*	*5th*	*50th*	*95th*	*5th*	*50th*	*95th*
12	2	4	6	11	16	20	4	8	11
13	3	5	6	14	18	23	5	8	11
14	4	5	7	16	20	25	6	9	12
15	4	6	8	18	23	27	6	10	13
16	5	7	9	20	25	29	7	10	13
17	6	8	10	22	27	31	8	11	14
18	7	9	10	24	29	33	8	11	15
19	8	9	11	26	31	33	9	12	15
20	8	10	12	28	33	37	10	13	16
21	9	11	13	30	35	39	10	13	16
22	10	11	13	32	36	41	11	14	17
23	10	12	14	34	38	43	11	14	17
24	11	13	15	35	40	44	12	15	18
25	12	13	15	37	42	46	12	15	19
26	12	14	16	39	43	47	13	16	19
27	13	15	16	40	45	49	13	16	19
28	13	15	17	42	46	51	14	17	20
29	14	16	17	43	48	52	14	17	20
30	14	16	18	45	49	53	15	18	21
31	15	17	18	46	50	55	15	18	21
32	15	17	19	47	52	56	15	19	22
33	16	17	19	49	53	57	16	19	22
34	16	18	20	50	54	58	16	19	22
35	16	18	20	51	55	60	16	20	23
36	17	19	20	52	56	61	17	20	23
37	17	19	21	53	57	62	17	20	23
38	17	19	21	54	58	63	17	21	24
39	18	20	21	55	59	64	18	21	24
40	18	20	22	56	60	64	18	21	24

Source: Mayden, K. L., Tortora, M., Berkowitz, R. L. Orbital diameters: A new parameter for prenatal diagnosis and dating. *Am J Obstet Gynecol* 144:289–297, 1982. With permission.

Appendix 20.
Ultrasound Measurement* of the Fetal Liver From
20 Weeks' Gestation to Term

Gestational Age (wk)	Number of Measurements	Arithmetic Mean (mm)	±2 SD (mm)
20	8	27.3	6.4
21	2	28.0	1.5
22	4	30.6	6.7
23	13	30.9	4.5
24	10	32.9	6.7
25	14	33.6	5.3
26	10	35.7	6.3
27	20	36.6	3.3
28	14	38.4	4.0
29	13	39.1	5.0
30	10	38.7	5.0
31	13	39.6	5.7
32	11	42.7	7.5
33	14	43.8	6.6
34	11	44.8	7.1
35	14	47.8	9.1
36	10	49.0	8.4
37	10	52.0	6.8
38	12	52.9	4.2
39	5	55.4	6.7
40	1	59.0	—
41	2	49.3	2.4

SD = standard deviation

*Mean length ± 2 SD.

Source: Vintzelios, A. M., et al. Fetal liver ultrasound measurements during normal pregnancy. *Obstet Gynecol* 66(4):477–480, October, 1985. With permission.

Appendix 21.

Detection of Fetal Ossification Centers by Weeks of Gestational Age

Gestational Age (Weeks)	Number of Fetuses Examined (n = 295)	Calcaneal	Talar	Distal Femoral Epiphyseal	Proximal Tibial Epiphyseal
22	12	—	—	—	—
23	14	—	—	—	—
24	9	4	—	—	—
25	10	9	—	—	—
26	8	8	2	—	—
27	12	12	10	—	—
28	9	9	9	—	—
29	10	10	10	—	—
30	15	15	15	—	—
31	14	14	14	—	—
32	17	17	17	5	—
33	19	19	19	10	—
34	15	15	15	14	—
35	21	21	21	19	—
36	29	29	29	27	8
37	25	25	25	23	19
38	22	22	22	22	20
39	18	18	18	17	16
40	16	16	16	16	16

Source: Gentili, P., Trasimeni, A., Giorlandino, C. Fetal ossification centers. *J Ultrasound Med* 3:193–197, May 1984. With permission.

Appendix 22.
Normal Ultrasonic Fetal Weight Curve (g)

Gest. Age	−2 S.D.	−1.5 S.D.	Mean	+1.5 S.D.	+2 S.D.
15	100	106	123	141	146
16	134	141	161	182	188
17	174	182	206	230	238
18	222	232	259	287	296
19	278	290	321	353	363
20	344	356	392	428	440
21	418	432	472	514	523
22	502	518	562	609	624
23	595	613	663	715	732
24	698	718	773	833	851
25	811	833	895	961	981
26	933	958	1026	1101	1123
27	1065	1092	1169	1252	1277
28	1205	1236	1321	1414	1442
29	1354	1388	1483	1588	1619
30	1510	1548	1655	1772	1808
31	1673	1716	1837	1968	2008
32	1843	1892	2027	2174	2219
33	2018	2073	2225	2391	2441
34	2198	2260	2431	2617	2673
35	2381	2451	2644	2852	3094
36	2567	2646	2864	3097	3168
37	2755	2844	3088	3350	3429
38	2944	3043	3318	3610	3699
39	3133	3244	3552	3877	3977
40	3320	3444	3788	4151	4262
41	3506	3643	4027	4430	4554
42	3688	3841	4268	4715	4852

Source: Ott, W. J. The diagnosis of altered fetal growth. *Obstetrics and Gynecology Clinics of North Am.* 15(2):237–263, June 1988.

Appendix 23.

Patterns of Sequential Dilatation for the Right and Left Maternal
Kidneys in Pregnancy

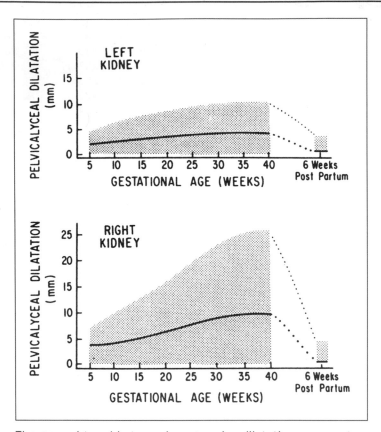

The general trend is toward progressive dilatation, more extensive on the right but with broad ranges for both. Dotted lines
merely extend mean and maximum values to the postpartum.

Source: Fried, A. M., Woodring, J. H., Thompson, D. J. Hydronephrosis of pregnancy: A
prospective sequential study of the course of dilatation. *J Ultrasound Med* 2(6):255–259,
June 1983. With permission.

Appendix 24.

Ovarian Volume and Changes in Ovarian Morphology as
Determined by Ultrasonography From Ages 2–13

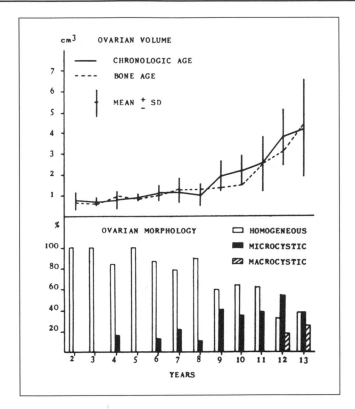

Source: Orsini, L. F., Salardi, S., Gianluigi, P., Bovicelli, L., Cacciari, E., Pelvic organs
in premenarchal girls: Real-time ultrasonography. *Radiology* 153:113–116, 1984.
With permission of the Radiologic Society of America.

Appendix 25.
Effects of Drugs on the Fetus

Drug	Central nervous system	Cardiovascular	Skeleton
Acetaminophen (overdose)			
Acetazolamide			Sacrococcygeal teratoma
Acetylsalicylic acid		Intracranial hemorrhage	
Albuteral		Fetal tachycardia	
Alcohol	Microcephaly		Short nose, hypoplastic maxilla, micrognathia, occasional features of skeleton
Amantadine		Single ventricle with pulmonary atresia	
Aminopterin*	Meningoencephalocele, hydrocephalus, incomplete skull ossification, brachycephaly, anencephaly		Hypoplasia of thumb and fibula, clubfoot, syndactyly, hypognathia
Amitriptyline			Micrognathia
Amobarbital	Anencephaly	Congenital heart malformations	
Antithyroid drugs*			
Azathioprine*		Pulmonary valvular stenosis	
Betamethasone	Reduced head circumference		
Bromides			
Busulfan			
Caffeine			Musculoskeletal defects
Captopril			
Carbon monoxide*	Cerebral atrophy, hydrocephalus		
Carbamazepine	Meningomyelocele	Atrial septal defect, patent ductus arteriosus	Nose hypoplasia, hypertelorism
Chlordiazepoxide	Microcephaly	Congenital defects of heart	
Chloroquine			
Chlorpheniramine	Hydrocephalus		
Chlorpropamide	Microcephaly		
Clomiphene	Meningomyelocele, hydrocephalus, microcephaly, anencephaly		
Codeine	Hydrocephalus	Congenital cardiac defects	Musculoskeletal malformations
Cortisone	Hydrocephalus	Ventricular septal defect, coarctation of aorta	
Coumadin*	Encephalocele, anencephaly, spina bifida	Congenital heart disease	Nasal hypoplasia, scoliosis, skeletal deformities
Cyclophosphamide*	Tetralogy of Fallot		Flattened nasal bridge
Cytarabine*	Anencephaly	Tetralogy of Fallot	
Daunorubicin*	Anencephaly	Tetralogy of Fallot	
Dextroamphetamine	Exencephaly	More cardiac defects than controls, atrial septal defect	

Extremities	Gastrointestinal	Genitourinary	Miscellaneous	Source
			Polyhydramnios	CR
				CR
			Growth retardation	CR
				RS
				PS
				PS
			Growth retardation	CR
				RS
				PS
				CR
				CR
Limb reduction, swelling of hands and feet		Urinary retention		CR
Severe limb deformities, congenital hip dislocation, polydactyly, clubfoot	Oral cleft	Intersex	Soft tissue deformity of neck	CR
				PS
				RS
			Goiter	CR
				RS
Polydactyly				CR
				AS
Polydactyly, clubfoot, congenital dislocation of hip				CR
				PS
	Pyloric stenosis, cleft palate		Microphthalmia, growth retardation	CR
		Hydronephrosis		PS
Leg reduction				CR
			Stillbirth	CR
				CR
Congenital hip dislocation	Cleft lip			PS
	Duodenal atresia			RS
				RS
Polydactyly, congenital dislocation of hip			Hemihypertrophy	CR
				PS
Dysmorphic hands and fingers				CR
Syndactyly, clubfoot, polydactyly	Esophageal atresia			CR
				RS
Dislocated hip	Pyloric stenosis, oral cleft		Respiratory malformations	PS
Clubfoot	Cleft lip			RS
				CR
Stippled epiphysis, chondroplasia punctata, short phalanges, toe defects	Incomplete rotation of gut		Growth retardation, bleeding	CR
				RS
Four toes on each foot, hypoplastic midphalanx, syndactyly				CR
				CR
Lobster claw of 3 digits, missing feet digits, syndactyly				
Syndactyly			Growth retardation	CR
				CR
				RS

(*continued*)

Appendix 25.
Effects of Drugs on the Fetus (continued)

Drug	Central nervous system	Cardiovascular	Skeleton
Diazepam	Spina bifida	More cardiac defects than controls	
Diphenhydramine			
Disulfiram			Vertebral fusion
Diuretics			
Estrogens		Congenital cardiac malformation	
Ethanol*	Microcephaly	Ventral septal defect, atrial septal defect, double outlet of right ventricle, pulmonary atresia, dextrocardia, patent ductus arteriosus, tetralogy of Fallot	Short nose, hypoplastic philtrum, micrognathia, pectus excavatum, radioulnar synostosis, bifid xyphoid, scoliosis
Ethosuximide	Hydrocephalus		Short neck
Fluorouracil			
Fluphenazine			Poor ossification of frontal bone
Haloperidol			
Heparin*			
Hormones, progestogenic	Anencephaly, hydrocephalus	Tetralogy of Fallot, truncus arteriosus, ventral septal defect	Spina bifida
Imipramine	Exencephaly		
Indomethacin			
Isoniazid	Meningomyelocele		
Lithium	Hydrocephalus, meningomyelocele	Ventral septal defect, Ebstein's anomaly, mitral atresia, patent ductus arteriosus, dextrocardia	Spina bifida
Lysergic acid diethylamide	Hydrocephalus, encephalocele, meningomyelocele		
Meclizine		Hypoplastic left heart	
Meprobamate		Congenital heart malformations	
Methotrexate*	Oxycephaly, absence of frontal bone, large fontanelles	Dextrocardia	Hypoplastic mandible
Methyl mercury*	Microcephaly, asymmetric head		
Metronidazole			Midline facial defects
Nortriptyline			
Oral contraceptives	Meningomyelocele, hydrocephalus, anencephaly	Cardiac anomalies	Vertebral malformations
Paramethadione		Tetralogy of Fallot	
Penicillamine		Ventral septal defect	
Phenobarbital	Hydrocephalus, meningomyelocele		
Phenothiazines	Microcephaly		
Phenylephrine			Eye and ear abnormalities
Phenylpropanolamine	Microcephaly, wide fontanelles	Congenital heart malformation	Pectus excavatus
Phenytoin*			Rib-sternal abnormalities, short nose, broad nasal bridge, wide fontanelle, broad alveolar ridge, short neck, hypertelorism, low-set ears

Extremities	Gastrointestinal	Genitourinary	Miscellaneous	Source
Absence of arm, syndactyly, absence of thumbs	Cleft lip-palate			CR
				RS
Clubfoot	Cleft palate			PS
Clubfoot, radial aplasia, phocomelia	Tracheoesophageal fistula			CR
				CR
			Respiratory malformations	PS
Limb reduction				CR
				PS
	Oral cleft		Growth retardation, diaphragmatic hernia	RS
				PS
	Oral cleft			CR
Radial aplasia, absent thumbs	Aplasia of esophagus and duodenum		Hypoplasia of lungs	CR
	Oral cleft			CR
				RS
Limb deformities			Bleeding	CR
				RS
Absence of thumbs				CR
Limb reduction	Cleft palate	Renal cystic degeneration	Diaphragmatic hernia	CR
Phocomelia			Stillbirth, hemorrhage	CR
				CR
				CR
				PS
Limb deficiencies				CR
				RS
			Respiratory defects	RS
Bilateral defects of limbs				RS
				CR
Long webbed fingers			Growth retardation, low-set ears	CR
				RS
				CR
Limb reduction				CR
Limb reduction	Tracheoesophageal malformations		Growth retardation	CR
				CR
			Growth retardation	RS
	Pyloric stenosis		Growth retardation	CR
Digital anomalies	Cleft palate, ileal atresia		Growth retardation, pulmonary hypoplasia	CR
Syndactyly, clubfoot	Omphalocele, abdominal distention			CR
				PS
Syndactyly, clubfoot, congenital dislocation of hip	Umbilical hernia			PS
Polydactyly, congenital dislocation of hip				PS
				CR
Hypoplastic distal phalanges, digital thumb, dislocated hip	Cleft palate-lip		Growth retardation	RS

(*continued*)

Appendix 25.

Effects of Drugs on the Fetus (*continued*)

Drug	Central nervous system	Cardiovascular	Skeleton
Polychlorinated biphenyls*			Spotted calcification in skull, fontanelle and sagittal suture
Primidone		Ventral septal defect	Webbed neck, small mandible
Procarbazine*	Cerebral hemorrhage		
Quinine	Hydrocephalus	Congenital heart defects	Facial defects, vertebral anomalies
Retinoic acid*	Hydrocephalus, microcephaly	Various congenital heart defects	Malformations of cranium, ear, face, ribs
Spermicides			
Sulfonamide			
Tetracycline			
Thalidomide*		Congenital heart malformations	Spine malformation
Thioguanine			
Tobacco			
Tolbutamide			
Trifluoperazine		Transposition of great arteries	
Trimethadione*	Microcephaly	Atrial septal defect, ventral septal defect	Low-set ears, broad nasal bridge
Valproic acid*	Lumbosacral meningomyelocele, microcephaly, wide fontanelle	Tetralogy of Fallot	Depressed nasal bridge, hypoplastic nose, low-set ears, small mandibles

Since only malformations that can be visualized by current ultrasonographic techniques are listed, the guide cannot be used as a complete list of drug-induced teratogenicity. CR = Case reports; RS = retrospective studies; PS = prospective studies; AS = animal studies. *Proved to be teratogenic.

Source: Koren, G., Edwards, M. B., Miskin, M. Antenatal sonography of fetal malformations associated with drugs and chemicals: A guide. *Am J Obstet Gynecol* 156:79–85, January 1985. With permission.

Extremities	Gastrointestinal	Genitourinary	Miscellaneous	Source
			Stillbirth, growth retardation	PS
				RS
				CR
Oligodactyly				CR
Dysmelias				CR
Limb deformities			Stillbirth	RS
				PS
Limb reduction				RS
Hypoplasia of limb or part of it, foot defects		Urethral obstructions		PS
				CR
Hypoplasia of limb or part of it, clubfoot				PS
Limb reduction (amelia, phocomelia), hypoplasia	Duodenal stenosis or atresia, pyloric stenosis		Microtia	RS
				PS
Missing digits			Growth retardation	CR
				PS
Finger-toe syndactyly, absent toes, accessory thumb				RS
				CR
Phocomelia				CR
			Growth deficiency	CR
Malformed hands, clubfoot	Esophageal atresia			PS
	Oral cleft		Growth deficiency	CR

Appendix 26.
Four-Quadrant Amniotic Fluid Index

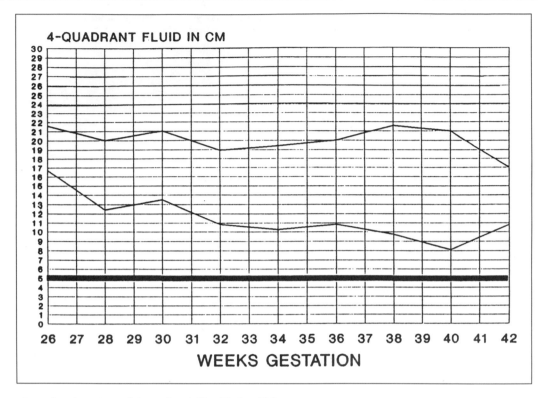

Source: Reproduced courtesy of the author, Jeffrey Phelan, M.D.

Appendix 27.
Umbilical Artery Doppler Resistance Index

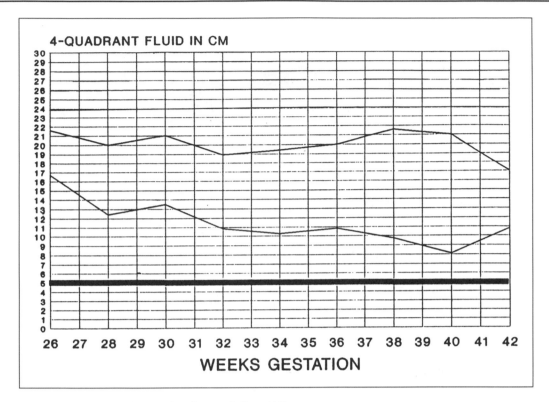

Source: Reproduced courtesy of the author, Gregory DeVore, M.D.

Appendix 28.
Fetal Heart Rate Versus Gestational Age

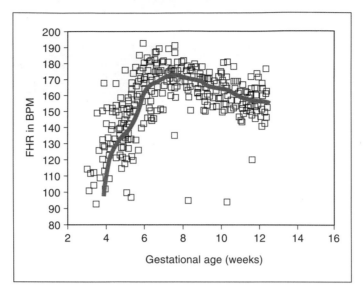

Source: Laboda et al. *J Ultrasound Med* 8:561–563, 1989. With permission.

Appendix 29.
Cerebellar Diameter Versus Age

**ESTIMATED VARIABILITY ASSOCIATED WITH DETERMINING
GESTATIONAL AGE FROM THE TRANSVERSE CEREBELLAR DIAMETER**

Gestational age (wk)	Variability* (wk)
12–17	±0.5
18–23	±0.9
24–29	±1.01
30–35	±1.2
≥36	±1.6

*Standard deviation of regression.

Source: Hill, et al. *Obstet Gynecol* 75:983, 1990. Reprinted with permission from The American College of Obstetrics and Gynecologists.

Appendix 30.
Thyroid Size Versus Age In Utero

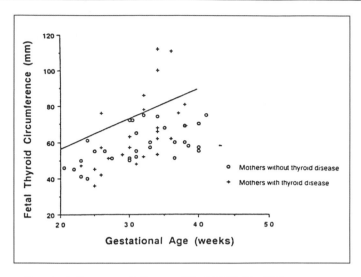

Source: Bromley & Berecerra, *J Ultrasound Med* 11:25–28, 1992.

Appendix 31.
Pounds to Kilograms

POUND TO KILOGRAM CONVERSION*

Pounds	0	1	2	3	4	5	6	7	8	9
0	0.00	0.45	0.90	1.36	1.81	2.26	2.72	3.17	3.62	4.08
10	4.53	4.98	5.44	5.89	6.35	6.80	7.25	7.71	8.16	8.61
20	9.07	9.52	9.97	10.43	10.88	11.34	11.79	12.24	12.70	13.15
30	13.60	14.06	14.51	14.96	15.42	15.87	16.32	16.78	17.23	17.69
40	18.14	18.59	19.05	19.50	19.95	20.41	20.86	21.31	21.77	22.22
50	22.68	23.13	23.58	24.04	24.49	24.94	25.40	25.85	26.30	26.76
60	27.21	27.66	28.12	28.57	29.03	29.48	29.93	30.39	30.84	31.29
70	31.75	32.20	32.65	33.11	33.56	34.02	34.47	34.92	35.38	35.83
80	36.28	36.74	37.19	37.64	38.10	38.55	39.00	39.46	39.91	40.37
90	40.82	41.27	41.73	42.18	42.63	43.09	43.54	43.99	44.45	44.90
100	45.36	45.81	46.26	46.72	47.17	47.62	48.08	48.53	48.98	49.44
110	49.89	50.34	50.80	51.25	51.71	52.16	52.61	53.07	53.52	53.97
120	54.43	54.88	55.33	55.79	56.24	56.70	57.15	57.60	58.06	58.51
130	58.96	59.42	59.87	60.32	60.78	61.23	61.68	62.14	62.59	63.05
140	63.50	63.95	64.41	64.86	65.31	65.77	66.22	66.67	67.13	67.58
150	68.04	68.49	68.94	69.40	69.85	70.30	70.76	71.21	71.66	72.12
160	72.57	73.02	73.48	73.93	74.39	74.84	75.29	75.75	76.20	76.65
170	77.11	77.56	78.01	78.47	78.92	79.38	79.83	80.28	80.74	81.19
180	81.64	82.10	82.55	83.00	83.46	83.91	84.36	84.82	85.27	85.73
190	86.18	86.68	87.09	87.54	87.99	88.45	88.90	89.35	89.81	90.26
200	90.72	91.17	91.62	92.08	92.53	92.98	93.44	93.89	94.34	94.80

*Numbers in the farthest left column are 10-pound increments; numbers across the top row are 1-pound increments. The kilogram equivalent of weight in pounds is found at the intersection of the appropriate row and column. For example, to convert 34 pounds, read down the left column to 30 and then across that row to 4: 34 pounds = 15.42 kilograms.

GRAMS TO POUNDS AND OUNCES CONVERSION FOR WEIGHT OF NEWBORNS

Pounds	Ounces 0	1	2	3	4	5	6	7	8	9	10	11	12	13	14	15
0	—	28	57	85	113	142	170	198	227	255	283	312	430	369	397	425
1	454	482	510	539	567	595	624	652	680	709	737	765	794	822	850	879
2	907	936	964	992	1021	1049	1077	1106	1134	1162	1191	1219	1247	1276	1304	1332
3	1361	1389	1417	1446	1474	1503	1531	1559	1588	1616	1644	1673	1701	1729	1758	1736
4	1814	1843	1871	1899	1928	1956	1984	2013	2041	2070	2098	2126	2155	2183	2211	2240
5	2268	2296	2325	2353	2381	2410	2438	2466	2495	2523	2551	2580	2608	2637	2665	2693
6	2722	2750	2778	2807	2835	2863	2892	2920	2948	2977	3005	3033	3062	3090	3118	3147
7	3175	3203	3232	3260	3289	3317	3345	3374	3402	3430	3459	3487	3515	3544	3572	3600
8	3629	3657	3685	3714	3742	3770	3799	3827	3856	3884	3912	3941	3969	3997	4026	4054
9	4082	4111	4139	4167	4196	4224	4252	4281	4309	4337	4366	4394	4423	4451	4479	4508
10	4536	4564	4593	4621	4649	4678	4706	4734	4763	4791	4819	4848	4876	4904	4933	4961
11	4990	5018	5046	5075	5103	5131	5160	5188	5216	5245	5273	5301	5330	5358	5386	5415
12	5443	5471	5500	5528	5557	5585	5613	5642	5670	5698	5727	5755	5783	5812	5840	5868
13	5897	5925	5953	5982	6010	6038	6067	6095	6123	6152	6180	6290	6237	6265	6294	6322
14	6350	6379	6407	6435	6464	6492	6520	6549	6577	6605	6634	6662	6690	6719	6747	6776

1 pound = 453.59 grams. 1 ounce = 28.35 grams. Grams can be converted to pounds and tenths of a pound by multiplying the number of grams by .0022.

Appendix 32.
Sonographic Renal Length Plotted Against Age

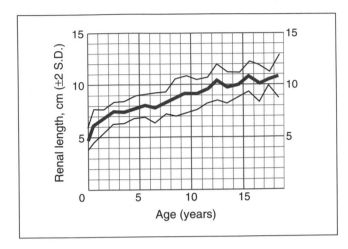

Source: Rosenbaum, D. M., Korngold, E., Teele, R. L. Sonographic assessment of renal length in normal children. *AJR* 142:467–469, 1984. Reprinted with permission from the American Roentgen Society.

Appendix 33.
Report for Cleaning and Preparing Endocavitary Ultrasound Transducers Between Patients

In response to the need for a universal policy on cleaning and preparing endocavitary ultrasound transducers between patients, the AIUM's Ultrasound Practice Committee led by Steven R. Goldstein, M.D., with the help of a multidisciplinary task force, as outlined on page one, has developed the following report:

In general, transvaginal and transrectal ultrasound are considered relatively noninvasive procedures and therefore at low risk for infection. However, since the probes are placed in contact with mucous membranes, guidelines for preparation and cleaning between patients are necessary.

Medical instruments fall into different categories with respect to potential for infection transmission. The most critical level of instruments are those that are intended to penetrate skin or mucous membranes. These require sterilization. Less critical instruments that simply come into contact with mucous membranes such as fiber optic endoscopes require a lower level of disinfection than sterilization. Of the latter, endocavitary ultrasound probes are even less critical because they are routinely covered with a single use disposable barrier.

Fortunately, only the lowest level of disinfection is required for hepatitis, cytomegalovirus, HIV, and herpes (all considered lipid viruses), vegetative bacteria (e.g., pseudomonas, salmonella staphylococci) and fungi such as candida and cryptococcus. A slightly higher level of disinfection is required for non-lipid viruses such as polio. The highest level of disinfection is required only for highly resistant spore-forming organisms.

There are several integral concepts to these guidelines. It should be emphasized that all sterilization/disinfection represents a statistical reduction in the number of microbes present on a surface. Meticulous cleaning of the instrument is the essential key to an initial reduction of the microbial/organic load by at least 99%. This cleaning is followed by a disinfecting procedure to ensure a high degree of protection from infectious disease transmission, even an if the instrument is NOT covered by a disposable barrier during use.

The following specific recommendations are made for the use of endocavitary ultrasound transducers:

1. Cleaning

After removal of the probe cover, use running water to remove any residual gel or debris from the probe. Use a damp gauze pad or other soft cloth and a small amount of mild nonabrasive liquid soap (household dishwashing liquid is ideal) to thoroughly cleanse the transducer. Consider the use of a small brush especially for crevices and areas of angulation depending on the design of your particular transducer. Rinse the transducer thoroughly with running water, then dry the transducer with a soft cloth or paper towel.

2. Disinfection

Cleaning with a detergent/water solution as described above is clearly the cornerstone of disinfection. However, additional use of liquid chemical germicides may help to ensure further statistical reduction in microbial load. Because of the vagaries of the cleaning process and the potential disruption of the barrier sheath, additional disinfection with chemical agents may be desirable. Examples of such chemical agents include but are not limited to

- 2.4–3.2% glutaraldehyde products (a variety of available proprietary products including "Cidex," "Metricide," or "Procide."

- common household bleach (5.25% sodium hypochlorite) diluted to yield 500 parts per million chlorine (10 cc in one liter of tap water).

- iodophor disinfectant/detergents (hard surface disinfectants diluted for use per manufacturer's instruction [e.g., "Westcodyne"]). Antiseptic-type iodophors (e.g., "Betadine") are not acceptable for use as disinfectants.

- quaternary ammonium compounds (e.g., "Coverage Spray" and a wide variety of other proprietary "quats"). NOTE: Benzalkonium chloride ("Zepharin") should not be used as a disinfectant under any circumstances . . . it is not only ineffective, but will readily serve as culture medium for a variety of bacteria, including Pseudomonas aeruginosa, an overt clinical pathogen.

Practitioners should consult the labels of proprietary products for specific instructions. They should also consult instrument manufacturers regarding compatibility of these agents with probes. Note that such agents are potentially toxic and many require adequate precautions such as proper ventilation, personal protective devices (gloves, face/eye protection, etc.) and thorough rinsing before reuse of the probe.

3. Probe Covers

The transducer should be covered with a barrier, usually a latex condom. These should be non-lubricated and non-medicated. Practitioners should be aware that condoms have a six-fold enhanced AQL (acceptable quality level) when compared to standard examination gloves. They have an AQL equal to that of surgical gloves. Occasionally, patients may be latex-sensitive, and alternative barriers (vinyl) should then be used.

4. Aseptic Technique

Obviously, for the protection of the patient and the health care worker, all endocavitary examinations should be performed with the operator properly gloved throughout the procedure. Gloves should be used to remove the condom or other barrier from the transducer and to wash the transducer as outlined above. As the barrier (condom) is removed, care should be taken not to contaminate the probe with secretions from the patient. At the completion of the procedure, hands should be thoroughly washed with soap and water. Note: Obvious disruption in condom integrity does NOT require modification of this protocol. These guidelines take into account possible probe contamination due to a disruption in the barrier sheath.

In summary, all disinfection processes are an attempt to statistically reduce the microbial load. Adherence to the above guidelines will help optimize the level for protection of both patients and health care providers.

Reprinted with permission from the American Institute of Ultrasound in Medicine (AIUM Reporter 11:7, 1995).

Appendix 34.
Ultrasound Professional Organizations

A.I.U.M.
American Institute of Ultrasound in Medicine
14750 Sweitzer Lane, Suite 100
Laurel, MD 20707-5906
(301) 498-4100
Fax Number: (301) 498-4450
Journal of Ultrasound in Medicine

S.D.M.S.
Society of Diagnostic Medical Sonographers
12225 Greenville Ave., Suite 434
Dallas, Texas 75243
(214) 235-7367
Journal of Diagnostic Medical Sonography

A.R.D.M.S.
American Registry of Diagnostic Medical Sonographers
600 Jefferson Plaza, Suite 360
Rockville, MD 20852-1150
(301) 738-8401

S.V.T.
Society of Vascular Technology
1101 Connecticut Ave., N.W., Suite 700
Washington, D.C. 20036
(202) 857-1149
Journal of Vascular Technology

A.S.E.
American Society of Echocardiography
4101 Lake Boone Trail, Suite 301
Raleigh, N.C. 27607
(919) 787-5181
Journal of the American Society of Echocardiography

C.S.D.M.S.
Canadian Society of Medical Sonographers
Lois Pon, R.D.M.S. - Executive Director
P.O. Box 2235
Orillia, ON, Canada L3V6S1
(705) 487-0184
Interface, Quarterly Newsletter

B.M.U.S.
British Medical Ultrasound Society
36 Portland Place
London, England W1N4AT
011-44-71-580-4189

Appendix 35.
AIUM Guidelines

The following guidelines have been approved by the AIUM and are published here as a service to our readers. Additional copies of *Guidelines for Performance of the Abdominal and Retroperitoneal Ultrasound Examination* (order #GA) and *Guidelines for Performance of the Scrotal Ultrasound Examination* (order #GS) can be ordered from the AIUM. The cost is $6 for AIUM members and $20 for nonmembers. Mail your order to AIUM Publications Department, 14750 Sweitzer Lane, Suite 100, Laurel, MD 20707–5906; or phone (301) 498–4100 or (800) 638–5352; Fax (301) 498–4450. Prepayment is required.

GUIDELINES FOR PERFORMANCE OF THE SCROTAL ULTRASOUND EXAMINATION

The following are proposed guidelines for ultrasound evaluation of the scrotum. The document consists of two parts:

Part I: Equipment and Documentation Guidelines

Part II: Guidelines for a General Examination of the Scrotum

These guidelines have been developed to provide assistance to practitioners performing ultrasound studies in the scrotum. In some cases, additional and/or specialized examinations may be necessary. While it is not possible to detect every abnormality, adherence to the following guidelines will maximize the probability of detecting most of the abnormalities that occur in the scrotum.

PART I
Equipment and Documentation

Equipment

Scrotal studies should be conducted with a real-time scanner, preferably using a linear or a curved linear transducer. The transducer or scanner should be adjusted to operate at the highest clinically appropriate frequency, realizing that there is a trade-off between resolution and beam penetration. With modern equipment, these frequencies usually are 5 MHz or greater. For pediatric applications, 7–10 MHz is preferable. Doppler frequencies used should be the highest possible to optimize resolution and flow detection. With modern equipment, Doppler frequencies range from 3.5–7 MHz. Stand-off pads can be used, if necessary, to improve imaging.

COMMENT: Resolution should be of sufficient quality to routinely differentiate small cystic from solid lesions.

Documentation

Adequate documentation is essential for high quality patient care. This should be a permanent record of the ultrasound examination and its interpretation. Images of all appropriate areas, both normal and abnormal, should be recorded in any image format. Variations from normal size should be accompanied by measurements. Images are to be labeled with the examination date, patient identification and image orientation. A report of the ultrasound findings should be included in the patient's medical record, regardless of where the study is performed. Retention of the ultrasound examination should be consistent both with clinical need and with relevant legal and local health care facility requirements.

PART II
Guidelines for the Scrotal Ultrasound Examination

The testes should be studied in at least two projections, long axis and transverse. Views of each testicle should include the superior, mid, and inferior portions as well as its medial and lateral borders. The adjacent epididymis should be evaluated. The size and echogenicity of each testicle and epididymis should be compared to its opposite side, when possible. Scrotal skin thickness should be evaluated.

Blood flow in the testis and surrounding scrotal contents should be evaluated using color Doppler and pulsed Doppler where there is a question of torsion versus epididymitis in the clinical setting of the "acute scrotum." The flow in the symptomatic scrotum should be compared with the non-symptomatic side and variations form normal should be noted. Low flow detection settings should be used when needed to document testicular blood flow. Flow in intratesticular arteries cannot always be established with certainty by color Doppler sonography. If flow cannot be demonstrated in the asymptomatic testis, testicular scintigraphy should be considered to corroborate the presence or absence of testicular perfusion.

The contents of the scrotal sac should be examined for the detection of extratesticular masses, fluid collections, or other abnormalities. Measurements should be obtained when appropriate. Additional techniques such as the valsalva maneuver or upright positioning can be used as needed.

GUIDELINES FOR PERFORMANCE OF THE ABDOMINAL AND RETROPERITONEAL ULTRASOUND EXAMINATION

The following are proposed guidelines for the ultrasound evaluation of the abdomen and retroperitoneum. The document consists of two parts:

Part I: Equipment and Documentation Guidelines

Part II: Guidelines for the Abdominal and Retroperitoneal Examination

These guidelines have been developed to provide assistance to practitioners performing ultrasound studies of the abdomen and retroperitoneum. In some cases, additional and/or specialized examinations may be necessary. While it is not possible to detect every abnormality, adherence to the following guidelines will maximize the probability of detecting most of the abnormalities that occur in the abdomen and retroperitoneum. Pediatric abdominal ultrasound examinations should adhere to the guidelines for adults, except as specified in this document.

PART I
Equipment and Documentation

Equipment

Abdominal and retroperitoneal studies should be conducted with a real-time scanner, preferably using sector or curved linear transducers. The transducer or scanner should be adjusted to operate at the highest clinically appropriate frequency, realizing that there is a trade-off between resolution and beam penetration. With modern equipment, these frequencies usually are between 2.25 and 5.0 MHz. In appropriate clinical situations, duplex or color Doppler may be incorporated into the examination. For pediatric applications, higher frequency transducers (5 MHz or greater) usually provide more optimal images.

Documentation

Adequate documentation is essential for high-quality patient care. There should be a permanent record of the ultrasound examination and its interpretation. Comparison with prior relevant imaging studies may prove helpful. Images of all appropriate areas, both normal and abnormal, should be recorded in imaging or storage format. Variations from normal size should be accompanied by measurements. Images are to be labeled with the examination date, patient identification, and image orientation. A report of the ultrasound findings should be included in the patient's medical record, regardless of where the study is performed. Retention of the ultrasound examination should be consistent both with clinical need and with relevant legal and local health care facility requirements.

PART II
Guidelines for the Abdominal and Retroperitoneal Examination

The following guidelines describe the examination to be performed for each organ and anatomic region in the abdomen and retroperitoneum. A complete examination of the upper abdomen would include the liver, gallbladder and biliary tract, pancreas, spleen, and limited views of both kidneys. A complete retroperitoneal examination would include images of the aorta, inferior vena cava, retroperitoneal abnormalities such as lymphadenopathy, masses or fluid collections, views of the kidneys, and in the case of neonatal retroperitoneal examinations, imaging of the adrenal glands. A complete renal/urinary tract examination would include several views of both kidneys and perirenal structures (longitudinal and transverse), attempts to visualize the ureters, and views of the urinary bladder. The liver, gallbladder, biliary tract, pancreas, spleen, kidneys, urinary bladder, adrenal gland, aorta, and inferior vena cava also may be imaged separately or in combination.

Liver

The liver survey should include both long axis (coronal or sagittal) and transverse views. The liver parenchyma should be evaluated for focal or diffuse abnormalities. If possible, views comparing the echogenicity of the liver to the right kidney should be performed. The major vessels (aorta/inferior vena cava) in the region of the liver should be imaged, including the position of the inferior vena cava where it passes through the liver.

The regions of the ligamentum teres on the left, the dome of the right lobe, right hemidiaphragm, and right pleural space should be imaged. Hepatic veins should be visualized in both lobes.

The right and left branches of the portal vein should be identified. Spectral Doppler or color Doppler may be used to document blood flow and blood flow direction in the hepatic artery, hepatic veins, and portal veins, as well as to identify collateral venous pathways. Analysis of waveforms may be useful.

Gallbladder and Biliary Tract

When possible, routine gallbladder and biliary tract examinations should be done with the patient fasting for at least 8 hours prior to the examinations. The gallbladder evaluation should include long axis (coronal or sagittal) and transverse views obtained in the supine position. Left lateral decubitus, erect, or prone positions also may be necessary to allow a complete evaluation of the gallbladder and its surrounding area. The gallbladder should be assessed for the presence of stones and other masses and their mobility. The gallbladder wall thickness and tenderness to transducer compression should be assessed.

The intrahepatic ducts can be evaluated by obtaining views of the liver demonstrating the right and left hepatic branches of the portal vein. Doppler may be used to differentiate hepatic artery from biliary ductal dilatation. The extrahepatic ducts can be evaluated in supine, left lateral decubitus and/or semi-erect positions. The intrahepatic and extrahepatic bile ducts should be evaluated for dilatation and other abnormalities. With these views, the relationship between the bile ducts, hepatic artery and portal vein can be shown. When possible, the common bile duct in the pancreatic head should be visualized.

Pancreas

The pancreatic head, uncinate process, and body should be identified in transverse and, when possible, long axis (coronal or sagittal) projections. The gastroduodenal artery and distal common bile duct should be assessed in the region of the pancreatic head. If possible, the pancreatic tail should be imaged. The pancreatic duct should be assessed for dilatation and any other abnormalities. The peripancreatic region should be assessed for adenopathy, fluid collections, and vascular abnormalities.

Spleen

Representative views of the spleen in long axis (sagittal or coronal) and in transverse projection should be performed. An attempt should be made to demonstrate the left pleural space. When possible, the echogenicity of the left kidney should be compared to that of the spleen. Doppler may be used to determine the presence and direction of flow in the splenic vein and artery.

Kidneys and Urinary Tract

Representative long axis (coronal or sagittal) views of each kidney should be obtained, visualizing the cortex and the renal pelvis. A maximum measurement of renal length should be recorded for both kidneys. Prone or upright positioning may be used when necessary to provide more optimal images of the kidney. Transverse views of both the left and right kidneys should include the upper pole, middle section at the renal pelvis, and the lower pole. When possible, comparison of renal echogenicity with the adjacent liver and spleen should be performed. The perirenal regions should be assessed for abnormality.

Spectral and color Doppler should be used when clinically indicated to assess renal arterial and venous patency. Doppler may be of value in the differentiation of minor degrees of dilatation of the collecting system from blood vessels. Flow wave-form analysis may be used to evaluate medical renal disease and follow response to therapy.

Images of the urinary bladder lumen and the bladder wall should be obtained when possible. The wall should be assessed for thickness and the presence of focal lesions should be documented. Dilatation or other visible abnormalities of the distal ureters should be documented. Transverse and longitudinal scans may be used to demonstrate any post-void residual.

Pediatric and neonatal images should include longitudinal and transverse images of the kidneys to assess renal parenchymal detail, collecting system dilatation, and demonstrate a comparison of liver/kidney and spleen/kidney echogenicity. The highest possible frequency transducer for optimal imaging should be used.

Aorta and Inferior Vena Cava

The aorta and inferior vena cava should be imaged in long axis (sagittal or coronal) and transverse planes. Scans of both vessels should be attempted from the diaphragm to the bifurcation. If possible, images of the abdominal aorta should include the origin of the common iliac vessels. Aneurysmal dilatation of the aorta should be measured in the AP and transverse dimensions. The surrounding soft tissue should be evaluated for abnormalities. Duplex and color Doppler may be of value in evaluating luminal flow in the aorta and inferior vena cava, as well as distinguishing vascular from nonvascular causes of pulsatile abdominal masses. In the case of possible aortic rupture or dissection, ultrasound may not be the initial examination of choice.

Adrenal

The adrenal gland can be imaged in the neonate and, to a lesser extent, in the infant. The adrenal gland can be evaluated for hemorrhage, masses, and other abnormalities.

The following guideline has been approved by the AIUM and is published here as a service to our readers. Additional copies of *Guidelines for Performance of the Vascular/Doppler Ultrasound Examination* (order #GVD) can be ordered from the AIUM. The cost is $6 for AIUM members and $20 for nonmembers. Mail your order to AIUM Publications Department, 14750 Sweitzer Lane, Suite 100, Laurel, MD 20707-5906; or phone 301-498-4100 or 800-638-5352; Fax (301) 498-4450. Prepayment is required and there is a $10 minimum for credit card orders.

GUIDELINES FOR PERFORMANCE OF THE ULTRASOUND EXAMINATION OF THE EXTRACRANIAL CEREBROVASCULAR SYSTEM

The following are proposed guidelines for the ultrasound evaluation of the neck arteries. The document consists of two parts:

Part I: Equipment and Documentation

Part II: Ultrasound Examination of the Extracranial Carotid and Vertebral Arteries

These guidelines have been developed to provide assistance to practitioners performing ultrasound examination of the carotid and vertebral arteries. In some cases, additional and/or specialized examinations may be complementary or necessary. These include, but are not limited to, hemodynamic studies such as oculoplethysmography, orbital and periorbital Doppler, and transcranial Doppler. While it is not possible to document every abnormality, adherence to the following will maximize the probability of detecting most abnormalities.

PART I
Equipment and Documentation

Equipment

The sonographic evaluation of the carotid and vertebral arteries should include both real-time imaging of the arteries and their contents and analysis of the flow signals generated within the lumen of the artery.

Real-time imaging should be conducted at the highest clinically appropriate frequency. Realizing that there is a trade-off between resolution and beam penetration, this will most likely be done at a frequency of 5 MHz or above, preferably with a linear or curved linear transducer.

Analysis of the flow signals generated from within the artery should be conducted with a carrier frequency of 3 MHz or above. A real-time display of the velocity (or frequency shift) distribution should be available for analysis of the appropriate velocity (or frequency shift) parameters. This is currently achieved with either continuous wave Doppler or duplex sonography (using range gating). Color flow imaging can be used to help with the placement of the range gate, thus facilitating the examination.

Documentation

Adequate documentation is essential for high quality patient care. There should be a permanent record of the ultrasound examination and its interpretation. Images of all appropriate areas, both normal and abnormal, should be recorded on any appropriate imaging or storage format. Appropriate velocity (or frequency shift) parameters should be recorded as well, with the site at which velocity (or frequency shift) signals are being analyzed clearly indicated.

Variations from normal size or flow dynamics should be accompanied by measurements. All images are to be appropriately labeled with the examination date, patient identification, and image location and orientation. A report of the ultrasound findings should be included in the patient's medical record, regardless of where the study is performed. Retention of the ultrasound examination should be consistent both with clinical need and with relevant legal and local health care facility requirements.

PART II
Ultrasound Examination of Extracranial Carotid and Vertebral Arteries

The extracranial cerebrovascular examination should always include an evaluation of the extracranial carotid system, including the common, internal, and external carotid arteries on both sides. When indicated, the vertebral arteries should be examined as well.

Carotid

Real-time imaging of the common carotid and its external and internal branches should be performed in both long axis and transverse planes. Images to be recorded on each side should include at least one long axis view of each of the common, internal, and external carotids. The extent, location, and characteristics of any atherosclerotic plaque should be recorded. Transverse images can be recorded as needed when they more clearly demonstrate an abnormality.

Blood flow velocity (or frequency shift) should be examined along the accessible portions of the common, internal, and external carotid arteries. The angle between the direction of motion and the applied ultrasound signal should be kept between 0 degrees and 60 degrees, as the reliability of such measurements decreases at angles above 60 degrees, and angle correction should be applied when needed to determine blood flow velocity. A record of the velocity (or frequency shift) spectrum should be kept for each of the internal and external carotid arteries at the site of maximal peak-systolic velocity (or frequency shift) in each of these vessels. Velocity (or frequency shift) measurements should also be recorded in the common carotid at a point upstream from the carotid bulb. If there are sites of hemodynamically significant stenosis, the velocity (or frequency shift) spectrum should be recorded proximal to, at, and distal to each such site. The location of the site(s) should be documented.

Vertebral

The vertebral artery should be studied in at least the long axis view. A record should be made of the velocity (or frequency shift) distribution and direction of blood flow within the vertebral artery at its accessible portions.

GUIDELINES FOR PERFORMANCE OF THE ULTRASOUND EXAMINATION OF THE PERIPHERAL ARTERIES

The following are proposed guidelines for the ultrasound evaluation of the peripheral arteries. The document consists of two parts:

Part I: Equipment and Documentation
Part II: Ultrasound Examination of the Peripheral Arteries

These guidelines have been developed to provide assistance to practitioners performing ultrasound examination of the peripheral arteries. In many cases, particularly for the evaluation of peripheral arterial occlusive disease, physiologic tests including pressure measurement and plethysmography are used in conjunction with ultrasound. In some cases, an additional and/or specialized examination may be necessary. While it is not possible to document every abnormality, adherence to the following will maximize the probability of detecting most abnormalities.

PART I
Equipment and Documentation
Equipment

The sonographic evaluation of the peripheral arteries should include real-time imaging of the arteries and of their contents as well as analysis of the flow signals detected within the lumen of the arteries and in the contiguous tissues.

Real-time imaging should be conducted at the highest clinically appropriate frequency. Realizing that there is a trade-off between penetration and resolution, this will most likely be at a frequency of 3 MHz or above. In most cases, a linear or curved linear transducer is preferred.

Analysis of the flow signals originating from within the artery should be conducted with an appropriate frequency, in general 2.5 MHz or above. A real-time display of the velocity distribution should be available for analysis of appropriate velocity parameters. This is currently achieved with either continuous wave Doppler or duplex sonography (using range gating). Color flow imaging can be used to facilitate the examination.

Documentation

Adequate documentation is essential for high quality patient care. There should be a permanent record of the ultrasound examination and its interpretation. Images of all appropriate areas, both normal and abnormal, should be recorded on any appropriate imaging or storage format. Appropriate velocity parameters should be recorded as well, with the site at which velocity signals are being analyzed clearly indicated. Variations from normal size or flow dynamics should be accompanied by measurements. All images are to be appropriately labeled with the examination date, patient identification, and image location and orientation. A report of the ultrasound findings should be included in the patient's medical record, regardless of where the study is performed. Retention of the ultrasound examination should be consistent both with clinical need and with relevant legal and local health care facility requirements.

PART II
Ultrasound Examination of the Peripheral Arteries

These guidelines describe the examination of the femoropopliteal arteries. Analogous techniques can be used to evaluate other peripheral arteries, including calf or upper extremity arteries.

Real-time imaging of the femoral and popliteal arteries should be performed in both the long axis and transverse planes. Images to be recorded should include a long axis view of the femoral artery centered on the bifurcation, and a long axis view of the mid-popliteal artery. Additional long axis and transverse views should be recorded whenever they help to delineate the character and extent of any abnormality (e.g., aneurysm, pseudoaneurysm, dissection, atherosclerotic plaque).

Blood flow velocity should be sampled along the full length of the femoral and popliteal arteries. Velocity spectra should be obtained near the center stream of flowing blood, using an appropriately sized range gate. The angle between the direction of moving blood and the ultrasound signal should be between 0 degrees and 60 degrees, as the reliability of such measurements decreases at angles above 60 degrees, and angle correction should be applied when needed to determine blood flow velocity. A record of the velocity spectrum should be kept for each of the following segments: common femoral, profunda femoral, mid- and distal superficial femoral, and proximal as well as distal popliteal arteries. At any site of hemodynamically significant stenosis, the velocity spectrum should be recorded both at the site as well as at a point located 2–4 cm proximal to the site. The location of any such site should be documented. All sites with absent flow signals should also be documented both as to location and extent.

When using pressure measurements in conjunction with ultrasound for the evaluation of peripheral arterial occlusive disease, systolic pressures should be determined using a Doppler device and a blood pressure cuff appropriate in size for the extremity in question. Accepted diagnostic techniques and criteria should be employed, which may involve comparisons between upper and lower extremities (e.g., ankle-to-brachial ratio) or between the extremity in question and the contralateral extremity.

Any cystic or solid perivascular mass should be recorded as to location, size, and presence and nature of flow signals within. The caliber and flow dynamics of the adjacent artery and vein should be measured and documented.

GUIDELINES FOR PERFORMANCE OF THE ULTRASOUND EXAMINATION OF THE PERIPHERAL VEINS

The following are proposed guidelines for the ultrasound evaluation of the peripheral veins. The document consists of two parts:

Part I: Equipment and Documentation
Part II: Ultrasound Examination of the Peripheral Veins

These guidelines have been developed to provide assistance to practitioners performing ultrasound examination of the peripheral veins. In some cases, an additional and/or specialized examination may be necessary. While it is not possible to document every abnormality, adherence to the following will maximize the probability of detecting most abnormalities.

PART I
Equipment and Documentation
Equipment

The sonographic evaluation of the peripheral veins should include both real-time imaging of the veins and of their contents and evaluation of the flow signals originating from within the lumen of the veins. Real-time imaging should be conducted at the highest clinically appropriate frequency, realizing that there is a trade-off between resolution and beam penetration. This should usually be at a frequency of 5 MHz or above, with the occasional need for a lower frequency transducer. In most cases, a linear or curved linear transducer is preferable. Evaluation of the flow signals originating from within the lumen of the vein should be conducted with a carrier frequency of 2.5 MHz or above. A display of the relative amplitude and direction of moving blood should be available.

Imaging and flow analysis are currently performed with duplex sonography, using range gating. Color flow imaging can be used to facilitate the examination.

Documentation

Adequate documentation is essential for high quality patient care. There should be a permanent record of the ultrasound examination and its interpretation. Images of all appropriate areas, both normal and abnormal, should be recorded on any appropriate imaging or storage format. A record should also be kept of any site of abnormal blood flow dynamics. Variations from normal size should be accompanied by measurements. All images are to be appropriately labeled with the examination date, patient identification, and image location and orientation. A report of the ultrasound findings should be included in the patient's medical record, regardless of where the study is performed. Retention of the ultrasound examination should be consistent with both clinical need and with relevant legal and local health care facility requirements.

PART II
Ultrasound Examination of the Peripheral Veins

The guidelines below describe the examination of the lower extremity veins. Analogous techniques can be used to evaluate the upper extremity veins.

The ultrasound examination of the lower extremity veins should always include an evaluation of the femoral and popliteal veins. When indicated, the contralateral leg, calf veins, saphenous veins, and/or iliac veins should be evaluated.

Femoral and Popliteal Veins

The nature of the examination depends in part on the clinical indication for the study. In particular, an examination for deep venous thrombophlebitis should include real-time imaging with compression and/or other accepted techniques involving imaging or blood flow.

The femoral and popliteal veins should be imaged in at least the transverse projection. The full extent of these veins should be examined, and images should be recorded at each of the following levels: common femoral, mid-superficial femoral and mid-popliteal veins. Additional transverse or long axis views can be included if they more clearly demonstrate any abnormality of the veins or adjacent tissues (e.g., lymph node, hematoma, pseudoaneurysm, or other masses). When using compression as a diagnostic criterion for deep venous thrombophlebitis, real-time imaging should be performed in the transverse plane along the full length of the femoral and popliteal veins, with and without pressure applied to the skin in an effort to completely appose the venous walls. Images with and without compression should be recorded at each of the three levels listed above. The extent and location of sites where the veins fail to compress should be clearly recorded.

Blood flow signals should be examined at the level of the common femoral, proximal superficial femoral, proximal profunda femoral, mid superficial femoral, and popliteal veins both at rest and during augmentation of blood flow using calf or thigh compression. When indicated, additional maneuvers such as Valsalva and forced respiration should be attempted. When evaluating for venous insufficiency, the level and extent of reversed flow should be determined during the performance of accepted maneuvers.

Calf Veins

The calf veins should be imaged in at least the transverse view. Real-time imaging should be performed with and without pressure applied on the skin in an effort to completely appose the walls of the vein. Imaging of the full extent of these veins should be attempted. Views of the lower extremity veins should include transverse images of the peroneal, posterior tibial, anterior tibial, and when possible, muscular veins. The extent and location of sites where the veins fail to compress should be clearly recorded. Additional transverse or long axis views can be obtained if they more clearly demonstrate any abnormality.

Blood flow signals should be obtained at the mid calf in the posterior tibial and peroneal veins.

The following guidelines have been approved by the AIUM and are published here as a service to our readers. Additional copies of *Guidelines for Performance of the Thyroid and Parathyroid Ultrasound Examination* (order #GT), *Guidelines for Performance of the Prostate (and Surrounding Structures) Ultrasound Examination* (order #GP), or *Guidelines for Performance of the Antepartum Obstetrical Ultrasound Examination* (order #GAOB) can be ordered from the AIUM. The cost is $5 for AIUM members and $10 for non-members, shipping and handling additional. To order, phone the AIUM Publications Department at (301) 498–4100 or (800) 638–5352.

GUIDELINES FOR PERFORMANCE OF THE THYROID AND PARATHYROID ULTRASOUND EXAMINATION

The following are proposed guidelines for ultrasound evaluation of the thyroid and parathyroid glands. The document consists of two parts:

Part I: Equipment and Documentation Guidelines

Part II: Guidelines for the Thyroid and Parathyroid Ultrasound Examination

These guidelines have been developed to provide assistance to practitioners performing ultrasound studies of the thyroid and parathyroid glands. In some cases, additional and/or specialized examinations may be necessary. While it is not possible to detect every abnormality, adherence to the following guidelines will maximize the probability of detecting many of the abnormalities that occur in these glands.

PART I
Equipment and Documentation

Equipment

Thyroid and parathyroid studies should be conducted with a real-time scanner, preferably using a linear or curved linear array transducer. The transducer should be selected to utilize the highest clinically appropriate frequency, realizing that there is a trade-off between resolution and beam penetration. With modern equipment, these frequencies usually are 5 MHz or greater. For pediatric applications, 7–10 MHz is preferable. Doppler frequencies used should be the highest possible to optimize resolution and flow detection. With modern equipment, Doppler frequencies range from 3.5–7 MHz.

COMMENT: Resolution should be of sufficient quality to routinely distinguish between small cystic and solid lesions.

Documentation

Adequate documentation is essential for high quality in patient care. There should be a permanent record of the ultrasound examination and its interpretation. Images of all appropriate areas, both normal and abnormal, should be recorded in an appropriate format. Variations from normal size should be accompanied by measurements. Images are to be labeled with the examination date, patient identification, and image orientation. A report of the ultrasound findings should be included in the patient's medical record. Retention of the ultrasound examination should be consistent both with clinical need and with relevant legal and local health care facility requirements.

PART II
Guidelines for the Thyroid and Parathyroid Ultrasound Examination

A. The Thyroid Examination

The right and left lobes of the thyroid should be imaged in at least two projections, long axis and transverse. Transverse views of the thyroid should include images of the superior, mid, and inferior portions of the right and left lobes. Longitudinal images should include the medial, mid, and lateral portions of each lobe. The thyroid isthmus should be imaged in a transverse plane. Visualized thyroid abnormalities should be documented and the location, size, and number of abnormalities should be recorded. Incidentally detected abnormalities of the adjacent soft tissues such as enlarged lymph nodes, thrombosed veins, etc., should be documented.

Whenever possible, comparison should be made with other imaging studies such as radionuclide studies. Color flow imaging and pulsed Doppler sonography may be useful to evaluate the vascularity of the thyroid gland and of localized masses. Color Doppler sonography can distinguish prominent thyroid vessels from cystic masses. In addition, color Doppler sonography can be used to identify vascular abnormalities adjacent to the thyroid.

Ultrasound guidance may be used to biopsy thyroid masses.

B. The Parathyroid Examination

Examination for suspected parathyroid enlargement should include images in the region of the anticipated parathyroid gland location. These should include longitudinal images through the medial and lateral aspect of the right and left lobes of the thyroid gland, as well as transverse images through the upper, mid, and lower poles of the right and left lobes of the thyroid. Although the normal parathyroid glands usually are not visualized using currently available sonographic technology, enlarged parathyroid glands in the neck may be visualized. The size, number, and location of visualized parathyroid glands should be documented. Measurements of the parathyroid gland should be made in at least two and preferably three dimensions.

Ultrasound guidance may be used to biopsy parathyroid glands or to direct ablative interventional procedures.

GUIDELINES FOR PERFORMANCE OF THE ULTRASOUND EXAMINATION OF THE PROSTATE

The following are proposed guidelines for the ultrasound evaluation of the prostate and surrounding structures. The document consists of two parts:

Part I: Equipment and Documentation

Part II: Ultrasound Examination of the Prostate and Surrounding Structures

These guidelines have been developed to provide assistance to practitioners performing an ultrasound study of the prostate. In some cases, an additional and/or specialized examination may be necessary. While it is not possible to detect every abnormality, adherence to the following will maximize the detection of most abnormalities.

PART I
Equipment and Documentation

Equipment

A prostate study should be conducted with a real-time transrectal (also termed endorectal) transducer using the highest clinically appropriate frequency, realizing that there is a trade-off between resolution and beam penetration. With modern equipment, these frequencies are usually 5 MHz or higher.

Documentation

Adequate documentation is essential for high quality patient care. There should be a permanent record of the ultrasound examination and its interpretation. Images of all appropriate areas, both normal and abnormal, should be accompanied by measurements. Images are to be appropriately labeled with the examination date, patient identification, and image orientation. A report of the ultrasound findings should be included in the patient's medical record. Retention of the permanent record of the ultrasound examination should be consistent both with clinical need and with the relevant legal and local health care facility requirements.

Care of the Equipment

Transrectal probes should be covered by a disposable sheath prior to insertion. Following the examination, the sheath should be disposed, and the probe soaked in an antimicrobial solution. The type of solution and amount of time for soaking depends on manufacturer and infectious disease recommendations. Following the examination, if there is a gross tear in the sheath, the fluid channels in the probe should be thoroughly flushed with the antimicrobial solution. Tubing and stop cocks should be disposed after each examination.

PART II
Ultrasound Examination of the Prostate and Surrounding Structures

The following guidelines describe the examination to be performed for the prostate and surrounding structures.

Prostate

The prostate should be imaged in its entirety in at least two orthogonal planes, sagittal and axial or sagittal and coronal, from the apex to the base of the gland. In particular, the peripheral zone should be thoroughly imaged. The gland should be evaluated for size, echogenicity, symmetry, and continuity of margins. The periprostatic fat and vessels should be evaluated for asymmetry and disruption in echogenicity.

Seminal Vesicles and Vas Deferens

The seminal vesicles should be examined in two planes from their insertion into the prostate via the ejaculatory ducts to their cranial and lateral extents. They should be evaluated for size, shape, position, symmetry, and echogenicity. Both vas deferens should be evaluated.

Perirectal Space

Evaluation of the perirectal space, in particular the region that abuts on the prostate and perirectal tissues, should be performed. If rectal pathology is clinically suspected, the rectal wall and lumen should be studied.

GUIDELINES FOR PERFORMANCE OF THE ANTEPARTUM OBSTETRICAL ULTRASOUND EXAMINATION

The following are proposed guidelines for the antepartum obstetrical ultrasound examination. The document consists of three parts:

Part I: Equipment and Documentation Guidelines

Part II: Guidelines for First Trimester Sonography

Part III: Guidelines for Second and Third Trimester Sonography

These guidelines have been developed for use by practitioners performing obstetrical ultrasound studies. They represent minimum guidelines for the performance and documentation of obstetrical sonograms. A limited examination may, however, be performed in clinical emergencies or if used as a follow-up to a complete examination. In certain cases, particularly those in which a purpose of the study is to identify, characterize, or exclude structural congenital anomalies, an additional targeted examination may be necessary. Adherence to the following guidelines will increase the chance of detecting many fetal abnormalities, but even with more detailed examinations, it is not possible to detect all fetal anomalies.

PART I
Equipment and Documentation

Equipment

These studies should be conducted with real-time equipment, using an abdominal and/or vaginal approach. A transducer of appropriate frequency should be used. Fetal ultrasound should be performed only when there is a valid medical reason. The lowest possible ultrasonic exposure settings should be used to gain the necessary diagnostic information.

COMMENT:

(1) Real-time sonography is necessary to confirm the presence of fetal life through observation of cardiac activity and active movement.

(2) The choice of transducer frequency is a balance between beam penetration and resolution. With modern equipment, 3 to 5 MHz abdominal transducers allow suffi-

cient penetration in most patients, while providing adequate resolution. A lower frequency transducer may be needed to provide adequate penetration for abdominal imaging in an obese patient. Vaginal scanning usually is performed at a frequency of 5 to 7.5 MHz.

Documentation

Adequate documentation of the study is essential for quality patient care. This should include a permanent record of the ultrasound images, incorporating whenever possible the measurement parameters and anatomical findings proposed in the following sections of this document. Images should be appropriately labeled with the examination date, patient identification, and, if appropriate, image orientation. A report of the ultrasound findings should be included in the patient's medical record. Retention of the ultrasound examination should be consistent both with clinical need and with relevant legal and local health care facility requirements.

PART II
Guidelines for First Trimester Sonography

OVERALL COMMENT: Scanning in the first trimester may be performed either abdominally, vaginally, or using both methods. If an abdominal examination is performed and fails to provide diagnostic information, a vaginal scan should be done when possible. Similarly, if a vaginal scan is performed and fails to image all areas needed for diagnosis, an abdominal scan should be performed.

1. The uterus and adnexa should be evaluated for the presence of a gestational sac. If a gestational sac is seen, its location should be documented. The presence or absence of an embryo should be noted and the crown-rump length recorded.
   COMMENT:
   (1) Crown-rump length is a more accurate indication of gestational age than gestational sac diameter. If the embryo is not identified, the gestational sac should be evaluated for the presence of a yolk sac. The estimate of gestational age should then be based on either the

mean diameter of the gestational sac or on the morphology and contents of the gestational sac.
   (2) Identification of a yolk sac or an embryo is definitive evidence of a gestational sac. Caution should be used in making a definitive diagnosis of gestational sac prior to the development of such structures. Without these findings an intrauterine fluid collection can sometimes represent a pseudogestational sac associated with an ectopic pregnancy.
   (3) During the late first trimester, biparietal diameter and other fetal measurements also may be used to establish fetal age.
2. Presence or absence of cardiac activity should be reported.
   COMMENT:
   (1) Real-time observation is critical for this diagnosis.
   (2) With vaginal scans, cardiac motion should be appreciated by a crown-rump length of 5 mm or greater. If an embryo less than 5 mm in length is seen with no cardiac activity, a follow-up scan may be needed to evaluate for fetal life.
3. Fetal number should be documented.
   COMMENT: Multiple pregnancies should be reported only in those instances where multiple embryos are seen. Occasionally, more than one sac-like structure may be seen early in pregnancy and incorrectly thought to represent multiple gestations, owing to incomplete fusion between the amnion and chorion, or elevation of the chorionic membrane by intrauterine hemorrhage.
4. Evaluation of the uterus, adnexal structures, and cul-de-sac should be performed.
   COMMENT:
   (1) This will allow recognition of incidental findings of potential clinical significance. The presence, location, and size of myomas and adnexal masses should be recorded. The cul-de-sac should be scanned for presence or absence of fluid. If there is fluid in the cul-de-sac, the flanks and subhepatic space should be scanned for intraabdominal fluid.
   (2) Because differentiation of normal pregnancy from abnormal preg-

nancy and ectopic pregnancy can be difficult, the correlation of serum hormonal levels with ultrasound findings often is helpful.

PART III
Guidelines for Second and Third Trimester Sonography

1. Fetal life, number, presentation, and activity should be documented.
   COMMENT:
   (1) Abnormal heart rate and/or rhythm should be reported.
   (2) Multiple pregnancies require the documentation of additional information: number of gestational sacs, number of placentas, presence or absence of a dividing membrane, fetal genitalia (if visible), comparison of fetal sizes, and comparison of amniotic fluid volume on each side of the membrane.
2. An estimate of amniotic fluid volume (increased, decreased, normal) should be reported.
   COMMENT: Physiologic variation with stage of pregnancy should be considered in assessing the appropriateness of amniotic fluid volume.
3. The placental location, appearance, and its relationship to the internal cervical os should be recorded. The umbilical cord should be imaged.
   COMMENT:
   (1) It is recognized that apparent placental position early in pregnancy may not correlate well with its location at the time of delivery.
   (2) An overdistended maternal urinary bladder or a lower uterine contraction can give the examiner a false impression of placenta previa.
   (3) Abdominal, transperineal, or vaginal views may be helpful in visualizing the internal cervical os and its relationship to the placenta.
4. Assessment of gestational age should be accomplished at the time of the initial scan using a combination of cranial measurement such as the biparietal diameter or head circumference, and limb measurement such as the femur length.

COMMENT:

(1) Third trimester measurements may not accurately reflect gestational age. If one or more previous studies have been performed, the gestational age at the time of the current examination should be based on the earliest examination that permits accurate measurement of crown-rump length, biparietal diameter, head circumference, and/or femur length by the equation: current fetal age =estimated age at time of initial study +number of weeks elapsed since first study.

(2) Measurements of structurally abnormal fetal body parts (such as the head in a fetus with hydrocephalus or the limbs in a fetus with a skeletal dysplasia) should not be used in the calculation of estimated gestational age.

4A. The standard reference level for measurement of the biparietal diameter is an axial image that includes the thalamus.

COMMENT: If the fetal head is dolichocephalic or brachycephalic, the biparietal diameter measurement may be misleading. Occasionally, computation of the cephalic index, a ratio of the biparietal diameter to fronto-occipital diameter, will be needed to make this determination. In such situations, other measurements of head size, such as the head circumference, may be necessary.

4B. Head circumference is measured at the same level as the biparietal diameter, around the outer perimeter of the calvarium.

4C. Femur length should be routinely measured and recorded after the 14th week of gestation.

COMMENT: As with head measurements, there is considerable biological variation in normal femur lengths late in pregnancy.

5. Fetal weight should be estimated in the late second and in the third trimesters and requires the measurement of abdominal diameter or circumference.

5A. Abdominal circumference should be determined on a true transverse view, preferably at the level of the junction of the left and right portal veins.

COMMENT: Abdominal circumference measurement is necessary to estimate fetal weight and may allow detection of growth retardation and macrosomia.

5B. If previous fetal biometric studies have been performed, an estimate of the appropriateness of interval growth should be given.

6. Evaluation of the uterus (including the cervix) and adnexal structures should be performed.

COMMENT: This will allow recognition of incidental findings of potential clinical significance. The presence, location, and size of myomas and adnexal masses should be recorded. It is frequently not possible to image the maternal ovaries during the second and third trimesters. Vaginal or transperineal scanning may be helpful in evaluating the cervix when the fetal head prevents visualization of the cervix by transabdominal scanning.

7. The study should include, but not necessarily be limited to, assessment of the following fetal anatomy: cerebral ventricles, posterior fossa (including cerebellar hemispheres and cisterna magna), four-chamber view of the heart (including its position within the thorax), spine, stomach, kidneys, urinary bladder, fetal umbilical cord insertion site and intactness of the anterior abdominal wall. While not considered part of the minimum required examination, when fetal position permits, it is desirable to examine other areas of the anatomy.

COMMENT:

(1) It is recognized that not all malformations of the abovementioned organ systems can be detected using ultrasonography.

(2) These recommendations should be considered a minimum guideline for the fetal anatomic survey. Occasionally some of these structures will not be well visualized, as occurs when fetal position, low amniotic fluid volume, or maternal body habitus limit the sonographic examination. When this occurs, the report of the ultrasound examination should include a notation delineating structures that were not well seen.

(3) Suspected abnormalities may require a targeted evaluation of the area(s) of concern.

The following guideline has been approved by the AIUM and is published here as a service to our readers. Additional copies of *Guidelines for Performance of the Ultrasound Examination of the Female Pelvis* (order #GFP) can be ordered from the AIUM. The cost is $5 for AIUM members and $10 for nonmembers plus $1 shipping and handling fee. Mail your order to AIUM Publications Department, 14750 Sweitzer Lane, Suite 100, Laurel, MD 20707–5906; or phone (301) 498–4100 or (800) 638–5352; Fax (301) 498–4450. Prepayment is required.

GUIDELINES FOR PERFORMANCE OF THE ULTRASOUND EXAMINATION OF THE FEMALE PELVIS

The following are proposed guidelines for ultrasound evaluation of the female pelvis. The document consists of two parts:

Part I: Equipment and Documentation Guidelines

Part II: Guidelines for the General Examination of the Female Pelvis

These guidelines have been developed to provide assistance to practitioners performing ultrasound studies of the female pelvis. In some cases, additional and/or specialized examinations may be necessary. While it is not possible to detect every abnormality, adherence to the following will maximize the probability of detecting most of the abnormalities that occur.

PART I
Guidelines for Equipment and Documentation

Equipment

Ultrasound examination of the female pelvis should be conducted with a real-time scanner, preferably using sector or curved linear transducers. The transducer or scanner should be adjusted to operate at the highest clinically appropriate frequency, realizing that there is a trade-off between resolution and beam penetration. With modern equipment, studies performed from the anterior abdominal wall can usually use frequencies of 3.5 MHz or higher, although a lower frequency transducer may occasionally be necessary to provide adequate penetration in an obese patient. Scans performed from the vagina should use frequencies of 5 MHz or higher.

Care of the Equipment

All probes should be cleaned after each patient examination. Vaginal probes should be covered by a protective sheath prior to insertion. Following each examination, the sheath should be disposed and the probe wiped clean and appropriately disinfected. The type of antimicrobial solution and the methodology for disinfection depends on manufacturer and infectious disease recommendations.

Documentation

Adequate documentation is essential for high quality patient care. A permanent record of the ultrasound examination and its interpretation should be kept by the facility performing the study. Images of all appropriate areas, both normal and abnormal, should be recorded. Variations from normal size should be accompanied by measurements. Images are to be appropriately labeled with the examination date, facility name, patient identification, image orientation, and whenever possible, the organ or area imaged. A report of the ultrasound findings should be included in the patient's medical record. Retention of the permanent record of the ultrasound examination should be consistent both with clinical need and with the relevant legal and local health care facility requirements.

PART II
Guidelines for Performance of the Ultrasound Examination of the Female Pelvis

The following guidelines describe the examination to be performed for each organ and anatomic region in the female pelvis. All relevant structures should be identified by the abdominal and/or vaginal approach. If an abdominal examination is performed and fails to provide the necessary diagnostic information, a vaginal scan should be done when possible. Similarly, if a vaginal scan is performed and fails to image all areas needed for diagnosis, an abdominal scan should be performed. In some cases, both an abdominal and a vaginal scan may be needed.

General Pelvic Preparation

For a pelvic sonogram performed from the abdominal wall, the patient's urinary bladder should, in general, be distended adequately to displace small bowel and its contained gas from the field of view. Occasionally, overdistention of the bladder may compromise evaluation. When this occurs, imaging should be repeated after the patient partially empties the bladder.

For a vaginal sonogram, the urinary bladder is preferably empty. The vaginal transducer may be introduced by the patient, the sonographer, or the physician. A female member of the physician's or hospital's staff should be present, when possible, as a chaperone in the examining room during vaginal sonography.

Uterus

The vagina and uterus provide anatomic landmarks that can be used as reference points when evaluating the pelvic structures. In evaluating the uterus, the following should be documented: (a) uterine size, shape, and orientation; (b) the endometrium; (c) the myometrium; and (d) the cervix.

Uterine length is evaluated on a long axis view as the distance from the fundus to the cervix. The depth of the uterus (anteroposterior dimension) is measured on the same long axis view from its anterior to posterior walls, perpendicular to its long axis. The width is measured on the axial or coronal view.

Abnormalities of the uterus should be documented. The endometrium should be analyzed for thickness, focal abnormality, and the presence of fluid or mass in the endometrial cavity. Assessment of the endometrium should allow for normal variations in the appearance of the endometrium expected with phases of the menstrual cycle and with hormonal supplementation. The myometrium and cervix should be evaluated for contour changes, echogenicity, and masses.

The endometrial thickness measurement should include both layers, measured anterior to posterior, in the sagittal plane. Any fluid within the endometrial cavity should be excluded from this measurement.

Adnexa (Ovaries and Fallopian Tubes)

When evaluating the adnexa, an attempt should be made to identify the ovaries first since they can serve as a major point of reference for assessing the presence of adnexal pathology. Although their location is variable, the ovaries are most often situated anterior to the internal iliac (hypogastric) vessels, lateral to the uterus, and superficial to the obturator internus muscle. The ovaries should be measured and ovarian abnormalities should be documented. Ovarian size can be determined by measuring the ovary in three dimensions (width, length, and depth), on views obtained in two orthogonal planes. It is recognized that the ovaries may not be identifiable in some women. This occurs most frequently after menopause or in patients with a large leiomyomatous uterus.

The normal fallopian tubes are not visualized in most patients. The para-adnexal regions should be surveyed for abnormalities, particularly fluid-filled or distended tubular structures that may represent dilated fallopian tubes.

If an adnexal mass is noted, its relationship to the uterus and ipsilateral ovary should be documented. Its size and echopattern (cystic, solid, or mixed; presence of septations) should be determined. Doppler ultrasound may be useful in select cases to identify the vascular nature of pelvic structures.

Cul-de-Sac

The cul-de-sac and bowel posterior to the uterus may not be clearly visualized. This area should be evaluated for the presence of free fluid or mass. When free fluid is detected, its echogenicity should be assessed. If a mass is detected, its size, position, shape, echopattern (cystic, solid, or complex), and its relationship to the ovaries and uterus should be documented. Identification of peristalsis can be helpful in distinguishing a loop of bowel from a pelvic mass. In the absence of peristalsis, differentiation of normal or abnormal loops of bowel from a mass may, at times, be difficult. A transvaginal examination may be helpful in distinguishing a suspected mass from fluid and feces within the normal rectosigmoid. An ultrasound water enema study or a repeat examination after a cleansing enema may also help distinguish a suspected mass from bowel.

The following guideline has been approved by the AIUM and is published here as a service to our readers. Additional copies of *Guidelines for Performance of the Ultrasound Examination of the Infant Brain* (order #GPN) can be ordered from the AIUM. The cost is $5 for AIUM members and $10 for non-members plus $1 shipping and handling fee. Mail your order to AIUM Publications Department, 14750 Sweitzer Lane, Suite 100, Laurel, MD 20707–5906; or phone (301) 498–4100 or (800) 638–5352; Fax (301) 498–4450. Prepayment is required.

GUIDELINES FOR PERFORMANCE OF THE ULTRASOUND EXAMINATION OF THE INFANT BRAIN

The following are proposed guidelines for ultrasound evaluation of the infant brain. The document consists of two parts:

Part I: Equipment and Documentation Guidelines

Part II: Guidelines for a General Examination of the Infant Brain

These guidelines have been developed to provide assistance to practitioners performing ultrasound studies on the infant brain. In some cases, additional and/or specialized examinations may be necessary. While it is not possible to detect every anomaly, adherence to the following guidelines will aid in the detection of those abnormalities of the infant brain that can be evaluated by ultrasound.

PART I
Guidelines for Equipment and Documentation

Equipment

Pediatric neurosonographic examinations should be conducted with a real-time scanner, preferably with a high resolution transducer suitable to the size of the anterior fontanelle. The transducer or scanner should be adjusted to operate at the highest clinically appropriate frequency, realizing that there is a trade-off between resolution and beam penetration. With modern equipment, these frequencies are usually between 5.0 and 7.5 MHz. Occasionally, a frequency of 10 MHz may be preferable. Doppler sonography or color flow imaging may be used to evaluate intracranial blood flow in selected cases. Doppler power output should be kept as low as possible to gain necessary diagnostic information. Scanning equipment should be cleaned after each use.

Documentation

Adequate documentation is essential for high quality patient care. A permanent record of the ultrasound examination and its interpretation should be kept by the facility performing the study. Images of all appropriate areas, both normal and abnormal, should be recorded in an image or storage format. Variations from normal should be assessed and compared to previous examinations, if any. Images are to be appropriately labeled with the examination date, facility name, patient identification, and image orientation. A report of the ultrasound findings should be included in the patient's medical record. Retention of the permanent record of the ultrasound examination should be consistent both with clinical need and relevant legal and local health care facility requirements.

PART II
Guidelines for Performance of the Ultrasound Examination of the Infant Brain

The following guidelines describe the complete sonographic examination to be performed for the infant brain. It is recognized that some examinations, particularly those performed in a neonatal intensive care unit, may be limited by patient condition, IV site placement, as well as life support equipment.

Imaging should primarily be performed through the anterior fontanelle. If the anterior fontanelle cannot be used, imaging may be performed through alternate acoustic windows such as other sutural openings, or directly through the squamosal portion of the temporal bone. Appropriate positioning of the transducer over the scanning window is essential. Imaging should be performed using the minimum transducer pressure necessary to acquire diagnostic information.

Ventricular System and Brain Parenchyma

Representative coronal and sagittal views should be obtained of the brain parenchyma and extra-axial fluid spaces. The transducer should be systematically angled laterally and medially in sagittal planes and anteriorly and posteriorly in coronal planes, in order to image as much of the brain parenchyma, ventricular system, and extra-axial spaces as possible.

Representative coronal views should be obtained by systematically angling the transducer from the front to back of the calvarium. Anteriorly angled images should include the frontal lobe and frontal horns of the lateral ventricles. Nonangled images should include the imageable portions of the frontal, parietal and temporal lobes, the basal ganglia, and the body and atria of the lateral ventricles. Posteriorly angled images should attempt to include the posterior portions of the temporal lobes, the occipital lobes and the subtentorial area, the cerebellum, as well as the posterior portions of the ventricular system.

Representative sagittal views with appropriate degrees of leftward or rightward angulation should attempt to include the Sylvian fissures, the lateral ventricles, including the surrounding white matter, the choroid plexus, and the germinal matrix region including the caudothalamic groove. A midline sagittal view should, when possible, include the corpus callosum, cavum septi pellucidi and cavum vergae extension (if present), the third ventricle, the area of the aqueduct of Sylvius, the fourth ventricle, the vermis of the cerebellum, and the cisterna magna.

The presence or absence of hemorrhage, parenchymal abnormalities, ventricular dilatation, extraaxial fluid collections, and congenital anomalies should be noted.

Additional views, if necessary, may be taken through the posterior fontanelle, any open suture, or through thin areas of the temporoparietal bone.

The following guideline has been approved by the AIUM and is published here as a service to our readers. Additional copies of *Guidelines for Performance of the Ultrasound Examination of the Breast* (order #GB) can be ordered from the AIUM. The cost is $6 for AIUM members and $20 for nonmembers. Mail your order to AIUM Publications Department, 14750 Sweitzer Lane, Suite 100, Laurel, MD 20707–5906; or phone (301) 498–4100 or (800) 638–5352; Fax (301) 498–4450. Prepayment is required.

GUIDELINES FOR PERFORMANCE OF THE ULTRASOUND EXAMINATION OF THE BREAST

The following are proposed guidelines for the ultrasound evaluation of the breast. The document consists of two parts:

Part I: Equipment and Documentation

Part II: Ultrasound Examination of the Breast

These guidelines have been developed to provide assistance to practitioners performing the ultrasound examination of the breast.

PART I
Equipment and Documentation
Equipment

Ultrasonographic examination of the breast should be conducted with a real-time scanner, preferably using high-resolution linear, curved linear, or sector transducers. The transducer should be operated at the highest clinically appropriate frequency, realizing that there is a tradeoff between resolution and beam penetration. Ordinarily, transducer frequencies of 7.5–10 MHz are used for breast imaging. A transducer frequency of 5 MHz is needed occasionally for beam penetration in a large breast or for a deep lesion.

COMMENT: The resolution of the transducer should be sufficiently high to allow differentiation of small cystic from solid lesions.

At least annually, equipment performance should be monitored.

Documentation

Adequate documentation of the study is essential for high quality patient care. Images of all appropriate areas, both normal and abnormal, should be recorded on an appropriate imaging or storage format.

1. The images should be labeled with examination date, patient name and identification number, image orientation, and anatomic location using a clock notation or labeled diagrammatic scheme of the breast. It is advisable to include the sonographer's or sonologist's identification number, initials, or other symbol on the image.
2. A report of the ultrasonographic findings should be placed in the patient's medical record.
3. Retention of the breast ultrasonographic images should be consistent with clinical need, the accompanying mammograms, and in compliance with legal and local health care facility requirements.

PART II
Ultrasound Examination of the Breast
Indications

Breast ultrasound should not be performed as a screening study in lieu of mammography but should be directed to identification and characterization of palpable abnormalities, ambiguous mammographic abnormalities, and the guidance of interventional procedures. In addition to the preceding applications, breast ultrasonography may be used to evaluate breasts containing silicone implants for implant leakage. Ultrasound is not indicated to screen breasts for occult masses or microcalcifications.

Characterization of Masses and Ambiguous Mammographic Abnormalities

1. The image should be labeled as to right or left breast, the lesion's location and the orientation of the probe with respect to the mass (e.g., transverse or longitudinal). The location of the lesion should be recorded using clock notation or shown on a schematic diagram of the breast.
2. At least two sets of images of a lesion should be obtained. One set of images should be without measuring calipers. The images without calipers are necessary because calipers obscure marginal detail. The mass should be measured in at least two, but preferably three, dimensions, and the dimensions should be recorded on the image. The reference points used for measurements should be shown on the images of the mass. For clarity, the units of measurement should be consistent, i.e., all measurements in either millimeters or centimeters.
3. Regardless of where the breast sonogram is performed, it should be correlated with physical examination and with mammography if it has been performed.

4. Mass characterization with ultrasonography is highly dependent upon technical factors. Transducer selection should be appropriate to the size and depth of the abnormality; frequency of the transducer should be sufficiently high to permit distinction of fluid-filled from solid masses. The focal zone should be set at the depth of the lesion. Gain settings should be adjusted to allow differentiation of simple cysts and solid masses. Gain settings should not be so high that artifactual echoes are placed within simple cysts. By the same token, power and time gain compensation settings should not be too low to prevent recognition of internal echoes that are truly present in a mass.

5. When using a 7.5 or 10 MHz transducer to image the skin and the superficial tissues of the breast within the first 1.5 cm of the skin surface, it may be necessary to use an offset between the transducer face and the surface of the skin. Some transducers have built-in waterpaths, but other transducer adaptations or standoff materials also may be used.

6. Unlike abdominal and pelvic sonography where the organs are scanned in their entirety, breast sonography is a directed examination. Nevertheless, the anatomic landscape in which the lesion is located should be recognized and commented upon to enable restudy of the same area in future examination. For example, a cyst scanned transversely from the six o'-clock location of the right breast also might be related to its distance from the visualized pectoral muscle layer.

Guidance of Interventional Procedures

1. The interventional procedures that can be performed with sonographic guidance include but are not limited to cyst aspiration, presurgical needle hookwire localization, and fine needle or core biopsy.
2. A full ultrasonographic examination should first be completed of the mass or area of the breast in which the procedure is planned.
3. There is no single correct method for accomplishing interventional procedures with ultrasound imaging guidance. Both freehand technique with direct ultrasound visualization and use of a probe with a needle guide are suitable for breast interventions. The type of equipment on hand and the experience of the physician performing the procedure will determine selection of a technique.

High-frequency transducers of 7.5 and 10 MHz used for imaging breast tissues also are suitable for guiding interventional procedures. With these transducers, continuous visualization of the needle path is possible. Depending upon the probe configuration, the geometry of the acoustic beam, and the route of needle entry, either a small portion of the needle may be visible as an echogenic dot or, if the needle entry is aligned with the acoustic beam and nearly perpendicular to it, the entire shaft, including the needle tip, may be visible.

Appendix 36.
Society of Diagnostic Medical Sonographers: Code of Ethics and Code of Professional Conduct

CODE OF ETHICS FOR THE PROFESSION OF DIAGNOSTIC MEDICAL ULTRASOUND

Preamble

The goal of this code of ethics is to promote excellence in patient care by fostering responsibility and accountability and thereby help to ensure the integrity of professionals involved in all aspects of diagnostic medical ultrasound.

Objectives

- To create and environment where professional and ethical issues are discussed
- To help the individual practitioner identify ethical issues
- To provide guidelines for individual practitioners regarding ethical behavior

Principles

Principle I: In order to promote patient well-being, professionals shall:

A. Provide information about the procedure and the reason it is being done. Respond to patient's concerns and questions.
B. Respect the patient's self-determination and the right to refuse the procedure.
C. Recognize the patient's individuality and provide care in a non-judgmental and non-discriminatory manner.
D. Promote the privacy, dignity and comfort of the patient and his/her family.
E. Protect the confidentiality of acquired patient information.
F. Strive to ensure patient safety.

Principle II: To promote the highest level of competent practice, professionals shall:

A. Obtain the appropriate education and skills to ensure competence.
B. Practice according to published and recognized standards.
C. Work to achieve and maintain appropriate credentials.
D. Acknowledge personal limits and not practice beyond their capacity and skills.

E. Perform only those procedures that are medically indicated, restricting practice to validated and appropriate tests. For research studies, follow established research protocol, obtaining (and documenting) informed patient consent as needed.
F. Ensure the completeness of examinations and the timely communication of important information.
G. Strive for excellence and continued competence through continuing education.
H. Perform ongoing quality assurance.
I. NOT compromise patient care by the use of substances that may alter judgment or skill.

Principle III: To promote professional integrity and public trust, the professional shall:

A. Be truthful and promote honesty in interactions with patients, colleagues and the public.
B. Accurately represent their level of competence, education and certification.
C. Avoid situations which may constitute a conflict of interest.
D. Maintain appropriate personal boundaries with patients including avoidance of inappropriate conduct, be it verbal or nonverbal.
E. Promote cooperative relationships within the profession and with other members of the health care community.
F. Avoid situations which exploit others for financial gain or misrepresent information to obtain reimbursement.
G. Promote equitable access to care.

CODE OF PROFESSIONAL CONDUCT FOR DIAGNOSTIC MEDICAL SONOGRAPHERS

Preamble

The Code of Professional Conduct of the Society of Diagnostic Medical Sonographers is a statement of the high standards of conduct toward which sonographers are committed to strive. Sonographers, as members of a health care profession, acknowledge their responsibilities to their patients, to other health care professionals, and to each other.

I. **Sonographers** shall act in the best interests of the patient.
II. **Sonographers** shall provide sonographic services with compassion, respect for human dignity, honesty, and integrity.
III. **Sonographers** shall respect the patient's right to privacy, safeguarding confidential information within the constraints of the law.
IV. **Sonographers** shall maintain competence in their field.
V. **Sonographers** shall assume responsibility for their actions.

For further information contact:

Society of Diagnostic Medical Sonographers
12770 Coit Road, Suite 708
Dallas, TX 75251
Ph: (972)239-7367 Fax: (972)239-7378

INDEX

Page numbers followed by *f* refer to figures.